Intravenous Therapy in Nursing Practice

Edited by

Lisa Dougherty OBE MSc RGN RM ONCCert
Nurse Consultant Intravenous Therapy
The Royal Marsden Hospital NHS Foundation Trust, London

Julie Lamb BSc (Hons) DPSN RGN
General Manager, Cancer Services
Barts and The London NHS Trust

Foreword by

Tom Elliott
Divisional Director and Deputy Medical Director
University Hospital Birmingham NHS Foundation Trust

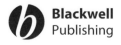

Blackwell
Publishing

Blackwell Publishing editorial offices:
Blackwell Publishing Ltd, 9600 Garsington Road, Oxford OX4 2DQ, UK
Tel: +44 (0)1865 776868
Blackwell Publishing Inc., 350 Main Street, Malden, MA 02148-5020, USA
Tel: +1 781 388 8250
Blackwell Publishing Asia Pty Ltd, 550 Swanston Street, Carlton, Victoria 3053, Australia
Tel: +61 (0)3 8359 1011

First published 1999 Harcourt Publisher Ltd
Second edition published 2008 by Blackwell Publishing Ltd

2   2009

Library of Congress Cataloging-in-Publication Data

Intravenous therepy in nursing practice/edited by Lisa Dougherty and Julie Lamb. – 2nd ed.
        p. cm.
    Includes bibliographical references and index.
    ISBN: 978-1-4051-4647-0 (pbk. : alk. paper)
    1. Intravenous therapy.   2. Nursing.   I. Dougherty, Lisa.   II. Lamb, Julie.
    [DNLM: 1. Infusions, Intravenous– nursing. 2. Home Infusion Therapy–nursing. WY 100 16125 2008]

    RM170.I595 2008
    615′ .6–dc22
    2007018853

A catalogue record for this title is available from the British Library

Set in 9.5/11.5 pt Sabon
by Newgen Imaging Systems (P) Ltd, Chennai, India
Printed and bound in Singapore by COS Printers Pte Ltd

The publisher's policy is to use permanent paper from mills that operate a sustainable forestry policy, and which has been manufactured from pulp processed using acid-free and elementary chlorine-free practices. Furthermore, the publisher ensures that the text paper and cover board used have met acceptable environmental accreditation standards.

For further information on Blackwell Publishing, visit our website:
www.blackwellnursing.com

Intravenous Therapy in Nursing Practice

Contents

Contributors

Liz Bishop RGN, BSc (Nurs) MSc (Adv Cli Prac)
Consultant Nurse (Haemato-oncology), Guy's Hospital, London

Karen Bravery RN RSCN BSc (Hons)
Nurse Practitioner/Practice Development Nurse, Elephant Day Care, Great Ormond Street Hospital for Children, NHS Trust, London

Lisa Dougherty OBE MSc RGN RM ONCCert (Advanced Clinical Practice – Cancer Nursing)
Nurse Consultant Intravenous Therapy, The Royal Marsden NHS Foundation Trust, London

Teresa Finlay RGN OncNC BSc (Hons) MSc PGDip HPEd
Senior Lecturer, School of Health and Social Care, Oxford Brookes University, Oxford

Janice Gabriel MPhil PgD BSc (Hons) RN FETC ONC, Cert MHS
Nurse Director, Central South Coast Cancer Network, Southampton

Sarah Hart MSc BSc (Hons) RGN FETC Infection Control Certificate
Clinical Nurse Specialist – Infection Control/Radiation Protection, The Royal Marsden NHS Foundation Trust, Surrey and London

Lorraine Hyde RGN ONc Diploma in Nursing Studies, BSc (Hons) Nursing
Senior Nurse Manager, Day Care Services, The Royal Marsden NHS Foundation Trust, Surrey

Jill Kayley MSc (Autonomous Health Care Practice) RN DN Certificate
Independent Nurse Consultant – Community IV Therapy, Reading, Berks

Julie Lamb BSc (Hons) DPSN RGN
General Manager, Cancer Services, Barts and The London NHS Trust, London

Michèle Malster BA (Hons) RGN FETC
Specialist Peri-operative Practitioner, David Beevers Day Unit, St James' University Hospital, Leeds

Chris Quinn MBA PgDMS RGN FETC ENB100
Patient Safety Advocate, Cardinal Health Basingstoke

Katie Scales PGDip (Ethics) BEd (Hons) HDQC Physiology DPSN RNT RN ENB 100, ENB 400, Charing Cross Hospital, London
Consultant Nurse Critical Care, Charing Cross Hospital, Hammersmith Hospitals NHS Trust, London

Clare Shaw BSc (Hons) PhD RD (Registered Dietitian)
Consultant Dietitian, The Royal Marsden NHS Foundation Trust, London

Zoe Whittington BSc (Hons) Dip Clin Pharm DMS MRPharmS
Pharmacy, The Royal Marsden NHS Foundation Trust, Surrey

Foreword

Intravenous therapy is an important component of patient care and is part of the role of both doctors and nurses. It is therefore essential that easy to read and informative texts are available for training of these healthcare workers. The second edition of this book offers such a text.

The book is conveniently divided into three sections: fundamentals, practice and finishes, with a review of four specialty areas. The chapters assume no previous knowledge and offer a comprehensive view point on all areas related to intravenous therapy.

The first chapter deals with the legal and professional aspects of intravenous therapy. The professional and legal accountability are reviewed, together with the responsibility of nurses and duty of care. Useful sections on record-keeping and consent to treatment compliment an excellent review of the guiding principles. Anatomy and physiology and fluid electrolyte balance are dealt with in chapters two and three. They are informative and well illustrated.

The text is augmented by useful tables identifying the important veins for vascular access. The various electrolyte inbalances are also clearly summarised in tables.

An important aspect of intravenous therapy is the risk of associated catheter related sepsis. Chapter four reviews all the major risk factors related to infections associated with catheters and summarises the approach to both prevention and treatment. A section outlining the additional risks to healthcare workers, such as needlestick injuries, is also presented. The pharmacological aspects of intravenous therapy are next discussed and include methods of administering medicine.

Section two deals with the practice associated with intravenous therapy and contains chapters on peripheral intravenous therapy, local and systemic complications, types of infusion devices, vascular access and long-term central venous access. This section includes a chapter on how to obtain peripheral venous access. This is a comprehensive and practical review including psychological effects on the patient, methods to reduce anxiety and pain, how to improve venous access, skin preparation and choice of veins. An excellent summary describes the procedure for cannulation and also gives an approach to problem solving techniques.

The text concludes with the review of four specific areas which include blood transfusion therapy, parental nutrition, paediatric intravenous therapy in practice and the safe handling and administration of intravenous cytotoxic drugs. The review of these different specialities will be essential reading for healthcare workers involved in any of these areas.

Without doubt this text provides an excellent update for any healthcare worker whose role includes intravenous therapy. It should be essential reading for nurses and also doctors and will enable them to obtain an excellent knowledge base. The book is well referenced and written by authors' expert in their different areas. This book should become a standard reference text in the area.

Professor Tom Elliott
Divisional Director & Deputy Medical Director
University Hospital Birmingham NHS Foundation Trust
Birmingham, UK
November 2007

Preface

The administration of intravenous (i.v.) therapy is now a common part of most nurses' roles. The profession has moved a long way since the Breckenridge report in 1976 which first outlined nurses' responsibilities regarding the addition of drugs to infusion bags and their hanging—the sum total of a nurse's involvement in i.v. therapy in the United Kingdom at the time. Since then, i.v. therapy has become increasingly more complex, and as technology has advanced, so too has the degree of nursing involvement.

Nurses now not only prepare and administer drugs, but also assess, insert and remove both peripheral and central venous access devices; evaluate, select and purchase access devices and infusion equipment; and provide education and training in the many facets of this challenging area of practice.

There has also been a shift away from the hospital setting to the community, where i.v. therapy involves not only the healthcare professional, but also the patient and carer. As well as healthcare professionals in nursing and medicine, i.v. therapy also involves pharmacists, nutritionists and microbiologists. This has led to a demand for knowledge about i.v. therapy and its applications in all types of settings.

Over recent years The Royal College of Nursing Intravenous Therapy Forum has published guidance and standards for i.v. practice in the UK. The first definitive textbook written specifically for nurses in the UK was published in 1999; it is now time to provide an up-to-date comprehensive text based on recent evidence-based practice that includes practical procedures and problem-solving techniques.

The aim of this book is to provide the fundamental principles that underpin i.v. therapy, and any associated procedures, in a comprehensive and practical way.

Intravenous therapy is relevant to almost all areas of nursing, and features in specialities such as critical care and oncology. The book will help a wide range of healthcare professionals, including nurses and junior doctors. It will provide the student nurse with information on how to prepare and administer i.v. drugs for the first time, as well as informing the specialist nurse who wishes to expand her practice and insert peripherally inserted central catheters.

The book starts with the history of i.v. therapy and provides a comprehensive view of the development of the nurse's role and how practice has expanded. Professional, legal and ethical issues, including accountability and training, are also covered. No textbook on i.v. therapy would be complete without foundation chapters on anatomy and physiology, fluid and electrolyte balance and infection control.

The chapters on the pharmacology and safe administration and management of i.v. therapy are preparatory chapters for those healthcare professionals starting out in i.v. therapy. They set out the practicalities of how to prepare and administer i.v. therapy safely, along with the factors that influence the methods of drug administration and the responsibilities of each healthcare professional involved in the process. Another vital chapter concerns local and systemic complications: each complication associated with i.v. therapy is discussed, covering the recognition, prevention and treatment of each type. The chapter on flow control takes the reader from the simple gravity drip to the various complex electronic infusion devices, and includes guidance provided by the Medicines and Healthcare products Regulatory Agency on all intravenous equipment.

Venepuncture and cannulation are two of the most commonly performed invasive procedures and are now an integral part of many nurses' roles. The chapter on obtaining vascular access provides step-by-step instructions for performing these tasks, along with background on how these procedures impact on the patient.

Vascular access has always been a feature in the acute care setting, and there is a chapter to address the common issues related to the care and maintenance of central venous catheters, as well as complications of insertion. This theme is continued in the chapter on long-term central venous access, which provides readers with a step-by-step guide to the insertion and removal of peripherally inserted central catheters, and addresses the quality-of-life issues for patients living with a central venous access device. Most of these patients will be cared for in their own homes—hence the chapter on i.v. therapy in the community, which focuses on the advantages and disadvantages for patients and emphasizes the requirements for good information and teaching.

Finally, the last four chapters of the book focus on more specialist subjects. Blood transfusion and parenteral nutrition therapy are short but comprehensive chapters which provide the reader with a broad overview of the subjects. Paediatric i.v. therapy provides a view of many of the subjects covered throughout the book but from the paediatric perspective. The safe administration of cytotoxic drugs focuses specifically on the i.v. administration of these hazardous drugs and the problems associated with extravasation.

Many practices of i.v. therapy such as dressings and maintaining patency, still lack sufficient scientific evidence to support them. The aim of this book is to provide a balanced view of the available research and opinions of experts, which should enable the reader to come to his or her own conclusions regarding i.v. practice.

The contributing authors were selected for their expertise in the area covered in their chapters. They were felt to be clinically based practitioners with up-to-date knowledge and involvement in research and practice development in the field of i.v. therapy. The result is a book that will suit healthcare professionals, at every level and in almost every speciality, whose desire is to provide safe and evidence-based intravenous practice, with positive outcomes for the patient or client.

London, 2007

Lisa Dougherty
Julie Lamb

Acknowledgements

We were both delighted that the first edition was so well received and over the last few years we were asked when we were going to update the book. It is thanks to Blackwell Publishing that a second edition has become a reality and we would like to thank Beth Knight and Katharine Unwin for their support throughout the process.

We would also like to thank all the contributors—those who returned to update their chapters and the new authors who edited the remaining chapters. We feel that the book has been improved upon not only in content but also in layout.

I would like to again thank Val Speechley for inspiring me to become involved in the field of intravenous therapy—I never dreamt that I would still be excited by it 22 years on! I would also like to thank Liz who has supported me through all my writing and patiently waited 2 years for me to reappear from behind the computer screen!

Lisa Dougherty

My love and gratitude to my family; Mike for his enduring tolerance and patience and Beth and Tom, my *raison d'être*.

Julie Lamb

Section 1
Fundamentals

CHAPTER 1

Legal and Professional Aspects of Intravenous Therapy

Lorraine Hyde

Introduction

It is estimated that the majority of patients admitted to hospital at the beginning of the 21st century will require a vascular access device during some part of the patient journey (Petersen 2002). Technological advances and the vast range of vascular access used in different clinical settings have professional and legal implications for nursing practice. Infusion therapy is an integral aspect of nursing practice and can range from caring for a peripheral cannula to managing multiple and complex infusions and equipment (RCN 2005). Nurses must be aware of the law and how it relates to practice, especially in the dynamic arena of the NHS (*See* Box 1.1 for a history of intravenous therapy).

BOX 1.1

History of intravenous therapy

The recorded history of i.v. therapy began in 1492 when a blood transfusion from two Romans to the dying Pope Innocent was attempted. All three died.

In 1628, Sir William Harvey's discovery of the blood circulatory system formed the basis for more scientific experimentation. In 1658 Sir Christopher Wren predicted the possibility of introducing medication directly into the bloodstream, although it was Dr Robert Boyle who used a quill and bladder to inject opium into a dog in 1659, with J D Major succeeding with the first injection into a human in 1665.

A 15-year-old Parisian boy successfully received a transfusion of lamb's blood in 1667. However, subsequent animal to human transfusions proved fatal and eventually, in 1687, the practice was made illegal.

In 1834, James Blundell proved that only human blood was suitable for transfusion, and later that century Pasteur and Lister stressed the necessity for asepsis during infusion procedures.

In 1900 Karl Landsteiner led the way in identifying and classifying different blood groups, and in 1914 it was recognized that sodium citrate prevented clotting which opened the gate for the extensive use of blood transfusions.

Intravenous therapy was being used widely during World War II, and by the mid-1950s was being used mainly for the purposes of major surgery and rehydration only. Few medications were given via the i.v. route, with antibiotics more commonly being given intramuscularly.

(Continued)

> **BOX 1.1** (*Continued*)
>
> Throughout the 1960s and 1970s, intermittent medications, filters, electronic infusion control devices and smaller plastic cannulae became available. Use of multiple electrolyte solutions and medications increased along with blood component therapy, and numerous i.v. drugs and antibiotics were being added to i.v. regimens.
>
> The use of i.v. therapy has expanded dramatically over the last 35 years. This expansion continues to accelerate and can be attributed to the following factors:
>
> * the understanding of hazards and complications
> * improvement in i.v. equipment
> * increased knowledge of physiological requirements
> * increased knowledge of pharmacological and therapeutic implications
> * increased availability of nutrients and drugs in i.v. solutions
> * changes in the traditional roles of doctors and nurses, allowing nurses to develop skills that were traditionally the remit of the medical profession (e.g. insertion of central venous access devices).
>
> In November 1992, the Department of Health's (DH's) Research & Development Division commissioned Greenhalgh & Company Ltd to undertake a 12-month research study into the interface between junior hospital doctors and ward nurses. The aim of the study was 'to contribute to the improvement in patient care' by examining the interface between junior hospital doctors and ward nurses with a view to enhancing the role of nurses and reducing the inappropriate workload of junior hospital doctors.
>
> Within its terms of reference, three core questions were posed (Greenhalgh 1994):
>
> 1. What do junior doctors and nurses currently do?
> 2. What work is transferable between junior doctors and nurses for the benefit of patient care?
> 3. What model or exemplars of good practice in this interface between junior doctors and nurses can be identified and disseminated for the benefit of patients and the service?
>
> At the end of the study, the report identified key findings and recommendations which showed an obvious need to look at current nursing and medical practice based upon technological advances in medical/nursing treatments and to move forward in partnership to provide an environment of care in which 'good practice' can flourish.

The expanding responsibility of nurses practising in intravenous (i.v.) therapy has both advantages and disadvantages. The nurse's emerging role offers rewards such as intellectual stimulation and professional satisfaction. However, the increase in responsibility brings with it the increased capacity for liability and the added potential of legal risks.

The nursing profession seeks to maintain and improve upon standards of care, and nurses on the register are accountable for an increasing range of responsibilities. Such responsibilities are increasingly complex in nature and some were traditionally the responsibility of the medical profession, such as insertion of central venous catheters. Therefore, nurses do require a working knowledge of the professional and legal responsibilities as it applies to their practice since it contributes towards best practice and enhances the therapeutic nurse–patient relationship (Cox 2001).

This chapter will focus upon the law as it applies to the nursing profession and the NHS. The professional dimension is discussed, focusing upon the Nursing and Midwifery Council (NMC) guidelines and principles for practice. The legal and professional dimension of intravenous therapy is explored using examples of practice issues.

Law and the Legal System

There are two main sources of law. The first is Acts of Parliament and Statutory Instruments which are enabled by the powers given to parliament (also known as statute law). 'Since 1688 the Crown in Parliament has been the supreme legislative body in

England, and subsequently in the United Kingdom' (Hodgson 2002, page 3). Statutes are formed in two ways. Firstly a statute is presented to the House of Commons as a bill. If this is sponsored by the government it will become legislation since it has government support. Private Members' Bills do not have the sponsorship of the government and will therefore only become law if they have government support (McHale 2001b). This type of law takes precedence over all other laws (Dimond 2005). There are many statutes which apply to nursing, such as the Nurses Midwives and Health Visitors Act 1997, the National Health Service Act 1977 and the Health Act 1999, to name but a few (Dimond 2005).

The second source of law is the common law (also known as case law), which is derived from decisions by judges in individual cases; these are often interpretations of statute law (Dimond 2005). Common law operates through a system of precedent. Therefore, a judge, in deciding upon an individual case, may be obliged to follow the decision of an earlier court. Decisions in the House of Lords, the highest court of the land, are binding in all lower courts (McHale 2001c).

In addition, English law is sometimes governed by laws laid down in Europe through our participation in the European Union (McHale 2001c, page 11). The European Union operates an agreement by member states to cooperate and collaborate in aspects of criminal justice and home affairs.

The legal system in England is divided into two main branches, criminal and civil law. Criminal law concentrates on crime and breaches can lead to prosecution, whilst civil law deals with all other cases (Hodgson 2002). Civil law is the branch of law whereby a negligence claim against a nurse would be heard. A patient who has suffered harm as a consequence of inadequate care whilst being treated by the nurse can claim compensation for a breach of duty of care. It is therefore important for the nurse to understand liability in relation to civil action. The legal aspects of nursing and the professional responsibilities of the nurse will now be explored.

Professional Guidelines

The main codes for nurses practising in the UK are:

- the International Council for Nurses (ICN) *Code of Ethics for Nurses* (ICN 2000)
- the NMC *Code of Professional Conduct: Standard for Conduct, Performance and Ethics* for nurses, midwives and specialist community public health nurses (NMC 2004a).

The first code of ethics was adopted by the ICN in Sao Paulo, Brazil, in July 1953. This code was subsequently revised at the ICN meetings in Frankfurt and Germany, and again in Mexico City in 1973, and further revised in 2000 (Tschudin 2003).

The first ICN code (1953) described the fundamental responsibility of the nurse as threefold:

- to conserve life
- to alleviate suffering
- to promote health.

Twenty years later, this duty was seen as fourfold:

- to promote health
- to prevent illness
- to restore health
- to alleviate suffering.

The ICN code (ICN 2000) is comprehensive in terms of ethical care and has four principal elements: nurses and people, nurses and practice, nurses and the profession, nurses and co-workers. It acknowledges the universal need for nursing, the inherent respect for life and dignity, and the rights of humankind (Tschudin 2003).

Each man and woman who, following appropriate education and training, becomes a registered nurse, midwife or health visitor also becomes a member of one of the regulated health professions. The Nurses, Midwives and Health Visitors Act 1979 had empowered the then United Kingdom Central Council (UKCC) and the national boards to maintain the register and regulate nurses. A review of the statutory regulation of nurses was undertaken in 1999 and recommendations were made in the Health Act (1999). The UKCC was replaced by the Nursing and Midwifery Council (NMC) and new procedures for fitness to practice emerged (Dimond 2005). The NMC states that its principal function is 'to protect the public by ensuring that nurses and midwives provide high standards of care to their patients and clients'. To achieve its aims, the NMC:

- maintains a register of qualified nurses, midwives and specialist community public health nurses
- sets standards for conduct, performance and ethics
- provides advice for nurses and midwives
- considers allegations of misconduct, lack of competence or unfitness to practice due to ill health (NMC 2006).

In order to ensure that practitioners are fit for purpose and are able to provide relevant and evidence-based nursing interventions the NMC issued guidance to all practitioners as set out below.

'As a registered nurse, midwife or specialist community public health nurse, you are personally accountable for your practice. In caring for patients and clients, you must:

- respect the patient or client as an individual
- obtain consent before you give any treatment or care
- protect confidential information
- co-operate with others in the team
- maintain your professional knowledge and competence
- be trustworthy
- act to identify and minimise risk to patients and clients.'

These are the shared values of all the United Kingdom health care regulatory bodies' (NMC 2004a).

The document further states that there is a duty on all registrants to be aware of their personal accountability within the clinical context which means that the practitioner is 'answerable for their actions and omissions, regardless of advice or directions from another professional' (NMC 2004a). It is vital, therefore, that nurses maintain their knowledge and skills and embrace the notion of lifelong learning since health care is dynamic and nursing interventions need to be responsive and relevant. The code is requiring the nurse to apply clinical judgement which ensures safe practice and this can only be achieved through continuous learning and updating. Nurses are required by the NMC to maintain a professional portfolio which demonstrates knowledge and skill acquisition, and the document can be requested for scrutiny by the council at any time. In 2002, the NMC issued the *Code of Professional Conduct* which infers that the individual practitioner should be directed to recognizing and serving the interests of patients. Its purpose was to:

'inform the professions of the standard of professional conduct required of them in the exercise of their professional accountability and practice; inform the public, other professions and employers of the standard of professional conduct that they can expect from a registered practitioner' (NMC 2002).

It leaves no room for uncertainty or ambiguity, stating clearly that nurses are personally responsible for their practice. In 2004, the NMC reproduced the code, changing its name to *The NMC Code of Professional Conduct: Standards for Conduct, Performance and Ethics*. All references to 'nurses, midwives and health visitors' were replaced with 'nurses, midwives and specialist community public health nurses'. A new section was added to include indemnity insurance which reflects the growing culture of litigation within health-care today (NMC 2004b).

Professional Registration

The Nursing Midwifery Order 2001 requires the NMC to have specific statutory functions and committees (Dimond 2005). One of the fundamental aspects of the NMC's functions is the maintenance of the register. The professional register is a means of declaring, to all those interested, that a reasonable standard of competence and conduct is expected from those named in it. Additionally, it is stating that these are the people to whom the NMC has declared its expectations, given its advice and presented its standards, and whom it can call to account.

Removal from the register

Under article 21 of the Nursing and Midwifery Order 2001, the Council is required to establish and review the standards of conduct, performance and ethics of registrants and prospective registrants and to give guidance on these matters and keep under review effective arrangements to protect the public from persons whose fitness to practice is impaired (Dimond 2005) (*See* Box 1.2). Fitness to practice implies a registrant's suitability to be on the register without restrictions. The NMC will deal with allegations that fitness to practice is impaired due to:

- misconduct
- lack of competence
- a conviction or caution (including a finding of guilt by a court martial)
- physical or mental ill health
- a finding by any other health or social care regulator or licensing body that a registrant's fitness to practice is impaired
- a fraudulent or incorrect entry in the NMC's register (NMC 2004b).

BOX 1.2

Issues that the NMC are regularly asked to consider (NMC 2004b)

- Physical, sexual or verbal abuse.
- Theft.
- Failure to keep proper records.
- Failure to provide adequate care.
- Deliberately concealing unsafe practice.
- Committing criminal offences.
- Continued lack of competence despite opportunities to improve.
- Impairment of fitness to practice due to physical or mental ill health include:
  - alcohol or drug dependence
  - untreated serious mental illness.

Anyone can make a complaint about a registrant to the NMC. The NMC committees that deal with all allegations of unfitness to practice are:

- the Screeners and Practice Committees who consider the allegation and establish if the complaint is well founded but who may refer the matter to the other committee for consideration
- the Investigating Committee (IC)
- the Conduct and Competence Committee (CCC)
- the Health Committee (HC).

When a complaint is received and the registrant is involved in a criminal investigation in relation to the allegations made against them, the NMC will wait for the outcome before proceeding. Fitness to practice procedures operate upon the principle that the individual is innocent until proven guilty, which means that a registrant can continue to practice until a judgement has been made. However, if patients, clients or the public would be exposed to an unacceptably high level of risk if the registrant continued to practice then the IC can impose an interim order. Interim orders are imposed for a maximum of 18 months. They must be reviewed for the first time within 6 months and thereafter every 3 months until the order is revoked or the case concluded (NMC 2004b).

Where the IC considers that there is a case to answer it may undertake mediation or refer the case to screeners for them to undertake mediation to the HC or the CCC. The CCC operates to the same high standard of proof as a court and hearings are generally held in public to encourage transparency and reflect the NMC's public accountability. The panel has a range of powers which include:

- issuing a caution
- suspension from the register or
- removal from the register.

Health Commitee proceedings are usually held in private because of the confidential nature of the medical evidence being considered. They can:

- issue a caution
- suspend from the register
- remove from the register.

When an HC panel removes a registrant's name from the register they may not apply for restoration to the register for 5 years from the date of the removal. Anyone who has been removed from the register has the right to apply to be restored to it. Restoration cases are considered by panels of either the CCC or the HC as appropriate.

Professional Accountability

It is important for the nurse to appreciate the differences in terms of accountability within the four arenas in Figure 1.1 since there can be an overlap between professional accountability and legal accountability. An example of this may be the situation where a nurse fails to stop at the scene of a road accident. This is not a violation of the law but from a professional perspective the NMC may call her to account since there was a breach of its code of professional conduct (Dimond 2005). The code states: '8.5 In an emergency, in or outside the work setting, you have a professional duty to provide care. The care provided would be judged against what would reasonably be expected from someone with your knowledge, skills and abilities when placed in those particular circumstances' (NMC 2004a).

Accountability must be regarded as implicit within any area of practice where the professional practitioner delivers care. The practitioner has to make judgements and be answerable for those judgements. The NMC define accountability as 'responsible for something or to someone' which means that the nurse has an obligation or duty of care to the patient. To be responsible, however, it is necessary to have knowledge, and this includes knowledge of the law. Ignorance of the law is no defence, and therefore the nurse should be aware of the limits that the law imposes upon her as well as the power it gives (Dimond 2005).

Clark (2000) describes accountability as meaning 'the professional takes a decision or action not because someone has told him or her to do so, but because, having weighed up the alternatives and consequences in the light of the best available knowledge, he or she believes that it is the right decision or action to take'.

The NMC assert that although a nurse can be responsible for an action, accountability means being able to explain why. In exercising their professional duty nurses must be able to justify their actions and decisions, and clearly this is not possible unless a nurse has the necessary knowledge. Therefore, accountability requires knowledge (Cox 2001). As well as knowledge this means accountability is concerned with how far the nurse can be held in law to account for her actions. Certainly any profession will use the term accountability as a fundamental measure of its status as a profession.

Because of its dependence on such issues as authority and autonomy, the concept of accountability is closely related to the concept of professionalism. The modern concept of accountability, applied to nursing, assumes that the nurse is a member of a profession (McGann 2004). Watson (2004) maintains that 'accountability is the hallmark of a profession' since it is a framework for exercising the professional aspects of the work of nurses and midwives: those parts of their roles and jobs for which they have been trained.

Nursing has some of the features of a profession in that training and a registered qualification are both required in order to practise. By virtue of this, nurses become accountable to the general public for their practice and this accountability is regulated by a statutory body, the NMC, which as stated earlier is responsible for the training of nurses and holds the authority to remove individuals from the register and thereby their right to practise (Watson 2004).

The NMC states that registrants have a duty to the profession to behave in a manner which upholds codes of conduct, maintains the reputation of the profession and justifies public trust and confidence (NMC 2004a). This principle applies whether the nurse is on duty or not, or indeed is in employment or not. Therefore nurses have personal accountability in terms of their values and belief system. For example, if a nurse is negligent then he or she has to come to terms with the decision taken and be able to justify the misconduct if required.

Tschudin (2003) discusses accountability not only as meaning having to answer for an action when something goes wrong, but also as a continuous process of monitoring how a nurse performs professionally. The responsibility differs in different situations, but there is a need to be aware that one is constantly accountable. A distinction needs to be made between legal and moral accountability. This viewpoint is shared by Tingle (2004, page 56) who states 'accountability is a worthy pursuit for nurses and that the periodic exercising of accountability—when things go wrong—is only really possible if nurses learn to be accountable continually.'

Legal Accountability

Legal accountability is the principal form of accountability for every citizen, and nurses like all other professionals are personally accountable through the law for their actions or omissions. This individual legal accountability is channelled through the criminal and civil law in the courts (Tingle 2004). The law assumes that ignorance of accountability will not be an excuse should a legal action result. Consequently, it is imperative that nurses are aware of the legal aspects of their role (Figure 1.1).

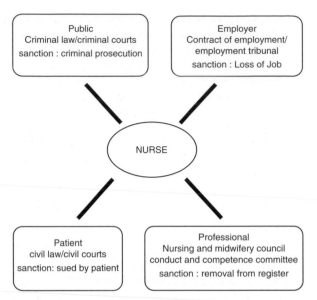

Figure 1.1   The four areas of accountability.

Litigation within healthcare in the United Kingdom (UK) has increased over the years and has huge financial implications for the NHS (Dougherty 2003). It has been estimated that almost £4 million is required to settle the actual and potential claims from events that have occurred within healthcare (Dimond 2005). Many nurses are becoming involved in providing expert advice to the courts when a clinical negligence claim is being pursued by a patient or relative. Since most judges have no medical or nursing expertise they rely on information provided by expert witnesses in order to come to a decision about an individual case. An expert witness is defined as 'a non-lawyer specialist in a particular field who is asked by a solicitor to give an independent opinion on a particular case' (Dougherty 2003, page 29). The expert witness uses their knowledge and expertise to provide non-biased information on the case to the solicitor and therefore requires good analytical, writing and communication skills.

The reality of nursing within an increasingly complex healthcare delivery system, with its risks of litigation, is reflected in the NMC Code of Conduct which suggests that healthcare professionals ensure that they have indemnity insurance (NMC 2004a).

Nursing Responsibility

The increase in knowledge and technological advances in i.v.-related equipment within i.v. therapy and the expanding use of toxic drugs have led to a growing appreciation of the need for accuracy and vigilance in the administration of i.v. drugs and fluids. Organizations are now concerned with clinical risk, and there are many strategies advocated by organizations such as the National Patient Safety Agency (NPSA), to reduce the potential for error—for example, standardizing i.v. infusion devices to avoid the healthcare worker becoming confused by the range of different pumps. The NPSA was set up in response to the government report *An Organisation with a Memory* (DH 2000a) and its prime function was to improve patient safety by reducing the risk of harm through error. The report states that every year 400 people die or are seriously injured in adverse events involving medical devices. One of the targets identified in the report was to reduce serious error in the use of medicines by the end of 2005.

The NPSA links in with the The Reporting of Injuries, Diseases and Dangerous Occurences Regulations 1995 (RIDDOR 95) reporting scheme. It examines the extent to which the NHS organizations learn from untoward incidents and service failures to ensure that similar situations are avoided in the future, draws conclusions and makes recommendations. The premise is that the NHS moves away from the culture of 'blame' and embraces a true understanding of the root causes of failures and errors (Dimond 2005). This type of transparency ensures that healthcare is responsible and accountable for its functions but is responsive to the ever changing arena of healthcare. Nurses must be aware of their responsibility to ensure that their practice is safe and to report untoward incidents immediately. The NMC states that it is important that an open culture of reporting medication errors is encouraged, and the nurse is responsible for immediately reporting errors or incidents in the administration of medicines (NMC 2004c).

The concept of responsibility can be divided into:

- the personal aspect of being responsible
- the legal aspect of having responsibility (Tschudin 2003).

There may be circumstances where a nurse could be held morally responsible but where there is no legal liability. For example, if a nurse fails to volunteer her services at the scene of a road accident, the law at present recognizes no legal duty to volunteer help and thus any legal action brought against the nurse would fail. However, many would hold that there is a moral duty to use her skills to help a fellow human being. Obviously the law and ethics overlap, but each is both wider and narrower than the other (Dimond 2005).

Nurses, however, have responsibilities not only to their patients, but also to the profession and to society as a whole. They have a responsibility not only to improve their own knowledge and skills, but also to contribute to the development of knowledge and skills within the profession as a whole (NMC 2004a).

Responsibility is not complete without accountability. Many responsibilities and duties are only seen clearly when something goes wrong. Values are only discovered through challenges. The NMC code is essentially a document outlining nurses' responsibilities.

Duty of Care

All nurses owe their patients a duty of care. Liability is likely to follow if that duty is breached. A breach will consist of a failure to meet the requisite standard of care. Difficulties can occur as to whether a duty of care exists, especially in circumstances outside the employment situation. A duty of care is not owed universally and the claimant bringing the action has to show that a duty of care was owed to him or her personally (Dimond 2005). However, if the nurse at the scene of an accident declares she is a nurse and helps, then from the professional context she has taken on a duty of care (NMC 2004a , page 11). However, in law there is no duty required of her unless there is 'a pre-existing relationship between the parties' (Dimond 2005, page 40).

The standard of care required is determined by the Bolam test: 'the standard of the ordinary skilled man exercising and professing to have that special skill. A man need not possess the highest expert skill at the risk of being found negligent. It is a well-established law that it is sufficient if he exercise the ordinary skill of an ordinary man exercising that particular art' (Bolam v Fern Hospital Management Committee 1957). This standard is a well-established principle (Dimond 2005, page 42). However Bolitho (1997) asserted that when challenged, if expert opinion could not withstand logical analysis then the judge has the right to conclude that the body of opinion is not reasonable or responsible (Foster 2002). Therefore, when justifying a clinical decision practitioners would be expected to acknowledge the risks and benefits in the particular situation. The competencies of the individual as well as their ability to consider national and local clinical guidelines in order to make a decision would be scrutinized, if the practitioner's clinical judgement was the subject of litigation. Healthcare practitioners would also be required to demonstrate that their knowledge was relevant and up to date, a principle which is reflected by the NMC Code of Conduct which embraces the notion that lifelong learning and being fit for purpose are fundamental to the role of the nurse (NMC 2004a).

Lord Aitkin laid down the basis of the duty of care that we owe to others in Donaghue v Stevenson (1932) (Dimond 2005). A person must take reasonable care to avoid acts or omissions that he can reasonably foresee would be likely to injure a person directly affected by those acts. This concept forms a cornerstone of the civil wrong of negligence where a breach of duty with resultant harm constitutes liability, and later cases have only served to refine this (Dimond 2005).

For a successful litigation outcome, the plaintiff must establish three principles based on the balance of probabilities:

- that a duty of care is owed by the defendant to the plaintiff
- that there has been a breach of that duty
- that, as a result of that breach, the plaintiff has suffered harm of a kind recognized in law and which is not too remote.

For example, a litigation claim could be evoked if in the course of her duty, a nurse made a drug administration error which caused the patient distress and injury.

Vicarious Liability

NHS trusts and other employers have two forms of liability: (1) direct liability, i.e. the Trust itself is at fault; and (2) vicarious or indirect liability, i.e. the Trust is responsible for the faults of others, mainly its employees (Dimond 2005). It is a necessary requirement that the employee was acting within the course of their employment when the incident occurred and that the employee was authorized to perform the procedure (Tingle 2001a). For example, a nurse is employed on a surgical unit and obtains a blood sample from a patient. However, she has not had the training to undertake the task and has not been authorized to perform the task by the hospital. The patient could then sue the nurse. If a nurse commits a negligent act then he or she is personally responsible and accountable for the negligence. It is possible that the employer could seek to recover any compensation which may be paid out. However, the Department of Health (DH) advises against this in practice (Tingle 2001a; Dimond 2005).

Indemnity insurance is provided for the nurse via professional organizations or trade unions. In a consultation paper (2002) the NMC considered making it a compulsory requirement for nurses but decided against it (Dimond 2005). It recommended instead that a registered nurse, midwife or specialist community public health nurse, in advising, treating and caring for patients/clients, has professional indemnity insurance. This is in the interests of clients, patients and registrants in the event of claims of professional negligence (NMC 2004a; Dimond 2005).

Legal Aspects of Medicines

The main legislation controlling the supply, storage and administration of medicines is the Medicines Act 1968 (DH 1968) and the Misuse of Drugs Act 1971. Nurse should be familiar with subsequent statutory instruments such as the Misuse of Drug Regulations (2001) which makes provision for the classification of controlled drugs, their possession, supply and manufacture. The previous Medicines Control Agency has now been incorporated into the Medicines and Healthcare products Regulatory Agency (MHRA) (Dimond 2005). Guidance on the administration of medicines is provided by the NMC's document *Guidelines for the Administration of Medicines* (2004c) and whilst this has no legal force it is the standard by which the nurse would be measured in terms of her professional accountability. Nurses should be familiar with the *British National Formulary* as an excellent resource for accurate information on medicines.(Before administering each drug, the nurse should complete the following checklists.

- Correct patient—consent, information.
- Correct drug—side-effects, reconstitution, diluent.
- Correct dose.
- Correct site and method of administration—check patency of venous access device if to be given intravenously.
- Correct procedure—level of competence of nurse, safe reconstitution, safe equipment, asepsis.
- Correct record-keeping.

One such document, the *Guidelines for the Administration of Medicines* (NMC 2004c) states clearly that the Council has prepared these standards to assist practitioners to fulfill the expectations it has of them, to serve more effectively the interests of patients and clients, and to maintain and enhance standards of practice. It continues to list a number of principles in which the practitioner must exercise their professional judgement (*See* Box 1.3).

Nurse Prescribing

The history of nurse prescribing is a long one. It began in 1978 when the Association of Nursing Practice (ANP) and the Royal College of Nursing (RCN) presented a report to its parent body entitled *District Nurses' Dressings* (RCN 1978) which had raised concerns over the reliance on GP prescriptions in order for the district nurse to deliver care (Jones 1999, page 6). At that time the government had commissioned a review of community nursing provision in England under the chairmanship of Julia Cumberledge.

BOX 1.3

Guidelines for the administration of medicines (NMC 2004c, page 4)

Principles in relation to the prescription

- Be based, whenever possible, on the patient's informed consent and awareness of purpose of the treatment.
- Be clearly written, typed or computer-generated and be indelible.
- Clearly identify the patient for whom the medication is intended.
- Record the weight of the patient on the prescription sheet where the dosage of medication is related to weight.
- Clearly specify the substance to be administered, using its generic or brand name where appropriate and its stated form, together with the strength, dosage, timing, frequency of administration, start and finish dates and the route of administration.
- Be signed and dated by the authorized prescriber.
- Not be for a substance to which the patient is known to be allergic or otherwise unable to tolerate.
- In the case of controlled drugs, specify the dosage and the number of dosage units or total course; if in an out-patient or community setting, the prescription should be in the prescriber's own handwriting; some prescribers are subject to handwriting exemption but the prescription must be signed and dated by the prescriber.

Nurse prescribing is an acknowledgement and endorsement of the current contribution of nurses to patient care and a recognition of the need to supply items necessary for effective nursing treatment.

To prescribe effectively, nurses need:

- an increased awareness of professional accountability
- a full understanding of the process of assessment and diagnosis that results in the act of prescribing
- knowledge of therapeutics and practical prescribing (Andrews 1994).

It was the Cumberledge Report (Cumberledge 1986) that first identified the need for limited nurse prescribing:

> The DHSS should agree a limited list of items and simple agents which may be prescribed by nurses as part of a nursing care programme and issue guidelines to enable nurses to control drug dosage in well defined circumstances.

The report was positively received by government, and Dr June Crown was asked to lead an advisory group to report back to government by 1 October 1987. Following a number of subsequent reports which recommended that nurses should prescribe from a limited formulary, the Nurse Prescribing Advisory Group (DH 1989) Crown Report ('the First Crown Report') made 27 recommendations addressed to the DH, the UKCC, health authorities and the professions. These recommendations relate to six core areas:

- practice
- education
- administration
- legal issues
- communication
- public safeguards.

The nurse's prescribing powers have developed dramatically in recent years. Following the publication of the First Crown Report, legislation has been passed to allow nurses to prescribe (DH 1992). There are currently four pieces of legislation that define the legal situation for nurses involved in the supply and administration of 'prescription-only medicines' (Dimond 2005).

- The Medicines Act 1968—this is the starting point; Section 58 describes current requirements.
- The Medicines Order (1983)—this legislation explains in further detail particular aspects of the Medicines Act 1968 and gives legal definitions of the terms used.
- Medicinal Products: Prescribing for Nurses Act 1992 (DH 1992)—this provides legal authorization to nurses to be involved in the supply and administration of 'prescription-only medicines' and states in Section 1 that 'registered nurses, midwives and health visitors … who comply with such conditions as may be specified' could become appropriate practitioners.
- Medicines Order (1994)—this outlines the conditions to be met by nurses who are to be prescribing practitioners.

On page 2 of the DH document *Improving Patients' Access to Medicines: A Guide to Implementing Nurse and Pharmacist Prescribing within the NHS in England* (DH 2006) independent prescribing is defined as 'Prescribing by a practitioner responsible and accountable for the assessment of patients with diagnosed or undiagnosed conditions and for decisions about clinical management required, including prescribing'. The document emphasizes the fundamental requirement for all healthcare professionals involved in prescribing to have relevant education, experience and competence according to professional codes of practice. Among other issues, the document is a guide on levels of responsibility, educational requirements and clinical governance issues.

In summary, nurse prescribing has developed rapidly and the law now allows nurses in hospitals and primary care to issue prescriptions from the BNF for any drug within their area of competence (DH 2006). These additional responsibilities must, however, be coupled with the necessary education and competence as well as a systematic approach to maintaining knowledge.

Record-keeping

Record-keeping is an integral part of nursing, midwifery and specialist community public health nursing practice. It is a tool of professional practice and one that should help the care process. It is not separate from this process and it is not an optional extra to be fitted in if circumstances allow (NMC 2005). The NMC guidelines on record-keeping was revised in 2004 to bring it in line with changes brought about by the Nursing and Midwifery Order 2001, and was further revised in 2005 to clarify information supplied regarding current legislation (NMC 2005).

Accurate, accessible and comprehensive documentation of the care given to and condition of a patient is essential for effective and high-quality patient care, and continuity of care between different health practitioners (Cox 2001). In 2000 the Health Service Commissioner stated that poor record-keeping was a feature of many of the complaints that he investigated. Consequences of poor record-keeping are threefold:

- patient care is compromised
- the practitioner and employer lose protection against negligence claims
- the practitioner is acting contrary to her professional code of practice (Cox 2001).

Furthermore, the NMC states that the quality of record-keeping is also a reflection of the standard of a practitioner's professional practice. Good record-keeping is a mark of the skilled and safe practitioner, whilst careless or incomplete record-keeping often highlights wider problems with the individual's practice (NMC 2005). The NMC also states that it is good practice to retain records in relation to the Human Rights Act 2001 and the Caldicott Report 1997 (DH 1997).

The government's commitment to computerized record-keeping and investment in computer technology means that these types of record will become the norm and it is important that the nurse is familiar with good practice guidelines. Clarity of records as well as legibility and avoiding use of abbreviations will help ensure high standards of record-keeping. The DH document *Winning Ways: Working together to reduce Healthcare Associated Infection in England* (DH 2003) gives guidelines on documenting details regarding the vascular access device including date and time of insertion and removal of device. Accurate record-keeping in terms of infection control is viewed as pivotal to the reduction in catheter-related infections.

The Caldicott Committee was established to undertake a review of the information sources for patient data within the NHS organizations and other agencies for purposes other than direct care or medical research or where there is a statutory requirement for information (DH 1997). It recommended that guardians should be appointed to ensure that shared information between healthcare providers should be given on 'a need to know' basis with confidentiality health checks performed each year (McHale 2001b). These principles help ensure that patient details are recorded, stored and disseminated appropriately.

The importance of nurses keeping accurate and thorough records can never be underestimated, and to neglect this area of practice is to open oneself to professional and legal complications. Failure to maintain reasonable standards of record-keeping could be evidence of professional misconduct and subject to professional conduct proceedings. Furthermore, any documents produced in a court of law will be subject to close scrutiny and therefore any weaknesses in record-keeping would compromise the professional when they came to give evidence (Dimond 2005).

Consent to Treatment

The notion of informed consent stems from the 1947 Nuremberg trials of 23 Nazi doctors accused of crimes involving human subjects. The Nuremberg Code (1947) laid down 10 standards to which doctors must conform when carrying out experiments on human subjects. Subsequently, guidance in the Declaration of Helsinki 1964, updated in 2000, states 'the ethical principles to provide guidance to physicians and other participants in medical research involving human subjects' (Tschudin 2003, page 94).

The idea of consent is based on the principle of respect for the person and thus on the concept of human rights of life and liberty (Tschudin 2003). Central to thinking about the nursing care of the patient is the philosophical concept of autonomy. On the premise that people know what is in their best interest, the ethical principle states that the choices of mature people must be respected and, reflecting this principle, the law insists that consent is, in the vast majority of cases, a prerequisite to the care of the patient (Cox 2001).

As a registered nurse, midwife or specialist community public health nurse, you must obtain consent before you give any treatment or care. Furthermore, when obtaining valid consent you must be sure it is:

- given by a legally competent person
- given voluntarily
- informed

(NMC 2004a)

Consent can be given in a variety of ways and, as far as the law is concerned, there is no specific requirement that consent for treatment should be given in any particular way. Verbal, implied, written and expressed consent are all equally valid; however, they can vary in their value as evidence in proving that consent was given (Dimond 2005). Consent is not just about the patient saying 'yes', but also about them saying 'no', which can be a challenge for some healthcare professionals (Tschudin 2003).

Some examples of different types of consent follow.

Verbal consent, for example, would be where the nurse asks the patient's permission to obtain a blood sample and the patient agrees to the procedure.
Implied consent is given if the nurse asks the patient for permission to insert a peripheral cannula and the patient holds out their arm for the procedure.
Written consent is obtained by asking the patient to sign a document to state that they understand the procedure, for example, insertion of a central venous catheter.

The DH updated its guidance on consent to examination and treatment in 2001, the intention being that it was a reference document which should be regularly updated (Dimond 2005).

Essentially, most nursing actions are invasions of a person's privacy. Most of these actions are considered necessary and consent is given implicitly by going into hospital. This, however, should never be taken for granted. Giving full explanations of what is being done, and why, how and when, is essential for the patient to remain a free agent and exercise the right to say no (Tschudin 2003).

Refusal to consent to treatment

It is often difficult for nurses to accept a patient's refusal to give consent, particularly when the treatment being offered is life-saving. However, the nurse must remember that the patient has the right to choose and her role is to support the patient in this right. An action of battery may be brought if treatment is given in the face of an explicit refusal of consent (McHale 2001a).

While a clear refusal should be respected, there are situations in which a patient's refusal may be overridden. General guidance for healthcare professionals was laid down in Re T (*See* McHale 2001a). This case concerned a patient who was 34 weeks pregnant and who, when taken to hospital following a road traffic accident, refused a blood transfusion. This decision had been reached after she had spent some time alone with her mother, who was a Jehovah's Witness—T herself was not a Jehovah's Witness. However, T's condition deteriorated following the birth and she required a blood transfusion. The hospital caring for T sought a declaration on the legality of their administering a transfusion if required – a declaration that was granted by the court.

In delivering judgement in this case, Lord Donaldson laid down a number of guidelines to assist healthcare professionals faced with patients who were refusing treatment (McHale 2002).

- If a patient had refused consent this could lead those treating him to ask whether he was capable of refusing consent to treatment.
- The implications of treatment refusal vary tremendously and the nurse should consider whether the refusal of treatment means that the patient will only suffer pain and discomfort at one extreme or whether refusal means almost certain death.
- The scope of the refusal should also be considered—whether it applies in all situations and whether it is based upon assumptions which have not been realised.

In addition, the nurse should consider whether the patient's decision has been reached without undue influence being applied. Where a patient is clearly refusing medication, it is essential for staff to record detailed accounts of the patient's attitude and level of competence, and the advice given to the patient and, preferably, where the patient takes his own discharge contrary to professional advice, to obtain the patient's signature to that effect (Dimond 2005).

Expansion of Nursing Roles

The role of the nurse has developed in a far more fundamental way than simply taking on previously medical tasks. Advances in medical knowledge and technology have contributed towards the effective management of disease and illness. These advances have increased the complexity of healthcare systems. 'Their unique combination of processes, technologies and human interactions means that modern healthcare systems are among the most complex in the world' (DH 2000a, page 5). Nursing has been responsive to these developments and the role of the nurse has expanded to include roles such as nurse specialist and nurse consultant which embrace professional practice from a more holistic perspective than that of the traditional medical model of task orientation.

The modern healthcare system with all its complexities required a radical modernization and in July 2000 The National Plan for the NHS was published (DH 2000b). The vision that the NHS would embrace the notion of protocol-based care meant that nurses had to be empowered to undertake a wide range of clinical skills that had traditionally been the remit of the medical profession (Dimond 2005). Role expansion is inextricably linked with the risk of legal and professional complications for the nurse.

BOX 1.4

The NMC code of professional conduct: standards for conduct, performance and ethics (NMC 2004a)

As a registered nurse, midwife or specialist community public health nurse, you must maintain your professional knowledge and competence.

- You must keep your knowledge and skills up to date throughout your working life. In particular, you should take part regularly in learning activities that develop your competence and performance.
- To practice competently, you must possess the knowledge, skills and abilities required for lawful, safe and effective practice without direct supervision. You must acknowledge the limits of your professional competence and only undertake practice and accept responsibilities for those activities in which you are competent.
- If an aspect of practice is beyond your level of competence or outside your area of registration, you must obtain help and supervision from a competent practitioner until you and your employer consider that you have acquired the requisite knowledge and skill.
- You have a duty to facilitate students of nursing, midwifery and specialist community public health nursing and others to develop their competence.
- You have a responsibility to deliver care based on current evidence, best practice and, where applicable, validated research when it is available.

Nurses have a responsibility to maintain their knowledge and skill through continuing education in order that the care they provide is relevant and does not happen outside their limits of competence. Post-registration education and practice (PREP) is a fundamental requirement of professional practice, and nurses have a duty to have at least 5 refresher days every 3 years. The NMC's expectations of its registrants in terms of education and competence are shown in Box 1.4.

With regard to achieving best practice within i.v. therapy, the RCN document *Standards for Infusion Therapy* (RCN 2005) can help maintain good-quality care and directs the practitioner towards evidence-based practice. It includes information relating to infusion-related complications, infection control, placement, care and maintenance of vascular access devices, most appropriate infusion devices and infusion-related equipment, and infusion therapies, including chemotherapy, analgesia, transfusion and epidural administration.

Other quality measures within the NHS have been created by the 1999 Health Act. One of these was the creation of the Commission for Health Improvement (CHI), now known as the Healthcare Commission (HC), which presents an annual report on 'the provision of healthcare by or for NHS bodies' to Parliament. Its functions include providing advice and information on the monitoring and improving of healthcare provided by NHS trusts and primary care trusts (Cox 2001). In July 2005 it reported for the first time on the experiences of patients, who had commented upon the quality of the care they received.

The HC operates alongside the National Institute for Health and Clinical Excellence (NICE). These organizations were set up by government to ensure that healthcare policy moved towards the rights of patients and their relationship with health carers.

The administration of intravenous drugs was probably the most well known area of medical to nurse delegation, and is now an integral part of nursing practice. To address this issue, in 1976 Lord Breckenridge was asked to chair a working party to look at the addition of drugs to intravenous infusion fluids. Evidence presented to the working party, from the nursing viewpoint, identified that the addition and administration of drugs via i.v. infusion fluids was increasingly carried out by nurses (DHSS 1976). The working party recognized that nurses' authority and responsibility in this area of practice were not clearly defined and were made more confusing by local policies and standards of training which varied widely. There was no further guidance until the British Intravenous Therapy

Association (BITA) guidelines in 1987, and then a statement from the RCN and BMA (RCN/BMA 1993) which set out principles to guide healthcare professionals developing i.v. practices (Box 1.5).

More recently, in 2003 the RCN published the first-ever *Standards for Infusion Therapy* in the UK which was updated in 2005 (RCN 2005). The standards were originally sent to 17 RCN groups and forums and seven multiprofessional organizations for an extensive peer review. Professor Elliott in his foreword wrote that 'without doubt this book should become a standard in itself and be of value to all healthcare workers involved in infusion therapy' (Elliott 2005).

It could be argued that the expansion and development of nursing roles have been driven by a political force, in the main through the reduction of junior doctors' hours, but also through the 10 key roles listed in the NHS Plan 2000 (DH 2000b) (*See* Box 1.6). Nurses would like to believe that they have exploited this directive to their professional advantage and satisfaction as well as to the benefit of patient care.

BOX 1.5

Intravenous drug therapy—RCN and BMA guiding principles (RCN/BMA 1993)

- Patients' interests are paramount.
- Practitioners have a responsibility to draw attention to areas where local protocols conflict with the patient's best interests.
- Intravenous therapy administration must be viewed as a partnership responsibility with standards consistent amongst the healthcare team.
- The intravenous route is only to be used when there are no other alternatives.
- All healthcare staff involved with intravenous therapy administration have a responsibility to ensure that they have attained the appropriate knowledge and skills to enable the delivery of safe and effective care.
- Healthcare professionals should actively participate in minimizing the risks associated with i.v. therapy.
- Policies and protocols should be developed at local level which should reflect the active contributions of experienced healthcare professionals.
- Consistent standards must apply across the healthcare team.
- Each practitioner is considered as responsible and personally accountable for their practice.
- Intravenous therapy should be audited.

BOX 1.6

Ten key roles for nurses in the NHS plan (DH 2000b)

1. To order diagnostic investigations such as pathology tests and X-rays.
2. To make and receive referrals direct, say, to therapist or pain consultant.
3. To admit and discharge patients for specified conditions and within agreed protocols.
4. To manage patient caseloads, say for diabetes or rheumatology.
5. To run clinics, say for opthamology or dermatology.
6. To prescribe medicines and treatments.
7. To carry out a wide range of resuscitation procedures, including defibrillation.
8. To perform minor surgery and outpatient procedures.
9. To triage patients to the most appropriate health professional using the latest IT.
10. To lead in the way local health services are both organized and run.

Standards of Training

It is crucial in an area of clinical practice such as the administration of i.v. therapy that the practitioner has the appropriate knowledge base on which to underpin practice. Currently there is no national standard of i.v. training, and trusts and employers are in the position of having to draw up local policies and education packs, the standard and content of which vary widely (RCN 2005).

However, due to the emergence of dedicated i.v. nurses and with i.v. therapy becoming more commonplace, it is imperative that recommendations for standards of practice, which were first identified in the 1980s and have been evolving since then, are adhered to.

The British Intravenous Therapy Association was established in 1980 in response to a call from interested nurses who were concerned about the standards of i.v. practice and the preparation of nurses for this practice. The aim of the association was to promote, for the public benefit, investigation into i.v. practice, nurse education and research with concomitant dissemination of knowledge through publication.

In order to achieve these aims, the following objectives were identified:

- to establish codes of practice for nurses engaged in i.v. therapy
- to provide information and promote education related to i.v. therapy
- to establish and develop bursaries/grants for the pursuance of research into i.v. therapy.

If an i.v. training programme is to gain national recognition and acceptance, it is important that the content and standard of that programme are consistent and relevant to clinical practice, and are coordinated and facilitated by clinical experts.

All practitioners have a duty to provide safe standards of i.v. care to all patients. Healthcare staff involved in i.v. therapy must be able to demonstrate a sound knowledge of:

- legal, professional and ethical issues
- anatomy and physiology
- fluid balance and blood administration
- mathematical calculations related to medications
- pharmacology and pharmaceutics related to reconstitution and administration
- local and systemic complications
- infection control issues (*See* the DH Infection Controls Assurance Standard 2003)
- use of equipment, including infusion equipment
- drug administration
- risk management/health and safety
- care and management of vascular access devices
- infusion therapy in specialist areas covered separately (paediatrics, oncology, parenteral nutrition, transfusion therapy) (Delisio 2001; RCN 2005).

Nurses who wish to expand their skills beyond drug administration, that is, to venepuncture, cannulation and placement of central venous access devices, need to attend additional competency and education programmes relevant to that area of practice. It is essential that practitioners keep abreast of clinical advances and changes in practice, and it is therefore recommended that training updates be attended at least every 2 years, or earlier if the practitioners deem it necessary.

Conclusion

Within the modern healthcare system nursing practice has become more autonomous as nursing knowledge and professional roles have expanded. The complexities of healthcare delivery require nurses to maintain their knowledge and expertise in order to appropriately respond to the needs of their patients and therefore be fit for purpose. With increased autonomy, however, comes a need to improve the nurse's understanding of the implications of expanding nursing practice and the legal and professional parameters of such progression. Finally to be a skilled and safe practitioner, who is responsive to the needs of the patient, a nurse requires the application of legal and ethical principles related to nursing.

References

Andrews S (1994). Nurse Prescribing. In: Hunt G, Wainright P, eds. *Expanding the role of the nurse*, ch 5, 74–78. Blackwell Science, Oxford.

Bolitho v City and Hackney Health Authority (1997) 3 WLR 115.

British Medical Association/Royal Pharmaceutical Society of Great Britain (BMA/RPSGB) (2007) *British National Formulary*. RPS Publishing, London. bnf.org

Clark J (2000) *Accountability in Nursing, Second WHO Ministerial Conference on Nursing and Midwifery in Europe*. Munich, 15–17 June 2000.

Cox C (2001) *The Legal Challenges Facing Nurses*. Discussion paper. Royal College of Nursing, London.

Cumberledge J (1986) *Neighbourhood Nursing—A Focus for Care. Report of the Community Nursing Review*. HMSO, London.

Delisio NM (2001) Intravenous nursing as a speciality. In: Hankins J, Lonsway RA, Hedrick C, Perdue MB, eds. *Infusion Therapy in Clinical Practice*, 2nd edn, 6–14. WB Saunders, Philadelphia.

Department of Health (DH) (1968) *The Medicines Act*. HMSO, London.

Department of Health (1989) *Report of the Advisory Group on Nurse Prescribing (Crown Report)*. HMSO, London.

Department of Health (1992) *Medicinal Products: Prescription by Nurses Act*. HMSO, London.

Department of Health (1997) *Report on the Review of Patient Identifiable Information (Caldicott Report)*. HMSO, London.

Department of Health (2000a) *An Organisation with a Memory: Report of an Expert Group on Learning from Adverse Events in the NHS*. TSO, London.

Department of Health (2000b) *The NHS Plan: a Plan for Investment, a Plan for Reform*. Department of Health, London.

Department of Health (2003) *Winning Ways. Working together to reduce Healthcare Associated Infection in England*. Department of Health, London.

Department of Health (2006) *Improving Patients' Access to Medicines: A Guide to Implementing Nurse and Pharmacist Independent Prescribing within the NHS in England*. Gateway reference 6429. www.dh.gov.uk

Department of Health and Social Security (1976) *Health Service Development, addition of drugs to intravenous infusion fluids. HC (76) 9 (Breckenridge Report)*. HMSO, London.

Dimond B (2005) *Legal Aspects of Nursing*, 4th edn. Pearson Education Ltd.

Dougherty L (2003) The expert witness. Working within the legal system of the United Kingdom. *Journal of Vascular Access Devices*, 8 (2): 29–35.

Elliot TSJ (2005) *Standards for infusion therapy*. Royal College of Nursing. London.

Foster C (2002) Negligence: the legal perspective. In: Tingle J, Cribb A, eds. *Nursing Law and Ethics*, 75–89. Blackwell Science, Oxford.

Greenhalgh AF (1994) *The Interface Between Junior Doctors and Nurses: A Research Study for the Department of Health*. Greenhalgh & Co, Macclesfield.

Health Act (1999) ISBN 1 10 540899 9. TSO, London.

Hodgson J (2002) The legal dimension: legal system and method. In: Tingle J, Cribb A, eds. *Nursing Law and Ethics*, 3–18. Blackwell Science, Oxford.

Human Rights Act (Amendment) Order (2001) ISBN 011029267 7. TSO, London.

International Council of Nurses (2000) *Code of Nursing Ethics*. International Council of Nurses, Geneva.

Jones M (1999) Nurse Prescribing. The history, the waiting, the battle. In: Jones M ed. *Nurse Prescribing. Politics to practice*, 5–27. Bailliere Tindall, London.

McGann S (2004) Development of Nursing as an accountable profession. In: Tilley S, Watson R, eds. *Accountability in Nursing and Midwifery*, 9–20. Blackwell Science, Oxford.

McHale J (2001a) Consent to treatment I: general principles. In: McHale J, Tingle J, eds. *Law and Nursing*, 2nd edn, 89–109. Butterworth-Heinemann, Oxford.

McHale J (2001b) Confidentiality and access to health records. In: McHale J, Tingle J, eds. *Law and Nursing*, 2nd edn, 137–163. Butterworth-Heinemann, Oxford.

McHale J (2001c) Introduction: the nurse and the legal environment. In: McHale J, Tingle J, eds. *Law and Nursing*, 2nd edn, 1–26. Butterworth-Heinemann, Oxford.

McHale J (2002) Consent and the capable adult patient—the legal perspective. In: Tingle J, Cribb A, eds. *Nursing Law and Ethics*, 99–120. Blackwell Science, Oxford.

Medicines (Pharmacy and General Sale—Exemption) Amendment Order (1994) SI 1994 no. 2409. HMSO, London.

Medicines (Products other than Veterinary Drugs) (Prescription only) Order (1983) S1 1983 no 1212. HMSO, London.

The Misuse of Drug Regulations (2001) SI 2001 no. 3998.

Nursing and Midwifery Council (2002) *Code of Professional Conduct*. Nursing and Midwifery Council, London.

Nursing and Midwifery Council (2004a) *Code of Professional Conduct: Standards for Conduct, Performance and Ethics*. Nursing and Midwifery Council, London.

Nursing and Midwifery Council (2004b) *Complaints about Unfitness to Practice: A Guide for Members of the Public*. Nursing and Midwifery Council, London.

Nursing and Midwifery Council (2004c) *Guidelines on the Administration of Medicines*. Nursing and Midwifery Council, London.

Nursing and Midwifery Council (2005) *Guidelines for Records and Record-keeping*. Nursing and Midwifery Council, London.

Nursing and Midwifery Council (2006) *About the NMC* [www document]. www.nmc-uk.org [accessed 29 January 2007]

Petersen B (2002) *Stepping into the future: who will care for healthcare?* Presentation at the NAVAN Conference, San Diego.

Royal College of Nursing (1978) *District Nurses' Dressings*. Unpublished report to RCN Council from the Community Nursing Association of the RCN. Copy in RCN archives, London.

Royal College of Nursing (2005) *Standards for Infusion Therapy*. Royal College of Nursing, London.

Royal College of Nursing/British Medical Association (1993) *Intravenous Drug Therapy: a Statement*. Royal College of Nursing/British Medical Association, London.

Tingle J (2001a) Nursing negligence: general issues. In: McHale J, Tingle J, eds. *Law and Nursing*, 2nd edn, 27–47. Butterworth-Heinemann, Oxford.

Tingle J (2001b) Legal aspects of expanded role and clinical guidelines and protocols. In: McHale J, Tingle J, eds. *Law and Nursing*, 2nd edn, 68–88. Butterworth-Heinemann, Oxford.

Tingle J (2004) The legal accountability of the nurse. In: Tilley S, Watson R, eds. *Accountability in Nursing and Midwifery*, 47–63. Blackwell Science, Oxford.

Tschudin V (2003) *Ethics in Nursing. The Caring Relationship*, 3rd edn. Butterworth-Heinemann, Oxford.

Watson R (2004) Accountability and clinical governance. In: Tilley S, Watson R, eds. *Accountability in Nursing and Midwifery*, 2nd edn, 38–46. Blackwell Science, Oxford.

CHAPTER 2

Anatomy and Physiology Related to Intravenous Therapy

Katie Scales

Introduction

The circulation is a collective term used to describe movement of blood around the body by the heart and blood vessels.

The purpose of this chapter is to discuss the structure and function of the components that comprise the circulation, and some of the mechanisms that control blood flow. Physiology that underpins the practice of intravenous (i.v.) therapy will be explained and made relevant to clinical practice. The information is presented in an integrated manner, in other words anatomy and physiology are combined to produce a more cohesive explanation of this complex science.

The Heart

The heart is a hollow muscular organ lying slightly left of the midline within the thorax. The superior surface (where the vessels enter the heart) is called the base and is wider than the inferior surface, which is called the apex. The heart provides the force for the propulsion of blood through the arterial and capillary system and for its return through the venous system.

The heart is, in essence, a single organ containing two pumps that complement each other. The pump on the right side of the heart pumps blood through the lungs (the pulmonary circulation), while the pump on the left side pumps blood to all other parts of the body (the systemic circulation). Blood flow through the heart is unidirectional and the flow control is achieved by a series of valves that, in a healthy person, only allow blood to flow in a forward direction (Morton *et al.* 2005) (Figure 2.1).

From Figure 2.1 it can be seen that two major veins, the superior and inferior vena cava (SVC, IVC), enter the right atrium; these are also known as the great veins (Guyton & Hall 2006). These vessels contain the systemic venous return, i.e. the SVC conveys venous blood from the head, neck, arms and upper thorax, while the IVC conveys blood from the rest of the thorax, the abdomen and the lower limbs.

Venous return to the heart is passive and relies on negative pressure in the thorax to attract blood back to the heart, as well as local muscle activity in the limbs. Because there are no valves separating the SVC and IVC from the right atrium, the pressure is the same in the SVC/IVC as it is in the right atrium. When measuring central venous pressure,

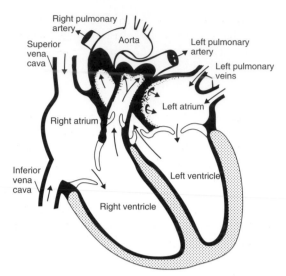

Figure 2.1   The heart in vertical cross-section with blood flow indicated by arrows. (From Wilson & Waugh 1996. Reproduced with kind permission from Churchill Livingstone.)

catheters are usually located in the subclavian vein or SVC. Mortality is increased when catheters are placed in the heart itself (Collier & Goodman 1995). Some catheters such as pulmonary artery catheters are designed for cardiac placement.

Blood flows from the right atrium down into the right ventricle; it is then pumped into the pulmonary artery and pulmonary capillaries for gas exchange. Venous return from the lungs delivers oxygenated blood to the left atrium; blood flows down into the left ventricle and is pumped out into the aorta for systemic distribution.

Closer inspection of the structure of the ventricle reveals finger-like projections of muscle arising from the apex of each ventricle; these are called papillary muscles. From the top of the papillary muscle, tendon-like cords connect with the cusps of the atrioventricular valves. These structures provide stability for the atrioventricular valves that might otherwise prolapse from the force of the ventricular contraction. There are reported cases of pulmonary artery catheters becoming entangled in these anatomical structures (Arnaout *et al.* 2001). This is often only discovered when the catheter fails to be removed by simple, gentle traction. Force should not be used as this will result in rupture of the structures within the ventricle. The management of an entangled pulmonary artery catheter is not easy, and cardiac surgery to visually remove the device may be the only solution (Perreas *et al.* 1999). To prevent trauma to the valves or the chordae it is important to ensure that the balloon at the tip of the pulmonary artery catheter has been completely deflated before removing the pulmonary artery catheter.

The rhythmical contraction and relaxation of the heart is termed the cardiac cycle, consisting of two phases: systole, when the heart contracts, and diastole, when the heart relaxes. Because of the systolic and diastolic activity of the heart, the cardiac output is intermittent, a pulsatile rather than a continuous flow. When the left ventricle contracts, it ejects its volume into the aorta. The resting arterial pressure of the aorta creates a resistance to ejection, which is termed afterload. The volume of blood returning to the heart to fill the ventricles is termed preload. Preload is affected by overall blood volume and the resting tone of the blood vessels. If peripheral vessels become excessively dilated, blood will begin to pool in the periphery, reducing venous return to the heart. The converse is also true: peripheral constriction inhibits pooling and increases venous return. Preload and afterload can both be manipulated by the use of drugs that affect vascular tone; these drugs can vasoconstrict or vasodilate and are classified as vasoactive agents. The effects of these drugs are assessed using haemodynamic monitoring (Morton *et al.* 2005) and their use is usually restricted to critical care areas.

Serum levels

Correct serum levels of sodium, potassium and calcium are required for normal function of the heart. Too high a calcium level causes the heart to stop in systole, and too high a potassium level causes the heart to stop in diastole (Green 1985). This is of practical importance when undertaking i.v. therapy. If concentrated solutions containing potassium or calcium are infused rapidly via a central venous catheter directly into the heart, it is possible to cause cardiac arrest (Green 1985). This situation can occur unintentionally during the transfusion of cold, stored blood. When blood is cooled and stored, potassium leaches out of the red blood cells, causing a significant elevation in the serum potassium concentration. If this is transfused rapidly via a central venous catheter, asystole can be induced.

Blood Vessel Structure

There are five classifications of blood vessel: arteries, arterioles, capillaries, venules and veins. All blood vessels (with the exception of the capillary) have a similar construction. There are three layers to the vessel wall and the differences are determined by the location and function of each vessel.

The internal layer (tunica intima)

This is a layer of simple squamous epithelial cells known as endothelium together with a basement membrane and a layer of elastic tissue known as the internal elastic lamina (Tortora & Derrickson 2006). Endothelium is a continuous layer of cells that lines the entire cardiovascular system; it extends from the blood vessels to form the internal lining of the heart. Endothelium facilitates blood flow along the vessel, preventing the adhesion of blood cells to the vessel wall. Any trauma which roughens the lining encourages platelets to adhere to the vessel wall and may result in thrombus formation (Weinstein 2007) and the inflammatory process of phlebitis (Hadaway 2001). Endothelial cells can easily be damaged (Box 2.1).

BOX 2.1

Factors which may result in damage to endothelial cells

- Rapid advancement of a cannula.
- Poor technique when advancing a cannula, i.e. not maintaining adequate traction on skin and vein.
- Using a cannula which is too large for the lumen of the vein.
- Using a cannula which remains relatively rigid after insertion.
- Siting a cannula near to areas of flexion such as over joints.
- Inadequate securement, which may result in movement of the cannula.
- Poor skin preparation and incorrect use of dressings, which can lead to contamination of the site.
- Infusion of any of the following irritant solutions:
    — hypertonic
    — hypotonic
    — very low or high pH.
- Infusion of particulate matter.
- Rapid infusions of large quantities of fluid which may be too great for the vessel to accommodate.

Clinical Skills Laboratory 2007

The middle layer (tunica media)

This layer is composed of elastic tissue and smooth muscle fibres that run in a circular pattern around the lumen. The tunica media also has an external elastic lamina made up of elastic tissue (Tortora & Derrickson 2006). The amount of elastic tissue can vary within vessels. For example, the largest-diameter arteries (> 1 cm) are referred to as elastic arteries because the tunica media contains a high proportion of elastic fibres. In comparison, medium-sized arteries (1 mm–1 cm) are classified as muscular arteries because the tunica media contains more smooth muscle and less elastic fibre than an elastic artery (Tortora & Derrickson 2006). The amount of smooth muscle found in the tunica media also varies between vessels. Arteries have a thicker muscle layer than veins and the quantity and arrangement of the smooth muscle fibres within an artery provides a relatively rigid structure. By comparison, veins have less smooth muscle and elastic tissue, and as a result are more prone to collapse if venous pressure is low (Green 1985). Sympathetic nerves from the autonomic nervous system innervate the smooth muscle of the tunica media (Tortora & Derrickson 2006). The sympathetic fibres control the tone of the vessel. Increased sympathetic stimulation causes the muscle layer to contract and the lumen of the vessel is reduced; this narrowing of the vessel is termed vasoconstriction. The opposite is also true: reduced sympathetic stimulation causes the smooth muscle fibres to relax and the vessel lumen increases; the increased diameter of the vessel is termed vasodilation. The smooth muscle layer is sensitive to changes in temperature, and mechanical or chemical irritation can cause spasm of the vessel. In veins, this can impede blood flow, resulting in pain which can often be relieved by heat. Arterial spasm from chemical irritation may have serious consequences; the artery can become damaged, leading to ischaemia, and this may cause necrosis and gangrene (Weinstein 2007).

Smooth muscle may also undergo what is called the stress relaxation phenomenon (Hadaway 2001). When a tourniquet is placed on the limb to aid distension of the peripheral veins, the muscle fibres elongate to accommodate the increased volume of blood in the veins. The pressure increases and then falls back to normal in spite of the increased volume. If the tourniquet is then removed, the volume and pressure suddenly fall, and within several minutes normal pressure is re-established. This can be helpful for deciding the length of time that a tourniquet is left in place, particularly when advancing long cannulae into veins, as obstruction may be encountered if not enough time has been left for the vein to return to normal (Hadaway 2001).

Smooth muscles can also react to excessive stretching. The muscles contract to resist the stretch; this is illustrated when a tourniquet has been left in place for a long period of time and the veins can no longer be palpated (Hadaway 2001).

The outer layer (tunica adventitia)

This layer is composed of connective tissue, collagen and nerve fibres. It surrounds and supports the vessel. The nerve fibres are mainly fibres of the sympathetic nervous system. Nerve impulses keep the vessel in a state of tonus—an increase in the rate of impulses will cause the vessel to constrict further, while a decrease in impulses will cause it to relax more. The amount of fibrous tissue varies between vessels. As a generalization, this layer is thicker in arteries than in veins; however, the vena cava and aorta have similar quantities (Tortora & Derrickson 2006).

Dynamics of Blood Flow

The movement of a fluid through a tube can occur in a turbulent or a streamlined manner; the streamlined movement of a fluid is termed laminar flow. Blood flow around the

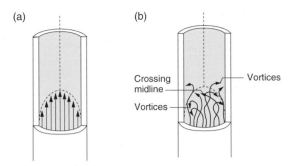

Figure 2.2 (a) Laminar blood blow; (b) turbulent blood flow.

circulation, in a healthy person, is considered to be laminar, i.e. non-turbulent flow that demonstrates a spearhead appearance when analysed. The blood in the centre of the vessel (around the axis of the vessel) travels faster than the blood in contact with the walls of the vessel. Friction forces cause the layer of blood in contact with the vessel wall to slow down; indeed, the velocity (speed) of blood in contact with the vessel is measured at zero (Berne *et al.* 2004), while the blood in the centre of the vessel moves the fastest (Figure 2.2). More pressure is required to move a turbulent fluid than is required to move a fluid whose flow is laminar.

In turbulent flow, the elements of the fluid move in all directions, flowing crosswise and lengthwise along the vessel (Guyton & Hall 2006). Turbulent flow can occur when blood flow is required to make a sharp turn, for example when blood vessels branch, when the inner surface of a vessel becomes roughened, if the diameter of a vessel changes abruptly (i.e. obstruction), or if the flow is greatly increased. In health, turbulent flow is only seen at the branches of large arteries (Guyton & Hall 2006) and in the sinuses of Valsalva in the aorta and pulmonary artery. The sinuses of Valsalva are small outpocketings in the walls of the aorta and pulmonary artery adjacent to the aortic and pulmonary valves (Berne *et al.* 2004).

Turbulence is usually accompanied by audible vibrations. Flow through diseased heart valves can be heard and is called a murmur. Profound anaemia causes a significant increase in cardiac output and a reduction in the viscosity of the blood; this can also produce audible turbulence. Turbulent flow can predispose patients to thrombus formation (Berne *et al.* 2004).

For the body tissues to survive, there must be adequate blood flow within the circulation. In order to maintain adequate flow, there must be an adequate head of pressure within the vessels that supply the tissues. Blood is like any other fluid—the only reason it will move from A to B is if the pressure at A is greater than the pressure at B (Green 1985). From the perspective of blood flow around the circulation, pressure in the aorta must be greater than the pressure in the right atrium if blood is to flow through the tissues and return to the heart.

The tone of the venous system is the most influential feature of venous return, because of the capacity that the venous system can hold. The average blood volume of an adult is about 7 mL/kg so a 70-kg man will have approximately 5 L of blood in circulation (Guyton & Hall 2006). At any given time, 9% of the blood volume or 0.5 L will be found in the pulmonary circulation, 20% or 1 L in the heart and arteries, 7% or 0.4 L in the arterioles and capillaries and 3 L in the venous system (Guyton & Hall 2006). The veins are described as 'capacitance vessels' because of their ability to distend and accommodate greater volume (Berne *et al.* 2004). The veins provide a 'reservoir function' to store large quantities of blood (Guyton & Hall 2006). In comparison, the arterial system has far less ability to change its capacity. The blood from the ventricles is ejected into the arterial system and it is arterial pressure that the ventricle has to overcome to eject the stroke volume. The arteries are therefore described as resistance vessels, because they produce resistance to blood flow (Berne *et al.* 2004).

Despite cardiac output being intermittent (pulsatile), peripheral blood flow is continuous. This is due to aortic distension during ventricular contraction and elastic recoil of the aortic wall causing forward propulsion of blood during ventricular relaxation (Berne *et al.* 2004). This is mainly due to the fact that the aorta is an elastic artery. As blood is ejected from the left ventricle into the aorta, the aortic wall is stretched by the impact of the blood flow. The aortic wall stores this mechanical energy briefly and then as the elastic fibres recoil the stored energy is released and the blood is propelled onwards down the aorta (Tortora & Derrickson 2006). As the aortic wall recoils the volume of blood displaced by that recoil maintains the arterial diastolic pressure and ensures a continuous flow to the periphery even during the diastolic phase of the heart (Berne *et al.* 2004; Figure 2.3).

This ability of the aortic wall to distend and recoil is termed compliance. Compliance deteriorates with age and with diseases that reduce the elasticity of the aorta, such as atherosclerosis and calcification. As compliance reduces, systolic pressure rises because the pressure is not being absorbed by the wall of the aorta. At the same time, diastolic pressure appears to become lower because there is no recoil phase to maintain the flow during diastole. Hence the pulse pressure (the difference between systolic and diastolic blood pressures) appears to become progressively wider in the elderly and in people with atherosclerotic disease (Tortora & Derrickson 2006).

The section of the aorta that receives the stroke volume from the left ventricle undergoes continual pressure, and the higher the blood pressure, the greater the shearing forces to which it is exposed. Local degeneration of the endothelium can occur, along with tearing of the arterial wall (Berne *et al.* 2004). This is known as a dissecting aneurysm. Aneurysms can dissect upwards, causing dissection of the coronary arteries and tamponade, or downwards leading to dissection of the renal and hepatic arteries. The condition is potentially life-threatening and is a vascular emergency.

Blood moves rapidly through the aorta and its branches, which become narrower as they progress towards the periphery. The composition of the vessel wall also changes as the arteries become smaller. The aorta is predominantly an elastic structure—the property that facilitates distension and recoil and thus aids blood flow and pressure control.

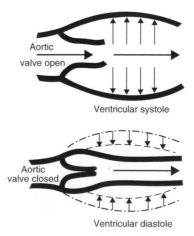

Figure 2.3 Distension and recoil of the aorta. (From Wilson & Waugh 1996. Reproduced with kind permission from Churchill Livingstone.)

In contrast, small arteries are quite muscular. The pressure in the arteries is usually referred to as blood pressure, while the pressure in the great veins is usually referred to as venous pressure (Morton *et al.* 2005).

The Arterial System

Blood leaves the left side of the heart via the ascending aorta. This is the largest arterial structure of the body, measuring 2.5 cm in diameter with a wall thickness of 2 mm (Tortora & Derrickson 2006). The aorta curves to form an arch which passes behind the heart and descends vertically through the thorax and abdomen (Figure 2.4). The aortic arch gives rise to three major arteries: the brachiocephalic trunk, the left common carotid

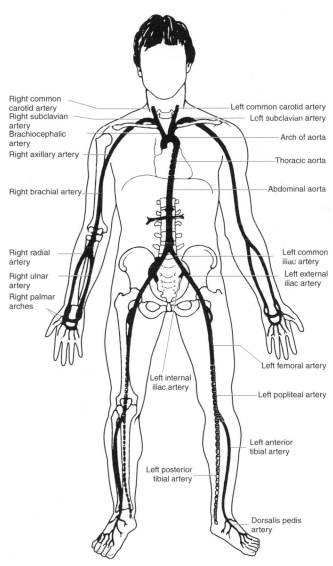

Figure 2.4   The aorta and the main arteries of the limbs. (From Wilson & Waugh 1996. Reproduced with kind permission from Churchill Livingstone.)

artery and the left subclavian artery. The brachiocephalic trunk further divides to form the right subclavian artery and the right common carotid artery (Moore & Dalley 2006).

Each subclavian artery arches laterally, passing behind the clavicles and over the superior surface of the first ribs before entering the axilla area where they become known as the axillary arteries. The first part of the artery lies deeply; then it runs more superficially and becomes the brachial artery. The brachial artery runs down the medial aspect of the upper arm and passes to the front of the elbow in the area known as the cubital fossa. The median nerve lies close to the brachial artery within the cubital fossa (Guyton & Hall 2006).

About 1 cm below the cubital fossa the brachial artery divides to form the radial and ulnar arteries, although the bifurcation may occur much higher in the arm, even in the axilla (Drake *et al.* 2005). The radial artery runs along the lateral (thumb side) of the forearm and produces the pulse commonly felt at the wrist, just in front of the radius bone. Superficial branches of the radial artery do occur and can be found on the dorsal surface of the hand (Drake *et al.* 2005). The radial artery is commonly punctured to obtain a sample of arterial blood for blood gas analysis.

The ulnar artery runs along the opposite side of the forearm and passes across the palm of the hand. The ulnar nerve runs alongside the ulnar artery in the distal half of the forearm (Drake *et al.* 2005). Anastomoses (connections) are found between the radial and ulnar arteries and are called the deep and superficial palmar arches. From these vessels arise the palmar metacarpal and palmar digital arteries which supply the structures of the hand and fingers (Drake *et al.* 2005).

Because the brachial artery is the main arterial structure supplying the upper limbs, it is considered imprudent to site an intra-arterial device in the brachial artery unless no other access is available. Loss of brachial arterial supply would result in loss of blood flow to the forearm. Use of a more distal artery such as the radial artery is better practice, as collateral circulation to the forearm can be provided by the ulnar artery. The brachial artery does provide useful access to the arterial system for procedures such as cardiac catheterization. However, the proximity of the median nerve can result in iatrogenic injury which is a poorly recognised complication of this procedure (Kennedy *et al.* 1997). It is good practice to perform an Allen test before cannulating either the radial or the ulnar artery to ensure that collateral circulation exists (Morton *et al.* 2005).

From the aortic arch, the aorta descends down through the thorax and abdomen, giving off branches to supply the organs and structures that surround it. The aorta bifurcates in the lumbar region to form the common iliac arteries which in turn bifurcate to form the internal and external iliac arteries. The external iliac artery passes under the inguinal ligament to enter the femoral triangle in the anterior aspect of the thigh; at this point it becomes the femoral artery (Drake *et al.* 2005). The femoral triangle is the junction between the upper thigh and the abdominal wall and contains the femoral vein and femoral nerve as well as the femoral artery. The femoral artery is palpable within the femoral triangle, which is an important clinical feature because the femoral vessels remain useful for both venous and arterial access when other sites are unavailable. The femoral artery runs vertically through the femoral triangle and continues to descend down the thigh before running behind the knee where it becomes known as the popliteal artery (Drake *et al.* 2005). The popliteal artery divides just below the knee to form the anterior and posterior tibial arteries. The anterior tibial artery runs over the top of the foot, forming the dorsalis pedis artery. The dorsalis pedis artery can be palpated on the dorsal surface (top) of the foot approximately 2–3 cm from the base of the second toe. It is important to be able to locate the dorsalis pedis pulse in order to assess perfusion of the feet, for example after vascular interventions have been performed through the femoral artery or if an intra-aortic balloon pump (IABP) is *in situ* within the femoral artery

(Morton *et al.* 2005). The posterior tibial artery runs down the back of the leg and passes behind the medial malleolus and into the sole of the foot. The posterior tibial artery can be palpated behind the medial malleolus and is an alternative method of assessing perfusion to the distal limb when arterial observations are required.

Drug administration

It is rare to administer drugs into the arterial system. The main exception to this is the instillation of thrombolytic agents to thrombosed arteries. The most common occurrence is the direct instillation of streptokinase or a similar agent into the pulmonary artery for the treatment of massive and life-threatening pulmonary embolism (Wong *et al.* 1999). This is usually done via a pulmonary artery catheter. There are also case reports of intracranial thrombolysis for the management of acute stroke using intra-arterial microcatheters that are inserted directly into the thrombus (Jungreis *et al.* 1989). More recently intra-arterial chemotherapy has been introduced to directly target tumours through their arterial blood supply. The most established therapies are for liver and pancreatic carcinomas (Irie 2001) and clinical trials are taking place involving other organs.

Drug administration via arteries is usually contraindicated because it can lead to arterial spasm and ischaemia of the distal limb. Accidental intra-arterial drug administration most commonly occurs because a cannula has been incorrectly placed (Chin & Singh 2005) or because an arterial cannula has been inadequately labelled (Soni 1989). In conscious patients, arterial drug administration can cause severe pain (but not always). In the unconscious patient, blanching of the limb may be the initial sign and there can be continued discoloration distal to the injection site (Soni 1989; Kessell & Barker 1996). This is a vascular emergency and a physician must be called to treat the situation as quickly as possible.

Capillaries

As arterioles diverge into capillary structures, precapillary sphincters occur. Proportionally these structures have the most smooth muscle fibre of any vessel. This is the part of the vascular system that generates peripheral resistance. A single arteriole can divide into several capillaries, producing a significant drop in pressure. As a result, flow through capillaries is intermittent rather than pulsatile and it is only when the arterioles are extremely dilated that pulsations can be observed in the capillaries, for example in sepsis (Guyton & Hall 2006).

The capillary is responsible for blood flow to the cells and for nutrient supply and gas exchange. Capillary flow is sometimes termed nutritional flow (Berne *et al.* 2004). The more highly active the tissue structure, the more extensive is the capillary network. For example, cardiac and skeletal muscle have a higher capillary density than subcutaneous tissue or cartilage. Not all capillaries are the same diameter; in fact, some are smaller than the diameter of a red blood cell. The red cell is obliged to manipulate its shape to facilitate passage through the capillary (Berne *et al.* 2004).

Capillaries are thin-walled vessels composed of a single layer of endothelial cells. The thin capillary wall allows the passage of nutrients and oxygen out of the blood and, in exchange, takes up waste products of cell metabolism. Permeability of the capillary wall varies between tissue structures (capillaries of the gut and liver are more permeable than those of skeletal muscle); it also varies along the length of the capillary (the venous end is more permeable than the arterial end). Capillary permeability can be altered by certain chemicals, e.g. histamine (Berne *et al.* 2004).

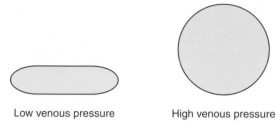

Low venous pressure   High venous pressure

Figure 2.5   Change in cross-sectional area of vein with increase in venous pressure.

The Venous System

Veins convey the blood from the capillary bed back to the heart. Usually they are larger in diameter and thinner walled than their corresponding arteries. There are on average about four times as many veins as the corresponding arteries, because the blood is travelling more slowly than it does in the arteries (Guyton & Hall 2006).

As the venous ends of the capillaries converge to form venules, the diameter of the vessels progressively increases. The cross-sectional area of a vein at low-to-moderate venous pressure is elliptical. Veins that are distended and under higher venous pressure demonstrate a more rounded cross-section (Green 1985; Figure 2.5). This is of clinical importance when using ultrasound to locate veins during central venous catheter insertion. If ultrasound reveals an elliptical or flattened vein it may be necessary to improve the intravascular volume by fluid filling or increased head-down positioning in order to locate and successfully cannulate a central vein.

As the venules converge to form veins, the diameter of the vessels continues to increase. As the vessel diameter increases, the pressure continues to fall. Between the capillary and the right atrium, the venous pressure falls from 12 to 0 mmHg. The pressure of blood entering the right side of the heart is usually the same as atmospheric pressure (Guyton & Hall 2006).

When pressure is very low over long distances, there is little incentive for the blood to return to the heart. The venous return is assisted by two main mechanisms: negative pressure within the thorax and muscular activity in the limbs.

Valves

One feature of veins not seen in the arterial system is the presence of valves. A valve is a fold of the tunica intima, strengthened by connective tissue (Berne *et al.* 2004). Valves in veins are bicuspid and the cusps are crescentic in shape. The occurrence of valves is more plentiful in the veins of the limbs than in any other part of the venous system. Valves are sparse in the veins of the abdomen, thorax and neck (Woodburne & Burkel 1994). The head and neck have the advantage of gravity to assist the return of blood to the heart. Valves help to support the column of blood above the valve; the more frequent the valve, the smaller the column of blood it must support. This assists blood flow back to the heart and prevents pooling of blood in vessels most affected by gravity.

In a healthy person, the valves only allow blood flow in one direction and are effective in preventing venous distension from gravity. Blood in the saphenous vein, for example, is at a low pressure and a long way from the heart. Gravity is exerted on the vessel and its contents. Without skeletal muscle activity and the presence of valves, blood would pool in the periphery, veins would distend, and venous return would be reduced.

As an individual moves their limbs, the skeletal muscle contracts and relaxes. As the skeletal muscle contracts, it compresses the vein next to it and causes the blood in the

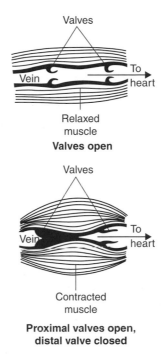

Figure 2.6   Flow of blood through vein aided by the contraction of skeletal muscle. (From Wilson & Waugh 1996. Reproduced with kind permission from Churchill Livingstone.)

vessel to be displaced. The valve below the muscle prevents the blood from being displaced downwards; the valve above the muscle is forced open and the blood moves upwards into the next valve compartment (Figure 2.6). As in the heart, blood flow through the valves is unidirectional in the healthy individual. When a person has varicose veins, the veins have usually become distended, often due to persistently raised venous pressure, caused for example by pregnancy, obesity, or hepatic or right heart failure. As the vessel diameter increases, the valve cusps no longer close correctly, the valves are rendered incompetent and blood flow ceases to be unidirectional. Individuals are at increased risk of venous thrombosis from stasis of blood in these distended veins, although this risk does diminish with age (Heit *et al.* 2000).

Knowledge of the presence of valves in the hand and arm veins is important when considering cannulation or venepuncture. If valves can be identified they should be avoided as they may prevent blood withdrawal and cannula advancement (Dougherty 2004).

Venous return

From the lower limbs

The lower limbs contain both deep and superficial veins. Deep veins generally follow the path of the arteries and have similar names. Superficial veins are located in the superficial fascia and they interconnect with the deep veins; they do not usually accompany the arteries (Guyton & Hall 2006).

There are two main superficial veins of the leg—the saphenous veins. The small saphenous vein begins at the ankle where the small veins that drain the top of the foot converge. It runs superficially up the back of the leg and enters the popliteal space where it joins the deep popliteal vein. The great popliteal vein begins on the inner aspect of the

(a)

(b)

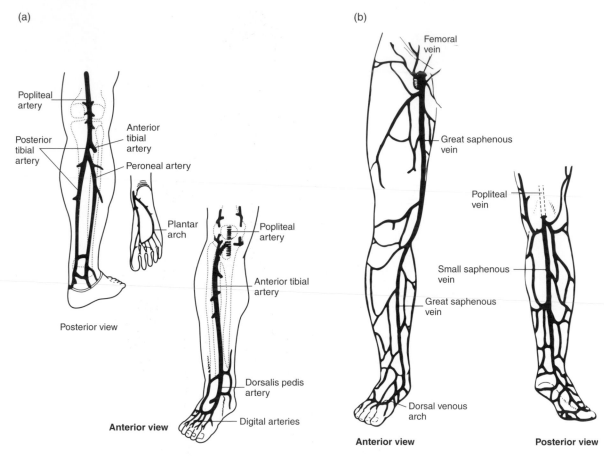

Figure 2.7 (a) Right popliteal artery and its main branches; (b) superficial veins of the leg. (From Wilson & Waugh 1996. Reproduced with kind permission from Churchill Livingstone.)

top of the foot and runs upwards along the inner aspect of the thigh. It joins the deep femoral vein just below the inguinal ligament (Figure 2.7).

As the femoral vein reaches the level of the inguinal ligament, it becomes known as the external iliac vein and lies medially to the femoral artery. The femoral nerve lies laterally to the artery.

At the level of the sacroiliac joint, the external iliac vein is joined by the internal iliac vein and forms the common iliac vein. The right and the left common iliac veins combine to form the inferior vena cava (Drake *et al.* 2005) (Figure 2.8).

As small veins converge to form larger veins, the blood flow within the vessel increases. By the time the blood reaches the SVC or IVC, it will have a flow rate of approximately 2–3 L/min. (The circulation flows at 5 L/min and there are only two vessels entering the left side of the heart.)

The blood flow within the vessel is an important factor when selecting the vascular access for a patient. If the access is for an infrequently administered non-irritant drug then a vessel with a low blood flow in the periphery is quite appropriate. If the access is for irritant solutions such as parenteral nutrition or for drugs with extremes of pH or osmolarity then access must be into a central vein with a high blood flow to ensure that the agents are diluted and distributed rapidly before they can injure the vein (Bard 2006).

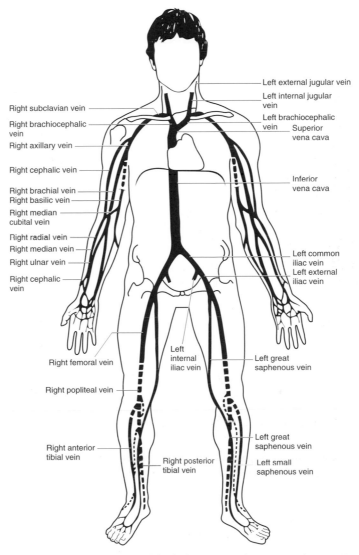

Figure 2.8   Vena cava and the main veins of the limbs. (From Wilson & Waugh 1996. Reproduced with kind permission from Churchill Livingstone.)

From the upper limbs

Like the veins of the leg, arm veins are classified as deep or superficial. Deep veins follow the course of the major arteries, drain the areas supplied by the arteries and have similar names (Guyton & Hall 2006). The fingers are drained by the digital veins; these are small and rarely used for cannulation (Scales 2005). The digital veins converge to form the dorsal metacarpal veins which end in the dorsal venous arch, a relatively prominent structure on the back of the hand that is easily visualized and palpated (Scales 2005). Despite this, there are reports in the literature of accidental cannulation of both the superficial radial artery and the superficial ulnar artery during attempted cannulation of the dorsal venous arch (Chin & Singh 2005). Chin and Singh (2005) postulate that the use of a tourniquet may contribute to the absence of arterial pulsation during vein selection.

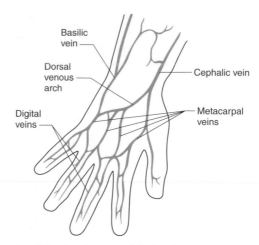

Figure 2.9   Superficial veins of the dorsal aspect of the hand.

The radial end of the dorsal venous arch continues to form the cephalic vein, also fed by the dorsal veins of the thumb, and ascends up the radial side of the wrist (Woodburne & Burkel 1994). The superficial branch of the radial nerve is sensory and runs along the ante-rolateral aspect of the forearm. As it approaches the wrist the nerve passes laterally around the radial side of the forearm where it continues onto the dorsum of the hand (Drake *et al*. 2005). Superficial branches of the radial artery are also found in this region and can be accidentally cannulated when attempting cephalic vein cannulation (Lirk *et al*. 2004).

The accessory cephalic vein emerges either from the dorsum of the forearm or from the ulnar end of the dorsal venous arch. It ascends diagonally across the dorsum of the fore-arm and joins the cephalic vein in the region of the elbow (Woodburne & Burkel 1994).

The ulnar end of the dorsal venous arch continues to form the basilic vein; it continues along the ulnar side of the forearm, being fed by tributaries from both the anterior and posterior surfaces of the forearm (Woodburne & Burkel 1994; Figure 2.9).

The median cubital vein, a large branch of the cephalic vein, runs diagonally across the anterior aspect of the elbow, connecting the cephalic and basilic veins. The median cubital vein is only present in 70% of the population (Woodburne & Burkel 1994). All these veins are superficial, generally palpable and usually visible when the arm is inspected. Three nerves are located in the cubital fossa, the superficial radial nerve run-ning along the outer aspect of the elbow, the median nerve running centrally in a similar location to the brachial artery and the ulnar nerve running along the inner aspect of the elbow (Drake *et al*. 2005).

As the cephalic vein leaves the cubital fossa, it runs upward and turns inward, piercing the brachial fascia. It continues along the upper arm, finally emptying into the axillary vein (Woodburne & Burkel 1994).

Having been joined by the median cubital vein, the basilic vein continues upward and turns inward, piercing the brachial fascia midway between the elbow and the shoul-der. At the level of the axilla, it joins with the brachial veins to form the axillary vein (Figure 2.10).

The median antebrachial vein lies in the middle of the anterior forearm, beginning in the palmar venous arch and terminating in either the median cubital or basilic vein. The median cubital vein also connects with the deep veins in the cubital fossa (Woodburne & Burkel 1994).

The brachial veins are the deep veins of the arm. They run parallel to the arterial struc-tures and are paired veins. The basilic vein joins with the brachial veins to form the distal

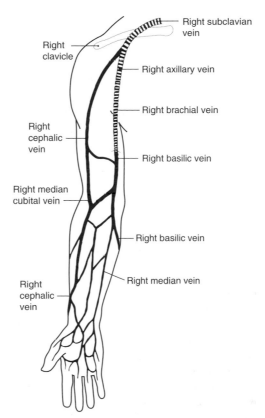

Figure 2.10 Main veins of the right arm. Broken line indicates deep veins. (From Wilson & Waugh 1996. Reproduced with kind permission from Churchill Livingstone.)

part of the axillary vein. The cephalic vein empties into the proximal portion of the axillary vein. As the axillary vein ascends and passes over the first rib, it becomes the subclavian vein (Drake *et al.* 2005). At this stage the subclavian vein is on the outside of the upper part of the thorax. Consequently there is a risk of pneumothorax if the pleura is accidentally injured during subclavian vein catheterization (Morton *et al.* 2005). Similarly, the subclavian artery runs parallel and slightly posterior to the subclavian vein (Drake *et al.* 2005) and accidental subclavian artery puncture is also a recognized complication of subclavian vein catheterization (Morton *et al.* 2005).

The venous drainage from the head and neck is via the internal and external jugular veins. The external jugular vein is formed posterior to the angle of mandible and lies parallel to the external carotid artery. The external jugular vein runs straight down the neck in the superficial fascia and crosses the sternocleidomastoid muscle as it descends (Drake *et al.* 2005). Once the external jugular vein reaches the lower part of the neck, just above the clavicle, it pierces the cervical fascia and enters the subclavian vein (Drake *et al.* 2005).

The internal jugular vein drains blood from the skull, brain, face and parts of the neck. It lies within the carotid sheath, a column of fascia that surrounds the internal jugular vein, the common carotid artery, the internal carotid artery and the vagus nerve (Drake *et al.* 2005). The internal jugular is initially posterior to the internal carotid artery. As it descends it becomes more lateral, eventually becoming lateral to the common carotid artery with the vagus nerve lying posterior and partially between the two vessels (Drake *et al.* 2005). The development of a haematoma within the carotid sheath, which may be secondary to carotid artery puncture, multiple needling of the internal jugular or as a result of coagulopathy, can lead to nerve injury with symptoms such as Horner's syndrome (Jarvis *et al.* 2005).

The paired internal jugular veins merge with the subclavian veins behind the sternal end of the clavicle to form the brachiocephalic veins, and the right and left brachiocephalic veins merge to form the SVC.

Numerous cranial and peripheral nerves pass through the anterior region of the neck. The cranial nerves of the anterior neck include the facial nerve (VII), the glossopharyngeal nerve (IX), the vagus nerve (X), the accessory nerve (XI) and the hypoglossal nerve (XII) (Drake *et al.* 2005). The carotid sinus is innervated by a branch of the glossopharyngeal nerve, and the carotid body is supplied by a branch of the vagus nerve (Drake *et al.* 2005). Both have the potential to be injured during internal jugular vein catheterization. The accessory and hypoglossal nerves do not branch as they pass down the anterior side of the neck but they do lie between the internal jugular vein and the internal carotid artery (Drake *et al.* 2005) which also makes them vulnerable to iatrogenic injury when neck veins are catheterized.

The peripheral nerves include the transverse cervical nerve and the upper and lower roots of the ansa cervicalis which is a loop of nerve fibres from cervical nerves C1 to C3 (Drake *et al.* 2005). As the hypoglossal nerve passes across the internal and external carotid arteries some of the cervical nerve fibres descend between the internal jugular vein and the internal carotid artery. These nerve fibres are the superior root of the ansa cervicalis (Drake *et al.* 2005). The inferior root of the ansa cervicalis descends medial or lateral to the internal jugular vein before joining the superior root (Drake *et al.* 2005). The phrenic nerves are also important peripheral nerves that pass through the anterior neck region. They pass down the neck and around the lateral border of each anterior scalene muscle (the muscle arises from the first rib and connects to the cervical vertebrae) and then pass between the subclavian vein and the subclavian artery to enter the thorax and innervate the diaphragm (Drake *et al.* 2005).

Also within the anterior neck structure are the thyroid and parathyroid glands, part of the endocrine system. The common carotid arteries pass behind the lateral borders of the thyroid gland next to the internal jugular veins (Drake *et al.* 2005) and consideration needs to be given to these structures when undertaking catheterization of the internal jugular veins.

Veins are the routine source of vascular access for parenteral drug and fluid administration, and the locations of important veins for this purpose (as well as advantages and disadvantages of using them) are shown in Table 2.1.

Arrangement of the vasculature

Arteries and veins usually run in parallel to each other in the limbs. Core body temperature is 37°C and peripheral temperature is usually the same as the environment. If cold blood from the peripheries were to return to the heart, it could cause a fatal dysrhythmia. The parallel arrangement of arteries and veins allows heat from arteries to pass across to veins. Thus the venous blood warms up as it returns to the heart and arterial blood gradually cools as it flows out towards the periphery. This process is known as 'countercurrent heat transfer' (Berne *et al.* 2004).

If blood is to be involved in temperature control, it has to flow close to the skin so that the heat can be radiated into the environment. Subcutaneous tissue, by definition, lies under the skin and can sometimes obscure the visibility of veins. This may well contribute to poor temperature regulation in obese people as the superficial nature of veins is lost and the subcutaneous tissue becomes an insulation through which radiation of heat becomes progressively more difficult.

Table 2.1   Important veins for vascular access.

Location	Advantages	Disadvantages
Peripheral veins of upper limb		
Dorsal venous network of the hand:		
Digital veins Metacarpal veins	Last resort for fluid Well adapted for i.v. use Bones of hand provide a natural splint Enables successive venepuncture/cannulation sites above previous puncture site	Small May be fragile or poorly supported in elderly Restricts the use of the hand Extravagation of blood may readily occur May be more painful
Radial and ulnar veins	Very superficial	Nerves close to surface of skin make this a more painful area, especially at the inner aspect of the wrist
Cephalic vein	Large vein	Movement at the wrist may cause discomfort and restrict movement
Accessory cephalic vein	Easy to visualize, stabilize and palpate Excellent for transfusion administration Position makes it a natural splint	May be obscured by tendons controlling thumb
Basilic vein	Large vein Found by flexing the elbow and bending the arm Best route for midline and PICC insertion as straightest route to central veins	Often overlooked Site may make it more awkward to assess and observe Tends to have more valves, making advancement of cannula difficult May only be able to palpate a small segment Haematomas form easily on removal of devices
Median cubital veins	Large, easily accessible veins for venepuncture well supported by muscular and connective tissue	Cannulation over a joint can lead to dislodgement, infiltration/extravasation or mechanical phlebitis Care needed to prevent accidental arterial puncture
Peripheral veins of lower limb		
Dorsal venous network of the foot	Easily accessible	More difficult to palpate Increased risk of complications due to impaired circulation Prone to DVT Difficult to stabilize Restricts ability to walk
Medial and lateral marginal veins of the foot	Larger veins Easy to palpate and visualize	Increased risk of complications due to impaired circulation Prone to DVT Difficult to stabilize Restricts ability to walk

(Continued)

Table 2.1 *(Continued)*

Location	Advantages	Disadvantages
Central veins		
Subclavian Infraclavicular	Easily accessible Easier to maintain dressing (flatter surface) Preferred in children	May require a longer needle for insertion Associated with a number of complications such as pneumothorax, brachial nerve plexus damage, haemothorax, etc.
Supraclavicular	Short distance from skin to vein, therefore easily accessible	Dressing may be more difficult to hollow above clavicle Associated with a number of complications such as pneumothorax, brachial nerve plexus injury, haemothorax, etc.
Jugular	Associated with fewer complications than subclavian Larger vein	Difficult to dress due to movement of neck and beard growth on male patients
Internal External	Easily accessible Superficial vein Usually visible and easy to palpate	May result in damage to carotid arteries Tip location in SVC not always as successful as internal
Femoral	Alternative site in emergency Tip location in IVC	Dressings difficult to maintain and associated with high infection risk, thrombosis

DVT, deep vein trombosis; IVC, inferior vena cava; PICC, peripherally inserted central catheter; SVC, superior vena cava.

Regulation of the Vascular System

There are two key control mechanisms for the peripheral circulation—control by the nervous system and local control influenced by the tissues around the vessels. In the skin and splanchnic regions, nervous control is dominant, whereas in the heart and brain, environmental conditions are more influential (Berne *et al.* 2004). Local control, known as autoregulation, is achieved by chemicals and by levels of oxygen and carbon dioxide.

The endothelial lining of arterioles and small arteries produces a number of vasoactive substances that can bring about localized vasodilation or vasoconstriction. Endothelium-derived relaxing factor (EDRF) is responsible for local vasodilation. EDRF is principally composed of nitric oxide (Guyton & Hall 2006). Endothelin, a large amino acid peptide that is present in the endothelial cells of most blood vessels, is a potent vasoconstricting agent. Endothelin is usually released in response to damage to the endothelium such as crush injuries to tissues or the injection of damaging chemicals into blood vessels (Guyton & Hall 2006). The release of endothelin and the subsequent vasoconstriction help to prevent haemorrhage from injured vessels.

Electrolytes also play a role in vascular tone. An increase in calcium ions causes vasoconstriction (hence the use of calcium channel blockers as a mechanism of blood pressure control) whilst an increase in potassium and magnesium ions can cause vasodilation

(Guyton & Hall 2006). Carbon dioxide can be a potent vasodilator, especially in cerebral vasculature, as can hydrogen ions (Guyton & Hall 2006).

The arterioles are mainly responsible for regulating blood flow throughout the body. Smooth muscle fibres make up a large proportion of the vessel structure. The vessel lumen can be varied from complete occlusion to maximum dilation (Berne *et al.* 2004). The vessel usually rests in a state of partial tone, i.e. it is neither fully relaxed nor fully contracted. It is therefore able to move in either direction in response to a stimulus.

Most of the body's arteries and veins are supplied solely by the fibres of the sympathetic nervous system (Berne *et al.* 2004). Different vessels have different amounts of sympathetic supply. It is the sympathetic activity that maintains the resting tone of the blood vessel. Changes in sympathetic activity cause changes in vascular tone. Increased sympathetic stimulation of a blood vessel causes contraction, whilst decreased stimulation causes relaxation (Berne *et al.* 2004). The alteration in lumen size creates a change in flow (or resistance). This mechanism is most highly active in the arteriole. A few vessels, mainly limited to the viscera and pelvic organs, have parasympathetic innervation. Increased parasympathetic activity in these regions causes relaxation of the blood vessels (Berne *et al.* 2004).

The regulation of vascular tone by the sympathetic nervous system is termed 'vasomotor' control. This means that the vasomotor centre (VMC) of the brain is sending instructions to the blood vessels. This is done in response to information received by the brain about the state of the blood pressure, the cardiac output, the venous return, body temperature and stress stimuli (Green 1985).

One of the most important mechanisms for control of vascular tone is the baroreceptor mechanism. This is a rapid mechanism that quickly restores blood pressure, and is utilized, for example, when an individual decides to move from a lying to a standing position (Guyton & Hall 2006).

Baroreceptors are nerve endings that are stimulated by the degree of stretch of the blood vessel. High blood pressure causes significant stretch (distortion) of the vessel wall, and low blood pressure reduces the stretch (Berne *et al.* 2004). The baroreceptors that influence the systemic circulation are located in the carotid sinuses and the aortic arch. The carotid sinus is the area of bifurcation of the common carotid artery (Berne *et al.* 2004).

The baroreceptors send signals to the VMC, conveying information about arterial blood pressure. When arterial blood pressure is high, frequent impulses are sent to the VMC. The response of the VMC is to reduce the amount of sympathetic stimulation of the capacitance vessels (peripheral veins), thus forcing peripheral pooling of blood to occur. At the same time, fewer signals are sent to the sinoatrial node and the heart rate subsequently slows. This has the effect of reducing venous return and cardiac output; blood pressure will subsequently be reduced. The opposite is also true. Low blood pressure reduces stimulation of the baroreceptors; they in turn send fewer impulses to the VMC. This is interpreted as low blood pressure and sympathetic stimulation of the blood vessels is increased, causing venoconstriction. This increases the venous return to the heart and, in conjunction with increased heart rate, brings about an increase in blood pressure.

Care must be taken when removing central venous catheters (CVCs) from the internal jugular site because of its close proximity to the carotid artery. In sensitive patients, when pressure is applied to the puncture site, the carotid sinus can be unintentionally stimulated and the VMC will respond by slowing the heart rate and creating venodilation. The more continued the pressure, the slower the heart rate will become. This unfortunate side-effect of CVC removal is easier to notice in a monitored patient; the unmonitored patient may present with fainting (Berne *et al.* 2004). Reducing the pressure on the neck will restore both the heart rate and blood pressure. Green (1985) reports that the mechanism can also be evoked by wearing a tight shirt collar.

Composition and Function of Blood

Blood is a complex liquid which performs a number of essential functions.

- Transport of:
  - oxygen from the lungs to the tissues
  - carbon dioxide from the tissues to the lungs
  - nutrients from the gut to the tissues
  - wastes from the tissues to the liver and kidneys
  - hormones from their site of production to their target tissues.
- Homeostasis:
  - regulation of blood pH by the use of buffers and proteins
  - regulation of body temperature by the distribution of heat
  - regulation of the composition and volume of the interstitial fluid compartment
  - control of blood loss by haemostatic mechanisms
  - immunity and control of infection.

Blood contains various chemicals in solution and a variety of cells in suspension (Table 2.2). The fluid component is termed plasma and makes up about 55% of the blood volume; blood cells make up the remaining 45%. The percentage of blood that is cells is called the haematocrit (Guyton & Hall 2006).

Blood is a viscous fluid. Viscosity is measured in relation to water, which is said to have a viscosity of 1.0. The viscosity of whole blood at normal haematocrit is about 3 (Guyton & Hall 2006). Viscosity relates to the thickness and adhesiveness of a liquid. Blood feels 'sticky' or adhesive when touched, and is heavier than water when the same volumes are compared. Viscosity is an important feature of blood and heart function, and is affected by the haematocrit (percentage of cells in the blood) and plasma proteins. Many factors can influence viscosity, for example alteration in the concentration of cells, abnormalities of the red blood cell, hydrational state and nutritional imbalance. Vessel diameter also influences apparent viscosity.

Blood is usually 8% of total body weight. On average, women have 4–5 L of blood, while men have 5–6 L. This reflects the differences in physical size between men and women (Guyton & Hall 2006). If blood volume is taken to be 5 L, then 3 L of that volume is plasma. There are many substances dissolved or suspended in plasma, including proteins, electrolytes, vitamins, lipids, hormones, nitrogenous wastes and gases. The concentration of each of these will depend upon health, metabolic activity and diet (Berne *et al.* 2004).

Haemostasis

The term haemostasis means the prevention of blood loss (Guyton & Hall 2006). Maintaining haemostasis is to balance the agents that cause blood to clot and the agents that inhibit the clotting of blood. For preservation of the human organism, any holes in the circulation must be quickly plugged, but the plug must not be so great as to obstruct the flow of blood along the vessel.

If a vessel is severed or damaged, the initial reaction is one of vascular spasm, partly from nervous reflexes and partly from spasm of the injured muscle in the vessel wall (Guyton & Hall 2006). The next phase in haemostasis is the formation of a platelet plug. When circulating platelets come into contact with the damaged surface of a blood vessel, they immediately undergo change. They alter their shape by swelling and developing projections on their cell surfaces. The cell membrane of the platelet is coated with glycoproteins which prevent adherence to normal endothelium and yet cause adherence to

Table 2.2 Cells present in blood.

Name of cell	Type of cell	Produced by	Life span	Normal range	Function
Red blood cells (erythrocytes)	Anuclear cell, i.e. no nucleus and no genetic material for reproduction	Bone marrow	120 days (Green 1985)	A normal haemoglobin level is 15 g/dL in men and 13.5 g/dL in women (Berne & Levy 1993)	Tissue oxygenation. Raised haemoglobin increases viscosity and impedes blood flow. Neutrophils migrate to sites of tissue injury in response to chemical signals from other cells (chemotactic) 'phagocytic' behaviour, i.e. they ingest and destroy foreign material
White blood cells (leukocytes)	Neutrophils, eosinophils, basophils (granulocytes due to granular nature of their cytoplasm)	Bone marrow	4–5 days	A normal white cell count is 4000–10000 cells/µL	Eosinophils travel rapidly to site of tissue injury (within 30 min) and appear to survive for weeks—phagocytic and chemotactic basophils are mobile phagocytic cells which can produce an anaphylactic response
	Monocytes	Mature in 24–48 hours and migrate to the liver; spleen and lymph nodes; remain for months or years - macrophages produced in the bone marrow, but T-lymphocytes mature in the thymus gland			Monocytes are the largest, mobile phagocytic cells capable of replication and have multiple functions—active in immune response
	Lymphocytes				Lymphocytes are non-granular cells—two main subgroups are the B- and T-lymphocytes. B-lymphocytes have immunoglobulins on their cell surfaces and can secrete specific immunoglobulins antibodies
					There are several types of T-cell: (1) the helper cell which assists B-lymphocytes to produce antibodies; (2) the suppressor cell which inhibits B-lymphocytes from producing antibodies; (3) cytotoxic T-cells which cause cell destruction of identified antigens; (4) null cells which appear to be neither B- nor T-lymphocytes by characteristic; and (5) the natural killer cells which appear capable of destroying tumour cells, virus-infected cells or cells coated with antibody
Platelets	Anuclear	Fragments of megakaryocyte cell in the bone marrow			Involved in clotting process

injured areas of the blood vessel wall (Guyton & Hall 2006). This is particularly true when collagen is exposed from deep within the vessel wall. The platelet membrane also contains phospholipids that activate various stages of the clotting process. As well as adhering to the collagen in the vessel wall, platelets also adhere to a clotting protein called von Willebrand factor that leaks into the traumatized tissue from the plasma (Guyton & Hall 2006). The activated platelets release adenosine diphosphate (ADP) and an enzyme called thromboxane A_2 into the blood (Guyton & Hall 2006). These agents act on nearby platelets and activate them too. This continues, and a platelet plug is formed.

If the vascular damage is small, a platelet plug may suffice to prevent blood loss. If the damage is more significant then thrombus formation will be required to achieve haemostasis. Platelet plugs are constantly being manufactured to repair minor wear and tear of blood vessels. Individuals with a low platelet count are unable to perform this vital task and subsequently develop hundreds of minor haemorrhagic areas which are visible on the skin. These haemorrhages will also be occurring in the internal tissues and organs. This classic haemorrhagic picture is called a petechial rash.

Thrombus formation involves the manufacture of a blood clot. The rapidity of clot formation depends on the severity of the vascular injury. Clot formation is slower in minor injury than in major injury (Guyton & Hall 2006). In order to manufacture a thrombus, prothrombin must be converted to thrombin and fibrinogen must be converted to fibrin. The conversion of prothrombin can be achieved by both intrinsic and extrinsic pathways, and the formation of thrombin acts as a trigger for the conversion of fibrinogen. Calcium is needed during the conversion of both proteins.

The final clot is a network of fibrin strands running in every direction. The strands entrap red cells, platelets, white cells and plasma. Once the clot is formed, it begins to retract. The retracting clot draws the vessel walls together and compresses the fibrin network further.

The development of the blood clot is self-regulated. An important plasma protein exists called plasminogen. This is an inactive anticlotting protein which, when triggered, converts to the active agent plasmin. Plasmin destroys the fibrin strands of the thrombus and has the ability to digest fibrinogen and several other clotting factors.

If plasmin were to develop unchecked, the entire blood clot could be dissolved and the risk of haemorrhage from the break in the vessel would recur. To combat plasmin a substance called alpha-2 antiplasmin exists, which binds with plasmin and neutralizes it (Guyton & Hall 2006). The balance between clotting and clot control is taking place all the time and involves a complex series of intrinsic and extrinsic pathways.

The Skin

The skin is made up of a surface layer (the epidermis) and an underlying thicker layer (the dermis). The epidermis is composed of stratified squamous epithelium. This layer is typically less than 1 mm deep and has many layers of cells (Woodburne & Burkel 1994). The epidermis contains no blood vessels but is penetrated by sensory nerve endings.

The dermis has several layers and is thicker than the epidermis. The deeper dermal layer, the reticular layer, is composed of a mass of collagenous and elastic connective tissue fibres. This accounts for the strength of the skin.

The dermis contains small quantities of fat, blood and lymph vessels, nerves and sensory nerve endings, hair follicles, and sweat and sebaceous glands; smooth muscle fibres are also present (Woodburne & Burkel 1994; Figure 2.11). The subcutaneous connective tissue is loose textured and is composed of fibrous connective tissue and elastic fibres; its correct name is the hypodermis (Woodburne & Burkel 1994). The distribution

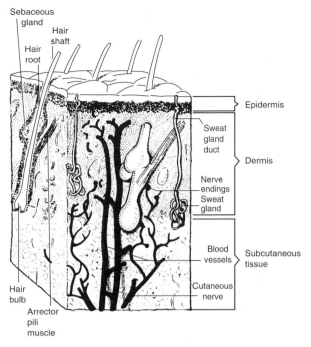

Figure 2.11   The skin, showing the main structures in the dermis. (From Wilson & Waugh 1996. Reproduced with kind permission from Churchill Livingstone.)

of subcutaneous fat varies in different parts of the body and is even absent in some regions, such as the eyelids. Where the fat layer is very prominent, it is termed adipose tissue. The hypodermis is generally thicker than the dermis (Woodburne & Burkel 1994).

The effects of ageing can alter the appearance and structure of the skin. The epidermis and dermis become thinner, loose and dry, with little subcutaneous tissue to support the vessels. In the elderly this may account for the fragility and increased risk of bleeding at venepuncture sites, shearing of skin layers when tape and dressings are removed, and skin dryness which increases with the use of alcohol-based cleaning solutions (Hadaway 2001; Whitson 1996).

Perception of pain

The skin is a highly innervated structure. The pain receptors in the skin and other tissues are all free nerve endings. Pain receptors are widespread in the superficial layers of the skin as well as certain internal tissues such as arterial walls and joint surfaces (Guyton & Hall 2006). Any single point on the skin surface will have at least three different networks of nerve fibres running across it (Nathan 1988), making the skin a highly sensitive organ. The skin relays three types of information:

- the nature of the stimulus (is the skin pricked or pressed?)
- the intensity of the stimulus (is a pain mild or severe?)
- the location of the stimulus (is the hand or the arm being palpated?).

There are two separate pathways for the transmission of pain signals into the central nervous system. Pain signals are either fast and sharp or slow and chronic. Fast sharp signals are transmitted by either thermal or mechanical pain stimuli and are transmitted in the peripheral nerves to the spinal cord by small type Aδ fibres. Slow chronic pain is transmitted mainly by chemical pain stimuli but can also be caused by persistent mechanical or thermal stimuli and is transmitted by C fibres (Guyton & Hall 2006).

During cannulation or phlebotomy, the sensation of pain experienced is information from the skin rather than from the vessel. The stretching of the skin surface, local tapping of the skin, rubbing with alcohol and palpation of the vessel all trigger sensory pathways from the skin to the brain. In some cases, the sensations are also triggering memories of previous experiences. Preparation for cannulation, for example, may cause individuals to anticipate pain as a result of previous experiences (Melzack & Wall 1996).

If the cause of the pain also results in cell damage, then local chemicals will be released by the injured tissues and the awareness or sensitivity of the area will be 'heightened'. For example, skin which has been sunburned becomes highly touch-sensitive; taking off a shirt can cause immense pain if the skin is sunburnt.

There is a clearly identified pain pathway which goes from the periphery to the spinal cord, through the spinothalamic tract, to the thalamus and into the sensory cortex. There are differing theories on the perception of pain, the most widely accepted being that postulated by Melzack and Wall in the 1960s, known as 'the gate theory' (Melzack & Wall 1965).

According to the gate theory, the place where the pain is generated and the place where the pain is interpreted are linked by a nervous pathway which contains a gate. The pain message passes along the pathway by opening the gate. The more pain there is, the wider the gate is opened. The gate can be closed, and the pain pathway blocked, from either the proximal or distal side of the gate. The proximal (brain) side can close the gate by the use of diversional techniques such as relaxation or meditation. The distal (peripheral) side can close the gate by sending different signals, for example by rubbing the affected area or by transcutaneous nerve stimulation. Often, when we knock into something and experience pain, the first thing we do is to rub the affected area. By stimulating different nerve pathways, the original pain sensation can be prevented from passing through the gate and reaching the sensory cortex.

The kind of pain experienced by an individual depends mainly on two things: the type of tissue being damaged, and the agent that is causing the pain. Blood can cause pain when it is in the wrong place, such as when it leaks out of blood vessels. Equally, a lack of blood (ischaemia) can cause pain. When blood flow to a tissue structure is blocked the tissue becomes painful within a few minutes. The greater the rate of metabolism the more rapidly the pain will develop. One of the suggested causes of pain during ischaemia is the accumulation of lactic acid as a consequence of anaerobic metabolism (Guyton & Hall 2006).

Pain reduction

When trying to reduce the pain of cannulation or phlebotomy, several techniques can be utilized. Assisting the individual to relax can lessen the awareness of pain. This can be done using diversional strategies, breathing techniques (Dougherty 1994) or other methods the individual may be familiar with. As little local stimulation of the area as possible before cannulation will reduce the hypersensitivity of the area. Routine 'tapping' of a vein before cannulation may increase the perception of pain.

Local anaesthetic agents may also be considered. These must be water-soluble, be non-irritant, have a rapid onset of action and a suitable duration of action for the technique being performed, be non-toxic when absorbed into the circulation and have no lasting side-effects (Laurence 1975). Spiers *et al.* (2001) demonstrated that the use of topical anaesthetic agents was effective in reducing the perceived anxiety of future cannulation.

Local anaesthetics work by preventing the local nerve fibres from generating or conducting impulses, thereby interrupting the ascending pathways to the brain. This is achieved by preventing the cell membrane of the nerve from taking in sodium ions from its environment. Without the influx of sodium, a nerve cell cannot generate an action potential and a nerve impulse cannot be generated (Guyton & Hall 2006).

Local anaesthesia for cannulation varies depending on the nature and site of the cannula. Subcutaneous infiltration with lignocaine is usually used for central venous catheter insertion. This has the effect of inhibiting nerve transmission of the cutaneous and subcutaneous sensory nerves. Topical application of local anaesthetic creams is more common for peripheral cannulation. (*See* Chapter 9).

Conclusion

A broad knowledge of the anatomy and physiology that underpin i.v. therapy is required by all practitioners who expand their practice to include this important skill. The range and depth of knowledge required will depend upon the specific area of practice and the role of the practitioner.

References

Arnaout S, Diab K, Al-Kutoubi A, Jamaleddine G (2001) Rupture of the chordae of the tricuspid valve after knotting of the pulmonary artery catheter. *Chest* 120: 1742–1744.

Bard (2006) www.accessabilitybybard [accessed 6 January 2006]

Berne RM, Levy NL, Koeppen B, Stanton B (2004) *Physiology*, 5th edn. Mosby, St Louis, Missouri.

Chin KJ, Singh K (2005) The superficial ulnar artery—a potential hazard in patients with difficult venous access. *British Journal of Anaesthesia* 94(5): 692–693.

Clinical Skills Laboratory (2007) www.clinicalskills.nhs.uk/education/cannulation2.asp [accessed 4 January 2007]

Collier PE, Goodman GB (1995) Cardiac tamponade caused by central venous catheter perforation of the heart: a preventable complication. *Journal of the American College of Surgeons* 181(5): 459–463.

Dougherty L (1994) *A study to Discover how Cancer Patients Perceive the Intravenous Cannulation Experience*. Unpublished MSc thesis, University of Surrey, Guildford.

Dougherty L (2004) Vascular access devices. In: Dougherty L, Lister S, eds. *The Royal Marsden Hospital Manual of Clinical Nursing Procedures*, 6th edn, 724–773. Blackwell Publishing, Oxford.

Drake RL, Vogl W, Mitchell AWM (2005) *Gray's Anatomy for Students*. Elsevier Inc., Philadelphia.

Green JH (1985) *An Introduction to Human Physiology*, 4th edn. Oxford University Press, Oxford.

Guyton AC, Hall JE (2006) *Textbook of Medical Physiology*, 11th edn. Elsevier Saunders, Philadelphia.

Hadaway LR (2001) Anatomy and physiology related to intravenous therapy. In: Hankins J, Lonsway RA, Hedrick C, Perdue MB, eds. *Infusion Therapy in Clinical Practice*, 2nd edn, 65–97. WB Saunders, Philadelphia.

Heit JA, Silverstein MD, Mohr DN, Petterson TM, O'Fallon WM, Melton LJ (2000) Risk factors for deep vein thrombosis and pulmonary embolism: a population-based case-control study. *Archives of Internal Medicine* 160: 809–815.

Irie T (2001) Intraarterial chemotherapy of liver metastases: implantation of a microcatheter–port system with use of modified fixed catheter tip technique. *Journal of Vascular Interventional Radiology* 12: 1215–1218.

Jarvis J, Watson A, Robertson G (2005) Horner's syndrome after central venous catheterization. *The New Zealand Medical Journal* 118: 1215.

Jungreis CA, Wechsler LR, Horton JA (1989) Intracranial thrombolysis via a catheter embedded in the clot. *Stroke* 20: 1578–1580.

Kennedy AM, Grocott M, Schwartz MS, Modarres H, Scott M, Schon F (1997) Median nerve injury: an underrecognised complication of brachial artery cardiac catheterisation. *Journal of Neurology, Neurosurgery, and Psychiatry* 63: 542–546

Kessell G, Barker I (1996) Leg ischaemia in an infant following accidental intra-arterial administration of atracurium treated with caudal anaesthesia: case reports. *Anaesthesia* 51(12): 1154–1156.

Lirk P, Keller C, Colvin J, Rieder J, Maurer H, Moriggl B (2004) Unintentional arterial puncture during cephalic vein cannulation: case report and anatomical study. *British Journal of Anaesthesia* 92(5): 740–742.

Laurence DR (1975) *Clinical Pharmacology*, 4th edn. Churchill Livingstone, Edinburgh.

Melzack R, Wall PD (1965) Pain mechanisms: a new theory. *Science* 150: 971–979.

Melzack R, Wall PD (1996) *The Challenge of Pain*. Penguin Books Ltd, Harmondsworth, Middlesex.

Moore KL, Dalley AF (2006) *Clinically Orientated Anatomy*, 5th edn. Lippincott Williams & Wilkins, Philadelphia.

Morton PG, Fontaine DK, Hudak CM, Gallo BM (2005) *Critical Care Nursing: a Holistic Approach*, 8th edn. Lippincott Williams & Wilkins, Philadelphia.

Nathan P (1988) *The Nervous System*, 3rd edn. Oxford University Press, Oxford.

Perreas KG, Kumar S, Khan Z, Rees A (1999) A knot in the heart—surgical removal of a pulmonary artery catheter entangled in the tricuspid valve chordae. *European Journal of Cardiothoracic Surgery* 15(1): 112–113.

Scales K (2005) Vascular access: a guide to peripheral venous cannulation. *Nursing Standard* 19(49): 48–52.

Soni N (1989) *Anaesthesia and Intensive Care: Practical Procedures*. Heinemann, London.

Spiers AF, Taylor KH, Joanes DN, Girdler NM (2001) A randomised, double-blind, placebo-controlled, comparative study of topical skin analgesics and the anxiety and discomfort associated with venous cannulation. *British Dental Journal* 190(8): 444–449.

Tortora GJ, Derrickson B (2006) *Principles of Anatomy and Physiology*, 11th edn. John Wiley & Sons. Inc, Hoboken, NJ, USA

Weinstein SM (2007) Anatomy and physiology applied to infusion therapy. In: Weinstein SM, ed, 53–62. *Plumer's Principles and Practice of Intravenous Therapy*, 8th edn. JB Lippincott, Philadelphia.

Whitson M (1996) Intravenous therapy in the older adult: special needs and considerations. *Journal of Intravenous Nursing* 19(5): 251–255.

Wilson KJW, Waugh A (1996) *Ross and Wilson: Anatomy and Physiology in Health and Illness*, 8th edn. Churchill Livingstone, Edinburgh.

Wong PSC, Singh SP, Watson RDS, Lip GYH (1999) Management of pulmonary thrombo-embolism using catheter manipulation: a report of four cases and review of the literature. *Postgraduate Medical Journal* 75: 737–742.

Woodburne RT, Burkel WE (1994) *Essentials of Human Anatomy*, 9th edn. Oxford University Press, Oxford.

CHAPTER 3

Fluid and Electrolyte Balance

Michèle Malster

Introduction

This chapter presents an overview of fluids and electrolytes, together with acid–base balance, and considers some of the common imbalances and their management. Each section starts by looking at normal balance and the homeostatic mechanisms that regulate it, before going on to describe the imbalances that can occur. The major imbalances of fluid, electrolytes and acid–base are presented in terms of their assessment and management. The more common causes of each imbalance are presented in tabular format, together with their physiological effects, in order to assist the reader's understanding of the rationale for interventions. The section on fluid and electrolyte replacement therapy gives details of the common crystalline and colloid solutions used in intravenous (i.v.) therapy, together with the indications for their use. The latter part of the chapter considers some of the more complex problems related to specific client groups.

Fluid Balance

Throughout the human life span, the water content and fluid compartments within the body alter. In infants, the fluid content represents 70–80% of their body weight, with the ratio of extracellular to intracellular fluid (ECF : ICF) being 3:2. This means that infants are particularly susceptible to dehydration, because extracellular fluid is more easily lost from the body than intracellular fluid. The percentage of total body water progressively decreases, reaching 60% of the body weight at 2 years of age. In the adult, the water content accounts for 60% of the body weight in males and 55% in females, and the ratio of ECF to ICF is approximately 1:2. From puberty there is evidence of sex differentiation in the total body water content; this occurs because of the greater percentage of body fat in females. Fat cells contain very little water and therefore the total body water (TBW) percentage decreases as the percentage body fat increases. It is important to remember this when managing i.v. therapy in obese patients. For example, if the requisite amount of fluid replacement for a lean person weighing 100 kg (TBW = 70%) were to be given to an obese person weighing 100 kg (TBW = 35%), this would result in the latter receiving twice the required amount of fluid (Statland 1963; *See* Figure 3.1).

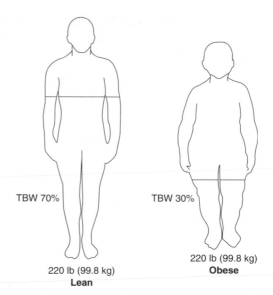

Figure 3.1   Body composition of a lean and an obese individual. TBW, total body water. (After Metheney 1992. Reproduced with permission from Lippincott, Williams and Wilkins.)

Fluid compartments

There are two main fluid compartments in the body:

- intracellular fluid—fluid in the cells
- extracellular fluid
  - plasma, i.e. intravascular fluid (IVF)
  - interstitial fluid (ISF)
  - transcellular fluid (TCF).

Transcellular fluid refers to fluid contained in body cavities, such as cerebrospinal fluid, intraocular fluid, synovial fluid, etc.

Composition

The body fluids are composed of water and dissolved particles (solutes). These solutes are referred to as electrolytes and non-electrolytes. When in solution, electrolytes can dissociate into either positively charged cations or negatively charged anions, which can conduct an electrical charge. In any solution, the number of cations must equal the number of anions; this is called electroneutrality. The major cations are:

- sodium (Na^+)
- potassium (K^+)
- calcium (Ca^{2+})
- magnesium (Mg^{2+}).

The major anions are:

- chloride (Cl^-)
- bicarbonate (HCO_3^-)
- phosphate (HPO_4^-)
- protein.

Within the ECF and ICF, there are large differences in the numbers of cations and anions. For example, within the cells potassium is the major cation, while outside the cells sodium predominates. The concentration of individual electrolytes is measured in millimoles per litre (mmol/L). Non-electrolytes are substances that do not dissociate in solution, including urea, glucose, creatinine and bilirubin.

Transport mechanisms

The fluid compartments are separated from one another by semipermeable membranes through which water and solutes may pass. While small solutes such as urea can pass easily through membranes, other large molecules such as proteins are confined to the intravascular fluid by the capillary membranes. The composition of each fluid compartment is maintained by the selectivity of its membrane. This ensures that nutrients can pass into the cells and waste products can pass out of the cells and ultimately to the plasma. The semipermeable membranes involved include:

- capillary membranes which separate IVF from ISF
- cell membranes which separate ISF from ICF
- epithelial membranes which separate ISF and IVF from TCF (Horne & Swearingen 1993).

The means by which fluid moves from one compartment to another involves both passive and active transport mechanisms.

Passive transport

Simple diffusion   Diffusion refers to the movement of solutes down a gradient from an area of high concentration (of solutes) to an area of low concentration until equilibrium is reached. Factors which affect the rate of diffusion include:

- concentration of solute
- size and molecular weight of solute
- surface area available for diffusion
- distance which the solute must diffuse
- temperature of the environment (Horne & Swearingen 1993).

Diffusion may also take place if there is a change in the electrical potential across the membrane. For example, anions will follow cations and the reverse will also happen. Movement of solutes will occur if they are lipid soluble or if the substances are small enough to pass through the cell wall. However, large lipid-soluble substances (e.g. glucose) require a carrier to enable them to diffuse into the cell. This process is called facilitated diffusion.

Facilitated diffusion   This method of diffusion also requires a concentration gradient, but the amount and rate of diffusion are dependent on the availability of carrier substance. After entering the cell, the carrier then releases itself and is available to aid diffusion of further substances. If the carrier becomes saturated (i.e. all the carrier is being used), even though a concentration gradient still exists, diffusion will be reduced.

Osmosis   This is the movement of solvent (e.g. water) from an area of low concentration of solutes (particles) to an area of high concentration of solutes across a semipermeable membrane. The forces involved relate to:

- oncotic pressure—the osmotic pressure exerted by proteins; for example, plasma proteins (albumin) exert pressure within the vasculature to hold fluid in the intravascular space
- osmotic pressure—the amount of hydrostatic pressure necessary to stop the osmotic flow of fluid

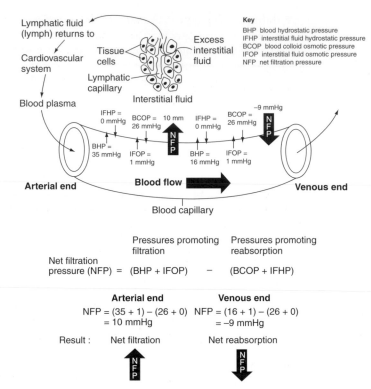

Net filtration pressure (NFP) =

Pressures promoting filtration		Pressures promoting reabsorption
(BHP + IFOP)	−	(BCOP + IFHP)

	Arterial end	**Venous end**
NFP =	(35 + 1) − (26 + 0)	NFP = (16 + 1) − (26 + 0)
	= 10 mmHg	= −9 mmHg
Result :	Net filtration	Net reabsorption

Figure 3.2   Capillary bed dynamics—dynamics of capillary exchange. (From Tortora & Grabowski 1996. Reprinted by permission of John Wiley & Sons, Inc.)

- hydrostatic pressure—the pressure exerted by the weight of the fluid (water) on the semipermeable membrane; this provides the principal force by which fluid moves out of the arterial end of capillaries (Figure 3.2).

Filtration   Filtration is used to describe the movement of solutes (particles) and solvent (fluid) from an area of high hydrostatic pressure to an area of low hydrostatic pressure.

Active transport
Where there is no electrical or concentration gradient, substances are unable to move by simple diffusion. Active transport, as its name suggests, requires the use of energy in the form of adenosine triphosphate (ATP) to move substances against a pressure or concentration gradient. This form of transport may involve the simultaneous movement of different substances. For example, as sodium ions move into the cell, potassium ions move out simultaneously. This is more commonly referred to as the 'sodium–potassium pump'. This pump is responsible for maintaining the intracellular fluid volume, by ensuring that the osmotic pressure exerted by the intracellular proteins (to pull water into the cells) is counterbalanced by the output of sodium ions (Paradiso 1995). As well as these transport mechanisms, other factors, such as osmolality and tonicity, also influence the movement of fluid.

Osmolality

Osmolality is a measurement of the concentration of the body's fluids, or the ratio of solutes to solvent, and its unit of measurement is the milliosmole/kilogram of water (mOsm/kg). Osmolality reflects the ability of a solution to create osmotic pressure and hence affect the movement of water. For example, an increase in the osmolality of the ECF will cause water to move from the ICF to the ECF, while decreased osmolality will have the reverse effect. The osmolality of each compartment is governed:

- in the ECF by sodium
- in the ICF by potassium
- in the IVF by plasma proteins.

Tonicity

Molecules that affect the movement of water (e.g. sodium, glucose, etc.) are called effective osmoles, while smaller molecules that move easily across most membranes (e.g. urea) are called ineffective osmoles (Horne & Swearingen 1993). Effective osmolality is also termed tonicity. Solutions that have the same tonicity as the body fluids (e.g. sodium chloride 0.9%) are called isotonic. Those solutions that have a lower tonicity (e.g. sodium chloride 0.45%) are called hypotonic, while those with a greater tonicity (e.g. sodium chloride 1.8%) are called hypertonic.

Regulation of body fluids

The body systems involved in regulating the body fluids are the renal, endocrine, cardiovascular, gastrointestinal (GI) and respiratory systems. They work interdependently to ensure that the homeostatic balance of fluid balance is maintained.

Renal system

The renal system is responsible for the regulation of sodium and water balance in the ECF. In response to a low serum sodium concentration, decreased plasma volume and increased sympathetic nervous stimulation, the cells in the juxtaglomerular apparatus in the glomerulus secrete a proteolytic enzyme called renin. Renin activates angiotensin 1, which is converted (by an enzyme from the lungs) to angiotension 2. Angiotensin 2 is a powerful vasoconstrictor and has two actions. Firstly, it causes vasoconstriction which increases peripheral resistance, thereby increasing arterial pressure. Secondly, it causes the release of a mineralcorticoid hormone called aldosterone from the adrenal cortex. Aldosterone acts on the distal convoluted tubule to increase the reabsorption of sodium; this retention of sodium leads to water retention and therefore the circulating volume is increased (*See* Figure 3.3).

Changes in the serum levels of sodium and potassium also affect the release of aldosterone. A decreased serum sodium or increased serum potassium will increase the release of aldosterone. As a result, sodium absorption from the renal tubules is enhanced in exchange for potassium and hydrogen ions, which are excreted in the urine.

Endocrine system

The thirst centre in the hypothalamus is the initial regulator of water intake. The urge to drink is stimulated by a decrease in the ICF in the thirst centre cells, together with feedback from the GI tract. Simultaneously, osmoreceptors in the hypothalamus detect changes in the osmolality of the ECF. When the osmolality of the plasma is increased, antidiuretic hormone (ADH) is released from the posterior pituitary gland. This hormone increases the permeability of the distal renal tubule to water and therefore more water is reabsorbed back into the circulation. As a result, only small amounts of concentrated urine are produced—sufficient to ensure the excretion of waste products. In contrast, if the osmoreceptors detect a decreased osmolality in the plasma, the secretion of ADH is inhibited, resulting in larger amounts of water being excreted as urine. At the same time, as the ICF volume in the thirst centre neurones increases, the thirst centre mechanism is inhibited (*See* Figure 3.4).

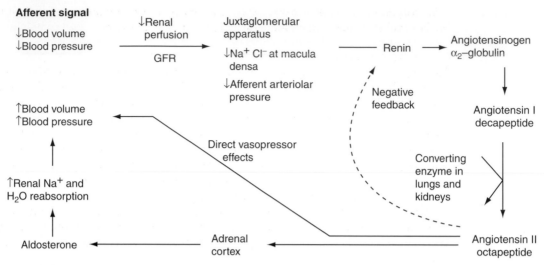

Figure 3.3 The renin–angiotensin–aldosterone system. GFR, glomerular filtration rate. (After Hinchcliff *et al.* 1997. Reprinted with permission from Elsevier.)

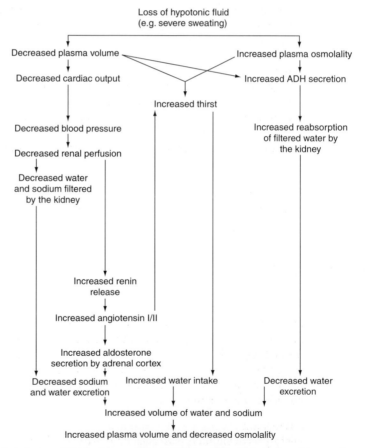

Figure 3.4 Regulation of fluid volume and osmolality: a clinical example. ADH, antidiuretic hormone. (After Horne & Swearingen 1993. Reprinted by permission of Elsevier.)

Sensory receptors in the GI tract provide feedback to the hypothalamus, so that ADH can be regulated to enhance water absorption from the intestines.

Cardiovascular system

Although large volume changes in the ECF interstitial fluid can occur with minimal change in body function, changes in the blood volume are less well tolerated. The function of the blood volume is to maintain tissue perfusion and therefore cell life. Approximately 25% of the cardiac output is pumped each minute to the kidneys at an optimal pressure, to maintain their perfusion, so that urine formation can occur. Changes in the blood volume have a direct effect on arterial blood pressure and therefore renal perfusion. This means that if the blood volume is increased, cardiac output and arterial pressure increase. An increase in renal arterial pressure leads to an increased glomerular filtration rate and ultimately increased urinary output.

Concurrently, baroreceptors and stretch receptors in the aorta and carotid arteries detect an increase in the arterial pressure and transmit inhibitory impulses to the sympathetic nervous system. This results in dilatation of the renal arterioles, which ultimately leads to an increase in urine formation.

Atrial natriuretic factor (ANF) is a polypeptide hormone secreted by the atria of the heart in response to increased stretching, brought about by an increased blood volume. ANF causes a decrease in the tubular reabsorption of sodium ions so that the osmolality of the filtrate is increased, which draws water into the tubule and consequently increases the volume of urinary output. It should be noted that ANF is only effective in the short-term control of blood volume.

Gastrointestinal system

Within the GI tract, the processes that help to regulate fluid volume are principally the processes of digestion and utilizing passive and active transport. Following digestive processes in the stomach, the chyme is mixed with GI secretions and moves through the small intestine. Here, approximately 90% of the water and nutrients are absorbed. A further 500–1000 mL of water are absorbed from the large intestine, so that there is only a minimal loss in the faeces.

Respiratory system

Approximately 400 mL/day of fluid is lost as expired water vapour. This amount will vary with respiratory rate and environmental humidity.

Fluid Volume Imbalances

Hypovolaemia

Hypovolaemia refers to a decrease in the ECF volume and is caused by excessive fluid loss or decreased fluid intake (Metheny 2000; Springhouse 2005). It occurs when the normal regulating mechanisms fail to cope adequately and may be accompanied by disturbances in osmolality, acid–base balance and electrolyte balance. If the hypovolaemia is very severe or prolonged, it may result in acute renal failure, because renal perfusion is not adequately maintained.

Assessment

History Severe fluid loss, such as diarrhoea, diaphoresis, vomiting, haemorrhage, etc. Decreased intake may be caused by starvation, unconsciousness, shock.

Physical evidence Third space loss (e.g. from ascites, bowel obstruction, etc.), diarrhoea, etc.

Clinical manifestations include evidence of compensation by the normal regulatory mechanisms, e.g. tachycardia, thirst, oliguria, etc. Reduced skin turgor, reduced jugular vein filling and furred tongue may be apparent. If hypovolaemic shock is present, the patient will appear pale with clammy skin and have a rapid, thready pulse and marked hypotension. As the dehydration progresses, the patient may exhibit signs of altered consciousness.

Tests include the following.

- Haematocrit:
  - increased in dehydration
  - decreased in haemorrhage.
- Serum electrolytes—will vary according to the type of fluid loss; for example hypernatraemia will occur with excessive diaphoresis. Electrolyte imbalances that may occur include hypernatraemia, hyponatraemia and hyperkalaemia (*See* Electrolyte imbalances on page 57).
- Blood urea nitrogen (BUN)—may be raised due to altered renal activity and reduced fluid intake.
- Arterial blood gas analysis:
  - metabolic acidosis: pH < 7.35; bicarbonate < 22 mmol/L
  - metabolic alkalosis: pH > 7.45; bicarbonate > 28 mmol/L.
    Metabolic acidosis is associated with shock, diabetic ketoacidosis, etc., while metabolic alkalosis results from diuretic therapy or excessive upper GI tract fluid loss.
- Urine specific gravity—increased to about 1.010, which indicates the action of ADH, trying to conserve fluid.

Management

If the patient is experiencing altered consciousness, measures to ensure their safety are required. Monitoring of the level of consciousness may be indicated. The management of hypovolaemia aims to replace the fluid loss, correct any electrolyte imbalance and treat the underlying cause. The hypovolaemia in shock occurs either from a sudden major loss or from loss of more than 25% of the intravascular volume. The type of fluid lost will determine the replacement fluid. For example, haemorrhage will require blood and blood products while water losses can be replaced with crystalline i.v. solutions such as sodium chloride 0.9% or dextrose 5%. The rate of i.v. infusion may need to be rapid in order to keep up with the loss and also to replace the deficit. The speed with which the replacement can be achieved will depend on the cardiac and renal function of the patient. For this reason, monitoring of the vital signs is essential and may require the insertion of a central venous catheter for haemodynamic monitoring. Other observations include skin colour, temperature and turgor.

Care is taken to ensure that the patient does not become overloaded, which could precipitate pulmonary oedema. Overloading can occur from infusing fluid too rapidly or infusing too much fluid.

Fluids used in replacement therapy include:

- compound sodium lactate
- human albumin, hetastarch or dextran solution
- fresh frozen plasma (Springhous 2006).

(*See* Crystalline solutions and Colloid solutions for details, pages 69 and 71).

The ultimate aim of fluid replacement therapy is to restore adequate tissue perfusion, so observations of the patient's status will relate to this, e.g. level of consciousness (CNS perfusion), fluid intake and output (renal perfusion) and peripheral pulses (peripheral perfusion). Further management will depend on the cause, e.g. diabetic ketoacidosis, which is described in the relevant section of this chapter.

Hypervolaemia

Hypervolaemia refers to an increase in the ECF volume and is generally caused by an overload of i.v. fluid administration, abnormal renal function (causing increased reabsorption of sodium and water) or the movement of fluid from the interstitial space to the intravascular fluid (Springhouse 2006). In susceptible patients, this may lead to pulmonary oedema and cardiac failure. However, usually the kidneys attempt to compensate by increasing the excretion of sodium and water and suppressing the release of aldosterone and ADH. Hypervolaemia is usually associated with alterations in acid–base balance, osmolality and electrolyte balance.

Assessment
History Intravenous fluid replacement therapy, cirrhosis, renal failure (oliguria), hypertonic i.v. fluid administration.
Physical evidence Oliguria, oedema, etc.
Clinical manifestations include bounding pulses, tachycardia, hypertension (compared to the patient's norm), neck vein distension and respiratory sounds associated with pulmonary oedema.
Tests include the following:

- Haematocrit—reduced because of haemodilution.
- Serum electrolytes—may reveal hyponatraemia due to excessive water retention.
- Serum osmolality—reduced.
- Blood urea nitrogen—decreased because the blood is diluted with excess water.
- Arterial blood gas analysis—may be altered in pulmonary oedema, showing a decreased Po_2 and alkalosis. A decreased Po_2 stimulates respiration, causing a decrease in Pco_2. The reduced ratio of Pco_2 to bicarbonate leads to an increased pH.
- Urine specific gravity—decreased, as the kidneys try to excrete the excess fluid.

Management
The main aim of treatment is to achieve a normal ECF volume. Management includes the use of diuretic therapy to aid excretion of the excess fluid, and restriction of sodium and water. The main risk is pulmonary oedema, so careful monitoring of respiration and breath sounds is necessary. Vital signs and fluid intake and output need to be monitored. Monitoring of blood gases will facilitate correction of alkalosis, and hypoxaemia will require oxygen therapy. The underlying cause of the hypervolaemia needs to be treated. Haemodialysis is indicated if renal failure is present.

Electrolyte Regulation and Imbalances

The concentration of individual electrolytes is measured in mmol/L. It should be noted that the normal ranges for serum electrolyte concentrations will vary slightly according to the method of laboratory assessment.

Sodium

Sodium is an important factor in maintaining the volume and osmolality of ECF. It influences the maintenance of potassium and chloride concentrations and is also essential for neuromuscular transmission (Innerarity & Stark 1990). It is regulated in relation to water and chloride and is the main cation that determines ECF osmolality. Changes in sodium concentration result in corresponding changes in the osmolality. As most of the sodium is outside the cells, its level can be measured by serum testing, normal ranging between 136 and 145 mmol/L.

The natural means of sodium loss from the body are via sweat, urine and faeces. The kidneys and endocrine systems are the main regulators of sodium balance. Two contrasting mechanisms in the kidneys try to ensure that excess or lack of oral intake of sodium can be accommodated with minimal changes in serum sodium concentration. One mechanism ensures that excess sodium (together with water) passes via the glomerular filtrate into the urine, while the other mechanism endeavours to retain sodium, by encouraging its reabsorption (together with water) from the renal tubules when intake of sodium is low. This occurs in the presence of aldosterone, which is released in response to decreased plasma levels of sodium. As well as the production of aldosterone, the role of the endocrine system also involves the production of ADH. If the level of sodium in the ECF is increased, it increases the osmolality of the ECF which stimulates the secretion of ADH, thereby enhancing the reabsorption of water from the tubular filtrate. As a result, ECF osmolality is reduced.

Hyponatraemia

Hyponatraemia is usually defined as a serum sodium less than 135 mmol/L. However, it should be noted that inpatients may have a serum sodium of up to 5 mmol/L less than outpatients. Hyponatraemia is common in the postoperative period, partly due to increased levels of ADH as a result of the stress of anaesthesia and surgery, and partly due to pain and nausea (Metheny 2000). Another cause may be overinfusion of dextrose 5%, commonly used to rehydrate patients. The two basic mechanisms that result in hyponatraemia are concerned with either an increase in ECF water or a decrease in ECF sodium. The causes are listed in Table 3.1.

However, it should be noted that some conditions may give rise to a reduced serum sodium concentration, although there is no true hyponatraemia. One typical example is in hyperglycaemia, where the elevated glucose level exerts an osmotic 'pull' of water out of the cells into the ECF, thereby diluting the sodium in the ECF. Other examples are hyperproteinaemia and hyperlipidaemia, which reduce the percentage of water in the plasma. The ratio of sodium to water remains the same but, because the plasma water content is reduced, the serum sodium level is reduced (Horne & Swearingen 1993).

Assessment

History   The medical history may identify the cause, such as a history of diuretic therapy, adrenal impairment or syndrome of inappropriate antidiuretic hormone (SIADH).

Physical evidence   Vomiting, diarrhoea.

Clinical manifestations   relating to impairment of the musculoskeletal system may be muscle cramps and twitching. Central nervous system impairment results from low ECF sodium causing water to move into the brain cells, which then swell. Symptoms may include headache, dizziness, convulsions and unconsciousness.

Diagnostic tests

- Serum sodium level < 135 mmol/L.
- Urine osmolality < 350 mOsm/kg (except SIADH).
- Serum osmolality < 285 mmol/kg, except in hyperglycaemia, etc.
- Urine sodium < 20 mmol/L, except in SIADH and adrenal impairment.

Management

Patient safety is paramount both in terms of ensuring that no injury is sustained if the patient has neurological disturbances, and in relation to the correction of the hyponatraemia. Serum sodium levels less than 120 mmol/L require urgent treatment to remove the patient from danger, while sodium levels of between 120 and 136 mmol/L need careful management to ensure that overcompensation does not occur. Generally the

Table 3.1 Causes of hyponatraemia.

Cause	Physiological process
Prolonged diuretic use	Sodium reabsorption from the loop of Henle is impaired
Excessive diaphoresis	Large amounts of sodium are present in sweat
Prolonged vomiting, diarrhoea	Large ECF loss
Extensive burns	Large volumes of ECF (and therefore sodium) are lost
Renal disease	Excessive consumption or infusion of hypotonic solutions
Salt-losing nephritis	Loss of sodium
Nephrotic syndrome	Water retained in excess of sodium
Overinfusion of i.v. dextrose 5%	Excess water in the ECF will move into the cell to reduce the sodium: water ratio
Psychogenic polydipsia	Excessive water consumption
Anorexia, alcoholism, fasting	Inadequate oral intake
Syndrome of inappropriate ADH (SIADH)	Water is retained and sodium becomes overdiluted
Adrenal impairment	Reduced levels of aldosterone result in sodium excretion
Cirrhosis	Water retained in excess of sodium
Congestive cardiac failure	Water retained in excess of sodium
Drugs	
Intravenous cyclophosphamide	Increases renal sensitivity to ADH
Carbamazepine	Induces ADH release
Amitriptyline	Water retention
'Ecstasy'	Increased sodium loss
Chlorpropramide	Increases action of ADH
Addison's disease	Increased sodium excretion

ADH, antidiuretic hormone; ECF, extracellular fluid.

management falls into two categories: hyponatraemia with reduced ECF volume and hyponatraemia with increased ECF volume. The first is concerned with replacing the sodium and fluid losses, together with other electrolytes as necessary. In extreme cases, a hypertonic solution of sodium chloride (e.g. 2.7%) may be required, if the patient is severely depleted.

The second category of management is concerned with reducing the increased ECF volume. This will vary according to the cause, but may also include diuretic therapy and water restriction. Serum electrolytes need to be monitored, together with fluid intake and output, to ensure optimal management of this imbalance.

Hypernatraemia

This is defined as serum sodium greater than 145 mmol/L. As sodium is the main cation determinant of osmolality of the ECF, an increase in its concentration will cause hypertonicity which will result in water being 'drawn' out of the cells. This means that the ICF volume is decreased in hypernatraemia. The main causes of hypernatraemia are water loss, dehydration or sodium gain in excess of water, but it may also be a complication of aggressive treatment of hyponatraemia, as previously mentioned. The specific causes of hypernatraemia are presented in Table 3.2.

Table 3.2 Causes of hypernatraemia.

Condition	Physiological process
Inadequate water intake	Decreased extracellular fluid water volume
Watery diarrhea	Excessive water loss
Severe insensible loss	Excessive water loss
Burns	Water and electrolyte loss
Osmotic diuretic therapy	Excessive water loss
Hyperglycaemia	Water loss due to osmotic diuresis
Diabetes insipidus	Excessive water loss due to lack of antidiuretic hormone
Near-drowning in salt water	Excessive sodium intake
Hypertonic i.v. saline	Increased sodium gain
Hyperaldosteronism (e.g. Conn's syndrome)	Sodium retention, due to excess aldosterone

Assessment

History   There may be a medical history of diabetes insipidus, osmotic diuretics or near-drowning.

Physical evidence   Water loss, e.g. from major burns, diarrhoea.

Clinical manifestations   will include those relating to water loss (e.g. intense thirst, hypotension, dry mucous membranes) and sodium gain (e.g. flushed skin, peripheral oedema, low-grade fever). Hyperactive reflexes, lethargy and seizures may occur in severe hypernatraemia because of its effect on neuromuscular conduction and the central nervous system.

Diagnostic tests

- Serum sodium > 145 mmol/L.
- Serum osmolality > 295 mmol/kg because of the increased serum sodium level.
- Urine osmolality > 525 mOsm/kg, except in diabetes insipidus when it is decreased.

Management   If the patient shows signs of neurological impairment, care must be taken to ensure that there is no risk of injury. Correction of the hypernatraemia will depend on the cause and it centres around reducing the sodium level. Cautious administration of i.v. hypotonic solutions is recommended, together with careful monitoring of vital signs, fluid intake and output, neurological status and serum sodium. The fluids of choice are dextrose 5% and hypotonic saline solutions. To minimize the risk of overcorrection and cerebral oedema (due to fluid overload and the shift of water into the cells, particularly in the brain), diuretics may also be given. Diabetes insipidus will require specific therapy using a vasopressin analogue.

Potassium

Potassium is the main cation in the ICF and is of vital importance in neuromuscular conduction, acid–base balance and cell function. It also has a direct effect on cardiac muscle conductivity. Although potassium ions continuously move in and out of the cells, most of the potassium is contained within the cells by the sodium–potassium pump, so that, by comparison with sodium, the serum level is low and ranges between 3.5 and 5.0 mmol/L. The distribution of potassium between the ICF and ECF is influenced by pH levels, aldosterone, adrenaline and insulin. In acidosis, when hydrogen ions move into the cells as part of the buffering mechanism, potassium ions move out in order to maintain electroneutrality: one positive ion (H^+) is exchanged for another (K^+). As a result, serum

Table 3.3 Causes of hypokalaemia.

Cause	Physiological process
Prolonged thiazide diuretic use	Increased loss in the urine
Parenteral nutrition	Inadequate potassium intake
Severe gastrointestinal fluid loss	High potassium levels in gastric fluid, bile, etc.
Hyperaldosteronism	Increased loss in urine in exchange for sodium
Severe diaphoresis	Potassium loss in sweat
Severe stress	Corticoid release promotes sodium retention in exchange for potassium
Alkalosis	Potassium shift into the cells in exchange for hydrogen ions
Increased insulin secretion or therapy	Potassium shift from ECF into cells; also insulin is a carrier
Burns	Potassium loss
Hypomagnesaemia	Magnesium is important in activating sodium potassium pump
Ectopic adrenocorticotrophic hormone	Increased urine loss

potassium rises in acidosis. In alkalosis, the ions move in the opposite direction and so serum potassium falls. It can therefore be seen that changes in serum potassium levels may not always indicate a loss of or increase in the total potassium level in the body, but only reflect changes in the ECF potassium levels.

Potassium levels in the body are regulated by the kidneys, which adjust the amount of potassium excreted in the urine. There is a reciprocal relationship between potassium and sodium, an illustration of which is provided by the action of aldosterone, which aids sodium reabsorption in exchange for the excretion of potassium.

Hypokalaemia

Hypokalaemia, defined as a serum potassium less than 3.5 mmol/L, occurs when there is loss of potassium from the body or a shift of potassium into the cells. Potassium is not stored in the body and serum levels are maintained within narrow limits. A low intake of potassium is rarely the cause of hypokalaemia, except in patients receiving parenteral nutrition who may have inadequate replacement of this electrolyte. The main loss of potassium is via the kidneys and a common cause is thiazide diuretic therapy. The main causes of hypokalaemia are presented in Table 3.3.

Assessment

History There may be a medical history of thiazide diuretic therapy, congenital adrenal hyperplasia or pyloric stenosis.

Physical evidence Major burns, gastrointestinal loss.

Clinical manifestations of neuromuscular impairment such as muscle weakness, cramps, fatigue, paraesthesiae and diminished reflexes are typical signs. Paralytic ileus may occur due to decreased gut motility. Cardiac dysrhythmias may also occur due to impaired myocardial conduction.

Tests include the following:

- Serum potassium < 3.5 mmol/L.
- ECG—may show ventricular dysrhythmias, ST segment depression, flattened T-wave or presence of U-wave (*See* Figure 3.5).

Hypokalaemia: Serum potassium <3.5 mmol/L

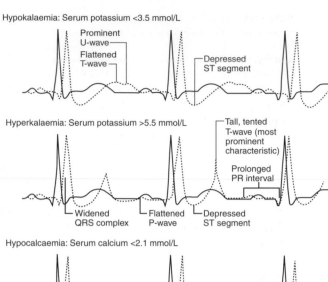

Hyperkalaemia: Serum potassium >5.5 mmol/L

Hypocalcaemia: Serum calcium <2.1 mmol/L

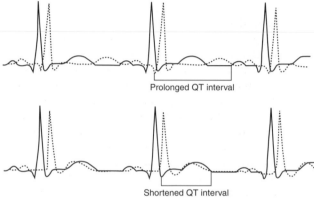

Prolonged QT interval

Shortened QT interval

Hypomagnesaemia: Serum magnesium <0.7 mmol/L

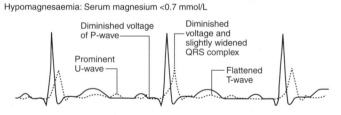

Hypomagnesaemia: Serum magnesium >2.1 mmol/L

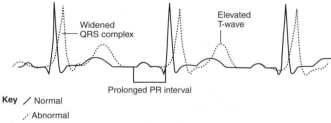

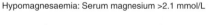

Key / Normal

.·` Abnormal

Figure 3.5 ECG changes associated with electrolyte imbalances. (Innerarity and Stark 1990. Reproduced with permission from Lippincott, Williams and Wilkins.)

- Arterial blood gas analysis—may detect metabolic alkalosis, with pH > 7.45 and increased bicarbonate levels.

Management   The aim of management is to treat the underlying cause and to replace the potassium by oral or i.v. supplements. If the i.v. route is used for replacement therapy, the patient requires careful monitoring during administration of the estimated amount of potassium (Joint Formulary Committee 2006). The most frequently used preparation is potassium chloride diluted in an isotonic solution (which will also provide some hydration). Use of a burette infusion set or syringe pump will assist in a more accurate rate of administration. If peripheral veins are used, the rate of infusion will need to be reduced to avoid irritation of the veins by the potassium chloride (Springhouse 2006). There is also a risk of damage to surrounding tissues if concentrated solutions extravasate, so delivery via a central venous access device may be preferable. Care should be taken to avoid rapid infusion of potassium, which could lead to cardiac arrest as a result of hyperkalaemia. ECG monitoring is recommended to detect abnormal rhythms or the development of hyperkalaemia due to overcorrection.

Hyperkalaemia

Hyperkalaemia is defined as a serum potassium greater than 5.5 mmol/L. There are four mechanisms that contribute to an increase in ECF potassium. The first relates to an increased potassium intake resulting from potassium replacement therapy by the oral or i.v. routes. Occasionally, however, an increased intake may be due to use of salt substitutes (which are high in potassium) by patients on a low sodium diet. Secondly, if excretion of potassium is inhibited (as in renal failure) or if there is failure of the control mechanisms (e.g. adrenocortical insufficiency leading to reduced aldosterone and cortisol associated with Addison's disease), serum levels will rise. Thirdly, since potassium is mainly found inside the cells, any condition which results in their breakdown will release potassium into the ECF, as the sodium–potassium pump fails. Finally, electrolyte shifts requiring the movement of a cation (e.g. potassium) out of the cell may result in an increased ECF potassium level. This can occur during hyponatraemia and metabolic acidosis, where sodium and hydrogen ions, respectively, move into the cell and potassium moves out of the cell to maintain electroneutrality. The causes of hyperkalaemia are presented in Table 3.4.

Assessment

History   There may be a medical history of prolonged or excessive salt substitute use, chemotherapy (cell lysis), hyponatraemia or diabetes mellitus.

Physical evidence   Crush injuries, burns, large-volume blood transfusion, diarrhoea.

Clinical manifestations   of neurological impairment may result in anxiety, irritability, muscle weakness, abdominal cramps and paraesthesiae. Cardiac dysrhythmias due to abnormal myocardial conduction will be accompanied by an irregular pulse. It should be noted that cardiac output is usually decreased as potassium is a myocardial depressant.

Tests include the following:

- Serum potassium > 5.5 mmol/L.
- ECG—may show dysrhythmias, elevated T-waves, depressed ST segment, flattened or absent P-wave (which may lead to asystole if not treated), prolonged PR interval and wide QRS complex (Figure 3.5).
- Arterial blood gas analysis—may indicate metabolic acidosis with a low bicarbonate level.

Management   Hyperkalaemia is a life-threatening condition and may lead to asystole. Prompt recognition of ECG changes is important and careful monitoring is necessary during treatment, which may need to be aggressive to prevent cardiac arrest.

Table 3.4   Causes of hyperkalaemia.

Cause	Physiological process
Potassium replacement therapy	Increased ECF potassium
Prolonged use of salt substitute	Increased potassium intake
Renal failure	Failure of tubules to balance potassium
Potassium-sparing diuretics	Retention of potassium
Bowel obstruction	Reduced potassium loss in faeces
Burns, trauma, etc.	Cell damage releases potassium into ECF
Large-volume blood transfusion	Cell lysis in donated blood increases with storage time
Hyponatraemia	Potassium ions move out of cell in exchange for sodium
Metabolic acidosis	Potassium ions move out of cell in exchange for hydrogen ions
Hyperglycaemia	Glucose osmotic diuresis causes potassium loss from cells
Hyperaldosteronism	Decreased potassium excretion
Addison's disease	Decreased potassium excretion
Chemotherapy	Cell lysis
Factors affecting accurate estimation:	
Prolonged tourniquet application during sampling	Haemolysis, releasing potassium from the cells
Fist clenching during blood sampling	May cause haemolysis
EDTA contamination	May lead to inaccurate reading
Haemolysed blood sample	Increased potassium estimation
Thrombocytosis	

ECF, extracellular fluid.

Potassium tends to cause depolarization of the cell membranes, but increasing the serum calcium levels helps to antagonize this effect and this is the rationale for administering i.v. calcium. Calcium is generally administered in the form of calcium gluconate, although calcium chloride may be used as an alternative. However, it is important to note that these two preparations are not interchangeable, because 10 mL of calcium gluconate contains 220 µmol/L (micromoles per litre) of calcium, while the same volume of calcium chloride contains 680 µmol/L. A slow i.v. infusion of calcium gluconate will help to negate the depressant effects of potassium on the myocardium. It acts rapidly, but its duration of action is not sustained.

Acute symptomatic hyperkalaemia (serum level > 5.5 mmol/L) may require treatment on a temporary basis with an i.v. infusion of dextrose 50% with insulin, which will assist the movement of potassium back into the cells.

Other forms of treatment include haemodialysis if renal function is impaired, and an i.v. infusion of sodium bicarbonate to correct the metabolic acidosis, if present.

Calcium

Calcium helps to maintain the structure and function of cell membranes and is essential in neuromuscular conduction and contraction in the heart and skeletal muscles. It is also required for hormonal secretions, enzyme activation and blood coagulation.

The skeletal system contains almost 99% of the body's calcium, while 1% is within the ICF and 0.1% within the ECF. Approximately 50% of the calcium is chemically active, ionized calcium and this represents the serum level that is measured. Normal serum ionized calcium levels range from 1 to 1.25 mmol/L, but this is not routinely measured. The remainder is bound to protein (e.g. albumin), which means that albumin levels need to be considered when assessing calcium levels. This is important as laboratories normally measure total calcium only (range 2.2–2.6 mmol/L); the result may include compensation for albumin levels.

Calcium balance is maintained by parathyroid hormone (PTH), calcitonin and calcitriol (1,2,5-dihydroxycholecalciferol, an active form of vitamin D). PTH, released in response to a low ECF calcium, enhances calcium reabsorption (the movement of calcium from bone into the plasma) and promotes intestinal and renal absorption of calcium (via calcitriol), thereby increasing the serum calcium level. In contrast, a high ECF calcium stimulates the thyroid gland to release calcitonin, which acts as a physiological antagonist to parathyroid hormone, inhibiting calcium release from bone and resulting in a decreased serum calcium.

The pH level of the serum will affect the ionized calcium level because, in alkalosis, more calcium is bound to protein. Another factor affecting serum calcium is the reciprocal relationship between calcium and phosphorus. A raised serum calcium leads to a lowered serum phosphorus, while a lowered serum calcium leads to a raised phosphorus level.

Hypocalcaemia

This is defined as a serum calcium less than 2.1 mmol/L and usually represents a reduced level of circulating ionized calcium. Hypocalcaemia is usually associated with vitamin D deficiency, abnormal parathyroid secretion, reduced calcium intake or increased calcium loss. It may cause skeletal abnormalities, impaired neuromuscular activity and defective clotting mechanisms. The causes of hypocalcaemia are presented in Table 3.5.

Table 3.5   Causes of hypocalcaemia.

Cause	Physiological process
Inadequate intake	Reduced total body calcium
Vitamin D deficiency	Reduced calcium absorption
Hypoparathyroidism	Inability to release calcium from bone
Hyperphosphataemia	Reduced serum calcium
Hypomagnesaemia	Decreased action of PTH
Alkalosis	Increased binding of calcium to protein
Acute pancreatitis	Decreased PTH hypoalbuminaemia
Hypoalbuminaemia	Reduces bound calcium only
Large-volume blood transfusion	Increased citrate intake binds with calcium

PTH, parathyroid hormone.

Assessment

History Hypoparathyroidism (may also be a surgical complication of thyroid surgery), chronic alcoholism, malnutrition.

Physical evidence Large-volume blood transfusion.

Clinical manifestations of neuromuscular impairment may be found, such as tetany, increased reflex responses, circumoral and finger tingling, and positive Trousseau's and Chvostek's signs, indicating latent tetany (*See* Box 3.1 and Figure 3.6). Other neurological signs include confusion, memory loss and seizures.

Tests include the following:

- Serum calcium < 2.1 mmol/L.
- Prolonged clotting times.
- ECG—changes may include dysrhythmias and prolonged QT interval and ST segment may be apparent (Figure 3.5).
- Serum phosphate and magnesium concentrations—these may assist in identifying the cause.

Management The initial aim of management is to prevent injury to the patient (if there is evidence of central nervous system impairment), and monitoring of neurological status is indicated. Hypocalcaemia may reduce myocardial contractility, leading to heart failure and pulmonary oedema, so vital signs and ECG should be monitored. Correction of hypocalcaemia is achieved in the short term by the cautious administration of i.v. calcium gluconate as an infusion. It should be noted that i.v. administration of calcium is a particular risk in patients who are receiving digoxin therapy, as calcium can sensitize the heart to digoxin. Longer-term treatment will depend on the cause (Metheny 2000; Springhouse 2006).

BOX 3.1

Trousseau's sign
This is a sign of carpal spasm induced by ischaemia. It can be elicited by placing a blood pressure cuff around the patient's arm and leaving it inflated for 2 minutes, at a pressure greater than the patient's systolic pressure.

Chvostek's sign
This is typified by unilateral contraction of eyelid and facial muscles. It results from irritation of the facial nerve which can be provoked by tapping the side of the face, just in front of the ear.

Kussmaul's respirations
A typical slow, deep breathing associated with respiratory acidosis.

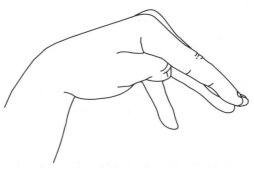

Figure 3.6 Trousseau's sign.

Table 3.6   Causes of hypercalcaemia.

Cause	Physiological process
Use of calcium supplements	Increased calcium intake
Increased vitamin D intake	Increased absorption of calcium
Medication	
Antacids	Containing calcium
Thiazides	Decreased calcium excretion
Lithium	Inhibits action of antidiuretic hormone
Hyperthyroidism	Increased calcitonin release
Hyperparathyroidism	Increased parathyroid hormone secretion leads to increased calcium release from bone
Renal tubule disease	Increased renal loss of calcium
Hypophosphataemia	Inverse reciprocal relationship with calcium
Malignancy	Humoral factors increase calcium release from bone
Tuberculosis, sarcoidosis	Increased calcium release from bone

Hypercalcaemia

Hypercalcaemia is defined as a serum calcium greater than 2.6 mmol/L and is caused by either an increased intake and absorption of calcium or a decreased excretion. Decreased loss of calcium in the urine may occur because of conditions that cause increased secretion of parathyroid hormone and calcitonin. Other causes of hypercalcaemia are presented in Table 3.6.

Assessment

History   Acute pancreatitis, bone deformity, hyperparathyroidism.

Physical evidence   Use of calcium substitutes.

Clinical manifestations   of neurological impairment of the central nervous system may be apparent, such as confusion, depression, etc. Hyperparathyroidism can lead to a reduced glomerular filtration rate and renal stone formation due to precipitation of calcium. Calcification of soft tissue may also occur.

Tests include the following:

- Serum calcium > 2.6 mmol/L.
- Bone density—reduced on X-ray.
- ECG—may show shortened ST segment and QT interval (*See* Figure 3.5).

Management   Protecting the patient from injury is of prime importance if there is neurological impairment. Correction of the hypercalcaemia can be achieved by the administration of loop diuretics (e.g. frusemide) to encourage calcium excretion, together with i.v. infusion of sodium chloride 0.9% to enhance the diuresis (by increasing the ECF volume). Careful monitoring of electrolyte levels is required to assess optimal correction. Other forms of treatment relate to the causative factors; for example, haemodialysis for renal failure, partial parathyroidectomy (for hyperparathyroidism) and the use of i.v. phosphates to correct hypophosphataemia.

Magnesium

Magnesium is mainly found in the ICF and bone and as sodium is related to potassium, so magnesium is related to calcium and phosphorus. Its concentration is largely regulated by the kidneys and ranges from 0.7 to 1.2 mmol/L. Magnesium influences neuromuscular irritability and is important in cardiac and skeletal muscle contraction. It also has an effect on peripheral vasodilatation and hence blood pressure and cardiac output.

Hypomagnesaemia

This is generally defined as a serum magnesium level less than 0.7 mmol/L and results from a loss of magnesium due to vomiting, diuretic therapy, etc. or from fluid and electrolyte changes associated with other imbalances, such as hypercalcaemia. The clinical presentation is usually one of altered neuronal activity similar to that seen in calcium disorders. Stridor is a major risk due to airway obstruction and ECG changes, and dysrhythmias may also occur (Figure 3.5). Management aims to protect the patient from injury and to replace the magnesium very slowly.

Hypermagnesaemia

Hypermagnesaemia usually occurs with a serum magnesium greater than 1.2 mmol/L, caused by a dietary increase in magnesium (supplements, antacids, etc.), fluid and electrolyte shifts, or inadequate excretion. The clinical presentation may be similar to hyperkalaemia, including cardiac dysrhythmias. Management includes good monitoring and the administration of calcium gluconate to counteract the cardiac effects of the increased magnesium.

Phosphorus

Phosphorus is the major anion of ICF, with a normal serum concentration of 0.8–1.5 mmol/L. As part of the phospholipid layer, it helps to maintain cell membrane integrity and is also an important component of teeth and bones. Phosphorus is essential for metabolism of fats, carbohydrates and protein, and for normal function of muscles, nervous system and red blood cells. It promotes energy transfer to cells (ATP) and acts as a urinary buffer to maintain acid–base balance.

Hypophosphataemia

Hypophosphataemia occurs when the serum phosphorus level falls below 0.8 mmol/L. It may be caused by inadequate intake, excessive loss (from the GI tract or diuretics), cation exchange (hypokalaemia, etc.) or endocrine disorders (e.g. hyperparathyroidism, aldosteronism). Neurological manifestations include muscle weakness, fatigue, nystagmus and seizures. Platelet dysfunction may also occur. Impaired oxygen release, due to a reduction in 2,3-diphosphoglycerate in erythrocytes, may lead to rapid, shallow breathing.

Management aims to replace the phosphate deficit. Monitoring for hypercalcaemia is indicated, as this can be a concomitant problem.

Hyperphosphataemia

Hyperphosphataemia exists when the serum phosphorus level exceeds 1.5 mmol/L. It should be noted that the reference range for children is higher. The main causes of hyperphosphataemia are renal failure, hypoparathyroidism, cellular destruction (with subsequent release of phosphates), vitamin D toxicity and enema use. Neuromuscular dysfunction may present as muscle spasms, tetany, circumoral paraesthesiae and positive Chvostek's and Trousseau's signs (Box 3.1). Soft tissue calcifications are associated with long-term hyperphosphataemia.

Care must be taken to protect the patient from harm, as seizures may occur. Aluminium hydroxide, a phosphate-binding drug, may be administered to decrease serum levels. Calcium supplements may be required to raise serum calcium levels, thereby reducing the level of phosphate (Kumar & Clark 2006). Serum electrolyte concentrations need to be monitored.

Fluid and Electrolyte Replacement Therapy

The aim of i.v. therapy is to restore or maintain normal fluid volume and electrolyte balance when the oral route is not possible. In this chapter nutritional needs will not be considered, and it should be noted that the normal i.v. crystalline fluids only provide sufficient kilocalories to limit starvation and catabolism. The infusion of i.v. fluids alters the composition of plasma by the addition of fluid and electrolytes and needs to be approached with caution, if fluid overload, fluid deficit, fluid shifts and unwanted alterations in electrolyte concentrations are to be avoided. The reader will appreciate that careful monitoring is essential, if the optimal outcome for the patient is to be achieved. While general guidelines are available for i.v. fluid and electrolyte replacement (e.g. Joint Formulary Committee 2006), it is essential that any regimen is tailored to the individual needs of the patient. The indications for i.v. fluid replacement include:

- replacement of abnormal fluid and electrolyte losses, some of which are described in this chapter
- maintenance of normal fluid and electrolyte balance, if the oral route cannot be used
- correction of fluid and electrolyte disorders
- promoting renal function.

Assessment of the patient's needs may involve visual observations of the patient, vital signs and laboratory tests as indicated in Box 3.2.

The fluids used for replacement therapy are of two main types: crystalline and colloid.

BOX 3.2

Assessment of need for intravenous fluid and electrolyte therapy

- Vital signs
- Fluid intake and output measurement
- Daily weighing
- Skin turgor
- Jugular vein filling
- Urinary specific gravity
- Central venous pressure measurement
- Serum electrolyte levels
- Arterial blood gas analysis

Crystalline solutions

Crystalline solutions are electrolyte solutions and are categorized according to their tonicity (compared with plasma osmolar concentration). There are three types:

- isotonic
- hypotonic
- hypertonic.

The contents of selected i.v. replacement solutions are presented in Table 3.7.

Isotonic solutions

Isotonic solutions have the same osmolality as plasma and, when infused, expand both the ICF and ECF equally. Such fluids do not alter the osmolality of the vascular compartment. Examples of isotonic solutions are dextrose 5%, sodium chloride 0.9%, dextrose 4% with sodium chloride 0.18%, compound sodium lactate and Plasma-Lyte 148 (Lund 1994; Joint Formulary Committee 2006).

Table 3.7 Contents of selected intravenous replacement solutions.

Solution	Tonicity	Contents
Dextrose 5%	Isotonic	Glucose 50 g
Sodium chloride 0.9%	Isotonic	Na$^+$ 150 mmol/L Cl$^-$ 150 mmol/L
Dextrose 4% with sodium chloride 0.18%	Isotonic	Glucose 40 g Na$^+$ 30 mmol/L Cl$^-$ 30 mmol/L
Compound sodium lactate	Isotonic	Na$^+$ 131 mmol/L Ca^{2+} 2.0 mmol/L K$^+$ 5.0 mmol/L Cl$^-$ 111 mmol/L Lactate 29 mmol/L
Plasma-Lyte 148	Isotonic	Na$^+$ 140 mmol/L K$^+$ 5 mmol/L Mg^{2+} 1.5 mmol/L Cl$^-$ 98 mmol/L Gluconate 23 mmol/L Acetate 27 mmol/L
Sodium chloride 0.45%	Hypotonic	Na$^+$ 75 mmol/L Cl$^-$ 75 mmol/L
Sodium chloride 1.8%	Hypertonic	Na$^+$ 300 mmol/L Cl$^-$ 300 mmol/L
Dextrose 10%	Hypertonic	Dextrose 100 g
Sodium bicarbonate 1.26%		Na$^+$ 150 mmol/L HCO$_3^-$ 150 mmol/L
Sodium bicarbonate 4.2%		Na$^+$ 500 mmol/L HCO$_3^-$ 500 mmol/L
Sodium bicarbonate 8.4%		Na$^+$ 1000 mmol/L HCO$_3^-$ 1000 mmol/L

Dextrose 5% It should be noted that even though the patient may only require water replacement, it is not possible to infuse distilled water, because it would cause haemolysis of erythrocytes where it entered the vein. Dextrose 5% is therefore used instead, as it is metabolized to water and carbon dioxide. It is used to replace water deficits, because it moves into all fluid compartments. It should never be used as the sole means of expanding ECF, because it can cause dilution of the sodium concentration.

Sodium chloride 0.9% (normal saline) This solution contains 150 mmol/L of sodium and 150 mmol/L of chloride, but is not a physiological solution, because the amounts are not equal to those of ECF. Indeed, the chloride is considerably greater than that in the ECF (105 mmol/L) and may pose an increased burden on the kidneys, with a risk of hyperchloraemic acidosis if excretion is impaired (Metheney 2000). Sodium chloride 0.9% should be used with caution in patients with renal disorders. It is, however, the solution of choice for expanding the ECF volume, because it does not enter the ICF.

Dextrose 4% with sodium chloride 0.18% This solution is commonly used for postoperative fluid maintenance. It is used to infuse water with a reduced sodium content.

Compound sodium lactate (Ringer's lactate, Hartmann's solution) This solution is designed to be a near-physiological solution of balanced electrolytes. It contains less chloride than sodium chloride 0.9%, and provides bicarbonate (when the lactate is metabolized), which may be useful in treating metabolic acidosis. However, its use in the treatment of metabolic acidosis *per se* is now considered inappropriate (Joint Formulary Committee 2006) and it is contraindicated in patients with liver disease, who are unable to convert lactate (Metheny 2000; Springhouse 2006).

Plasma-Lyte 148 This solution is another balanced electrolyte solution and the bicarbonate precursors are acetate and gluconate. It is used for fluid and electrolyte restoration.

Hypotonic solutions

These have a lower osmolality than plasma and contain fewer particles than plasma. As a result, fluid shifts from the ECF into the ICF to achieve equilibrium. In excess, this may cause the cells to swell and they may even rupture. An example of these solutions is sodium chloride 0.45% (or less).

Sodium chloride 0.45% This is half-strength normal saline and is a useful solution for replacing water in patients who have hypovolaemia with hypernatraemia. However, excessive use may lead to hyponatraemia due to dilution of sodium, especially in patients who are prone to water retention.

Hypertonic solutions

When compared with plasma, these solutions have a higher concentration of particles. Hypertonic solutions cause fluid to move out of the cells into the ECF in order to equalize the concentration of particles between the two compartments. This has the effect of causing the cells to shrink, which may disrupt their function. Meanwhile, the ECF volume expands and care is required to ensure that this does not precipitate a fluid volume excess and overload. It should be remembered that hypertonic solutions tend to irritate peripheral veins. The common hypertonic solutions are sodium chloride and dextrose solutions.

Sodium chloride 1.8% This solution is used to correct severe hyponatraemia. It needs to be infused very slowly to avoid the risk of overload, as previously mentioned, and some patients may require diuretic therapy to assist fluid excretion. Triple-strength saline (2.7%) is also available.

Dextrose 10% This may be used to provide kilocalories for the patient in the short term, but it is only sufficient to ward off the ketosis of starvation (Metheney 2000). One litre of dextrose 10% only provides 380 kcal. Hypertonic dextrose is also available in 20, 25 and 50% strengths, and the volume varies according to strength.

Colloid solutions

Colloid solutions are not electrolyte solutions, but rather fluids that contain solutes of a high molecular weight. They are hypertonic solutions which, when infused into the vascular compartment, exert an osmotic 'pull' on fluids from the interstitial and extracellular spaces. This means that they are particularly useful for expanding the intravascular volume and raising blood pressure. However, in susceptible patients this may lead to the risk of heart failure.

Colloid solutions are used to:

- correct hypotension
- expand intravascular volume
- mobilize third space fluids

- restore serum protein levels
- restore albumin levels.

The common colloid solutions include dextrans, etherified starches, gelatin, human albumin, plasma protein fraction and fresh frozen plasma. However, in view of the availability of other solutions, fresh frozen plasma should be reserved for specific situations other than intravascular fluid expansion. Its use is discussed in Chapter 13.

Dextrans   These are polysaccharides which act as colloids. They are available in two types: low-molecular-weight (LMW) dextrans and high-molecular-weight (HMW) dextrans. The molecular weight is denoted by the number, for example dextran 40 (LMW 40 000), dextran 70 or 110 (HMW 70 000 or 110 000). Both types are available in a solution of either sodium chloride 0.9% or dextrose 5%. LMW dextrans are used to improve the microcirculation in patients with poor peripheral circulation, while HMW dextrans are indicated in patients with hypovolaemia and hypotension. Patients require careful monitoring during infusion, and incidences of urticarial and anaphylactoid reactions have been reported (Joint Formulary Committee 2006).

Etherified starch   As the name suggests, these solutions are made from starch and examples include eloHAES, HyperHAES and Voluven. These solutions are used to increase the intravascular fluid, but may also interfere with coagulation. Haemodynamic monitoring is necessary to avoid the risk of circulatory overload. Close monitoring of electrolyte levels is indicated, so that levels can be adjusted according to individual patient need (Joint Formulary Committee 2006).

Gelatin (Haemaccel, Gelofusine)   This has a lower molecular weight than the dextrans and therefore remains in the circulation for a shorter period. Its haemodynamic action is about 2–3 hours and excretion is via the kidneys.

Human albumin   This solution is derived from plasma. There are two strengths: 4.5% (isotonic) and 20–25% (hypertonic: equivalent to five times the osmotic activity of plasma). The former is used to increase the circulating volume and restore protein levels (e.g. in hypoproteinaemia and hypoalbuminaemia) in conditions such as burns, acute pancreatitis and acute plasma loss. The latter is used, together with sodium and water restriction, to reduce excessive oedema (Joint Formulary Committee 2006).

Plasma protein fraction (PPF)   This is also prepared from plasma and, like albumin, is heat treated during preparation. It is recommended for slow infusion to increase the circulating volume.

Acid–Base Balance

For cells to function at an optimal level, they require an environment with a stable pH. The maintenance of a stable pH level is achieved by the regulation of acids and bases in the body fluids, particularly in the ECF. Acids are substances that can release hydrogen ions, while bases can accept hydrogen ions. The pH is a measure of hydrogen ion concentration; the main determinant is the ratio of acid (carbonic acid) to base (bicarbonate), the normal ratio in blood being 1 : 20. The pH level of blood, expressed as a numerical value, is inversely proportional to the number of hydrogen ions present. This means that the blood pH rises as the hydrogen ion concentration falls, and vice versa. Normal blood pH ranges from 7.35 to 7.45. If the pH falls below 6.8 or rises above 7.8, this is incompatible with life. A patient's acid–base balance can be determined by arterial blood gas analysis; in children, capillary blood may be used. Acidosis is defined as a blood pH below 7.35 and represents an increase in hydrogen ions or a decrease in bicarbonate ions. Alkalosis is defined as a blood pH above 7.45 and represents a decrease in hydrogen ions or an increase in bicarbonate ions. Changes in bicarbonate ion levels are associated with metabolic acid–base disturbances.

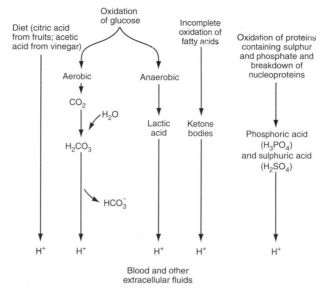

Figure 3.7   Production of human acids. (From Marieb 1989, p. 901. © 1989 by The Benjamin/ Cummings Publishing Company, Inc. Reprinted by permission of Pearson Education.)

Acids

Most of the acids in the body result from metabolic processes (*See* Figure 3.7). A metabolic process involves the conversion of either dietary or stored fuel to energy in the form of ATP or conversion of dietary fuel to an energy store such as glycogen and triglyceride (Halpcrin & Goldstein 1994). The increase in hydrogen ions generated by oxidation of fuel sources needs to be 'neutralized' in order to maintain the normal pH of body fluids. This is achieved when the excess hydrogen ions combine with either acids or bases, thereby forming substances which do not have an effect on the pH—this is otherwise known as 'buffering'.

Buffers

The main buffers include:

- protein
- bicarbonate
- phosphate
- ammonium.

Buffers occur in most body fluids and can respond immediately to changes in tissue fluid pH. The buffering systems involved include protein, bone, respiratory and renal systems.

Buffering systems

Respiratory system

The respiratory system provides the initial regulation of acid–base balance, by buffering and excreting carbonic acid (in the form of carbon dioxide and water). The lungs use carbon dioxide to regulate hydrogen ion concentration. Carbon dioxide combines with water to form carbonic acid; in the presence of carbonic anhydrase, this dissociates to carbon dioxide and water in the lungs, which can then be excreted during respiration. The following equation expresses this action:

$$CO_2 + H_2O \rightleftharpoons H_2CO_3 \rightleftharpoons H^+ + HCO_3^-$$

The free hydrogen ion generated with carbonic acid is buffered by haemoglobin.

The respiratory centre is directly affected by alterations in hydrogen ion concentration in the blood and within minutes can alter respiratory rate and depth to compensate. For example, an increase in hydrogen ions causes acidaemia, so respiration is increased to enhance carbon dioxide (acid) elimination. Conversely, if hydrogen ions are reduced (alkalosis), respiration is decreased to allow carbon dioxide (acid) retention. However, it should be noted that the respiratory system can only provide a short-term response; it is the renal system that provides longer term compensation.

Renal system

Ammonium buffering system   The metabolism of glutamine (an amino acid) in epithelial cells produces ammonia, which diffuses across the cell membrane into the tubule. Here it combines with actively secreted hydrogen ions to form ammonium sulphate, which is excreted in the urine. Hence hydrogen ions are excreted.

Bicarbonate buffering system   The kidneys can provide a more permanent regulation of changes in acid–base balance, by adjusting the acidity or alkalinity of the urine, but the rate of response varies from hours to days. The primary buffering system is the use of bicarbonate ions, which involves the reabsorption of bicarbonate and secretion of hydrogen ions in response to acidosis, and the excretion of bicarbonate (together with sodium) when there is alkalosis.

Phosphate buffering system   This occurs in body fluids and the tubules. It aids excretion of hydrogen ions in the urine and is important for maintaining the pH of urine.

It is important to note that potassium can also be exchanged for hydrogen ions in order to alter pH. However, in renal disease this compensatory mechanism leads to hyperkalaemia, if oliguria or anuria are present.

Although the body's buffering systems are able to maintain optimal acid–base balance and therefore pH level in body fluids, imbalances can occur following trauma or during the disease process.

Protein buffer system

The protein buffer system is concerned with regulation of the pH in ICF. Haemoglobin is the major protein involved and acts as a buffer to carbonic acid, which is produced in large amounts as a result of metabolic activity in the tissues. In the lungs, the acid dissociates to carbon dioxide and water, which is excreted via respiration. Buffer of carbonic acid is important because, during the buffering process, haemoglobin loses its affinity for oxygen and therefore oxygen transport to the tissues is enhanced.

Phosphates are also important in maintaining the pH within erythrocytes, as well as renal tubular fluid.

Bone buffering system

Bone also takes part in buffering acids. However, prolonged acid loading causes an increased excretion of calcium from the bone, which may present in chronic renal failure due to metabolic acidosis.

Acid–Base Imbalances

Acid–base imbalances are usually referred to as respiratory or metabolic depending on the cause. Respiratory imbalances are caused by either inadequate or excessive respiration.

Metabolic imbalances are usually caused by excessive hydrogen ion production from metabolic processes, or disorders of the GI and renal systems.

Acidosis refers to an excessive increase in hydrogen ions or decrease in bicarbonate ions, while alkalosis is the reverse. The following imbalances will be considered:

- respiratory acidosis
- respiratory alkalosis
- metabolic acidosis
- metabolic alkalosis.

Respiratory acidosis

Respiratory acidosis is caused by decreased alveolar ventilation, which results in carbon dioxide retention. This increases carbonic acid and hydrogen ion levels with a concomitant drop in blood pH. Decreased alveolar ventilation may be due to inadequate respiration or intermittent positive pressure ventilation (IPPV), respiratory obstruction, inadequate respiratory effort or cardiovascular disorders. Specific causes are presented in Table 3.8.

Assessment
History   Bronchospasm, pulmonary oedema, head injury, drug overdose.
Physical evidence   Agitation, airway obstruction, flail chest, dyspnoea.
Clinical manifestations   include breathlessness, cyanosis and sweating. The increased carbon dioxide retention may lead to cerebral oedema and papilloedema; the patient may complain of headache and blurred vision.

Tests   include the following.

- Arterial blood gas analysis—$P_aCO_2 > 40$ mmHg or 5.3 kPa, pH < 7.4.
- Serum bicarbonate—in chronic acidosis, to assess level of compensation.
- Serum electrolytes—if hyperkalaemia is suspected.
- Chest X-ray—to identify extent of the trauma, disease, aspiration.

Management
This will vary depending on the cause, i.e. mechanical obstruction should be relieved, IPPV should be adjusted, etc. If breathlessness is severe or the patient is agitated, reassurance

Table 3.8   Causes of respiratory acidosis.

Cause	Contributing factors
Inadequate respiration	Hypoventilation (spontaneous) Inadequate intermittent positive pressure ventilation Abdominal distension Chest injury Pneumonia
Inadequate respiratory effort	CNS depression Drug overdose Neuromuscular impairment
Respiratory obstruction	Laryngospasm Bronchospasm Chronic obstructive airways disease Aspiration
Cardiovascular disorders	Cardiac arrest Pulmonary oedema

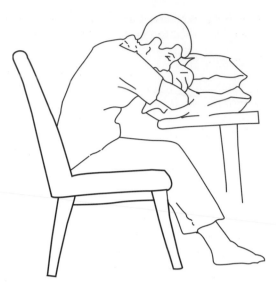

Figure 3.8   Modified Fowler's position.

should be given. Vital signs (particularly respiration) and arterial blood gases should be monitored. In chronic acidosis, i.v. fluids may be administered if fluid intake is reduced, in order to loosen secretions. Optimal positioning, e.g. Fowler's position, may assist respiration (*See* Figure 3.8). Physiotherapy and suction therapy may be required to manage impaired secretion removal. Oxygen therapy may be indicated if hypoxia is present. Caution is needed to avoid removing the hypoxic drive for respiration in chronic pulmonary disease.

Respiratory alkalosis

Respiratory alkalosis is caused by increased alveolar ventilation, leading to a reduction in serum carbon dioxide levels. Respiratory compensation is usually adequate, so the condition may have resolved in the time it takes for renal compensatory mechanisms to act. Acute respiratory alkalosis is often due to anxiety (with hyperventilation), but may result from pulmonary disorders or conditions leading to hypoxaemia. Chronic respiratory alkalosis may be caused by brain tumours, Gram-negative septicaemia and fever.

Assessment
History   Anaemia, pneumonia, cardiac failure, hyperventilation (IPPV), high altitude acclimatization.
Physical evidence   Anxiety with hyperventilation, fever.
Clinical manifestations   include confusion, fainting, tetany, paraesthesiae.
Tests include the following:

- ECG—to detect cardiac dysrhythmias.
- Arterial blood gases:
    - $P_aCO_2 < 40$ mmHg or < 5.3 kPa (acute)
    - $P_aCO_2 < 35$ mmHg or < 4.6 kPa (chronic)
    - pH > 7.4
    - P_aO_2 reduced, if hypoxia is present.
- Serum electrolytes—to assess compensation, if the condition is chronic.

- Serum phosphate—may drop, as phosphate moves into the ICF.
- Serum bicarbonate—decreased, as renal compensation occurs (7–9 days).

Management

The patient will require reassurance, particularly if anxiety is the cause; sedation or tranquillizers may be indicated. Carbon dioxide levels may be increased by encouraging the patient to breathe in and out of a paper bag, which promotes rebreathing.

In chronic respiratory alkalosis, renal compensation results in a decreased serum bicarbonate. The underlying cause needs to be treated. However, oxygen therapy may be required if hypoxia is also present, e.g. in heart disease associated with cyanosis. Monitoring blood gases is indicated.

Metabolic acidosis

Metabolic acidosis is caused by an excessive loss of alkali (base) or accumulation of acid. Loss of base in the form of bicarbonate occurs via the gastrointestinal tract or kidneys. Accumulation of acid is caused by anaerobic metabolism when cells are deprived of oxygen (e.g. in burns, trauma, etc.), and also when increased energy utilization necessitates the metabolism of fat stores (e.g. in starvation and diabetes mellitus). The resultant acidosis leads to a drop in serum pH and an increase in hydrogen ion concentration; the latter stimulates chemoreceptors, and respiration is increased. The increase in respiration, which is the initial compensatory mechanism, enhances carbon dioxide elimination and lowers the plasma carbon dioxide level. The kidneys also help to eliminate hydrogen ions by means of the bicarbonate buffering system. Some of the specific causes of metabolic acidosis are presented in Table 3.9.

It should also be noted that hydrogen ions enter the cell (to be buffered) in exchange for potassium, so alterations in potassium level are associated with acidosis.

Assessment

History   Salicylate poisoning, diuretic therapy.

Physical evidence   Diarrhoea, burns, trauma.

Clinical manifestations   include Kussmaul's respirations (Box 3.1) and peripheral vasodilation with flushed, warm dry skin. Hypotension and cold, clammy skin is also seen in shock. Acidotic effects on the nervous system may cause confusion, headache and loss of consciousness. Cardiac dysrhythmias may occur in response to altered potassium levels. Patients with diabetes may have 'fruity' breath which smells of 'pear drops'.

Table 3.9   Causes of metabolic acidosis.

Cause	Physiological process
Salicylate, alcohol poisoning	Formation of non-carbonic acid
Diuretic therapy	Loss of bicarbonate, hyperkalaemia (if potassium-sparing drugs)
Diarrhoea	Loss of bicarbonate
Diabetic ketoacidosis	Increased fat metabolism
Hyperalimentation solutions	Increased acid, if lactate not given
Acute and chronic renal failure	Inability to excrete acids
Burns, trauma, shock	Increased lactic acid production
Glaucoma	Carbonic anhydrase inhibitor therapy causes bicarbonate diuresis (Willatts 1987)

Tests   include the following.

- Arterial blood gas analysis:
  - pH < 7.35
  - (if compensated) P_aCO_2 < 35 mmHg or < 4.6 kPa.
- Serum bicarbonate < 22 mmol/L—also to assess metabolic compensation.
- Serum electrolytes—to detect any imbalance. For example, changes in potassium level are common, particularly hyperkalaemia (serum level > 5.5 mmol/L).
- ECG—to detect changes associated with alterations in potassium level (Figure 3.5).

Management

Alterations in level of consciousness put the patient at risk of injury, so protection is necessary. The main aim of treatment is to reduce the acidosis. However, if hypokalaemia is present, this should be treated first, as correction of the acidosis with sodium bicarbonate could cause severe hypokalaemia when potassium moves back into the cells in exchange for hydrogen ions (*See* Hypokalaemia on page 61). Close monitoring of ECG and vital signs is necessary.

Correction of the acidosis with sodium bicarbonate is indicated if the pH is less than 7.2, to avoid the threat of cardiac depression and dysrhythmias. The efficacy of treatment is monitored by arterial blood gas analysis, as there is no accurate means of estimating the dose required. It is important to ensure that, except in emergency situations, sodium bicarbonate is administered slowly to avoid overcompensation.

Interventions should also aim to treat the underlying cause. For example, the hyperglycaemic patient with metabolic acidosis will require the administration of insulin, which will also help to lower the concomitant hyperglycaemia associated with acidosis. The infusion of sodium chloride 0.9% will also enhance the reduction of potassium. In renal failure, haemodialysis will be required to correct any imbalance. Lactic acidosis in cardiovascular shock requires i.v. fluid replacement (to increase the blood volume and blood pressure) and management of tissue hypoxia. Treatment with sodium bicarbonate is controversial, because it may cause depression of the central nervous system. The reason is that when the sodium bicarbonate buffers the lactic acid, carbon dioxide is released which easily passes across cell membranes. Carbon dioxide can therefore enter the cerebrospinal fluid and cause depression of the central nervous system.

Metabolic alkalosis

Metabolic alkalosis is caused by an excessive loss of hydrogen ions or excessive retention of bicarbonate ions. The main mechanisms involved are loss of hydrogen ions from the GI tract, deficient bicarbonate excretion via the kidneys and diuretic therapy. The most common cause of hydrogen ion loss is from the GI tract via vomiting or nasogastric suction. Hydrochloric acid production in the stomach is associated with secretion of bicarbonate ions into the blood. These ions would then be used in the digestive juices to neutralize the chyme as it enters the duodenum. However, when gastric contents are expelled during vomiting, digestive juices are not stimulated, the bicarbonate ions are not utilized and so the serum bicarbonate level rises. Loss of acid increases the pH level in the blood and hydrogen ions are reduced. This inhibits chemoreceptor stimulation and reduces respiration. Hypoventilation allows carbon dioxide levels in the blood to rise in order to try to balance the excessive bicarbonate level. However, this compensation is limited, because a degree of hypoxia develops which then stimulates respiration (Springhouse 2003, 2006).

Reduction of hydrogen ions also causes an increased dissociation rate of carbonic acid (in an effort to increase the hydrogen ion level) and more bicarbonate is produced and conserved by the kidneys. The conservation of bicarbonate results in an increased loss of hydrogen, potassium and chloride ions. Both bicarbonate and chloride compete to

Table 3.10   Causes of metabolic alkalosis.

Cause	Physiological process
Vomiting, nasogastric suction	Loss of acid
Milk alkali syndrome	Excessive intake of alkali, hypercalcaemia
Diuretic therapy	Potassium loss
Cushing's syndrome	Potassium loss
Hyperaldosteronism	Potassium loss
Intravenous sodium bicarbonate	Overcompensation of acidosis
Large-volume blood transfusion	Citrate in donor blood is metabolized to bicarbonate

combine with sodium and, as chloride levels fall (during binding), bicarbonate levels rise in order to balance the sodium. Examples of specific causes of metabolic alkalosis are presented in Table 3.10.

Assessment

History   Primary aldosteronism, diuretic therapy.

Physical evidence   Vomiting, nasogastric suction.

Clinical manifestations   relate to changes in mental function, such as apathy, confusion and seizures. With severe hypokalaemia, neuromuscular changes may be apparent, such as tetany, and positive Trousseau's and Chvostek's signs (Box 3.1). The respiratory rate is decreased and the patient may experience dizziness.

Tests   include the following.

- Arterial blood gases
  - pH = 7.45–7.6
  - P_aCO_2 = 38–45 mmHg or 5.06–6.0 kPa
  - if acute: bicarbonate > 26 mmol/L
  - if chronic: bicarbonate > 45 mmol/L
  - (Note: values vary with level of compensation).
- Serum levels of potassium and chloride—decreased (relative to sodium).
- ECG—may show changes related to hypokalaemia (Figure 3.5).

Management

The patient's safety must be maintained if there are any signs of altered consciousness. Monitoring includes vital signs (particularly respiratory patterns), ECG, fluid intake and output, serum electrolyte levels and arterial blood gas analysis. The precipitating factors need to be addressed. For example, antiemetics and fluid replacement for vomiting may be indicated, while review of diuretic therapy will reduce the risk for those patients with fluid retention problems.

Fluid, Electrolyte and Acid–base Imbalances

Overview

Imbalances occur when the normal homeostatic mechanisms of the body are unable to operate. The main processes involved in fluid and electrolyte imbalances relate to:

- decreased intake and increased excretion which lead to deficiency
- increased intake and decreased excretion which lead to excess.

Acid–base imbalances are caused by metabolic conditions which affect the normal mechanisms of regulation.

Gastrointestinal loss

Gastrointestinal loss of fluid and electrolytes commonly results from vomiting, diarrhoea, fistulae, gastric suctioning, infection, inflammatory disease, etc. In the upper GI tract, the fluids contain high levels of potassium, sodium, chloride and hydrogen ions. For this reason, loss of fluid from the stomach and upper intestine often results in hypokalaemia and metabolic alkalosis. In contrast, fluids from the lower GI tract tend to be alkaline due to a high level of bases, which means that excessive loss due to diarrhoea may result in metabolic acidosis.

Management
Monitoring of serum electrolyte levels, together with fluid intake and output, is necessary. Correction of any imbalance is generally achieved by administering i.v. fluids and electrolyte replacements, as indicated. Estimation of the degree of metabolic disturbance may be achieved by arterial blood gas analysis.

Renal disease

The kidneys are the main regulators of fluid, electrolyte and acid–base balance in the body. Imbalances are due to failure of the buffering systems. Renal failure is often categorized into two types: acute and chronic. Acute renal failure is generally regarded as a reversible condition with a sudden onset, while chronic renal failure is generally considered as irreversible with a longer, more insidious onset. Other renal disorders contributing to disordered buffering include glomerulonephritis, pyelonephritis, acute tubular necrosis, renal calculi and tumours.

The main contributing factors to renal damage are decreased renal perfusion (e.g. major trauma, shock, third space losses), infection, damage to the renal parenchyma and nephrotoxic agents (e.g. sulphonamides, frusemide, lead, etc.). The imbalances resulting from inadequate renal compensation depend on the type of renal damage.

- If the glomerulus is defective, filtration into the capsule is altered so that excess fluid and electrolytes can pass. The buffering systems fail, resulting in metabolic acidosis.
- Tubular damage causes altered permeability, which results in abnormal excretion.
- Hormonal levels in the kidney are affected in renal disease. Low renal perfusion causes an increased renin release, which results in hypertension. Erythropoietin secretion is reduced and this leads to anaemia.
- High output of urine is associated with the polyuric phase of acute renal failure.
- Low output of urine is associated with electrolyte imbalance and uraemia. Oliguria and anuria result in hyperkalaemia, which may be asymptomatic up to a serum level of 6 mmol/L in acute renal failure and 7.5 mmol/L in chronic renal failure (Innerarity & Stark 1990).
- Hypervolaemia, due to oliguria, causes an excessive ECF volume which may precipitate peripheral and pulmonary oedema.
- Hypovolaemia may occur in the polyuric phase of acute renal failure, leading to hypotension.

The electrolyte imbalances that can occur in renal disease are presented in Table 3.11.

Management
The management will vary according to the type of renal disorder. Vital signs, fluid intake and output, and breathing (to detect the onset of pulmonary oedema)

Table 3.11 Electrolyte imbalances in renal disease.

Imbalance	Physiological process
Hyperkalaemia	Potassium excretion reduced
Hyperphosphataemia	Inability to excrete phosphorus
Hypocalcaemia	Reciprocal relationship between calcium and phosphorus
Hypermagnesaemia	Inability to excrete magnesium

should be monitored. Haemodynamic monitoring may be indicated in some patients, and ECG monitoring will facilitate detection of changes due to hyperkalaemia and hypocalcaemia. Serum levels of urea and electrolytes need close monitoring. Arterial blood gas analysis is necessary to assess the level of metabolic acidosis and the degree to which correction is achieved. Intravenous sodium bicarbonate may be administered with caution, bearing in mind the risk of hypocalcaemia (caused by calcium binding with the bicarbonate) and possible hypernatraemia from repeat doses of sodium bicarbonate (due to increased sodium load, which may also precipitate pulmonary oedema).

Patients whose kidneys still respond to fluid excess may be given diuretics; others, in whom this is not possible, will require haemodialysis.

Syndrome of inappropriate antidiuretic hormone (SIADH)

SIADH is associated with excessive release of ADH, even when plasma osmolality is low. The condition may be caused by damage to the pituitary gland or its hypothalamic control (e.g. from head injury or during surgery) and some central nervous system disorders which raise intracranial pressure. Other causative factors include respiratory disorders and malignant tumours which, by various means, increase the secretion of ADH. The normal action of ADH is to increase the permeability of the renal tubule to water, in response to a reduced circulating volume, thus conserving water and increasing the blood volume. However, in SIADH, water conservation occurs regardless of the amount of circulating volume. As a result, the serum osmolality and serum sodium are reduced. An increased IVF volume leads to an increased glomerular filtration rate and inhibits the release of aldosterone, so sodium is lost in the urine, resulting in hyponatraemia. As sodium levels drop in the ECF, water moves into the cells down an osmotic gradient. In the brain, this increase in ICF can lead to neurological impairment due to cerebral oedema.

Management
Observation of the patient for signs of cerebral oedema is indicated, together with maintenance of the patient's safety. Monitoring of the patient's serum sodium levels and osmolality, weight and fluid intake and output are indicated. Water intake should be restricted, while correction of the hyponatraemia with i.v. hypertonic saline can be achieved cautiously, using a volumetric infusion pump to avoid overload.

Diabetes insipidus

This is caused by either a deficiency in the production or release of ADH, or a reduced renal response to ADH. It may have an idiopathic origin or be due to brain injury or tumour. The onset may be gradual or sudden depending on the cause. The condition is characterized by polydipsia and polyuria (with copious amounts of very dilute urine). The fluid balance may remain in equilibrium, if the fluid intake matches the output. Otherwise, there is rapid depletion of the ECF with a concomitant rise in serum sodium and osmolality. The resultant hypovolaemia may lead to shock and may also precipitate seizures or coma.

Management

Patient safety must be maintained. The hypovolaemia is corrected with hypotonic i.v. fluids and the underlying cause needs to be treated. The hypernatraemia may resolve with adequate fluid replacement. Diabetes insipidus of cerebral origin may be treated with a vasopressin analogue.

Diabetic ketoacidosis

This relates to either partial or total insulin deficiency in a patient with diabetes mellitus, but may also occur in patients with undiagnosed diabetes. The condition is associated with an inability to produce the necessary amount of insulin to cope with a crisis (e.g. stress, surgery or infection) or may result from a failure to administer an adequate amount of insulin (e.g. omission of a dose). If insufficient insulin is available, glucose cannot be utilized for the production of energy, so alternative sources have to be found, such as fat. Metabolism of fat leads to the production of ketone bodies (as an acid waste product) and results in metabolic acidosis. Both hyperglycaemia and ketosis lead to increased osmolality of ECF, causing a shift of fluid out of the cells. As a result of the increased osmolality, an osmotic diuresis occurs which is typified by the polyuria commonly seen in this condition. This resultant dehydration, when it occurs in the brain cells, can lead to neurological disturbances.

It should be noted that serum electrolytes may appear normal, because continuing catabolism (breakdown of the tissues) releases cations and water into the ECF. However, potassium levels may rise because insulin deficiency inhibits potassium movement into the cells, while acidosis encourages potassium to leave the cell. Dehydration tends to exacerbate the hyperkalaemia, as further sodium and potassium are excreted in response to the release of aldosterone. Dehydration may lead to lactic acidosis, if tissue perfusion is decreased. Failure to correct this situation leads to respiratory and renal compensation. Respiratory compensation results in Kussmaul's respirations, in order to correct the acidosis by excreting carbon dioxide, while the kidneys try to excrete excess acid in the form of ketonuria. Kussmaul's respirations are the typical slow, deep breaths associated with respiratory acidosis.

Concomitant electrolyte imbalances include hypokalaemia, hyponatraemia and hypophosphataemia.

Assessment

History   Diabetes mellitus or signs and symptoms thereof, such as polyuria.
Physical evidence   Polyuria.
Clinical manifestations   include fruity breath typically associated with ketosis. Neurological impairment may take the form of confusion and loss of consciousness. Loss of skin turgor may be apparent, if dehydration has occurred, and Kussmaul's respirations (*See* Box 3.1) denote a respiratory attempt to correct acidosis.
Tests include the following:

- Serum electrolytes—to determine extent of imbalance.
- Arterial blood gases—to assess level of acidosis.
- Blood glucose level—elevated.
- Glycosuria and ketonuria are evident.

Management

The patient's safety is paramount. Correction of diabetic ketoacidosis is primarily concerned with correcting the dehydration and hyperglycaemia. Insulin needs to be titrated against blood glucose levels to ensure optimal correction. Intravenous sodium chloride 0.9% is often the solution of choice for rehydration, although hypotonic saline is useful to replace fluid loss, and compound sodium lactate may also be indicated to replace potassium 'loss' as it shifts from the ECF back into the cells. Fluid intake and output will need to be monitored, together with vital signs. Blood gas analysis is used to monitor the correction of the acidosis and to assess the need to administer i.v. sodium bicarbonate.

Hyperglycaemic hyperosmolar non-ketotic coma (HHNC)

This condition usually occurs with the onset of diabetes in middle-aged or elderly patients, but may occur in patients with non-insulin-dependent diabetes mellitus if there is a sudden progression in the disease state. It is a condition caused by an acute lack of insulin which results in hyperglycaemia, but is not severe enough to cause ketosis. As previously described, hyperglycaemia gives rise to an increased osmolality and osmotic diuresis, so there is risk of hypovolaemia, hyperkalaemia and hypophosphataemia. The water loss includes both ECF and ICF and, if severe, may cause the patient to lose up to 20% of the fluid volume. Depletion of the IVF volume causes increased viscosity of the blood, and in consequence the workload on the heart is increased. Increased blood viscosity, together with the patient's immobility, leads to the risk of blood stasis and the development of microemboli. Decreased perfusion of the kidneys and brain may lead to the possibility of fatal sequelae. The usual causes of this condition include inadequate secretion or action of insulin, excess dietary intake (i.e. inadequate insulin) and some drug therapies (e.g. phenytoin, thiazide diuretics) which may suddenly be exacerbated by stress.

Assessment

History   Diabetes mellitus.
Physical evidence   Polyuria, loss of skin turgor.
Clinical manifestations   of neurological deficit due to dehydration of brain cells may be apparent. Warm, dry, flushed skin and possible fever are associated with dehydration, together with a rapid pulse and hypotension. Respirations are increased but, unlike Kussmaul's respirations, are not deep.
Tests include the following:

- Serum blood glucose level > 30 mmol/L.
- Serum electrolytes—to assess imbalance.
- Arterial blood gas analysis—to assess extent of metabolic acidosis.
- Haematocrit—increased.
- Urinalysis—glycosuria evident.

Management

Neurological deficit may place the patient at risk of injury, so this is a primary concern. Treatment is concentrated on rehydrating the patient, usually with i.v. sodium chloride 0.9%, but care must be taken not to overload the patient. Fluid intake and output need to be monitored and skin turgor noted, in order to assess efficacy of fluid replacement therapy. Insulin is administered and titrated to blood glucose levels. Serum electrolyte levels should be monitored, and potassium and phosphate replacements, if indicated, will require cautious administration (*See* Hypokalaemia on page 61).

Burns

Burns may present one of the greatest challenges in terms of managing fluid, electrolyte and acid–base balances. This is because the extent and depth of burns vary greatly. The extent of burns is calculated by the 'rule of nines' (Figure 3.9), while their severity is classified as first, second or third degree. The main problem is the rapid loss of circulating volume, and one of the challenges of management is to replace fluid loss without causing oedema. Imbalances are caused by disruption of skin integrity and cellular destruction. Within the first 8 hours following the burn, plasma leaks from the damaged capillaries into the interstitial space to form local oedema. It is suggested that the movement of protein (in the plasma) to the burned area causes oedema in non-burned tissue, because of the resulting hypoproteinaemia (Horne & Swearingen 1993; Springhouse 2003). This shift of fluid may involve 10–50% of the circulating volume, resulting in severe hypovolaemia. Loss of skin also leads to fluid loss of up to 3 L/day via evaporation, depending on the environmental humidity. The increased capillary permeability gradually subsides over 48 hours.

Burns also decrease cell membrane potential, allowing sodium and water to enter the cell and potassium to leak out into the ECF and plasma. Tissue perfusion is decreased partly because of blood vessel damage, increased blood viscosity and erythrocyte aggregation, but also from hypoxia caused by metabolic acidosis following increased anaerobic metabolism. Respiratory compensation for the acidosis will be limited following inhalational injury, because of the resultant tissue oedema in the lungs. If the lung injury is severe, mechanical ventilation will be required to manage the hypoxaemia and respiratory acidosis.

The initial stage of imbalance in burns is characterized by a fluid shift from the plasma to the ECF, together with oliguria as the kidneys attempt to conserve fluid. The next stage (48 hours after the burn) is characterized by a shift of fluid from the ECF (as the oedema fluid is reabsorbed) and a diuresis to remove the excess fluid. At this stage, hypervolaemia

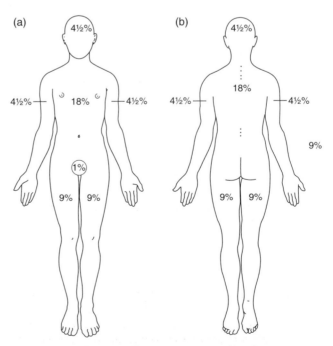

Figure 3.9   'Rule of nines' for assessment of burns: (a) anterior view; (b) posterior view. (After Thompson *et al.* 1989. Reprinted with permission of Elsevier.)

Table 3.12   Electrolyte imbalances associated with burns.

Imbalance	Cause
Hyperkalaemia	Cell lysis in the initial stage leads to release of potassium into ECF
Hypokalaemia	Increased excretion due to aldosterone
Hypernatraemia	Inadequate water replacement
Hyponatraemia	Large amounts of sodium lost in oedema
Hypocalcaemia	Loss of ECF from burn and shift of calcium to the wound
Hypophosphataemia	Associated with respiratory alkalosis

ECF, extracellular fluid.

may occur if i.v. fluid replacement is not adjusted or if renal damage has occurred. Electrolyte imbalances are common; the possible changes are presented in Table 3.12.

Assessment

History   Chemical, thermal or electrical burn.

Physical evidence of burn   The extent and degree need to be assessed.

Clinical manifestation   of tissue damage may include pain, hypoxia, etc. Evidence of fluid loss is characterized by shock, hypovolaemia, hypotension, oedema and blistering.

Tests   include the following.

- Serum electrolytes—to assess imbalances.
- Arterial blood gas analysis—to assess level of acidosis or alkalosis, or optimal mechanical ventilation.
- ECG—to monitor dysrhythmias associated with electrolyte imbalances.
- Chest X-ray—to assess damage from inhalational injury.

Management

In the initial stage, aggressive treatment of the hypovolaemia must be instituted. There are various formulae that can be used, as cited by Metheney (2000), Horne & Swearingen (1993) and Springhouse (2006). The usual fluids recommended are compound sodium lactate and colloid solutions, which need to be individualized for each patient. Compound sodium lactate is used to increase fluid levels (together with electrolytes), while colloid solutions are used to increase the circulating volume without increasing oedema. Optimal pain management will decrease the stress response and aid recovery. Monitoring includes haemodynamic monitoring, ECG, blood gas analysis, fluid intake and output, serum electrolytes and haematocrit. Acid–base and electrolyte imbalances will need to be corrected. Fluid replacement needs to be adjusted after the first 48 hours to avoid the risk of heart failure from hypervolaemia.

Conclusion

This chapter has reviewed the concepts of fluid, electrolyte and acid–base balance and considered some of the imbalances that can occur. These imbalances have been presented in terms of causes, assessment and management, which are designed to assist understanding of the rationale for interventions. The imbalances associated with specific client groups, towards the latter part of the chapter, give some indication of the complex nature of fluid, electrolyte and acid–base balance.

REFERENCES

Halperin ML, Goldstein MB (1994) *Fluid, Electrolyte and Acid–Base Physiology*, 2nd edn. WB Saunders, Philadelphia.

Hinchliff SM, Montague SE, Watson R (1997) *Physiology for Nursing Practice*, 2nd edn. Baillière Tindall, London.

Horne MM, Swearingen PL (1993) *Fluids, Electrolytes and Acid–Base Balance*, 2nd edn. Mosby, St Louis.

Innerarity SA, Stark JL (1990) *Fluids and Electrolytes*. Springhouse, Pennsylvania.

Joint Formulary Committee (2006) *The National Formulary*, 51st edn. The Pharmaceutical Press, Oxon.

Kumar & Clark (2005) *Medical Medicine*, 6th edn. Elsevier Saunders, London.

Lund W, ed. (1994) *The Pharmaceutical Codex*, 12th edn. The Pharmaceutical Press, London.

Marieb EN (1989) *Human Anatomy and Physiology*. Benjamin Cummings, Redwood City.

Metheny (1992) *Fluid & Electrolyte Balance*, 2nd edn. JB Lippincott, Philadelphia.

Metheny NM (2000) *Fluid and Electrolyte Balance*, 4th edn. JB Lippincott, Philadelphia.

Paradiso C (1995) *Fluids and Electrolytes*. JB Lippincott, Philadelphia.

Springhouse (2003) *Professional Guide to Pathophysiology*. Springhouse Publishing Co, Philadelphia.

Springhouse (2005) *Fluids and Electrolytes made Incredibly Easy*, 3rd edn. Springhouse Publishing Co, Philadelphia.

Springhouse (2006) *Fluids and Electrolytes: a 2-in-1 Reference for Nurses*. Springhouse Publishing Co, Philadelphia.

Statland H (1963) *Fluids and Electrolytes in Practice*, 3rd edn. JB Lippincott, Philadelphia.

Thompson JM *et al.* (1989) *Mosby's Manual of Clinical Nursing*, 2nd edn. Mosby-Year Book, St Louis.

Tortora GJ, Grabowski SR (1996) *Principles of Anatomy and Physiology*, 8th edn. John Wiley & Sons, Hoboeken, NJ.

Willats S (1987) Lecture notes on fluid and electrolyte balance Blackwell Scientific Publication Oxford.

CHAPTER 4
Infection Control in Intravenous Therapy
Sarah Hart

Introduction

Intravenous (i.v.) therapy is an integral part of patient care and management. Patients requiring i.v. therapy are often seriously ill and immunocompromised, and they are therefore especially susceptible to infection. Intravenous device-related infection leads to increased patient morbidity and mortality (Maki & Crnich 2003). In critically ill patients, i.v. devices are considered to be responsible for at least 80% of bloodstream infections (Eggimann *et al.* 2004). It has been estimated that every year almost 6000 patients in the UK acquire a catheter-related bloodstream infection, which prolongs the period of hospitalization and increases the cost of care. In 2000 the audit office estimated the additional cost of bloodstream infection to be £6209 per patient (DH 2005).

Intravenous systems are invaluable in enabling direct access to the patient's vascular system for monitoring and administration of drugs, and in providing a convenient means of obtaining blood. Unfortunately these advantages are matched by the risk of the patient developing an i.v.-related infectious complication, as an i.v. catheter disrupts the integrity of the skin and creates a pathway for organisms that are normally excluded by the skin's defence mechanisms to enter the body (Mermel 2000).

Infection has been identified as a potentially life-threatening complication of i.v. therapy, causing phlebitis, wound infections, bacteraemia, septicaemia and even death (Elliott *et al.* 1995). The care of patients with nosocomial catheter-related infections involves significant costs for both the hospital and the patients, including antibiotics, medical and surgical supplies, healthcare workers' time, delayed discharges and increased admission waiting times, as well as pain and anxiety for patients and their families. These significant risks and costs associated with i.v. catheter-related infections mean that prevention of infection is an important concern and objective for all healthcare workers involved in the care of patients (O'Grady *et al.* 2002).

A review of catheter-related infections conducted in the late 1990s indicated that catheter colonization ranged from 5.8% to 71.4% and catheter-related bloodstream infections ranged from 0.3% to 11.0% (Eggimann *et al.* 2004). A prospective study found that intravascular devices were the most common source of healthcare-associated bloodstream infections (Friedman *et al.* 2002). Between 1997 and 2001, 17 teaching and 56 non-teaching UK hospitals took part in a surveillance of hospital-acquired bacteraemia (HABS) using the Nosocomial Infection National Surveillance Scheme (NINSS). Device-related sources were responsible for 52.4% and 43.2% respectively of all HABS.

Central venous catheters (CVCs) were the commonest source, causing 38.3% of HABS in teaching hospitals compared to 22.3% in non-teaching hospitals (Coello *et al.* 2003). Box 4.1 provides a glossary of technical terms related to infection control.

Risk Factors for Acquiring Infections

A patient who has a decreased resistance to infection will have an increased susceptibility to developing an i.v.-related infection. There are a number of reasons why patients are more vulnerable to infection (Box 4.2).

Age

Patients are more susceptible to infection at the extremes of age. In the elderly, there are many reasons for this increased risk, including changes in cell-mediated immunity and humoral immunity (Srinivasan *et al.* 2005), physiological changes related to impaired circulation and cough reflex and less effective wound healing, and changes related to the absorption, distribution, metabolism and elimination of many antibiotics (Crossley & Peterson 2005). Young children also have an increased susceptibility to infection; although components of the immune system differentiate early in fetal life, functional maturity takes several years to complete. A baby's immature immune system is supported and augmented by maternal factors supplied by placental transfer, colostrum and breast milk. Premature babies have enhanced susceptibility to infection, not only because of their immunological immaturity but also because of the immaturity of many of their

---

BOX 4.1

Glossary of technical terms related to infection control

- *Bacteraemia*—bacteria present in blood as confirmed by culture with or without causing illness
- *Septicaemia*—as 'Bacteraemia' but implies greater severity
- *Sepsis*—clinical evidence of infection
- *Nosocomial infection*—hospital-acquired infection (HAI) not present or incubating at the time of admission; also referred to as 'healthcare-acquired infection'
- *Colonization*—persistent presence of microorganisms at a body site without causing infection
- *Endogenous*- originating from on or within the body
- *Exogenous*—originating from external causes
- *Immunocompromised patient*—an individual with impairment of either or both natural and speceific immunity to infection which increases the risk of infection by a variety of microorganisms

---

BOX 4.2

Factors that contribute to infection

- Age
- Genetics
- Immunosuppression
- Immunocompromised
- Loss of skin integrity
- Multiple invasive procedures
- Antibiotic therapy
- Presence of distant infection
- Poor nutrition

natural barriers to infection and because of the transgression of these barriers by the invasive monitoring and therapeutic techniques used in neonatal intensive care (Brady 2005).

Genetics

Familial patterns of susceptibility to infection suggest that resistance to acquiring an infection may be an inherited characteristic (Roitt *et al.* 2001).

Immunosuppression

A person may be immunosuppressed as a consequence of radiotherapy, chemotherapy or steroid therapy, and this subsequently causes granulocytopenia, cellular immune dysfunction and humoral immune dysfunction. A number of factors will determine the extent of the patient's immunosuppression, including the host defence defect caused by the disease itself and the dose and duration of immunosuppressive therapy, particularly corticosteroids.

The incidence of infection is directly related to the degree of immunosuppression; for example, the incidence of infection begins to rise once the granulocyte count falls below $1000/mm^3$, with the most severe infections occurring when the count falls below $100/mm^3$ (Glauser & Calandra 2000).

Immunocompromise

A person may have a defect in the immune system as a result of an underlying disease, notably those affecting the bone marrow. Patients with newly diagnosed leukaemia or myeloma are particularly susceptible to infection. In diseases such as chronic alcoholism or diabetes mellitus, the defect may not be so obvious as it is related to breaches in the first line of defence, such as injections, diabetic vascular disease or the high concentration of glucose in urine and secretions, which may promote colonization by microorganisms. These factors will predispose the person to infection (Calandra 2000).

Loss of skin integrity

The intact skin forms a very effective barrier to invasion by microorganisms, as few organisms have a natural ability to penetrate it. Skin has the added advantage of being relatively dry and having a mild acidity, and the regular desquamation of skin scale also assists in the elimination of microorganisms. Inflamed skin is more permeable to water, which can lead to greater colonization by microorganisms. Damaged skin provides an entry for microorganisms, which can lead to inflammation, cellulitis, wound infections and septicaemia (Calandra 2000).

Multiple invasive procedures

The skin and mucous membranes comprise the body's first line of defence against the entry of microorganisms (Tramont & Hoover 2005). Breaches in these barriers, such as by surgical intervention or intravenous and urinary catheters, allows access to microorganisms that may cause infection. Each procedure undergone by an immunocompromised patient must be evaluated to ensure that every effort is made to reduce the extent of damage and that an aseptic technique is adopted at all times.

Invasive procedures can also lead to a shift in microbial flora, for example, the minor trauma caused by shaving the skin before inserting a central catheter predisposes to invasion by the colonizing microorganisms of the skin and can be prevented by the use of hair clippers (Kjonniksen *et al.* 2002).

When the skin is moist, as in the groin and armpits, higher bacterial counts are found (Mims *et al.* 2004), which increases the risk of infection following invasive procedures.

Antibiotic therapy

The importance of effective antimicrobial therapy in the management of infection cannot be overemphasized. Unfortunately, antibiotics produce a shift in microbial flora. Alteration to normal microbial flora predisposes the patient to become colonized with organisms that are potentially more pathogenic. Such organisms may be acquired endogenously from the patient's own normal flora or exogenously from the hospital environment, visitors or healthcare workers, in particular from their hands. Beekmann and Henderson (2005) stated that alteration of the patient's skin flora as a result of antimicrobial therapy is a common event preceding catheter site infection.

Poor nutrition

Adequate nutrition is essential for the maintenance of an effective immune response (Ritz & Gardner 2006). Protein deficiency is associated with significant impairment of cell-mediated immunity, phagocyte function, complement system, secretory immunoglobulin and cytokine production (Chandra 2002). Fluid and electrolyte disturbances, in particular hyperglycaemia which is commonly found in critically ill patients, all impair immune responses and therefore increase the risk of infection (Butler *et al.* 2005).

Presence of distant infection

Recognizing the epidemiology of infection is important in establishing an approach to prevention. Colonization of the body by pathogenic microorganisms is a prerequisite for infection. Most patients with granulocytopenia who develop a *Staphylococcus aureus* infection carry this organism in their nose. Catheters can become infected from haematogenous seeding from other foci of infection (O'Grady *et al.* 2002). Beekmann and Henderson (2005) suggested that most sporadic nosocomial bacteraemias are not device related, but occur as a result of distant localized infection that goes on to seed the bloodstream. A small study examining catheter-related bacteraemias found that haematogenous seeding was strongly implicated in 24% of bacteraemias, although the patient's skin flora was the main source of catheter-related infection (Chan *et al.* 1998). All of these conditions depress the patient's immunological response to infection and may permit the invasion of organisms which can result in infection.

Factors Influencing the Survival of Microorganisms

The factors that can influence the survival of microorganisms include:

- the organism itself
- the number of organisms
- host resistance to infection
- environmental factors.

The organism itself may be pathogenic or non-pathogenic. Generally, only pathogenic organisms are capable of producing disease. This is related to the organism's natural capability to survive and proliferate in the environment; for example, Gram-negative bacteria such as *Klebsiella* and *Pseudomonas* thrive in damp conditions, which means they have the ability to contaminate and multiply in infusates. The rate of replication of the infecting organism is of central importance. Intravenous-related bacteraemias are usually caused by organisms that have the ability to multiply in 20–30 minutes. In a healthy person these organisms would be phagocytosed and removed, but in a neutropenic patient, uncontrolled replication can occur (Gabriel 2004). The risk of infection is directly related to the number of circulating neutrophils. The longer the length of neutropenia and/or a rapidly decreasing neutrophil count all increase the risk of infection (Glauser & Calandra 2000).

The emergence of antibiotic-resistant pathogenic organisms has increased the risk of serious infection by changing the balance of survival in favour of the resistant organism (Dancer *et al.* 2006; Oztoprak *et al.* 2006). Many organisms, and the infections caused by them, respond to an antibiotic of proven efficacy and safety; however, a resistant organism will not be susceptible to the antibiotic of choice. *Staphylococcus aureus* is one of the most common causes of soft tissue infections, and infections caused by this organism are treated with flucloxacillin. Methicillin-resistant *S. aureus* (MRSA), however, is resistant to flucloxacillin and can easily colonize i.v. insertion sites, providing a reservoir of infection which may go on to cause serious disease (Coia *et al.* 2006). There is a danger that MRSA will develop a resistance to other antibiotics, as recent reports of a vancomycin-resistant MRSA in Japan indicate (Bal & Gould 2005). Effective infection control policies are essential if these resistant organisms are to be contained.

Elliott (1993) studied the organisms responsible for bacteraemias associated with i.v. devices in England and Wales, as reported to the Communicable Disease Surveillance Centre (*See* Box 4.3). *Staphylococcus epidermidis* is the most common cause of i.v.-related infection, because it is a normal resident on the skin of both patients and healthcare workers. *S. epidermidis* also has the ability to grow and proliferate on catheters. Following attachment to a catheter surface the organism produces a glycocalyx slime-like substance which protects it from the patient's natural immune mechanisms and from antibiotics (Dunne 2002).

Many patients in hospital have diminished resistance to infection, which means that organisms that are relatively harmless to healthy people may cause disease in such patients. The greater the number of organisms, the greater is the risk; however, even a small number of organisms contaminating i.v. fluids, for example, is extremely dangerous and can cause serious infection (Moore *et al.* 2005).

A wide variety of microorganisms, including virulent strains, can be found in the hospital environment (Koerner *et al.* 1997). When a hospital department is physically clean, dust-free and dry, it is unlikely to be the main cause of exogenous infection. It is essential to maintain such an environment in order to provide the required surroundings for good hygiene and asepsis (DH 2003).

BOX 4.3

Organisms most commonly responsible for intravenous bacteraemias in decreasing order of total isolates

- *Staphylococcus epidermidis*
- *Staphylococcus aureus*
- *Streptococcus* spp.
- *Pseudomonas aeruginosa*
- *Escherichia coli*
- *Enterobacter* spp.
- *Klebsiella* spp.
- *Candida* spp.
- *Corynebacterium* spp.
- *Acinetobacter* spp.

Microorganisms will easily proliferate at room temperature. This means that the longer an infusion container is in use, the greater the proliferation of bacteria will be. If contamination of the infusate has inadvertently occurred, the likelihood of infection will increase. The pH, temperature and presence of nutrients in the infusion will influence the rate at which organisms multiply. Parenteral nutrition (PN) infusions, which are of a high nutritious value, are of particular concern (Beekmann & Henderson 2005) as they are commonly left hanging for 24 hours. To reduce the risk of contamination of PN fluids their production must be undertaken in a controlled clean environment as near to the time of administration as possible. If PN containers have to be stored before use, this must be in a designated refrigerator at 4°C to reduce the risk of contamination and multiplication of organisms (Rey *et al.* 2005).

Sources of Microorganisms

Sources of microorganisms include air and skin. Microorganisms present in the air come from two basic sources: humans and the environment. Individuals with a chest infection will, when coughing, liberate many bacteria-containing particles into the air. Similarly, skin scales, which are constantly eliminated from the skin during desquamation, can be liberated into the air by movements such as bed-making and pulling the bed curtains (Sexton *et al.* 2006).

The microorganisms on the skin are either resident or transient flora. Resident flora refers to permanent residents of the skin which are not readily removed by friction and includes *S. aureus* and *S. epidermidis*, both of which are major causes of i.v. infection. Resident flora play an important role in the prevention of colonization of the skin by other potentially pathogenic organisms. These organisms suppress the growth of many potentially pathogenic organisms by:

- the physical advantage of previous occupancy
- competing for essential nutrients
- producing inhibitory substances such as fatty acids which discourage other species of organisms from invading.

The disadvantage of resident flora found on the skin, and also in the gut, is that such flora can be spread into previously sterile parts of the body, e.g. when the skin is damaged or breached by an i.v. device. Resident flora can also be disturbed after administration of antibiotics which can lead to an overgrowth of potentially pathogenic resistant microorganisms (Dancer *et al.* 2006).

Transient flora are organisms that are not consistently found on the skin and that are loosely attached and easily removed when hands are properly washed. Unwashed hands, however, will readily transmit these organisms by direct contact onto whatever is being handled (DH 2001). This risk is particularly high during manipulation of the i.v. system.

Routes of Access of Microorganisms

Extraluminal

Extraluminal spread refers to the migration and entry of bacteria down the insertion site on the external surface of the catheter. The bacteria may originate from the air, the skin of the patient or healthcare workers, or contaminated dressings and lotions. Prevention includes hand-washing, aseptic technique, careful skin preparation, scrupulous hygiene by the patient and a clean environment (Safdar & Maki 2004).

Intraluminal

Intraluminal spread refers to the entry of organisms into the infusion system through contaminated fluids or additives into the infusion container or tubing. Similarly, if the catheter hub becomes contaminated during manipulation of the hub, migration of bacteria can occur. Prevention includes the use of sterile equipment, aseptic technique, hand-washing and keeping the number of i.v. catheter manipulations to a minimum (Safdar & Maki 2004).

Haematogenous spread

Haematogenous spread refers to the migration of organisms from a distant site of infection to the catheter, e.g. from the lungs, wound or bowel. This means that a catheter can be colonized from remote unrelated sites of infection. Prevention relies on fully evaluating the patient so that potential risks can be recognized and preventive measures commenced (Infusion Nurses Society (INS) 2006).

Contaminated infusates

The use of contaminated infusates can be avoided by careful inspection of the i.v. fluid to make sure that it is clear and free from particulate matter and that the container is intact with no cracks in the bottle or holes in the plastic bag. The label must be checked to verify that the container is not out of date. All containers must be labelled to indicate the time and date that the container was opened and when the infusion will be completed. Manufacturers' directions and local polices must be followed for all administration of infusion solutions (INS 2006).

Types of Infection

Infections can be grouped into two categories: exogenous and endogenous. Exogenous infection refers to organisms originating outside the patient's body and implies cross-infection from staff, other patients, visitors or the environment. Endogenous infection arises from organisms or factors already present in or on the patient's body before the onset of infection. An example of endogenous infection is the haematogenous spread of bowel flora by translocation (Carter 1994), where viable bacteria move from the gut of immunocompromised patients to other organs.

Exogenous and endogenous contamination of the i.v. system may have intrinsic or extrinsic causes (*See* Box 4.4).

BOX 4.4

Examples of how extrinsic sources of contamination can occur

- Additives to the i.v. fluids
- Infusion container changes
- Contaminated air
- Injections/flushes/specimen collection
- Contaminated skin disinfectants
- Hands of staff
- Patient's normal flora

Intrinsic contamination

Intrinsic contamination of i.v. equipment occurs before administration, due to a breakdown of asepsis, and is generally attributed to faults in the manufacturing and sterilization process or, more commonly, to damage sustained by the product during transit or storage of the i.v. system. Fortunately, this type of contamination seldom occurs, but when incidents do take place there are significant consequences for patients. Prevention is therefore an important objective, which means that all equipment must be closely inspected before use (INS 2006).

If intrinsic contamination is suspected, the product must not be used, and if signs of intrinsically acquired infection occur, the system must be discontinued immediately and comparable products of the same batch investigated for a similar fault; they should not be used until a satisfactory explanation has been found for the intrinsic contamination (MHRA 2005).

Staff must always be aware of the risk of intrinsic contamination. Prevention is assisted by purchasers vigorously assessing products to ensure reliability and suitability for the task for which they are intended. A hospital product review committee can assist with this process (Garcia 2005). The user of any product should be satisfied with the transportation and storage methods. This does not negate the need to carefully examine all equipment before use to detect and eliminate any faulty items. Items that are found to be of an unacceptable standard must be investigated. It may be appropriate to refer the problem to the MHRA who will investigate the complaint. Passing on complaints in this way allows the MHRA to have an accurate picture of the standard of products throughout the country. The MHRA can, if necessary, send out a hazard warning outlining the potential problem, which will help to prevent further incidents occurring (MHRA 2005).

Extrinsic contamination

Extrinsic contamination refers to contamination that occurs at any point during the use of the i.v. system and is generally due to improper operation, e.g. failure to maintain a sterile closed system. Hub-related contamination has been widely recognized as a precursor of catheter-related sepsis. Sitges-Serra *et al.* (1995) suggested that the microorganisms most commonly found on hubs are those varieties reflecting the hospital flora, with contamination occurring when a colonized hand is used to manipulate the catheter junction (Archibald *et al.* 1998).

Contamination of i.v. equipment, including items such as lotions, ointments and dressing packs, is prevented by maintaining aseptic technique at all times (*See* Box 4.5).

An example of extrinsic contamination was highlighted by Bauer & Denson's (1979) survey, which found high i.v. infection rates associated with the use of non-sterile Elastoplast on venepuncture sites. Similarly, Chodoff *et al.* (1995) reported seven cases

---

BOX 4.5

Principles of aseptic techniques

- Hand-washing
  - Surgical aseptic technique—antimicrobial liquid detergent and water
  - Non-touch aseptic technique—clean hands can be cleansed with an alcoholic hand-rub
- Sterile equipment. Single-use items not to be reused
- Clean equipment
- Clean environment—visibly clean, free from dust and soilage
- Cutaneous antisepsis—skin site cleaned with 2% alcoholic chlorhexidine gluconate which is allowed to dry before inserting the device

of nosocomial Gram-negative infections resulting from the use of contaminated saline solutions.

Intravenous practice has to take into consideration the risks of infection, and all policies and procedures should be designed to reduce these risks. If, however, contamination does inadvertently occur, the potential problem should be recognized by skilled nurses before complications have had time to set in (Lundgren & Ek 1996).

The following guidelines should be included in i.v. procedures.

- Replace intravenous administration sets used to administer blood and blood products every 12 hours or according to the manufacturer's or local policy instructions (Pratt *et al.* 2007). Replace intravenous administration sets used for total parenteral nutrition (TPN) at the end of the infusion or within 24 hours of initiating the infusion (Pratt *et al.* 2007). Change all intravenous tubing, stopcocks etc. no more frequently than at 72-hour intervals and replace all intravenous tubing when the vascular device is being resited (NICE 2003; Pratt *et al.* 2007).
- Infusion containers should not hang for more than 24 hours, except for those used for blood and blood product infusions which should be completed within 4 hours of removal from the blood fridge or hospital transfusion laboratory (Gray 2006).
- Maintain a closed system whenever possible.
- Hub manipulation should be kept to a minimum. Prevention of contamination during connection and disconnection involves the use of an aseptic technique and cleaning of the catheter and i.v. administration hub with an aseptic solution prior to disconnection.
- Use luer-lock connection fittings whenever possible to prevent accidental disconnection of the administration set (NICE 2003).
- Limit the number of connections (e.g. three-way taps and stopcocks) in the i.v. system (DH 2003) as these have been found to have a high contamination rate (Mehtar & Taylor 1981) due to the increased number of open ports that facilitate endoluminal contamination. These taps and stopcocks should be changed at the same time as the administration set (Goodinson 1990). When used, stopcocks must be capped (O'Grady *et al.* 2002).
- Local evaluation is required to establish whether or not to use i.v. filters. These are claimed to remove bacterial contaminants, particulate matter and air embolus and to reduce the incidence of phlebitis (van Lingen *et al.* 2004). No strong recommendations have been made regarding the use of in-line filters (O'Grady *et al.* 2002).
- When introducing the administration set into an infusion bottle, use an air inlet filter needle to prevent contamination of i.v. fluids by the influx of air.
- Some advice continues to state: rotate peripheral devices at 72-hour intervals (DH 2003) or immediately if contamination is suspected (INS 2006), although other guidance suggests that rates of phlebitis are not substantially different for peripheral catheters left in place for 72 hours compared to those left for 96 hours (O'Grady *et al.* 2002).
- The date of insertion and removal of all i.v. devices must be documented (DH 2003).
- Intravenous devices should only be inserted and manipulated by trained and competent staff using strict aseptic techniques (DH 2003).

It is essential that patients are told the importance of good hygiene. Patients should shower or bathe at least daily, and more often in hot weather. Studies have shown that there is no delay in healing if sutures become wet with soap and water during washing (Heal *et al.* 2006). The use of an occlusive dressing eliminates the potential problem of the suture line becoming damaged during washing. Showers are preferable to a bath, as the bath and bath hoists may easily become contaminated with bacteria, and during showering there is a reduced possibility of cross-infection from a previous user (Briggs & Wilson 1996).

Greaves (1985) reported that 'a bed bath can often leave a patient dirtier after the bath than before', as organisms can survive and multiply on items such as the wash bowl and wash cloths. If the only method of washing the patient is by a bed bath, they should be supplied with their own wash bowl and disposable wash clothes. On discharge of the patient, the bowl should be terminally disinfected before being put back into general use.

The risk of extrinsic contamination is reduced by strict adherence to aseptic technique, optimum patient hygiene and maintenance of a clean environment. An increasing number of patients are being discharged home with skin-tunnelled CVCs or implantable ports in place and these same principles and practices of infection control in i.v. care must be maintained in the home or alternative care setting (INS 2006).

Prevention of Catheter-Related Sepsis

Prevention of infection involves the adoption of techniques that incorporate the principles of asepsis and hygiene. The fundamental principles of infection control must be integrated into the design of the environment and influence the choice of all equipment used by patients and staff.

The principles of infection control are to protect the patient with systems that remove the potential source of infection, block the route of transfer of bacteria to susceptible patients and enhance the patient's resistance to i.v. device infection. Such methods must be research based and take into consideration the available information related to bacterial pathogenicity. These practices must be regularly evaluated and updated to take into account new research findings, as well as the more adventurous surgery and high-dose chemotherapy which is resulting in an ever-increasing number of patients being highly susceptible to infection.

Education programmes for those involved in i.v. care is essential, as inexperienced staff increase the risk of infection (O'Grady *et al.* 2002).

The general measures designed to protect patients from infection include meticulous attention to all aspects of i.v. therapy. Box 4.6 highlights factors that particularly influence the acquisition of i.v. catheter-related infection.

Aseptic technique

Aseptic technique is a method which has been evolved to prevent contamination of wounds and other vulnerable sites by ensuring that only sterile items come into contact with the site and that the environment in which the procedure is being carried out is as clean and safe as possible (Hart 2004). An aseptic technique must be used for all

---

BOX 4.6

Factors that influence acquisition of infection

- Type of catheter
- Insertion of device or catheter
- Prophylactic antibiotic at time of catheter insertion
- Purpose of catheter
- Duration of catheter
- Intravenous therapy teams
- Care of insertion site
- Dressing
- Catheter care
- Patient's underlying condition

vascular access device insertions, for site care and for accessing the system. There are two main types of aseptic technique: a full surgical aseptic technique and a non-touch aseptic technique.

Whilst a full surgical aseptic technique should be used for the placement of central venous access devices and includes sterile drapes, gown and gloves (Pratt *et al.* 2007), a non-touch sterile technique is suitable for administration of drugs, phlebotomy and insertion of peripheral devices (Larwood *et al.* 2000).

An infection control link nurse system provides a connection between clinical areas and the infection control team. Their role is to raise awareness and motivate staff to improve practice. Problems that occur are often related to a high turnover of staff and insufficient time for training and monitoring (Dawson 2003).

Whilst an aseptic technique can be undertaken in a variety of ways, there are basic principles that must be adhered to (Box 4.6).

Hand-washing

Hand-washing is the single most important procedure for preventing nosocomial infections. Many outbreaks of nosocomial infection have originated from the hands of healthcare workers, as transmission of microorganisms from one patient to another or from the environment to the patient can occur via unwashed hands (DH 2001). Hand-washing must be convenient and acceptable and its essential importance must be recognized. Hands must be washed when going on and off duty, before and after direct patient contact, and before and during aseptic techniques.

Before hand-washing sleeves should be rolled up, jewellery removed as rings inhibit hand-washing (Montville *et al.* 2002), cuts and abrasions covered with a waterproof plaster and fingernails kept short, clean and free from nail-varnish (NICE 2003).

The choice of hand-washing technique depends on the purpose of the hand-washing and is generally based on the infection risks of the patient being cared for. Social hand-washing involves washing hands with a non-medicated soap or detergent and will remove many transient microbial flora; it is suitable for when going on and off duty, and before and after brief patient care activities. Since soap can become contaminated it is important that it is supplied in a disposable dispenser which is replaced when empty (Brook & Brook 1993).

Hand-washing with an antimicrobial hand-washing product is required before all aseptic techniques and before contact with immunocompromised patients. Preparations containing chlorhexidine have be shown to be very effective in removing bacteria (DH 2001).

When hands are clean, a bactericidal alcoholic hand-rub can be used before and during patient contact, especially when undertaking aseptic techniques. Such preparations have the added advantage over soap of destroying transient microorganisms (DH 2001), as well as being quick and easy to use. A dispenser of the bactericidal alcoholic hand-rub should be fixed by every patient bed and treatment examination coach or chair as well as on the bottom shelf of all trolleys used for aseptic techniques, so that hands can be easily disinfected immediately before and during the procedure.

Correct and thorough drying of hands following hand-washing is equally important, as damp hands transfer bacteria much more readily than dry ones (Patrick *et al.* 1997). Similarly, hands that have not been dried properly are more likely to become cracked and sore, which will increase the risk of colonization by potentially pathogenic hospital-acquired organisms. An emollient handcream should be applied regularly to protect the skin (NICE 2003).

Hot air electric hand-dryers are being increasingly used in public areas and have proved useful as, unlike paper towels, they do not 'run out' and they do not have to be collected and disposed of. Nevertheless, in the clinical setting, a good-quality paper towel remains the product of choice, because the hand-dryer can warm the environment, can be noisy and can be slow, leaving hands damp (Taylor *et al.* 2000). This can result in busy staff wiping their damp hands on their clothes rather than waiting for the hand-dryer to dry their wet hands completely.

Patient hand-washing is equally important. Ill patients do not always wash their hands after using the toilet, urinal or commode, and could contribute to the transfer of organisms to other body sites. Nurses should stress the importance of good hygiene to their patients and offer help and support to allow patients to wash their hands, as studies have shown that debilitated patients are often not offered the opportunity to wash their hands (Mock & Olsen 2003).

Sterile equipment

All surgical instruments, dressings, lotions, solutions and drugs used for or introduced by injection must be provided sterile. This equipment must also have been protected against contamination during transit, storage and use.

Regardless of how sterilization has been achieved, all items must be inspected before use to ensure that sterilization has taken place, that the packaging is intact and that the shelf life has not expired.

Reusable surgical devices should be decontaminated in a sterile services department with requisite facilities and expertise. Single-use items must never be reused (DH 2003; MHRA 2005).

Clean equipment

Equipment that is not introduced into the i.v. system and does not come into contact with the i.v. site, but which is used during i.v. therapy, must be clean, including small items such as a splint and tape, and larger items such as pumps and drip poles. The items that are initially supplied clean and packaged must be stored in a dust-free, clean way. When a patient is being barrier-nursed, the minimum amount of equipment and medical and surgical supplies should be stored in the room, to eliminate the risk of unused items being used on subsequent patients. All equipment must be washed with detergent and wiped dry between every patient use and when spillage occurs, unless used for a known infected patient, when a chemical disinfectant must be used (Ayliffe *et al.* 2000).

Clean environment

The environment of a hospital plays an important part in the spread of hospital infection. For example, MRSA spread during bed-making can be redispersed into the air when the bedclothes or bedside curtains are handled (Shiomori *et al.* 2002). Cleaning programmes must be clearly defined and carefully monitored to ensure high standards of cleanliness are achieved (DH 2003). Properly trained and supervised domestic staff should clean the ward area thoroughly every day and damp dust areas such as bed frames and curtain rails weekly to ensure that microorganisms and the material on which they thrive will be removed.

Shelves and cupboards where surgical and medical supplies are stored must be dust-free, with a stock control system operating. It is essential that stock is not stored on the floor where it may become contaminated and, equally importantly, prevent thorough cleaning of the floor.

Type of catheter

Catheter design and composition contribute to the risk of infection. Catheters need to be made of materials that do not irritate the vascular intima. Similarly, catheters that inhibit the adherence of microorganisms probably reduce the risk of infection. The larger the catheter, the greater the entry site, which increases the risk of extraluminal contamination.

Multilumen catheters are generally inserted into critically ill patients or those who are expected to receive a large number of infusions. It is suggested that multilumen catheters are associated with a higher risk of infection, and single-lumen catheters should be used unless multiple access is required. When used for TPN one lumen must be kept exclusively for this purpose (Pratt *et al.* 2007).

Totally implantable vascular port systems are available and they are reported to have a low rate of complications (Wolosker *et al.* 2004). Implantable ports should be considered as a preferred device for paediatric oncology and stem cell transplantation patients (Adler *et al.* 2006). Sehirali *et al.* (2005) reported that ports resulted in minimal anxiety for the patient and his or her family.

A study to assess the risk of infection related to site of insertion found no significant difference between subclavian, internal jugular and femoral veins but concluded the need for insertion to be undertaken by experienced staff, strict aseptic technique used and trained nursing staff to undertake catheter care (Deshpande *et al.* 2005). Infection rates can be reduced by subcutaneous tunnelling for jugular (Timsit *et al.* 1996) and femoral veins (Timsit *et al.* 1999).

Peripherally inserted central catheters (PICCs) are widely used for intermediate and long-term venous access, supplementing conventional CVCs. A study to determine the risk of PICC-related bloodstream infections found them to be similar to CVCs, although the PICCs are more vulnerable to thrombosis and dislodgement (Safdar & Maki 2004).

A prospective study undertaken to determine the infection risk related to short-term non-cuffed, percutaneously inserted CVCs found that most infections were extraluminally acquired and originated from cutaneous microflora (Safdar & Maki 2004).

The use of a skin-tunnelled CVC reduces the risks associated with the percutaneous CVCs. With these catheters, the tip is placed in the superior vena cava or right atrium and enters the vascular system through the subclavian vein, via a subcutaneous tunnel. There is the added advantage of a Dacron cuff situated in the subcutaneous tunnel which stimulates growth of fibrous tissue to provide stability for the catheter and a barrier to ascending organisms (Dougherty 2004). Studies, in particular those where catheters were being handled by untrained staff, suggest that the incidence of catheter-related infection is reduced when skin-tunnelled catheters are used (Johnson & Oppenheim 1992).

Early studies demonstrate that antimicrobial impregnated/coated CVCs favourably influence the incidence of catheter colonization and bloodstream infections (Pratt *et al.* 2007). In view of the increasing use of long-term i.v. therapy, the reduction of the risk of infection by the use of a better material for catheters remains a desirable goal. Some studies found that antiseptic coating appears to reduce infection rates (Rupp *et al.* 2005), whilst others found no difference in infection rates (Osma *et al.* 2006). However, one study of CVCs with silver-impregnated cuffs found that insertion was more difficult which may have resulted in a higher incidence of CVC infection (Alderman & Sugarbaker 2005). Pratt and colleagues recommend the use of an antimicrobial impregnated CVC for adult patients who require short-term central venous access and who are at high risk for a catheter-related bloodstream infection (Pratt *et al.* 2007).

Insertion of intravenous devices

Placement of a device must be carried out by an experienced practitioner, as complication rates tend to be higher with inexperienced practitioners (Geddes *et al.* 1998). Infection is more likely to occur following a difficult insertion, possibly due to a deteriorating technique, tissue trauma or disruption of skin flora (Alderman & Sugarbaker 2005). In some hospitals, nurses have extended their role to the placement of tunnelled CVCs. This has been found to be both safe and effective (Boland *et al.* 2003). A study that assessed the incidence of infectious complications of CVCs in a critical care setting concluded that the frequency of this procedure ensured experienced staff inserted and provided care for i.v. devices which reduced complication rates (Deshpande *et al.* 2005). The site of insertion is significant, with catheters placed in the lower extremities, particularly the femoral vein, having an increased risk of infection (Beekmann & Henderson 2005).

Tunnelled catheters must be inserted in a controlled clean environment, ideally in the operating theatre or anaesthetic room. One study looked at the influence of microbial air quality during skin-tunnelled catheter insertion, in the operating theatre versus radiology suite. It found that the microbial contamination of air was 9.5 colony-forming units (cfu) in the operating room versus 27.5 cfu in the radiology suite. It concluded that the advances of the imaging guidance available in radiology outweighed the potential risk of inferior microbial air quality compared to the operating theatre. The main risk factor reported in this study was neutropenia, suggesting early insertion of i.v. devices prior to neutropenia reduces infection rates (Nouwen *et al.* 1999). Midline, peripherally inserted catheters and non-skin-tunnelled catheters must be inserted in a clean environment using theatre standards of aseptic technique. Peripheral devices are inserted in a wide range of environments, and aseptic techniques must be used (*See* Chapter 9) (RCN 2005).

The placement of all CVCs should be considered a minor operation, and therefore the skin and insertion field must be prepared for a surgical intervention using sterile drapes, with the person undertaking the insertion wearing sterile gloves and gown (Pratt *et al.* 2007).

Disinfection of the insertion site with an antiseptic solution prior to catheter insertion and during subsequent manipulation of the device is essential to prevent local catheter-associated infection. A 2% chlorhexidine-based preparation is recommended, although a tincture of iodine, an iodophor or 70% alcohol can be used (NICE 2003; Pratt *et al.* 2007).

Johnson and Oppenheim (1992) reviewed the literature relating to the administration of prophylactic antibiotics at the time of CVC insertion and found studies which demonstrated that these antibiotics had no effect on CVC infection. Routine antimicrobial prophylaxis before CVC insertion or during use of the CVC to prevent colonization or infection is not recommended (O'Grady *et al.* 2002; Pratt *et al.* 2007).

Patients' skin flora

The skin is the main source of bacteria responsible for i.v.-associated infection (Eggimann & Pittet 2002). Studies have shown a direct relationship between skin colonization and positive tip culture (Balakrishnan *et al.* 1991). Most transient microorganisms found on skin can be removed by washing with soap and water, whilst resident microorganisms will be reduced by washing with an antiseptic detergent (Ayliffe *et al.* 2000).

Different regions of the skin support different numbers and types of flora, which are largely determined by the degree of available humidity. Exposed dry areas have relatively low numbers of resident flora, whilst more moist areas, e.g. the axilla and groin, or as a result of sweating or fever, show larger numbers of resident flora (Wilson 2006).

It is essential to encourage the patient to shower daily and to wear clothing that is loose and light, which will keep them dry and cool. Clothing and bed linen must be changed regularly. All of these factors will help to keep the numbers of resident flora to a manageable level and so discourage endogenous infection. Loach (1997) provided a patient's view that, while cleanliness was a simple way of improving well-being, the task of washing used up so much energy that there seemed little point in making the effort. These comments reiterate the importance of nurses providing help and encouragement to the weak and vulnerable patients in their care.

Skin preparation is important in reducing the risk of site infection, and for all CVCs the patient should undergo routine preoperative care, which includes a shower or bath (Ayliffe *et al.* 2000).

Purpose of the catheter

The composition of the i.v. fluid influences the risk of acquiring an i.v. device-related infection. Different infusion fluids support the growth of differing pathogens. No infusate is free of risk, and even distilled water can support the growth of *Pseudomonas* species. Koerner *et al.* (1997) discussed an outbreak of Gram-negative septicaemia associated with contamination of infusions in a non-clinical area, and emphasized the importance of continuous staff training in infection control and the need to involve the infection control team in all structural planning for patient care areas.

Parenteral nutrition (PN) solutions are particularly good media for the growth of microorganisms. Prevention of infusion-related infection in PN can be achieved by having a PN team who make decisions on protocols for insertion, maintenance and delivery of the solutions. All PN solutions must be prepared in a laminar air flow hood using sterile techniques. Once prepared, the solution should be used immediately or stored following the manufacturer's and local instructions (INS 2006) (*See* Chapter 14).

The risk of bacterial proliferation during infusion of blood and blood products is particularly high as organisms will thrive in the ambient temperature of hospital wards. Infusion must be started within 30 minutes of removing blood from the refrigerator and must be completed within 5 hours of commencement. Blood should be infused through a blood administration set which must be changed at least 12-hourly or according to the manufacturer's or local policy instructions (Pratt *et al.* 2007). The controversy concerning the virological safety of blood and blood products continues. All donations of blood are tested to exclude hepatitis B, hepatitis C and antibody to HIV 1 and 2. A prospective study of 20 000 units of blood concluded the risk of transfusion transmission of infection is very small (Regan *et al.* 2000). This small risk continues to decrease (Soldan *et al.* 2003). There is a possibility that variant Creutzfeldt–Jakob disease can be transmitted by blood. This is due to the long incubation period which can be as long as 40 years and the absence of a reliable screening test which means this risk is unknown (Ironside 2006).

Prevention relies on donors understanding that they should not donate blood if they know they are, or suspect that they may be, infected. Alternatively, the use of autologous transfusions is an option for planned surgical procedures.

Duration of the catheter

The longer the device is *in situ*, the more likely it is that a patient will develop a catheter-related infection. The most recent advice from the Department of Health (2003) suggests that peripheral intravenous cannulae should be kept in place for the minimum time necessary and changed every 72 hours irrespective of the presence of infection. CVCs can be left in longer but should not be replaced over a guidewire if infection is present. The dates of insertion and removal must be documented in the clinical records in the usual manner (DH 2003).

A skin-tunnelled central catheter is the catheter of choice for planned long-term i.v. therapy as the tunnel separates the catheter entry site into the vein from the exit site on the skin, so providing a barrier to infection by inhibiting the extraluminal spread of organisms along the outside of the catheter (Dougherty 2004).

Intravenous teams

Studies have shown that an i.v. therapy team is effective in decreasing morbidity and mortality associated with i.v.-related bacteraemias (Miller 1998). Dougherty (1996) outlined the benefits of i.v. teams who, as well as developing the service, provide education, enhance patient care and reduce non-compliance with i.v. policies and infection rates. Scalley *et al.*'s (1992) 30-month study of i.v. cannulation, as performed by i.v. teams and non-i.v. team personnel, showed a significant cost saving in the case of the former, related to a reduction in the incidence of phlebitis.

Care of insertion site

If any excess hair needs to be removed, electric clipping or depilatory cream should be used immediately prior to insertion (Kjonniksen *et al.* 2002). Shaving is not recommended as it increases the risk of skin abrasions which can harbour bacteria. Cleaning and disinfection of the insertion site with an antiseptic solution is essential to prevent infection (Dank 2006). Skin must be cleaned before cannulation. Skin preparations are applied with friction, working outwards from the insertion site in a circular pattern on an area equal to the size of dressing. For the antimicrobial solution to be effective, it should be allowed to air dry (INS 2006). Maki *et al.*'s (1991) study of three antiseptics for skin site disinfection found that 2% chlorhexidine substantially reduced the incidence of i.v. infections. Chlorhexidine has the added advantage of continuing antibacterial activity for up to 6 hours after application to skin (Pereira *et al.* 1997). The addition of isopropyl alcohol 70%, which is effective and rapid acting, has the additional advantage of evaporating leaving the treated surface dry, but has poor penetration power and should only be used on visually clean skin surfaces (Ayliffe *et al.* 2000).

The insertion site must be kept clean and dry and inspected daily. Elliott *et al.* (1994) discussed how the application of antibiotic ointment to the insertion site has been proposed as a method of reducing contamination and subsequent colonization, but others have found no benefit from applying this type of ointment. Johnson and Oppenheim (1992) suggested that its use can alter the resident skin flora and lead to superinfection with organisms not affected by the ointment; therefore the use of antiseptic ointment is not recommended (Pratt *et al.* 2007)

If an occlusive dressing is to be used, it should be changed weekly unless there is evidence of infection or it becomes soiled. If a gauze dressing is being used to allow daily inspection of the site (Elliott *et al.* 1994), it will need to be changed daily, or more often if it becomes wet or soiled. During dressing changes an aseptic technique must be maintained (NICE 2003; RCN 2005; Pratt *et al.* 2007).

Two to three weeks after insertion of a skin-tunnelled catheter, the sutures may be removed. It is then only necessary to use a clean technique in the care of the catheter site. Dressings and applications of topical antiseptic are unnecessary, unless the patient prefers to have the site covered. Dressings do offer protection against friction from clothes and may make the patient feel more secure. However, it is essential to continue to use a full aseptic technique when opening the closed CVC system (NICE 2003; RCN 2005; Pratt *et al.* 2007).

Dressings

Catheter dressings must:

- be sterile
- secure the device to prevent dislodgement and trauma
- protect the wound from external contamination
- allow easy inspection of the site
- be comfortable and cost-effective
- not cause skin excoriation or irritation.

The choice of catheter dressing remains a controversial issue, with numerous studies yielding contradictory results (Lau 1996).

The type of catheter dressing applied does appear to influence the incidence of infection (Lau 1996). Hoffmann *et al.* (1992) reviewed the literature in this area and indicated that transparent dressings may significantly increase the risk of catheter infection compared with gauze dressings. They suggested that this may be due to the inadequate moisture vapour permeability of such dressings, as the collection of moisture under a dressing promotes the growth of bacteria (Callahan & Wesorick 1987). Treston-Aurand *et al.*'s (1997) review of the literature supported Hoffmann *et al.*'s speculation, but they argued that prospective randomized trials have not confirmed this suggestion.

Since these studies, new dressings have been developed with increased moisture permeability, which appears to prevent the accumulation of moisture on the skin surface (Keenlyside 1993). Treston-Aurand *et al.*'s (1997) study of transparent non-permeable standard polyurethane dressings, tape and gauze and transparent highly permeable polyurethane dressings resulted in a hospital in Michigan USA converting to the highly permeable dressing for use with CVCs, which eventually led to a 25% decrease in infection rates. These authors suggested that additional definitive randomized prospective investigations are needed to clarify the complex question of which dressing is the most suitable for i.v. use.

Transparent dressings have the added advantage of only needing to be changed every 5–7 days as well as allowing for immediate inspection of the i.v. site (Treston-Aurand *et al.* 1997). Transparent dressings also allow the patient to shower or bath normally. They provide a superior catheter fixation, thereby reducing the risk of catheter displacement as these flexible lightweight films allow freedom of movement.

All unused dressing material must be disposed of after completion of the dressing procedure as contamination may have occurred (Dietze *et al.* 2001).

Catheter care

Thrombolytic complications of catheters are often associated with catheter sepsis. It is unclear whether this is due to the occlusion requiring an increase in manipulations to unblock it, which allows the entry of microorganisms, or to the presence of the blood clot (O'Grady *et al.* 2002), which provides nutrients for pathogens to proliferate, leading to infection. Preventing the blood from clotting in the catheter is achieved by correct flushing between drugs and blood products, when the catheter is not in use (Pratt *et al.* 2007), and by restricting the times when the administration set is inadvertently turned off.

Diagnosis of Intravenous-Associated Infection

Intravenous catheter infection can be categorized as localized or systemic. Localized infection refers to the catheter site or catheter tunnel. The patient may complain of pain, tenderness, fever with erythema, oedema and cellulitis at the site or along the subcutaneous tunnel. Systemic infections are those which affect the body as a whole, and are not limited to a particular area. Bacteraemia and septicaemia are examples of i.v.-related systemic infections. *See* Box 4.7 for definitions.

Intravenous-associated sepsis is not always accompanied by phlebitis and the patient may have chills, fever, headaches, tremors, nausea, vomiting, abdominal pain, hyperventilation and shock (Maki *et al.* 1973).

Catheter site infection should not be confused with catheter-related sepsis. The presence of erythema or exudate at the site may indicate a localized infection and may not necessarily be a sign of catheter infection. Conversely, patients may be septic with no evidence at the catheter site. Fever in a person with a CVC should be attributed to the

---

BOX 4.7

Catheter-related infection definitions

- *Localized catheter colonization*—significant growth of a microorganism > 15 colony forming units (CFU) from the catheter tip
- *Exit site infection*—erythema or induration within 2 cm of the catheter exit site, in the absence of bloodstream infection
- *Tunnel infection*—tenderness, erythema, or site induration > 2 cm from the catheter site along the tunnelled tract in the absence of bloodstream infection
- *Pocket infection*—purulent fluid in the subcutaneous pocket of a totally implanted intravascular catheter, in the absence of bloodstream infection
- *Catheter-related bloodstream infection*—positive blood culture with no other source of infection

(Adapted from O'Grady *et al.* 2002)

---

catheter until proven otherwise. Cultures from blood, catheter site, urine, wound and sputum, plus an X-ray, should be obtained in order to diagnose unexplained pyrexia in immunocompromised patients.

Peripheral devices should always be removed when device infection is suspected. Similarly, skin-tunnelled CVCs with obvious tunnel infection should be removed as these infections are very difficult to treat without removal of the catheter. CVCs are not generally removed automatically as it can make management of sepsis more difficult by removing i.v. access for antibiotics. However, Clemence *et al.* (1995) suggested that removal of short-term CVCs where there is the suspicion of i.v. sepsis allows the catheter tip to be sent for microbiological culture, which can be helpful in diagnosing infection. Healing of the insertion site can occur once the catheter has been removed and thereby prevent reoccurrence of bacteraemia once the antibiotic therapy is completed. A number of febrile patients who are diagnosed as having a catheter-related infection may be septic with bacteraemia from other sources (Boktour *et al.* 2006).

Tunnelled catheters are generally left in place in an attempt to treat the bacteraemia with antibiotics. Similarly, a substantial number of patients can be cured if empirical anti-microbials are commenced. These will be chosen to include the possibility of a catheter-related infection based on the clinician's assessment of the patient, the likely bacterium responsible for the infection and the hospital's antibiotic policy. Microbiological results may take days to become available and a delay in treating an infection may be disastrous. As long as the clinician has prescribed treatment based on the best available information, adjustments to therapy can be made when laboratory results are available.

Patients with long-term CVCs who have a bacteraemia with no identified source and whose infection fails to respond to appropriate antibiotic therapy should have the catheter removed. The 5-cm distal tip should be cut off with sterile scissors, placed in a sterile universal container and sent for culture. The problem with tip cultures is that the results are difficult to interpret; it is difficult to discriminate between catheter contamination during removal, true catheter infection and contaminated i.v. fluids.

Quantitative microbiological studies of catheter tips can increase the reliability of distinguishing between catheter-related infection and bacteraemia from another source (Maki 1977).

Blood cultures taken from a separate peripheral vein and from the catheter can be compared in the process of diagnosing catheter sepsis. If blood cultures from the catheter are positive and the peripheral vein cultures are negative, this provides a reliable diagnosis of a catheter-associated infection. If the catheter blood cultures have a significant increase in bacterial colonies compared with the peripheral blood cultures, this also suggests a catheter sepsis (Elliott *et al.* 1994). Positive blood cultures with identical organisms can confirm a catheter as a source of infection. Rigors following the use of the catheter is generally considered highly suggestive of a catheter-related infection, although allergic reaction to the infusates has to be ruled out (Polyzos *et al.* 2001).

As diagnosis of infection is difficult, studies have been carried out on culturing catheters while they remain in position. This is achieved by passing a small sampling brush through the catheter and then culturing the brush (Kite *et al.* 1997). The aim is for the brush to pick up organisms from the tip of the catheter. Valves to prevent blood loss and air embolism are integral to the design of this sampling equipment (Dobbins *et al.* 2004). A great deal of skill and an aseptic technique is required during this procedure.

Surveillance cultures

The value of surveillance cultures of catheter hubs and exit sites is difficult to judge. It is accepted that patients generally acquire infections endogenously, which means that surveillance cultures are occasionally useful in identifying bacteria that may need additional or different antibiotic coverage from that recommended by the antibiotic policy. This is particularly important with regard to MRSA, which can easily colonize catheter sites (Oztoprak *et al.* 2006). MRSA screening should be carried out on all patients from risk groups and swabs should be taken from anterior nares, skin lesions, wounds, catheter sites and groin/perineum (Coia *et al.* 2006).

Treatment of Infection

If a patient is known or suspected to have an infection, the clinician must decide which organism is likely to be responsible and to which antibiotics it will or will not be sensitive.

There are now many different antibacterial drugs, which are classified by their chemical structure and their site of action on the bacterial cell. There are fewer antifungal and antiviral agents. Antimicrobial drugs are valuable in the treatment and, in some well-researched circumstances, the prevention of infection (Glauser & Calandra 2000). Unfortunately, their inappropriate use has the potential risk of toxicity and superinfection in a patient, as well as the problem of selection of resistant organisms. In view of the large number of antibiotics available, the clinician should refer to the hospital's antibiotic policy for guidance on treatment, and for complex treatment should consult the consultant microbiologist who will have a special interest in and knowledge of antibiotics (Health Protection Agency 2005a).

Beekmann and Henderson (2005) discuss at length how best to treat infection in a patient with a long-term central venous access device. They suggest that with the exception of true tunnel infections many infections may be successfully treated with the device in place. Careful observation for other related problems should be ongoing.

Education

Infection rates associated with intravenous catheters can be reduced if care is provided only by trained and competent staff (DH 2003). Dougherty (1996) not only outlines the importance of training, but emphasizes the need for continued support and skill maintenance for staff involved in i.v. work. Clarke (1994) described the value of an i.v. special interest group—including senior nursing, pharmacy, infection control, anaesthetic and dietetic staff—whose task is to develop specific protocols and guidelines (RCN 2005). It is essential that patients receiving i.v. therapy are instructed about the risk (and preventive measures required to reduce this risk) of acquiring an infection (NICE 2003).

Occupational Risk to Healthcare Workers

Nurses are at risk of acquiring infection in the workplace. Transmission of infection can occur through:

- skin puncture by blood-contaminated sharp objects such as needles, scalpels or scissors
- contamination of open wounds and skin lesions
- splashing of mucous membranes of the eye, nose or mouth
- human bites when blood is drawn.

Occupational exposure incidents reported to the Health Protection Agency between July 1996 and June 2004 showed that percutaneous injury was the most common injury (78%) reported, and of these 63% were by hollowbore needles. Forty five per cent of nurses and 37% of doctors and dentists reported the most number of injuries. It is thought that 38% of incidents could have been prevented with adherence to procedures for safe handling and disposal of sharps and clinical waste (Health Protection Agency 2005b).

It is not possible to calculate the risk to nurses, as it is not known how many people are infected with bloodborne infections in the UK. The UK Blood Transfusion Service screens all regular and new donors, but these results only provide information on a small section of the population (*See* Box 4.8).

It is this type of data, highlighting the number of undiagnosed carriers of infection, that gave rise to the suggestion that there is no safe patient, only safe technique; it reiterates the importance of treating all patients in the same way. This will result in staff becoming expert in undertaking procedures using a safe technique and will mean that when they are caring for a known infected patient, changes in practice will not be necessary, thereby avoiding the accidents that such changes provoke. The other advantage of using a safe technique for all patients is that when a known positive patient is treated, their confidentiality is maintained because there is no obvious change in practice between different patients on the ward. Unfortunately adherence to standard precautions is poor (Watterson 2005).

The degree of risk is directly related to the type of incident. The number of healthcare workers known to have become infected as a result of occupational exposure is small, considering the frequency of exposure to blood and body fluids in the clinical area (Hanrahan & Reutter 1997). The Health Protection Agency 2005 report records nine cases of hepatitis C seroconversion following an injury between July 1996 and June 2004. There is no record of hepatitis B seroconversion as it is assumed that all healthcare workers should now be vaccinated against hepatitis B. The first documented case in the UK of a healthcare worker seroconverting to HIV following an injury was in 1984; a further three cases occurred in 1992 to 1993. There was also reported a further seven probable cases of occupationally acquired HIV between 1984 and 1997 (Health Protection Agency 2005b).

BOX 4.8

Prevalence of bloodborne infection (Advisory Committee on Dangerous Pathogens 1995)

- 1 in 30 400 new blood donors found to be HIV+
- 1 in 287 000 regular blood donors found to be HIV+
- 1 in 1500 new blood donors found to be HBsAg-positive
- 1 in 2000 new blood donors found to be hepatitis C antibody-positive

All healthcare workers are subject to regulations under the Health and Safety at Work etc. Act 1974, whereby employers and employees have a duty to protect, as far as is reasonably possible, those at work. The Control of Substances Hazardous to Health Regulations (COSHH) (HSE 2002) provide a framework of action designed to reduce the risk from hazardous substances, including bloodborne viruses. The Management of Health and Safety at Work Regulations (DH 1999) cover an even broader range, involving assessment of risk, provision of health surveillance, information, instruction and training of employees. Reporting of exposure to, and incidents involving, pathogens that might jeopardize the health and safety of workers, including hepatitis B, falls within the Reporting of Injuries, Diseases and Dangerous Occurrence Regulations (Health and Safety Executive 1995). Similarly, the Industrial Injury Benefit Social Security Act 1975 lists viral hepatitis as one of a number of prescribed industrial diseases for which those affected may qualify for compensation.

Universal precautions

Universal precautions involve the appropriate use of barrier methods to prevent contamination by blood and body fluids of mucous membranes and non-intact skin, and the adoption of techniques to prevent inoculation accidents. Under these precautions, blood and body fluids of all patients are considered potentially infectious for bloodborne pathogens. Universal precautions are intended to supplement routine infection control policies such as hand-washing (DH 2001); *See* Box 4.9.

> **BOX 4.9**
>
> **Universal precautions**
>
> - Use of gloves
> - Use of aprons
> - Use of masks
> - Use of eye protection
> - Safe disposal of sharps
> - Avoiding needlestick injury
> - Covering breaks in skin with a waterproof dressing

Gloves

Gloves must be worn when the task to be undertaken involves or may involve contact with blood and body fluid; this includes phlebotomy. The use of gloves reduces the incidence of blood contamination of hands, but cannot prevent sharps injuries.

Clean gloves are adequate for most nursing tasks (Rossoff *et al.* 1993), as most tasks involve the use of a non-touch aseptic technique.

Gloves are a single-use disposable item and should be changed after each use. Regulations related to cleaning and reusing single-use medical devices apply to single-use gloves, which must not be decontaminated during use (DH 2003).

The likelihood of contamination depends on the following factors:

- skill and technique of the healthcare worker
- frequency with which the healthcare worker performs the procedure
- whether it is a routine or emergency procedure
- prevalence of bloodborne infections in the patient population
- terminal illness in the source patient
- the frequency and extent of blood and body fluid contact
- the number and extent of exposures

- inoculation accidents of increased risk
- skin integrity, i.e. whether it is visibly compromised
- the quality of infection control policies and procedures.

In 1991, the Medical Devices Directorate produced specifications for non-sterile, natural rubber latex examination gloves, requiring that gloves should be of a suitable strength and thickness to maximize protection whilst maintaining manual dexterity, be without perforations and be manufactured and lubricated with materials which will not harm the wearer (Medical Devices Directorate 1991). The use of poor-quality, low-cost gloves is neither safe nor cost-effective because glove changes during procedures would be required to ensure integrity. Gloves should be changed between patient contact. Wearing gloves does not replace hand-washing; hands and wrists should be washed thoroughly after glove removal (DH 2005).

Gloves should always be available for healthcare workers who wish to use them (DH 2003). Problems associated with the wearing of gloves do occur. Surveys have shown a high perforation rate for all gloves; this is mainly due to wear and tear in use, but unused gloves have also been found to be perforated (Malhotra *et al.* 2004). For these reasons, it is essential that breaks in the skin that are likely to be contaminated with blood and body fluids are covered with a waterproof dressing.

Prevention of needlestick injuries
Preventing sharps injuries is crucial.

The following list outlines good practice which should be adopted at all times.

- All employers must provide effective education and training on the safe use and disposal of sharps.
- All employees must work in accordance with health and safety procedures.
- Report any accidents, incidents or near misses immediately.
- Staff should ask for assistance when taking blood or giving injections to uncooperative patients.
- Wherever possible, replace sharps with other instruments or procedures.
- Never leave sharps lying around.
- Do not resheath used needles, unless there is a safe means of recapping (DH 1990). During 2004 a needlestick survey was undertaken by 20 self-selecting participating sites; 4% of injuries occurred during recapping of needles (Watterson 2005).
- Do not remove used needles from the syringe, but dispose of needles and syringes as a single unit.
- Do not bend, break or otherwise manipulate used needles by hand prior to disposal.
- Sharps should not be passed from hand to hand.
- Use needle-free or safety sharps device where possible after receiving education and training in their use (Trim & Elliott 2003).
- The person using the sharp should dispose of the used sharp. In the survey of self-selecting participating sites mentioned above just under a third of injuries were sustained by staff other than the original user of the sharp (Watterson 2005).
- Dispose of sharps immediately after use into a sharps container (British Standards Institution 1990).
- Follow the manufacturer's instructions when assembling, using and sealing sharps containers.
- Place the sharps container where sharps are being used.
- Do not overfill the sharps container or attempt to press down upon sharps to make more room in the sharps container.
- Filled sharps containers must be transported in a safe manner to an incinerator to be incinerated (ICNA/DH 2005).

Other factors that contribute to poor practice and which will increase the risk of sharps injuries include fatigue, stress, poor lighting, crowded working conditions, unsuitable furniture and working alone with a patient who may be agitated, abusive or confused (Ferguson *et al.* 2004; Suzuki *et al.* 2005).

Hanrahan and Reutter (1997) reported that modifying behaviour had failed to reduce sharps injuries and therefore it was necessary to seek other means of prevention, such as safer devices. Needleless administration and phlebotomy systems which eliminate the risk of a sharps injury are now available (Russo *et al.* 1999).

One of the frequently stated problems with inoculation accidents is underreporting. A confidential survey at a British district general hospital found that whilst 80% of respondents were aware that needlestick injuries should be reported only 51% of those that had received an injury reported the incident (Elmiyeh *et al.* 2004).

Houang and Hurley (1997) emphasized that knowledge of the risk alone is not sufficient to motivate correct behaviour, while McCoy *et al.* (2001) recommended a creative infection control programme based on modifiable factors to improve compliance with infection control policies and procedures. More recently preventative strategies have focused on needle protective devices which should reduce the incidence of sharp injuries (Trim & Elliott 2003).

Clinical waste

All waste arising from medical and nursing care which may cause infection to those exposed to it must be contained, transported and disposed of following the guidance contained in The Hazardous Waste (England and Wales) regulations (2005). Waste is divided into four categories: hazardous waste, non-hazardous waste, special waste to be treated as hazardous and special waste to be treated as non-hazardous.

The Department of Health Environment and sustainability Health Technical Memorandum 07-01: Safe management of Healthcare waste replaces Hazardous Waste (England and Wales) regulations (2005) replace the Special Waste Regulations 1996 following a review of the regulations by the Department of the Environment, Transport and the Regions which was published in June 2000 (DH 2006a).

There continues to be a requirement for the safe disposal of all waste in heavy-duty leak-proof bags and for all sharps to be disposed of in sharps containers which comply with the regulations.

It is essential that sharps are only placed in a designated sharps container. If they are inadvertently mixed with the general clinical waste, the many persons handling this waste during removal and eventual disposal could receive an inoculation injury. Postexposure care is much more complicated when the sharps source is unknown. Whilst all bags and containers must be labelled with the place of origin, it is still very difficult to accurately identify whom the sharp was used on. It must be remembered that HIV and hepatitis B protected by organic matter will survive in the environment for some time (Gould 1994).

Accident policy

When an inoculation accident or contamination of damaged skin occurs, action must be taken by:

- the injured person
- the microbiology department
- occupational health.

This is essential as an injury that leads to the injured person contracting HIV or hepatitis B or C will affect work and personal relationships (DH 2002).

Injured person

1. Encourage bleeding.
2. Wash area under running water.
3. Dry carefully and apply waterproof dressing.
4. Seek medical help for large wounds.
5. Obtain blood from patient on whom the needle had been used.
6. Arrange to give blood.
7. Fill in accident form.
8. Report incident to manager and occupational health.
9. Take bloods and accident form to microbiology department.

When contamination of skin occurs, the area must be washed under hot soapy water without the use of a nailbrush which could damage the skin and allow the entry of microorganisms. If contamination of eyes, nose or mouth occurs the area must be washed thoroughly with copious amounts of water and tasks 5–9 above must be undertaken (DH 2004).

Microbiology department

1. Test the patient's blood for hepatitis B and, if appropriate, hepatitis C and HIV. Store the remainder of blood in freezer.
2. Store the injured person's blood in freezer.

Occupational health

The patient's virology results coupled with the injured person's vaccination record will be used to decide the appropriate postexposure prophylaxis.

Hepatitis

Hepatitis B

The risk of a patient acquiring hepatitis B following a needlestick injury from a known hepatitis B-positive healthcare worker is 1 in 3 and with vaccination the risk reduces by 90%. However, vaccination must not replace good infection control practices (DH 1990).

Following all injuries, occupational health should evaluate whether the injured person needs vaccinations, booster vaccinations and a discussion on why the accident happened and how a similar incident could be avoided in future.

Persons who have received a needlestick injury or had contaminated eyes, mouth, fresh cuts or abrasions with blood from a known hepatitis B surface antigen (HBsAg)-positive patient will be offered the accelerated course of hepatitis B vaccine and hepatitis B immunoglobulin if the person has not been vaccinated. Previously vaccinated persons will receive a booster, while non-responders to hepatitis B vaccine will receive hepatitis B immunoglobulin and be considered for a booster dose of hepatitis B vaccine (DH 2006b).

Hepatitis C

The risk of acquiring hepatitis following a needlestick injury from a known hepatitis C-positive person is 1 in 30 (DH 2002). There is no available hepatitis C vaccine; infection can lead to a chronic carrier state and, in some cases, hepatocellular carcinoma (DH 2004). Treatment for hepatitis C is now available and effective in over 50% of cases, although success rates vary (DH 2004).

Human immunodeficiency virus (HIV)

The risk of a patient acquiring HIV following a needlestick injury from a known HIV-positive healthcare worker is 1 in 300 (DH 2002). The risk of a healthcare worker acquiring HIV following a needlestick injury from a known HIV-positive patient depends on the patient's viral load but is estimated to be 3 per 1000 (DH 2004). In the 2002 report viral load was never mentioned Antiretroviral prophylactic drugs are available following a significant injury. Help and support must also be immediately available following such incidents (DH 2004). Education and strict adherence to correct techniques and practices and infection control guidelines are essential to protect the patient from infection and to safeguard healthcare workers against exposure to bloodborne diseases.

Audit

Audit plays an important role in monitoring quality of care based on outcomes (e.g. infection rates) by the provision of useful information. Corrective action can be taken, followed by re-evaluation and, hopefully, resolution of problems.

The Hospital Infection Working Group of the Department of Health and Public Health Laboratory Service (1995) discussed the importance of audit of infection control policies in wards and departments. They mentioned the inclusion of i.v. catheterization as a topic for audit, suggesting that the results of such audits should be fed back to each ward, with educational programmes introduced as necessary to correct deficiencies (Hospital Infection Working Group of the Department of Health and Public Health Laboratory Service 1995).

Specific audit tools for hospital and community settings that include i.v. devices are available with recommendations on their use. The Infection Control Nurses Association along with the DH have produced audit tools for monitoring infection control guidelines in the hospital and the community setting (ICNA/DH 2004, 2005). The Department of Health 'Saving Lives' delivery programme is aimed at reducing healthcare-associated infection, and includes high impact interventions, included in this programme is the care of CVC and peripheral intravenous cannula care (DH 2005 updated 2007).

Research

The scope of i.v. therapy continues to become more complex and specialized. Nurses must be well versed in all aspects of care. Policies and procedures must be detailed, follow international guidelines and be kept abreast of new research. All nurses involved in i.v. care are required to know all of these policies and procedures, which are reviewed regularly.

Clinical research provides a basis for the practice of i.v. therapy by validating standards and by highlighting the practices that provide quality patient care. There are many issues related to i.v. practice which could be a focus for nursing research, including:

- evaluation of the effects of skill mix and staffing levels on:
    - infection rates
    - occlusion of catheters
    - sharps injuries
- evaluation of the impact of educational events on:
    - infection rates
    - occlusion of catheters
    - sharps injuries
- product evaluation research into:
    - i.v. safety devices, e.g. needleless systems
    - improved occlusive transparent dressings
    - catheter hubs which prevent endoluminal contamination.

The Department of Health state that a national research strategy is required to address gaps in current scientific and clinical knowledge about how to reduce healthcare-associated infections (DH 2003).

Conclusion

Remarkable clinical success has been achieved in the treatment of many diseases. It is inevitable that even greater changes will come in the future, with new developments in medical and nursing practice. Unfortunately, modern medical, surgical and immunosuppressive treatments have increased patients' susceptibility to infection. The provision of expert nursing care is the primary consideration, as vulnerable inpatients may have to be nursed in wards alongside patients with existing infections and be cared for by nursing and medical staff who care for both infected and vulnerable patients.

Intravenous catheter infection continues to be an important cause of mortality and morbidity for immunocompromised patients. One of the biggest challenges is the prevention of infection or, if this fails, the prompt diagnosis and treatment of the infection. It will never be possible to prevent all hospital-acquired infections, as the hospital environment, other patients and healthcare workers will expose the patients to exogenous infections during their stay in hospital. Similarly, many infections will be acquired endogenously. Nevertheless, every effort must be made to reduce the incidence of hospital-acquired infection.

Many issues related to the prevention of infection remain unresolved. This chapter has reviewed strategies in an attempt to help reduce the incidence of i.v.-related infection.

References

Adler A, Yaniv I, Stenberg R *et al.* (2006) Infectious complications of implantable ports and Hickman catheters in paediatric haematology-oncology patients. *Journal of Hospital Infection* 62(3): 359–365.

Advisory Committee on Dangerous Pathogens (1995) *Protection against Bloodborne Infections in the Workplace.* HMSO, London.

Alderman RL, Sugarbaker PH (2005) Prospective non-randomized trial of silver impregnated cuff central lines. *International Surgery* 90(4): 219–222.

Archibald LK, Ramos M, Arduino MJ *et al.* (1998) *Enterobacter cloacae* and *Pseudomonas aeruginosa* polymicrobial bloodstream infections traced to extrinsic contamination of a dextrose multidose vial. *Journal of Pediatrics* 133(5): 640–644.

Ayliffe GAJ, Fraise AP, Geddes AM *et al.* (2000) Physical and Chemical Disinfection. In: Ayliffe GAJ, Fraise AP, Geddes AM, Mitchell K, eds. *Control of Hospital Infection. A Practical Handbook*, 4th edn. pp. 75–91. Chapman & Hall Medical, London.

Bal AM, Gould IM (2005) Antibiotic resistance in *Staphylococcus aureus* and its relevance in therapy. *Expert Opinion on Pharmacotherapy* 6(13): 2257–2269.

Balakrishnan G, Simpkins C, Grieg M, Hallworth D (1991) Catheter related sepsis. *British Journal of Intensive Care* 1(1): 17–22.

Bauer E, Denson R (1979) Infection from contaminated elastoplast. *New England Journal of Medicine* 300(7): 370.

Beekmann SE, Henderson DK (2005) Infections caused by percutaneous intravenous devices. In: Mandell GL, Bennett JE, Dolin R, eds. *Principles and Practices of Infectious Diseases*, 6th edn, 2(300) pp. 3347–3361. Elsevier. Churchill Livingstone, New York.

Boktour M, Hanna H, Ansari S *et al.* (2006) Central venous catheter and *Stenotrophomonas maltophilia* bacteraemia in cancer patients. *Cancer* 106(9): 1967–1973.

Boland A, Haycox A, Bagust A, Fitzsimmons L (2003) A randomized controlled trial to evaluate the clinical and cost-effectiveness of Hickman line insertions in adult cancer patients by nurses. *Health Technology Assessment* 7(36): 1–99.

Brady MT (2005) Health care-associated infection in the neonatal intensive care unit. *American Journal of Infection Control* 33(5): 268–275.

Briggs M, Wilson S (1996) The principles of aseptic techniques in wound care. *Professional Nurse* 11(12): 805–810.

British Standards Institution (1990) *Specifications for Sharps Containers.* BS 7320. BSI, Milton Keynes.

Brook SJ, Brook I (1993) Contamination of bar soaps in a household setting. *Microbios* 76(306): 55–57.

Butler SO, Btaiche IF, Alaniz C (2005) Relationship between hyperglycemia and infection in critically ill patients. *Pharmacotherapy* 25(7): 963–976.

Calandra T (2000) Practical guide to host defense mechanisms and the predominant infections encountered in immunocompromised patients. In: Glauser MP, Pizzo PA, eds. *Management of Infections in Immunocompromised Patients*, pp. 3–17. WB Saunders Company Ltd, London.

Callahan JK, Wesorick B (1987) Bacterial growth under a transparent dressing. *American Journal of Infection Control* 15: 231–237.

Carter LW (1994) Bacterial translocation: nursing implications in the care of patients with neutropenia. *Oncology Nurses Forum* 21(5): 857–865.

Chan L, Ngeow YF, Parasakthi N (1998) Bacterial infection of central venous catheters in short term total parenteral nutrition. *The Medical Journal of Malaysia* 53(1): 10–15.

Chandra RK (2002) Nutrition and the immune system from birth to old age. *European Journal of Clinical Nutrition* 56 (Suppl 3): S73–S76.

Chodoff A, Pettis AM, Schoonmaker D, Shelly MA (1995) Polymicrobial Gram negative associated with saline solution flush used with a needleless intravenous system. *American Journal of Infection Control* 23(6): 357–363.

Clarke L (1994) Safety first. *The Journal of Infection Control Nursing* 21(1): 2–6 [in *Nursing Times* 90:5].

Clemence MA, Walker DN, Farr BM (1995) Central venous catheter practice: results of a survey. *American Journal of Infection Control* 23(1): 5–12.

Coello R, Charlett A, Ward V *et al.* (2003) Device-related sources of bacteraemia in English hospitals—opportunities for the prevention of hospital-acquired bacteraemia. *Journal of Hospital Infection* 53(1): 4657.

Coia JE, Duckworth GJ, Edwards DI *et al.* (2006) Guidelines for the control and prevention of methicillin-resistant *Staphylococcus aureus* (MRSA) in healthcare facilities. *Journal of Hospital Infection* 63(Suppl 1): 1–44.

Crossley KB, Peterson AB (2005) Infections in the elderly. In: Mandell GL, Bennett J E, Dolin R, eds. *Principles and Practice of Infectious Diseases*, 6th edn. 2(314) pp. 3517–3523. Elsevier Churchill Livingstone, New York.

Dancer SJ, Coyne M, Robertson C *et al.* (2006) Antibiotic use in association with resistance of environmental organisms in a teaching hospital. *Journal of Hospital Infection* 62(2): 200–206.

Dank LA (2006) Central venous catheter: a review of skin cleansing and dressings. *British Journal of Nursing* 15(12): 650–654.

Dawson SJ (2003) The role of the infection control link nurse. *Journal of Hospital Infection* 54(4): 251–257.

Department of Health (1990) *Guidance for Clinical Health Care Workers' Protection Against Infection with HIV and Hepatitis Viruses. Recommendation of the Expert Advisory Group on AIDS*. HMSO, London.

Department of Health (1999) *The Management of Health and Safety at Work Regulations* 1999, no. 3242. Department of Health, London.

Department of Health (2001) Standard principles for preventing hospital-acquired infections *Journal of Hospital Infection* 47(supplement): S21–S37.

Department of Health (2002) *Health Clearance for Serious Communicable Diseases*. Department of Health Publications.

Department of Health (2003) *Winning Ways. Working Together to Reduce Healthcare Associated Infection in England*. Department of Health Publications.

Department of Health (2004) *Hepatitis C. Essential information for professionals and guidance on testing*. Department of Health Publications, Gateway Reference 3234.

Department of Health (2005 updated last 2007) *Saving Lives. A Delivery Programme to Reduce Healthcare Associated Infection including MRSA*. Department of Health Publications, London.

Department of Health (2006a) *Environment and sustainability Health Technical Memorandum 07-01: Safe management of Healthcare waste*. HMSO, London.

Department of Health (2006b) *Immunisation Against Infectious Diseases*. HMSO, London.

Deshpande KS, Hatem C, Ulrish HL *et al.* (2005) The incidence of infectious complications of central venous catheters at the subclavian, internal jugular, and femoral sites in an intensive care unit population. *Critical Care Medicine* 33(1): 234–235.

Dietze B, Rath A, Wendt C, Martiny H (2001) Survival of MRSA on sterile goods packaging. *Journal of Hospital Infection* 49(4): 255–261.

Dobbins BM, Kite P, Catton JA, Wilcox MH, McMahon MJ (2004) In situ endoluminal brushing, a safe technique for the diagnosis of catheter-related bloodstream infection. *Journal of Hospital Infection* 58(3): 233–237.

Dougherty L (1996) The benefits of an IV team in hospital practice. *Professional Nurse* 11(11): 761–763.

Dougherty L (2004) Vascular access devices: insertion and management. In: Dougherty L, Lister S, eds. *The Royal Marsden Hospital Manual of Clinical Nursing Procedures*, 6th edn, pp. 724–773. Blackwell Publishing, Oxford.

Dunne WM (2002) Bacterial adhesion: seen any good biofilms lately. *Clinical Microbiology Reviews* 15(2): 155–166.

Eggimann P, Sax H, Pittet D (2004) Catheter related infections. *Microbes and Infection* 6(11): 1033–1042.

Elliott TS (1993) Line associated bacteraemias. *Public Health Laboratories Service Communicable Disease Report Review* 3(7): R91–R96.

Elliott TS, Faroqui MH, Armstrong RF, Hanson GC (1994) Guidelines for good practice in central catheterization. *Journal of Hospital Infection* 28(3): 163–176.

Elliott TS, Faroqui MH, Tebbs SE, Armstrong RF, Hanson G C (1995) An audit program for central venous catheter associated infections. *Journal of Hospital Infection* 30(3): 181–191.

Elmiyeh B, Whitaker IS, James MJ (2004) Needle-stick injuries in the National Health Service: a culture of silence. *Journal of the Royal Society of Medicine* 97(7): 326–327.

Ferguson KJ, Waitzkin H, Beekmann SE *et al.* (2004) Critical incidents of nonadherence with standard precautions guidelines among community hospital-based health care workers. *Journal of General Internal Medicine* 19(7): 726–731.

Friedman ND, Kaye KS, Stout JE, McGarry SA, Trivette SL *et al.* (2002) Healthcare-associated bloodstream infections in adults: a reason to change the accepted definition of community-acquired infections. *American Society of Internal Medicine* 137(10): 791–797.

Gabriel J (2004) *The Biology of Cancer*. Whurr Publishers Ltd, London.

Garcia R (2005) A selective role: infection control plays important part on product review committees. Interview by Robert Neil. *Materials Management in Health Care* 14(8): 13–14.

Geddes CC, Walbaum D, Fox JG, Mactier RA (1998) Insertion of internal jugular temporary hemodialysis cannulae by direct ultrasound guidance—a prospective comparison of experienced and inexperienced operators. *Clinical Nephrology* 50(5): 320–325.

Glauser MP, Calandra T (2000) Infections in patients with hematologic malignancies. In: Glauser MP, Pizzo PA, eds. *Management of Infections in Immunocompromised Patients*, pp. 141–189. WB Saunders Company Ltd, London.

Goodinson SM (1990) Good practice ensures minimum risks factors. *Professional Nurse* 6(3): 175–177.

Gould D (1994) Infection control in low risk environments. *Nursing Standard* 8(29): 30–32.

Gray A (2006) Blood component support. In: Grundy M, ed. *Nursing in Haematological Oncology*, 2nd edn, 2(12), pp. 245–265.

Greaves A (1985) We'll just freshen you up, dear. *Nursing Times Supplement* March 6: 3–8. Ballière Tindall. Elsevier, Edinburgh.

Hanrahan A, Reutter L (1997) A critical review of the literature on sharps injuries: epidemiology, management of exposure and prevention. *Journal of Advanced Nursing* 25 (1) 144–154.

Hart SM (2004) Aseptic technique. In: Dougherty L, Lister S, eds. *The Royal Marsden Hospital Manual of Clinical Nursing Procedures*, 6th edn, pp. 50–61. Blackwell Publishing, Oxford.

Heal C, Bruettner P, Raasch B *et al.* (2006) Can sutures get wet? Prospective randomized controlled trial of wound management in general practice. *British Medical Journal* 332(7549): 1053–1054.

Health and Safety Executive (1995) *The Reporting of Injuries, Disease and Dangerous Occurrences Regulations* (RIDDOR). Health and Safety Executive, London.

Health and Safety Executive (2002) *Control of Substances Hazardous to Health Regulations*. Health and Safety Executive, London.

Health Protection Agency (2005a) *Trends in Antimicrobial Resistance in England and Wales*. Health Protection Agency, London.

Health Protection Agency (2005b) *Eye of the Needle*. Health Protection Agency, London.

Hoffmann KK, Weber DJ, Samsa GP, William AR (1992) Transparent polyurethane film as an intravenous catheter dressing. *Journal of the American Medical Association* 267(15): 2072–2076.

Hospital Infection Working Group of the Department of Health and Public Health Laboratory Service (1995) *Hospital Infection Control Guidance on the Control of Infection In Hospitals*. Department of Health, London.

Houang ETS, Hurley R (1997) Anonymous questionnaire survey on the knowledge and practices of hospital staff in infection control. *Journal of Hospital Infection* 35(4) 301–306.

Infection Control Nurses Association (ICNA)/DH (2004) *Audit Tools for Monitoring Infection Control Standards*. Department of Health, London.

ICNA/DH (2005) *Audit Tools for Monitoring Infection Control Guidelines within the Community Setting*. Department of Health, London.

Infusion Nurses Society (2006) Infusion nursing standards of practice. *Journal of Infusion Nursing*. Supplement 10(29): S1–S92.

Ironside JW (2006) Variant Creutzfeldt–Jakob disease: risk of transmission by blood transfusion and blood therapies. *Haemophilia* 12 (Suppl 1): 8–15.

Johnson A, Oppenheim BA (1992) Vascular catheter related sepsis: diagnosis and prevention. *Journal of Hospital Infection* 20(2): 67–78.

Keenlyside D (1993) Avoiding an unnecessary outcome. *Professional Nurse* 8(5): 288–291.

Kjonniksen I, Anderson BM, Sondenaa VG, Segadal L (2002) Preoperative hair removal—a systematic literature review. *AORN Journal* 75(5): 928–938.

Kite P, Dobbins BM, Wilcox MH *et al.* (1997) Evaluation of a novel endoluminal brush method for in situ diagnosis of catheter related sepsis. *Journal of Clinical Pathology* 50(4): 278–282.

Koerner RJ, Morgan S, Ford M, Orr KE, McComb JM, Gould FK (1997) Outbreak of Gram-negative septicaemia caused by contaminated continuous infusions prepared in a nonclinical area. *Journal of Hospital Infection* 36(4) 285–289.

Larwood KA, Anstey CM, Dunn SV (2000) Managing central venous catheters: a prospective randomized trial of two methods. *Australian Critical Care* 13(2): 44–50.

Lau CE (1996) Transparent and gauze dressings and their effect on infection rates of central venous catheters: a review of past and current literature. *Journal of Intravenous Nursing* 19(5): 240–245.

Loach L (1997) Blue days. *Nursing Times* 93(32): 30–31.

Lundgren A, Ek A (1996) Factors influencing nurses' handling and control of peripheral intravenous lines. An interview study. *International Journal of Nursing Studies* 33(2): 131–142.

Maki DG (1977) A semi quantitative culture method for identifying intravenous catheter related sepsis. *New England Journal of Medicine* 296(23): 1305–1309.

Maki DG, Crnich CJ (2003) Line sepsis in the ICU: Prevention, diagnosis and management. *Seminars in Respiratory and Critical Care Medicine* 24(1): 23–36.

Maki DG, Goldman DA, Rhame FS (1973) Infection control in intravenous therapy. *Annals of Internal Medicine* 79(6) 867–887.

Maki DG, Ringer M, Alvarado CJ (1991) Prospective randomized trial of povidone-iodine, alcohol, and chlorhexidine for prevention of infection associated with central venous and arterial catheters. *Lancet* 338(8767): 339–342.

Malhotra M, Sharma JB, Wadhwa L *et al.* (2004) Prospective study of glove perforation in obstetrical and gynecological operations: are we safe enough? *The Journal of Obstetrics and Gynaecology Research* 30(4): 319–322.

McCoy KD, Beekmann SE, Ferguson KJ (2001) Monitoring adherence to standard precautions. *American Journal of Infection Control* 29(1): 24–31.

Medicines and Healthcare Products Regulatory Agency (MHRA) (2005) *Safeguarding Public Health*. MHRA, London.

Medical Devices Directorate (1991) *Specification for Non-sterile, Natural Latex Examination Gloves*, document no. TSS/3000.010/1. Department of Health, London.

Mehtar S, Taylor P (1981) A review of bacteriological observation in the care of IV cannulae. *British Journal of Intravenous Therapy* June: 16–22.

Mermel LA (2000) Prevention of intravascular catheter-related infections. *Annals of Internal Medicine* 132(5): 391–402.

Miller PK (1998) Downsizing. Use intravenous clinicians to maintain quality venous access care. *Journal of Intravenous Nursing* 21(2): 105–112.

Mims C, Dockrell HM, Goering RV, Roitt I, Wakelin D, Zuckermann M (2004) Infections of the skin, soft tissue, muscle and associated systems. In: Mims C, Dockrell HM, Goering RV, Roitt I, Wakelin D, Zuckermann M eds. *Medical Microbiology*, 3rd edn, (26) pp. 349–383. Elsevier Mosby, Edinburgh.

Mock V, Olsen M (2003) Current management of fatigue and anaemia in patients with cancer. *Seminars in Oncology Nursing* 19 (4 Suppl 2): 36–41.

Montville R, Chen Y, Schaffner DW (2002) Risk assessment of hand-washing efficacy using literature and experimental data. *International Journal of Food Microbiology* 73(2–3): 305–313.

Moore KL, Kainer MA, Badrawi N *et al.* (2005) Neonatal sepsis in Egypt associated with bacterial contamination of glucose-containing intravenous fluids. *The Pediatric Infectious Disease Journal* 24(7): 590–594.

National Institute for Health and Clinical Excellence (NICE) (2003) *Infection Control. Prevention of Healthcare-Associated Infection in Primary and Community Care*. Clinical Guideline 2. National Institute for Health and Clinical Excellence, London.

Nouwen JL, Wielenga JJ, van Overhagen H *et al.* (1999) Hickman catheter related infection in neutropenic patients: insertion in the operating theatre versus insertion in the radiology suite. *Journal of Clinical Oncology* 17(4): 1304–1311.

O'Grady NP, Alexander M, Dellinger JL, Heard SO, Maki DG *et al.* (2002) Guidelines for the prevention of intravascular catheter-related infections. *Morbidity and Mortality Weekly Report* 51 (RR–10): 1–29.

Osma S, Kahveci SF, Kaya FN *et al.* (2006) Efficacy of antiseptic-impregnated catheters on catheter colonization and catheter-related bloodstream infections in patients in an intensive care unit. *Journal of Hospital Infection* 62(2): 156–162.

Oztoprak N, Cevik MA, Akinci E (2006) Risk factors for ICU-acquired methicillin-resistant *Staphylococcus aureus* infections. *American Journal of Infection Control* 34(1): 1–5.

Patrick DR, Findon G, Miller TE (1997) Residual moisture determines the level of touch-contact-associated bacterial transfer following handwashing. *Epidemiology and Infection* 119(3): 319–325.

Pereira LJ, Lea GM, Wade K (1997) An evaluation of five protocols for surgical handwashing in relation to skin condition and microbial counts. *Journal of Hospital Infection* 36(1): 49–65 .

Polyzos A, Tsavaris N, Kosmas C *et al.* (2001) Hypersensitivity reactions to carboplatin administration are common but not always severe: a 10-year experience. *Oncology* 61(2): 129–133.

Pratt RJ, Pellowe CM, Wilson JA *et al.* (2007) ePIC 2 National evidence-based guidelines for preventing healthcare associated infection in NHS hospitals in England. *Journal of Hospital Infection* 655(Suppl): S1–S64.

Regan FA, Hewitt P, Barbara JA, Contreras M (2000) Prospective investigation of transfusion transmitted infection in recipients of over 20 000 units of blood. TTI study group. *British Medical Journal* 320(7256): 403–406.

Rey JB, Faure C, Brion F (2005) Stability of all-in-one standard formulae for paediatric parenteral nutrition. *PDA Journal of Pharmaceutical Science and Technology* 59(3): 206–220.

Ritz BW, Gardner EM (2006) Malnutrition and energy restriction differentially affect viral immunity. *Journal of Nutrition* 136(5): 1141–1144.

Roitt I, Brostoff J, Male D (2001) *Immunology*, 6th edn. 11 pp. 182–189. Mosby, Edinburgh.

Rossoff LJ, Lam S, Hilton E, Borenstein M, Isenberg HD (1993) Is the use of boxed gloves in an intensive care unit safe? *American Journal of Medicine* 94(6): 602–607.

Royal College of Nursing (2005) *Standards for Infusion Therapy*. Royal College of Nursing, London.

Rupp ME, Lisco SJ, Lipsett PA *et al.* (2005) Effect of a second-generation venous catheter impregnated with chlorhexidine and silver sulfadiazine on central-related infections: a randomized, controlled trial. *Annals of Internal Medicine* 143(8): 570–580.

Russo PL, Harrington GA, Spelman DW (1999) Needleless intravenous systems: A review. *American Journal of Infection Control* 27(5): 431–434.

Safdar N, Maki DG (2004) The pathogenesis of catheter-related bloodstream infection with non-cuffed short-term central venous catheters. *Intensive Care Medicine* 30(1): 62–67.

Scalley RD, Vans CS, Cochran RS (1992) The impact of an IV team on the occurrence of intravenous-related phlebitis. *Journal of Intravenous Nursing* 15(2): 100–109.

Sehirali S, Inal MM, Ozsezgin S *et al.* (2005) A randomized prospective study of comparison of reservoir port versus conventional vascular access in advanced stage ovarian carcinoma cases treated with chemotherapy. *International Journal of Gynecological Cancer* 15(2): 228–232.

Sexton T, Clarke P, O'Neill E *et al.* (2006) Environmental reservoirs of methicillin-resistant *Staphylococcus aureus* in isolation rooms: correlation with patient isolates and implications for hospital hygiene. *Journal of Hospital Infection* 62(2): 187–194.

Shiomori T, Miyamoto H, Makishima K *et al.* (2002) Evaluation of bedmaking related airborne and surface methicillin resistant *Staphylococcus aureus* contamination *Journal of Hospital Infection* 50(1): 30–35.

Sitges-Serra A, Pi-Suner T, Garces JM, Segura M (1995) Pathogenesis and prevention of catheter related septicemia. *American Journal of Infectious Disease* 23(5): 310–316.

Soldan K, Barbara JA, Ramsay ME, Hall AJ (2003) Estimation of the risk of hepatitis B virus, hepatitis C virus and human immunodeficiency virus infectious donations entering the blood supply in England 1993–2001. *Vox Sanguinis* 84(4): 274–286.

Srinivasan V, Maestroni GJ, Cardinali DP, Esquifino AI, Pandi-Perumal SR, Miller SC (2005) Melatonin, immune function and aging. *Immunity and Ageing* 2(1): 17.

Suzuki K *et al.* (2005) Daytime sleepiness, sleep habits and occupational accidents among nurses. *Journal of Advanced Nursing* 52(4): 445–453.

Taylor JH, Brown KL, Toivenen J, Holah JT (2000) A microbiological evaluation of warm air hand driers with respect to hand hygiene and the washroom environment. *Journal of Applied Microbiology* 89(6): 910–919.

Timsit JF, Sebille V, Farkas JC *et al.* (1996) Effect of subcutaneous tunneling on internal jugular catheter-related sepsis in critically ill patients: a prospective randomized multicenter study. *Journal of the American Medical Association* 276(17): 1416–1420.

Timsit JF, Bruneel F, Cheval C *et al.* (1999) Use of tunneled femoral catheters to prevent catheter-related infection. A randomized, controlled trial. *Annals of Internal Medicine* 130(9): 729–735.

Tramont EC, Hoover DL (2005) Innate (general or non-specific) host defense mechanisms. In: Mandell GL, Bennett JE, Dolin R, eds. *Principles and Practices of Infectious Disease*, 6th edn, 1(4) pp. 34–41. Churchill Livingstone, New York.

Treston-Aurand J, Olmsted RN, Allen-Bridson K, Craig CP (1997) Impact of dressing materials on central venous catheter infection rates. *Journal of Intravenous Nursing* 20(4): 201–206.

Trim JC, Elliott TS (2003) A review of sharps injuries and preventative strategies. *Journal of Hospital Infection* 53(4): 237–242.

Van Lingen RA, Baerts W, Marquering AC, Ruijs GJ (2004) The use of in-line intravenous filters in sick newborn infants. *Acta Paediatrica* 93(5): 658–662.

Watterson L (2005) Sharp thinking. *Nursing Standard* 20(5): 20–22.

Wilson J (2006) *Infection Control in Clinical Practice*. 2nd edn, 8, pp. 157–172. Baillière Tindall, London.

Wolosker N, Yazbek G, Munia MA, Zerati AE, Langer M, Nishinari K (2004) Totally implantable femoral vein catheters in cancer patients. *European Journal of Surgical Oncology* 30(7): 771–775.

CHAPTER 5

Pharmacological Aspects of Intravenous Therapy

Zoe Whittington

Introduction

Intravenous (i.v.) medicines are manufactured to extremely high standards. They must be sterile, non-pyrogenic and particle free, whilst also ideally being isotonic with body plasma (DH 2005). Medicines for i.v. administration are available as:

- ready-to-administer aqueous solutions, for example atropine or heparin
- sterile powders requiring reconstitution with or without further dilution before administration, for example flucloxacillin or ceftazidime
- ready-to-administer non-aqueous solutions, for example Diazemuls or propofol

Whilst other chapters deal with clinical aspects of i.v. therapy, the aim of this chapter is to:

1. describe the methods of i.v. medicine administration
2. detail important pharmacological considerations that impact on the administration of i.v. medicines
3. discuss the responsibilities of all those involved in the prescription, supply and administration of i.v. therapy
4. highlight areas of good practice in i.v. therapy.

The Administration of Medicines

A drug (or medicine) is any substance taken by mouth, injected into muscle, the skin, a blood vessel or body cavity, or applied topically to treat or prevent a disease or condition (Mosby 2005).

In the majority of cases, in order to reach the site of pharmacological action, medicines must be absorbed into the bloodstream. The method of administration determines the route taken to enter the bloodstream and the speed at which absorption occurs. Where different pharmaceutical formulations are available, for example tablet, injection, suppository or cream, the route of administration selected depends on a number of different factors. These include:

1. the severity of the patient's illness
2. the urgency with which the medicinal effect is needed

3. the part of the body requiring treatment
4. the patient's general state of health, perhaps most notably, their ability to swallow (Henry 2004).

Why use the intravenous route?

Intravenous therapy may be required for the treatment of acutely ill patients who are unable to take oral medicines or for medicines that have a low oral bioavailability. Some of the advantages and disadvantages of selecting this route are described in Figure 5.1.

Campbell (1996) estimated that 25 million patients per year in the NHS have some form of i.v. access during their hospitalization. The widespread use of i.v. therapy across a variety of healthcare settings is well recognized, and consequently the number of nurses caring for patients with i.v. therapy requirements is increasing (Jackson 2003). These i.v. therapy needs will, in the majority of cases, be met via peripheral i.v. access.

Peripheral i.v. access:

- is easy to achieve
- can be established quickly
- is relatively cheap and cost effective.

Advantages	Disadvantages
An immediate therapeutic effect is achieved through rapid delivery of the medicine to its target site	No facility to 'remove' a medicine once it has been intravenously administered
Pain +/– irritation caused by some substances if given subcutaneously or intramuscularly is avoided	Insufficient control of administration may result in speedshock or circulatory overload
Provides an alternative route of administration for patients who are unable to swallow or cannot tolerate medicines or fluids given orally	Additional complications can occur, such as microbial contamination, vascular irritation or medicine incompatibilities
	Needle phobia
Provides an alternative route of administration for medicines which are not absorbed at a sufficient dose from any other route, for example as a result of large molecular size or instability in gastric juices, or where erratic absorption occurs, for example following intramuscular administration	Altered body image resulting especially from central venous access devices
	Time taken for administration; must be performed slowly with constant monitoring of the patient's response
Allows a facility for control over the rate of administration of some medicines; prolonged action can be achieved by administering a dilute infusion over a prolonged period of time	

Figure 5.1 Advantages and disadvantages of the intravenous route. (Adapted from Dougherty 2002. Reprinted with permission of RCN Publishing Company.)

However, it also:

- risks complications of phlebitis, thrombophlebitis, infiltration or infection
- is not appropriate for therapy lasting more than a few days (Lister *et al.* 2004)
- does not allow simultaneous administration of several drugs or parenteral nutrition
- can only be used for infusions of isotonic, non-irritant, non-vesicant solutions (RCN 2005)
- is usually not appropriate for patients in the community (Kayley & Finlay 2003).

Fluid replacement

Body fluid volume, electrolyte concentration and acid–base balance are normally maintained within narrow limits despite wide variations in dietary intake, metabolic activity and environmental stresses. Homeostasis of body fluids is preserved primarily by the kidney and other interrelated physiological mechanisms (Horne *et al.* 1997). However, fluid replacement therapy may be indicated in the management of fluid or electrolyte imbalances which occur, for example, following surgery, from losses via fluid drains or as a result of dehydration, vomiting or diarrhoea (Hand 2001).

Sodium chloride

Sodium chloride in water is available in a variety of concentrations, and primarily acts as a source of electrolyte and fluid. Sodium chloride 0.9% is isotonic with physiological fluids, so that administration, therefore, will not create an osmotic movement of water across the cell membrane unless the intracellular fluid is more or less concentrated than usual. The extracellular fluid usually contains somewhere between 135 and 145 mmol of sodium chloride per litre. Sodium chloride 0.9% contains 150 mmol sodium per litre and will usually be administered to sustain extracellular fluid volume by compensating for losses resulting from dehydration or fluid drains following surgery (Horne *et al.* 1997).

Sodium chloride 3% (500 mmol sodium/L) or 5% (835 mmol sodium/L) are hypertonic solutions used to expand intravascular volume by pulling endothelial and intracellular water into the intravascular space; or used to restore sodium levels in severe sodium depletion, known as hyponatraemia. Hypertonic solutions must be used with extreme caution in the treatment of hyponatraemia though, as over-rapid correction can result in serious neurological adverse effects such as central pontine myelinolysis (Merck 1999). Hypertonic saline solutions can also cause irritation to peripheral veins and may result in fluid overload as a result of large fluid shifts from the intracellular fluid to the extracellular fluid.

Sodium chloride 0.45% (75 mmol sodium/L) is a hypotonic solution that is more useful than sodium chloride 0.9%, when the amount of fluid required for rehydration is unknown. It acts as a fluid and sodium replenisher (Horne *et al.* 1997).

Glucose

Administration of glucose in water is a useful means of replacing and maintaining fluid volume without altering existing electrolyte balance and provides a source of calories: 1 litre of glucose 5% provides approximately 170 kcal (Hand 2001). Whilst solutions of glucose 5% in water are classified as isotonic with physiological fluids, on administration they rapidly become hypotonic resulting from the rapid metabolism of glucose, leaving only water to be distributed across the fluid compartments (Cooper & Moore 1999).

Concentrations of greater than 5% glucose solutions are hypertonic and due to their low pH can result in peripheral vein irritation and thrombophlebitis. Dehydration can occur following rapid infusion as a result of osmotic diuresis.

Glucose and sodium chloride mixtures

A range of concentrations of glucose in sodium chloride solutions are readily available and combine the advantages of the separate fluids where there is both water and sodium depletion. A 1:1 mixture of isotonic sodium chloride 0.9% and 5% glucose allows some of the water (free of sodium) to enter the body cells that suffer most from dehydration. The sodium salt with a volume of water determined by the normal plasma sodium remains extracellular. Hypotonic solutions, for example glucose 2.5% in sodium chloride 0.9% drive fluid from the plasma into the interstitial space and are therefore used to rehydrate body cells.

Maintenance fluid should accurately reflect daily requirements and close monitoring is required to avoid fluid and electrolyte imbalance (Horne *et al.* 1997).

Clinical pharmacology

The interactions between a medicine and the body can be divided into two broad subheadings.

Pharmacodynamics: The actions of a *medicine* on the body, including pharmacological activity and adverse effects.

Pharmacokinetics: The actions of the *body* on a medicine, including its absorption, distribution, metabolism and excretion (Bennett & Brown 2003).

Absorption

Absorption is the process by which a medicine is taken into the body and is dependent on both the agent's properties and the route of administration. The term 'bioavailability' is a more useful concept when considering the amount of medicine present in the body available to have a pharmacological effect. Bioavailability is defined as the fraction of unchanged medicine reaching the systemic circulation following administration, regardless of route. When a medicine is injected intravenously, by definition, 100% of the dose administered reaches the systemic circulation and is available to exert its therapeutic effect. However, the bioavailability of orally administered medicines may be less than 100% for two main reasons.

Incomplete absorption   Most medicines taken by mouth are absorbed through the cells of the wall of the small intestine into the blood vessels supplying it. The medicine then enters the general systemic circulation via the liver and is carried around the rest of the body until reaching the site of its intended action. The oral bioavailability of aciclovir, an antiviral used in the treatment of herpes infections, is low because its chemical structure is too hydrophilic (having an affinity to water) to cross the lipid cell membrane of the gut. Conversely, the highly lipophilic (having an affinity to lipids) nature of the chemical structure of atenolol, a beta-blocker used in the treatment of hypertension, means that it is able to pass through the cells of the gut wall but is not soluble enough to cross the water layer adjacent to them (Katzung 2004).

First-pass elimination (Figure 5.2)   Following absorption across the gut wall, the blood vessels supplying the small intestine carry the medicine directly to the liver through the portal circulation before reaching the general systemic circulation. The liver is responsible for the metabolism of some, but not all, medicines. It breaks them down into smaller pieces which may or may not be pharmacologically active. Those medicines that are broken down into pharmacologically inactive components are said to undergo first-pass elimination. For example ranitidine, an H_2-receptor antagonist used in the treatment of duodenal or gastric ulcers, is broken down by the liver to inactive metabolites which are then absorbed into bile and excreted in the faeces. The dose of orally administered ranitidine must therefore exceed the amount the liver is capable of metabolizing in one go, such that some is able to pass through the liver and reach the general systemic circulation.

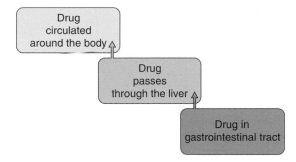

Figure 5.2 First-pass metabolism. Drugs absorbed into the bloodstream from the gastrointestinal tract undergo some metabolism in the liver before reaching the general circulation.

Medicines administered intravenously bypass the portal circulation and therefore do not undergo first-pass elimination (Katzung 2004).

Distribution

Distribution, in this context, is the movement of a medicine within the body. Most medicines are distributed widely, in part dissolved in water, in part bound to plasma and in part bound to tissues. The pattern of distribution will usually be uneven and reflects certain physiological and physiochemical properties of the medicine such as, for example, its ability to bind selectively to plasma or protein tissues or remain localized within particular organs. The site of a medicine's localization is likely to influence its action (for example, whether it crosses the blood–brain barrier to enter the brain), or the time it spends in the body and thereby its duration of action as a result of the amount or strength of plasma/tissue binding (Bennett & Brown 2003).

When protein bound, a medicine is largely inactive and hence unable to exert its pharmacological effect. However, in most cases, this binding is loose and medicines can be released as free drug down the concentration gradient as plasma levels of the drug fall or as a result of being displaced by a competing medicine with a higher affinity for that site. This is an important consideration for highly protein- or tissue-bound medicines (e.g. digoxin, warfarin or phenytoin), where displacement would result in sudden raised levels of free drug and hence lead to the risk of toxicity. For example, the administration of verapamil to a patient already receiving digoxin may result in toxic blood plasma levels of digoxin (McGavock 2005).

Two phases of distribution may be recognized and are shown in Figure 5.3.

1. The initial phase of distribution reflects the cardiac output and regional blood flow. The heart, liver, kidney, brain and other well-perfused organs receive most of the medicine during the first few minutes.
2. The second phase is slower and results in the delivery of medicine to muscle, most viscera, skin and fat. This may take several minutes to several hours (McGavock 2005).

Precise information about the concentration of a medicine attained in various tissues and fluids would be useful but can only be achieved through biopsy samples and is therefore usually unavailable for humans. However, blood plasma can be readily sampled. When considered with the dose administered, the drug concentration in blood plasma samples provides a measure of whether a drug tends to remain in the circulation or is distributed from the plasma into tissues (Bennett & Brown 2003).

However, it is not primarily the change in blood plasma levels that concerns practitioners but the effect of each individual dose of a medicine as noted by its onset,

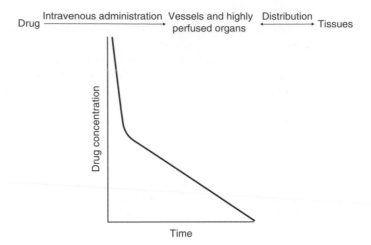

Figure 5.3   After intravenous administration, a drug reaches the blood vessels, and thus the most highly perfused organs in the central compartment, before affecting the peripheral tissues.

magnitude and duration of action. Unfortunately, accurate information about the time course of a medicine's effect is less readily available than information about the plasma levels achieved from individual doses. So, what is the relationship between effect and plasma levels, and when can responses be predicted by measuring drug concentration in plasma? It may be assumed that the effect of a medicine is related to its concentration at the receptor site and that in turn, the plasma concentration is likely to be constantly related to, but not necessarily the same as, tissue concentration. For many medicines, the correlation between plasma concentration and clinical effect is better than that observed between dose and effect. However, monitoring therapy by measuring plasma levels— 'therapeutic drug monitoring'—is only practical when plasma concentrations have been shown to correlate well with drug effect (e.g. gentamicin, theophylline and ciclosporin) and when therapeutic effect is inconvenient or impossible to measure (e.g. lithium) (Bennett & Brown 2003).

Therapeutic drug monitoring

When the dose of a medicine is increased progressively, the desired response achieved in a patient rises to a maximum point, beyond which further dose increases result only in an increase in adverse effects at the cost of no greater clinical benefit. This is because a medicine does not have a single dose–response curve but different curves for both its positive and negative effects (Bennett & Brown 2003).

The therapeutic index is the ratio between the median toxic dose and the median effective dose. The therapeutic range is defined as the lowest effective serum concentration to the maximum tolerable effective serum concentration. Often there is not a clear distinction between the maximum efficacy and the risk of toxicity. Examples of medicines with a wide therapeutic range include penicillins and cephalosporin antibiotics. Incremental increases in doses can be made within the normal dosing range without undue concern about the risk of developing toxicity under normal circumstances. However, dosage adjustment in medicines with a narrow therapeutic range, such as gentamicin, digoxin and theophylline, must be made cautiously as even small increases or decreases in dose would result in plasma levels falling outside of the therapeutic range and expose the patient to the risk of toxicity or loss of effect. This is important, for example, in the case of digoxin as the signs of its lack of therapeutic effect are difficult to distinguish from its signs of toxicity. Digoxin may be used in the treatment of supraventricular tachycardias (SVTs) but may also cause SVT at excessive doses (Bennett & Brown 2003).

Therefore, in the case of medicines with a narrow therapeutic index, optimization of therapy may involve plasma concentration measurements and monitoring in order to maintain the drug level within the therapeutic range, that is, at a high probability of desired clinical response and a relatively low probability of unacceptable drug toxicity (Winter 2004).

Therapeutic drug monitoring commonly includes patient-specific factors (age, weight, height, body mass index (BMI), sex, history of drug exposure, concurrent disease states), along with the medicine's pharmacology, dose, pharmacokinetic model, route of administration, potential drug interactions, sample processing and analysis. Whilst serum concentration monitoring can provide very useful information, frequent sampling may be detrimental to the patient's condition. The usefulness should always be assessed prior to sampling and should generally be restricted to therapy initiation, dosage alterations and prevention of drug toxicity (Winter 2004).

The proper timing for taking samples is a very significant factor and it varies for different agents and routes of administration. The blood sample should ideally not be taken from the same device through which the medicine has been infused. However, if it is necessary to use the device, then it should be thoroughly flushed with a suitable diluent such as 5–10 mL sodium chloride 0.9% or glucose 5% after drug infusion and before sampling. The choice of flush solution selected is dependent on drug compatibility but would usually be the same as the diluent used for reconstitution/dilution (Schulman *et al.* 1998).

Metabolism

Most medicines are treated by the body as foreign substances and become subject to its various mechanisms for ridding itself of chemical intruders—known as metabolism (Bennett & Brown 2003). The liver is the most important site of metabolism in the body, although the kidney, gut mucosa, lung and skin may also contribute. The processes of metabolism changes medicines in two major ways.

1. Reducing lipid solubility—metabolic reactions which make a drug molecule progressively more water soluble and so favour its elimination in the urine.
2. Altering biological activity—usually the conversion of a pharmacologically active to a pharmacologically inactive substance. However, this may occur in a number of different steps including conversion from one pharmacologically active to another active substance (e.g. the metabolism of codeine to morphine) or conversion of a pharmacologically inactive to an active substance (e.g. the metabolism of cyclophosphamide to 4-keto-cyclophosphamide).

Metabolism can be considered in two broad phases, described as phase 1 and phase 2.

Phase 1   Phase 1 metabolism brings about a change in the drug molecule by processes of oxidation, reduction and/or hydrolysis (Bennett & Brown 2003). Of these, the single most important group of reactions is oxidation, in particular those undertaken by a group of enzymes called the mixed function oxidases. The very large family of cytochrome P450 enzymes (CYP) are the most notable of the mixed function oxidases and are able to neutralize almost any given fat-soluble foreign substance ingested by the body (McGavock 2005). The many forms of CYP are grouped into families, of which the majority concerned with human metabolism belong to the groups CYP1, CYP2 and CYP3. These families are further subdivided, with the family CYP3A being involved in the biotransformation of the majority of all medicines (Bennett & Brown 2003).

However, some medicines disturb CYP function by either reducing (inhibiting) or enhancing (inducing) the enzymes' activity. These effects become important when two medicines are coprescribed, one of which induces or inhibits the CYP enzyme on which the other is dependent for its metabolism. It follows that the inhibition of a CYP will slow the metabolism of a second drug's metabolism, leading to an increase in plasma concentration and possibly to toxic levels (McGavock 2005). For example, clarithromycin is a potent inhibitor of CYP3A4, the CYP enzyme responsible for the metabolism of simvastatin. Coadministration can lead to a greater than 10-fold increase in the plasma levels of simvastatin and could expose the patient to the risk of developing serious adverse reactions such as myopathy and rhabdomyolysis (MSD 2005).

Alternatively, induction of a CYP enzyme will increase the rate of metabolism of the second drug and cause a reduction in the plasma concentration, potentially resulting in treatment failure. For example, rifampicin, an enzyme inducer, can increase the metabolism of oral contraceptives and lead to contraceptive failure (McGavock 2005).

Phase 2 Phase 2 metabolism almost invariably terminates the pharmacological activity of a medicine and involves its union with one of several water-soluble molecules to form a water-soluble conjugate which can be excreted in urine or, in the case of larger molecules, bile (Bennett & Brown 2003). Examples of these reactions include glucuronidation, acetylation and sulphation (McGavock 2005).

Excretion

The kidney represents the major route of elimination, with medicines and their metabolites carried out of the body in urine. Less frequently, medicines may be eliminated by the liver, carried out in the bile and excreted in faeces.

The main pharmacokinetic parameter used to describe the elimination of medicines from the body is 'clearance'. This is defined as the volume of plasma completely emptied of drug per unit time. For example, if the amount of medicine in a patient is equal to 1 gram per litre and the clearance of the medicine is 1 litre per hour then the rate of elimination will be 1 gram per hour (Katzung 2004). The rate of elimination can be expressed by the following equation:

$$\text{Rate of elimination } (k) = \text{clearance } (CL) \times \text{plasma concentration } (C)$$

For example, from the example given above:

$$\text{Rate of elimination } (k) = 1 \text{ L/h} \times 1 \text{ g/L}$$
$$= 1 \text{ g/h}$$

For most medicines clearance is a constant. This tells us, therefore, that as the concentration of a medicine in plasma increases, the rate of elimination increases. From the example given above, if C increases to 2 grams per litre:

$$\text{Rate of elimination } (k) = 1 \text{ L/h} \times 2 \text{ g/L}$$
$$= 2 \text{ g/h}$$

When the rate of administration is the same as the rate of elimination, i.e. the inputs balance the outputs, the plasma concentration becomes constant and the medicine has reached an equilibrium known as 'steady state'. At steady state, with continued scheduled administration the amount of medicine in all tissues remains relatively constant irrespective of the interval since the last dose was given (McGavock 2005).

Elimination half-life $(t_{1/2})$ is an important concept that is related to the rate of elimination and is defined as the time taken for the plasma concentration to decay by one-half. When the administration of a medicine stops, after the time taken for approximately five half-lives to pass, the concentration of the medicine in plasma will become approximately equal to zero. In other words, $5 \times t_{1/2} =$ approximately the time taken for all of an administered medicine to leave the body (Winter 2004). The half-life of some medicines is measured in minutes (e.g. epoprostenol) but for others it is a number of days (e.g. clonazepam).

How are medicines administered via the intravenous route?

Injections are sterile solutions, emulsions or suspensions which are prepared by dissolving or suspending the active ingredients and any added substances in water for injection, a suitable non-aqueous liquid, or a mixture of these vehicles (DH 2005). There are three main methods of i.v. medicine administration:

- continuous infusion
- intermittent infusion
- direct intermittent injection.

The method selected is dependent on the medicine being given, its desired effect and the patient's condition (Dougherty 2002). Sometimes i.v. infusion of a medicine is necessary because a direct intermittent injection would result in a toxic amount of drug in the bloodstream. For example, potassium chloride must not be administered at a rate greater than 20 mmol per hour or at a concentration greater than 40 mmol per litre. If a dose of 40 mmol was administered as a direct injection in a small volume it might cause painful vein irritation, potentially a serious extravasation injury and could result in cardiac arrest (Schulman *et al.* 1998).

Continuous infusions

Continuous infusions constitute the delivery of a medicine or fluid usually, but not always, within a large volume of solution at a constant rate over a prescribed period of time. The length of time over which a continuous infusion is administered will range from several hours to several days (Schulman *et al.* 1998). This method of i.v. administration may be selected if the medicine needs to be administered in a highly dilute form (e.g. to avoid the risk of chemical phlebitis), requires a constant plasma concentration to be maintained (as described in Figure 5.4), or needs large volumes of fluids or electrolytes to be given (Dougherty 2002). For example, in the case of medicines with very short half-lives as a result of their rapid metabolism or excretion (e.g. heparin or dopamine), direct injection or intermittent infusions would require repeated, very frequent administration. A continuous infusion of these medicines therefore avoids the need for repeated injections to be given. A comparison of the drug concentration profiles of intermittent infusion, continuous infusion and direct intermittent injection is given in Figure 5.5.

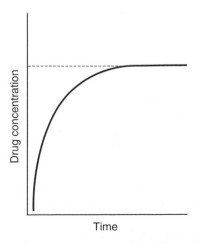

Figure 5.4 The steady-state drug plasma concentration achieved by continuous infusion.

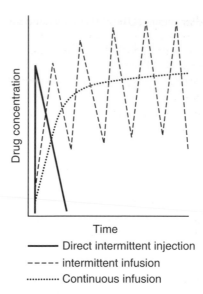

Figure 5.5 Serum drug levels of direct intermittent injection, intermittent injection and continuous infusion.

Continuous infusions are often delivered via an infusion device (pump or syringe driver; *See* Chapter 8) to ensure the accurate flow rate and even delivery of the medicine. The risk of fluctuating levels that could result from gravity infusion without a pump contradicts the aim of continuous administration. Care needs to be taken in monitoring a patient receiving a continuous infusion. The patient's physiological response to the medicine may need to be monitored and the insertion site of the cannula needs to be checked frequently for signs of phlebitis or infiltration (Dougherty 2002).

It is preferable that continuous infusions of medicines have dedicated i.v. access rather than being administered consecutively with a fluid infusion (or another drug infusion) through a single peripheral cannula. This avoids the risks associated with incompatibility. In addition, even when drugs and fluids are compatible, constant infusion of more than one fluid into the device cannot be monitored; fluids will flow along the path of least resistance if there is an obstruction to the flow in the system. Subsequent release of the obstruction will mean that a sudden delivery of a larger volume (and dose) of the drug and fluids through the cannula to the patient could occur (Finlay 2004).

Intermittent infusions

Intermittent infusion is the administration of a small-volume infusion (50–250 mL) over a period of between 20 minutes and 2 hours. This may be given as a single dose at one time or at repeated intervals during a 24-hour period (Pickstone 1999). An intermittent infusion may be used when a peak blood concentration is required at periodic intervals, when the pharmacology of a drug dictates this dilution, when the drug will not remain stable for the time required administering it in a more dilute volume, or where the patient is on a restricted fluid intake (Dougherty 2002).

The delivery of an intermittent infusion can be by one of the four following methods (Dougherty 2002).

Piggyback infusion The drug infusion is administered via the established pathway of a primary solution. The primary solution must be compatible and should only be attached by a specific piggyback injection port.

Simultaneous infusion The drug infusion is administered as a secondary infusion run concurrently with the primary infusion, attached to a lower secondary injection port.

Volume control set The drug infusion is administered via a volume control set such as a burette.

Directly via the venous access device The drug infusion is administered via an administration set connected to the venous access device. At the end of each infusion the drug container and administration set must be disconnected and discarded and the venous access device flushed.

Direct intermittent injection

Direct intermittent injection is also known as i.v. push or bolus injection and constitutes the administration of a medicine in a small volume of diluent, delivered directly into a venous access device or the injection site of an administration set using a needle and syringe. With the exception of those given in emergency situations such as cardiac arrest, most medicines must be administered slowly over a period ranging from 3 to 30 minutes (Dougherty 2002).

A direct injection can be used when: the maximum serum concentration of the medicine is required to reach vital organs rapidly, for example adrenaline (epinephrine) in the case of an emergency; the medicine cannot be further diluted for pharmacological or therapeutic reasons or does not require dilution; or a peak serum concentration is required and cannot be achieved by small-volume infusion (*See* Figure 5.6).

Too rapid administration can result in toxic levels and/or an anaphylactic-type reaction – speedshock (*See* Chapter 7). Administration of a compatible solution via the injection site of a fast-running drip might be advised to reduce the risk of venous irritation (Dougherty 2002).

What are the hazards associated with intravenous therapy?

> The administration of medicines by injection is a hazardous process that should be avoided whenever possible

(Clinical Research and Audit Groups (2002)

The Chief Medical Officers' report to ministers, *An Organisation with a Memory* (DH 2000), set out a challenging agenda to the NHS to improve patient care by

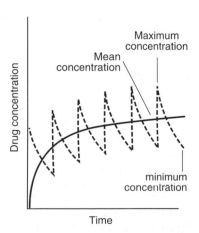

Figure 5.6 Variation of blood plasma concentration over time following multidose bolus injection.

reporting and learning from adverse events (DH 2004). This document resulted in the creation of the National Patient Safety Agency, tasked to spearhead patient safety efforts. In *Building a Safer NHS for Patients* (DH 2004), the government identified that our overriding aim is to embed a culture of safety in all NHS treatment. Ensuring that drug treatment is safe is central to this strategy, with the government directing at medicine use 50% of all its targets around reducing adverse healthcare events.

Intravenous therapy presents a potential risk to patient safety, with complications varying from minor to fatal (Ingram & Lavery 2005). To reduce these risks, all factors impacting negatively on the processes involved in i.v. therapy must be identified and managed. The Breckenbridge report (DH 1976) recommended that all aseptic preparation be undertaken in pharmacy aseptic units, a recommendation the Audit Commission (2001) subsequently reinforced in *A Spoonful of Sugar; Medicines Management in NHS Hospitals*. Preparation within pharmacy aseptic facilities is rigorously controlled, with explicit national guidance to assure the quality of the product (Beaney 2005). Although the abolition of all ward-based preparation may be an ideal situation, it cannot be realized within existing resources because shortages in pharmacy manpower and funding prevent its transfer to pharmacy-run i.v. additive services (Crowley *et al.* 2004). Therefore, as a practical solution, prioritized targeting has been suggested. High-risk products are prepared in pharmacy facilities, and risk reduction initiatives are employed to support the ward-based preparation of low-risk products (Cousins 1998).

It is also important to consider the hazards to staff undertaking the process of administering i.v. therapy and identify appropriate steps to minimize risk. The primary risks to nurses are injury and disease transmission due to needlestick incidents; spills and splashes which may result in the absorption of medicines through the skin or the development of skin irritation or sensitivity reactions; and the requirement for gloves as part of the universal precautions when dealing with blood and body fluids, potentially leading to the development of latex allergy (Dougherty 2002).

Adverse health outcomes for the patient resulting from i.v. therapy may come about as a result of:

- complications associated with the processes involved in administering medicines intravenously (*See* Chapter 6)
- drug instability and incompatibility
- human error.

Drug instability and incompatibility

A critical aspect of parenteral therapy is to ensure that the patient receives the intended dose in a pharmacologically active form. It is important to note that the expiry date printed on the pack relates to the medicine as it has been supplied by the manufacturer. Once the medicine has been removed from its original packaging (including the box it is supplied in) and reconstituted or diluted, its 'in-use' shelf-life is significantly shorter. Administering medicines in an unfavourable environment may render them unstable or inactive, and will have clinical implications for the patient in terms of lack of efficacy, increased side-effects or both (Allwood 1988). Information about the exact requirements for individual products is usually detailed in the package insert supplied by the manufacturer with the medicine. Individual trusts may also provide an 'i.v. guide' describing the details of i.v. administration for individual medicines.

As everything made by human hand is subject to decay it must be realized that a proportion of any dose prepared will be lost between the time of preparation and entry into the bloodstream (Cartensen & Rhodes 2000). The rate at which this occurs varies dramatically between medicines (Carstensen & Rhodes 2000) and may result from degradation, precipitation in a diluent or with a coadministered medicine, or an interaction with the delivery system (Allwood 1988).

Medicines supplied by the manufacturer as powders for reconstitution are, by definition, relatively unstable in aqueous solution. Degradation most commonly follows a process of hydrolysis but may also occur as a result of photodegradation or oxidation. It can be accelerated by an inappropriate pH change due either to the diluent or to the addition of a second drug, and in some cases may be noted to have occurred when the diluted drug solution develops a colour. For example, dopamine may change from a clear colourless to pink solution on dilution. In this case, mild discoloration represents only a minimal loss due to degradation and does not necessarily constitute a hazard. In practice, few medicines are sufficiently unstable in aqueous solutions within the pH range of 5–7.5 to lose significant activity under normal clinical conditions (Allwood 1988). Very rarely, however, degradation can result in the formation of toxic metabolites, for example the breakdown in the presence of light of sodium nitroprusside to cyanogens and toxic cyanide derivatives (Mayne Pharma Ltd 2005).

Photodegradation results from exposure to ultraviolet (UV) light of light-sensitive compounds such as dacarbazine, vitamin K (phytomenadione) and furosemide. UV light is present in daylight but is not a component of artificial fluorescent light. Whilst in practice no problems should occur provided light-sensitive drugs are not exposed to direct strong sunlight, in many cases light protection of the infusion bag and administration set may be advocated for light-sensitive medicines (Allwood 1988).

Precipitated medicines are pharmacologically inactive and constitute a hazard to patients. Precipitates of the medicine itself or an insoluble compound resulting from the reaction of two substances can block catheters and damage blood vessels and may theoretically lead to coronary or pulmonary embolism (Allwood 1988). The formation of a precipitate is time dependent, with some forming in less than 2 minutes whilst others may take several hours to become visible. Where precipitation is thought possible, regular inspection of infusions should be carried out, especially if the infusion is prescribed to be administered over several hours. Often the first sign that precipitation may have occurred is blockage of the administration set (Allwood 1988).

Causes of precipitation include the effects of pH, dilution, drug–drug coprecipitation, and temperature (Allwood 1988).

pH   A very large proportion of medicines in use are weak acids or weak bases. A weak acid is best described as a neutral molecule that can reversibly dissociate into a negatively charged molecule—an anion. Conversely, a weak base is a neutral molecule that can form a positively charged molecule—a cation, by combining with a proton (Katzung 2004). Most injections are formulated using a salt form of these acidic or basic moieties. So, for example, weak acids form alkali metal salts such as sodium or potassium, and weak bases form acid salts such as nitrate, hydrochloride or sulphate (Allwood 1988).

Salts of weak acids generally have an alkaline pH in solution. When these injections are diluted in water for injection, sodium chloride 0.9% or glucose 5% the pH of the resultant solution falls. If the pH falls below the pKa (the pKa tells us about the reactivity and solubility of a compound and is a measure of the extent of dissociation of hydrogen ions from an acid) of the drug and the aqueous solubility of the free acid is low, the free acid is likely to form a precipitate (Allwood 1988). Conversely, salts of weak bases are commonly formulated in solutions adjusted to an acidic pH. Dilution in an aqueous solution raises the pH and the free base may therefore precipitate if the pKa is exceeded (Allwood 1988). For example, when considering the administration of furosemide it is important to note that the pH of sodium chloride 0.9% and water for injection is neutral (approximately equal to 7) whereas glucose 5% has a pH of between 3.5 and 6.5.

Furosemide is an alkaline solution (pH 8.0–9.3) which must be administered in a diluent with a pH greater than 5.5. Therefore, glucose 5% solutions may not be suitable for diluting furosemide solutions (Trissel 2005).

Alternatively, the mixing of two medicines with very different pHs can result in precipitation. Ideally all medicines should be administered separately to minimize the risk of incompatibility. This is not always possible, however, especially for example in critically ill patients who may be on multiple i.v. therapies with limited i.v. access. In these situations medicines can be administered concurrently provided they are *known* to be compatible (Trissel 2005). It must never be assumed that medicines with the same pharmacological effect are therefore compatible. Further information about the safety of concurrent i.v. administration of medicines can be sought from the pharmacy department.

Dilution   Some medicines are poorly soluble in aqueous vehicles and are formulated using cosolvents such as ethanol, polysorbates and propylene glycol. If the injection is diluted in infusion fluid, the cosolvents are diluted out and the drug may then precipitate. Examples of such medicines include diazepam, digoxin and amiodarone (Allwood 1988).

Drug–drug coadministration   In this case, precipitation most commonly occurs following the mixing of an organic anion and cation to form an ion pair. Examples of medicines at risk of forming ion pairs with other medicines include gentamicin and heparin (Allwood 1988).

Temperature   Often any requirement to store reconstituted injection solutions at temperatures between 2 and 8°C aims purely to limit microbial growth and maintain sterility of the i.v. solution. In practice, injection solutions should be reconstituted/diluted immediately prior to administration. Generally, however, most compounds are more soluble as the solution temperature increases, although this is not always the case (Allwood 1988).

Administration of i.v. medicines now almost entirely depends on equipment made from plastics such as polyvinyl chloride (PVC), polyethylene and polyolefin (Allwood 1988). A small number of medicines bind to certain plastics by one of three mechanisms: adsorption (binding to the plastic surface), absorption (migration into the matrix of the plastic), or permeation (absorption and migration through the matrix of the plastic to the outer surface before evaporating into air) (Allwood 1988). Adsorption can occur at any solid surface irrespective of the plastic used, whereas absorption and permeation are a particular problem with PVC. It is impossible to predict quantitatively the extent of losses of any particular medicine but prevention is always the best approach (Allwood 1988). Some clinical examples of drug/administration set incompatibility are glyceryl trinitrate and paclitaxel.

Glyceryl trinitrate (GTN)   Administration of GTN via PVC-containing administration equipment will result in the adsorption of the drug, out of solution onto the PVC device. Thus, the amount of medicine available for administration to the patient is reduced. GTN must be administered in PVC-free bags and administration sets (Trissel 2005).

Paclitaxel DEHP   is a plasticizer used to increase the flexibility of PVC-containing bags or administration sets. One of the constituents in the formulation of paclitaxel, a cytotoxic used in the treatment of breast, ovarian and lung cancers, 'leaches' the DEHP out of the plastic into the solution being administered to the patient. In the long term, this may result in adverse health outcomes for patients and therefore paclitaxel is only administered using PVC-free bags and administration sets (Trissel 2005).

Human error

Building a Safer NHS for Patients (DH 2004) recognized that the accurate administration of medicines is critically dependent on the quality of all previous steps in the prescribing and dispensing processes. Safe administration cannot be entirely delegated to those actually giving a medicine, but risk management must be built into the whole medication process. In hospitals, drug administration is the final step in a multidisciplinary process in which professionals should work together to ensure that a patient receives a medicine safely (DH 2004). The government report identifies the following range of measures to ensure safe medication administration (DH 2004).

- Appropriate training for all staff involved in the handling of medication.
- Clear drug administration procedures in all settings where medicines are given.
- Double-checking by a second person in defined high-risk circumstances such as i.v. infusions, complex calculations.
- Discussion with patients or carers at the time of administration and involving them in checking where appropriate.
- Storing all medicines safely and in such a way that avoids the risk of drug selection errors and controlling the availability of high-risk medicines.
- Utilizing information technology to support prescribing, dispensing and administering medicines.

Intravenous therapy is a complex process usually requiring the preparation of medicines in clinical areas before administration to a patient. There have been reports of harm to patients and death following medication errors in i.v. therapy involving wrong drug, dose and diluent and cross-contamination errors (Cousins *et al.* 2005). A recent international study identified that in the UK the most frequent medication errors were associated with administration rate, usually higher than that recommended by manufacturers (Cousins *et al.* 2005).

Calculations

The basic information relating to drug calculations is given in Box 5.1. It is essential for healthcare professionals involved in drug prescribing, monitoring and administration to be familiar with the basic principles (RCN 2005).

BOX 5.1

Basic information

1 g (gram) = 1000 mg (milligrams)
1 mg (milligram) = 1000 mcg (micrograms)
1 L (litre) = 1000 mL (millilitres)
Note: microgram units must always be written in full to avoid confusion with milligrams.
Percentage (%) solution = grams in 100 mL
e.g. 1% w/v lignocaine = 1 g in 100 mL
A 1% w/v lignocaine solution means that there is 1 g of lignocaine in 100 mL of solution. Therefore, an ampoule of 10 mL lignocaine 1% contains 0.1 g or 100 mg of the active drug.
1 in 1000 = 1 g in 1000 mL (1 mg in 1 mL)
1 in 10 000 = 1 gram in 10 000 mL (0.1 mg in 1 mL)
For example, adrenaline 1 in 10 000 = 1 g in 10 000 mL (0.1 mg in 1 mL)
An ampoule of adrenaline 1 in 10 000 contains 1 gram or 1000 milligrams of drug in 10 000 mL. This is equivalent to 1 mg in 10 mL or 0.1 mg/mL.

Calculation of flow rates

Flow rates are expressed as volumes of fluid delivered per unit time, usually as millilitres per hour (mL/h) or drops per minute (drops/min) (*See* Box 5.2).

BOX 5.2

Calculation of flow rate in millilitres per hour (mL/h)

$$\text{Flow rate (ml/h)} = \frac{\text{Volume of fluid (mL)}}{\text{time of infuse (h)}}$$

Hence, to administer 500 mL of glucose 5% over 8 hours:

$$flow\ rate = \frac{500}{8} = 62.5\ mL/h$$

Calculation of flow rate in drops per minute (drops/min)

It is necessary to know:

- volume of fluid to be infused
- total infusion time
- calibration of the administration set used, i.e. number of drops/mL it delivers (this information is found on the administration set package), for example:
  - 15 drops/mL for blood sets
  - 20 drops/mL for solution sets
  - 60 drops/mL for burettes.

$$\text{flow rate (drops/min)} = \frac{\text{volume of fluid (mL)}}{\text{total infusion time (min)}} \times \text{calibration (drops/ml)}$$

To administer 1 litre of fluid over 12 hours using a burette:

$$Flow\ rate = \frac{1000\ (mL)}{12 \times 60\ (min)} \times 60\ (drops/mL) = \textbf{83}\ drops/min$$

Alternatively, use the following equations:

- For *a solution administration set*:

  drops/min = mL/h ÷ 3 (i.e. calibration of 20 drops/mL)

- For *a blood-administration set*:

  drops/min = mL/h ÷ 4 (i.e. calibration of 15 drops/mL)

- For *a burette microdrop set*:

  drops/min = mL/h (i.e. calibration of 60 drops/mL).

Examples

The following examples are included to demonstrate the use of different methods or equations for i.v. drug administrations. The calculation methods are dependent on the presentation of the drug (i.e. percentage weight in volume, mg/mL and so on) and on the dosing schedule on the prescription (i.e. prescribed as mg/min or mg/h, micrograms/kg patient weight per minute or per hour, units per day, and so on).

Example 1 Dopamine continuous infusion at 2.5 mcg/kg patient weight/min. The patient is fluid restricted, weighs 50 kg and has a central venous catheter. The drug is diluted as 200 mg (1 ampoule) in 50 mL sodium chloride 0.9% or dextrose (glucose) 5%. The following equation may be used for administration using a syringe pump.

$$\text{Administration rate (mL/h)} = \frac{\text{dose (mcg/kg/min)} \times \text{volume in syringe (mL)} \times 60 \text{ (to convert to h)}}{\text{amoun of drug in syringe} \times 1000 \text{ (to convert to mg)}}$$

$$= \frac{(2.5 \times 50) \times 50 \times 60}{200 \times 1000}$$

$$= 1.875 \text{mL/h}$$

Example 2 50 000 units of drug X in 50 mL of infusion fluid are to be administered at 600 units/h via a syringe pump. A quantity of 50 000 units in 50 mL solution means that 600 units/h is equivalent to:

$$\text{Administration rate (mL/h)} = \frac{\text{dose (iu/h)} \times \text{volume in syringe (mL)}}{\text{amount of drug in syringe (iu)}}$$

$$= \frac{600 \times 50}{50\,000}$$

$$= 0.6 \text{ mL/h}$$

Therefore, the syringe pump is set at 0.6 mL/h.

Example 3 A lignocaine infusion 0.4% w/v in dextrose 5% polyfusor needs to be given at 1 mg/min in a volumetric pump calibrated in mL/h.

$$\text{Administration rate (mL/h)} = \frac{\text{dose (mg/min)} \times 60 \text{ (to convert to h)}}{\text{concentration of solution (mg/mL)}}$$

$$0.4\% \text{ w/v} = 0.4 \text{ g in } 100 \text{ mL}$$

$$= 400 \text{ mg in } 100 \text{ mL}$$

$$= 4 \text{ mg/mL}$$

$$\text{Administration rate (mL/h)} = \frac{1 \times 60}{4}$$

$$= 15 \text{ mL/h}$$

Example 4 Magnesium sulphate 40 mmol is to be administered over 2 hours. Magnesium sulphate is available as 10 mL of 50% w/v concentration, equivalent to 2 mmol/mL. (The maximum concentration it should be administered at is 0.8 mmol/mL at a maximum rate of 0.6 mmol/min.)

$$\text{Number of mL of concentrate} = \frac{40 \text{ mmol}}{2 \text{ mmol/mL}}$$

$$= 20 \text{ mL}$$

$$\text{Minimum volume for infusion} = \frac{40 \text{ mmol}}{0.8 \text{ mmol/ml}}$$

$$= 50 \text{ mL}$$

Therefore remove 20 mL from a 50-mL sodium chloride 0.9% bag and add 20 mL magnesium concentrate to the remaining bag volume

$$\text{Maximum rate of infusion} = \frac{40 \text{ mmol}}{0.6 \text{ mmol/min}}$$

$$= 67 \text{ min}$$

Therefore it is safe to run this dose over 2 hours as prescribed

$$\text{Administration rate (mL/h)} = \frac{50 \text{ mL}}{2 \text{ h}}$$

$$= 2.5 \text{ mL/h}$$

What are the roles and responsibilities of each profession involved in intravenous therapy?

This section aims to give a brief overview of the roles and responsibilities of the health-care professionals involved in the practice of i.v. drug therapy. It is not intended to give a comprehensive review of the accountabilities, but to help introduce guidelines and raise awareness of the issues surrounding good clinical practice. It is recognized that with the newly evolving roles of the health professionals of all disciplines, such as nurse and pharmacist prescribers, there is scope for developing partnerships in caring for patients in an integrated multidisciplinary fashion.

Following the successful piloting of prescribing by district nurses and health visitors, Dr June Crowns' report *Review of Prescribing, Supply and Administration of Medicines* (DH 1999) proposed that prescribing responsibilities are extended to include new groups of health professionals. Initially, health ministers focused on extending the prescribing roles of nurses and pharmacists as these were considered the most numerous non-medical health professionals (NPC 2003), but subsequently the focus has been expanded to include a wide range of health professionals.

The report recommended the introduction of a distinction between two categories of prescribers.

- Supplementary prescribers—authorized to prescribe for patients whose condition has been diagnosed or assessed by an independent prescriber, within the parameters of an agreed clinical management plan.
- Independent prescribers—responsible for the initial assessment of a patient and drawing up a clinical management plan. The independent prescriber also has authority to prescribe the medicines required as part of the plan. As of 28 April 2006, qualified independent nurse and pharmacist prescribers have been able to prescribe any licensed medicine for any medical condition within their competence including, for nurses, some controlled drugs (DH 2006).

Following the successful completion of a formal course of training, independent and supplementary prescribers must be able to demonstrate sufficient knowledge and competence to:

- assess a patient/client's clinical condition
- undertake a thorough history, including medical history and medication history, and diagnose where necessary, including over-the-counter medicines and complementary therapies
- decide on management of presenting condition and whether or not to prescribe
- identify appropriate products if medication is required
- advise the patient/client on effects and risks
- prescribe if the patient/client agrees
- monitor response to medication and lifestyle advice (NMC 2006).

It is therefore now legal for a nurse to administer, via any route, medicines that have been prescribed by a qualified non-medical prescriber (supplementary or independent) to a patient in exactly the same manner as when prescribed by a doctor.

Responsibilities of the prescriber

Prescribers are urged to restrict the use of the i.v. route to situations where there is no alternative method of administration available, and to keep the period of i.v. administration to a minimum. This is to minimize the problems (clinical and practical) associated with i.v. drug therapy (Clinical Research and Audit Groups 2002).

Prescribing information should be clearly written on the prescription chart and include the following:

- *approved name* of the medicine to be administered intravenously
- *dose* of the medicine
- *method of administration* e.g. bolus into an administration set/cannula, intermittent infusion or continuous infusion
- *infusion fluid* in which the medicine is to be diluted
- *volume* of infusion fluid
- *final concentration* of the infusion
- *calculated rate* at which the infusion is to be administered, e.g. 'mg per minute', 'drops per minute', 'mL per minute', 'mL per hour', etc.
- *device* to be used for administration of drugs where more than one device is in use, e.g. peripheral or central venous catheter (NPSA 2007).

Responsibilities of the pharmacist

Pharmaceutical care has been defined as 'the responsible provision of drug therapy for the purpose of achieving definite outcomes that improve a patient's quality of life' (Hepler & Strand 1990). The outcomes desired are cure of disease, elimination or reduction of symptomology, arresting or slowing a disease process, or preventing a disease or symptomology (Hepler & Strand 1990). Pharmaceutical care was subsequently refined by Strand and coworkers to 'a practice in which the practitioner takes responsibility for a patient's drug-related needs and holds him or herself accountable for meeting these needs' (Maguire 2001).

Medicines management, perhaps a more familiar term than pharmaceutical care in England, encompasses a range of activities intended to improve the way in which medicines are used, both by patients and by the NHS (NPC 2002). It is used by some synonymously with pharmaceutical care, and by others as an umbrella term within which pharmaceutical care is only one aspect. Clinical medicines management services involve assessment, monitoring and review of prescribing for individuals (NPC 2002). Medicines management/pharmaceutical care is not specifically care by pharmacists, but care achieved through the administration of medicines and therefore requires a multidisciplinary approach (Maguire 2001). For pharmacists, this involves the process by which they cooperate with a patient and other professionals in designing, implementing and monitoring a therapeutic plan that will produce specific therapeutic outcomes for the patient. This in turn involves three major functions (Hepler & Strand 1990):

1. identifying potential and actual medicine-related problems,
2. resolving actual medicine-related problems, and
3. preventing potential medicine-related problems.

These functions can be achieved by alerting prescribers, nursing staff and other health professionals to any potential problems through the following.

- Checking for the appropriate selection of specific medicines and medicine regimens (dose, route, frequency, administration method, duration of therapy).
- Endorsing the prescription chart with relevant and necessary information such as preparation method, dilution details of infusions.
- Responding to specific enquiries raised by health professionals regarding all aspects of drug therapies, including methods of administration, diluents and infusion fluids, drug stability, delivery systems (e.g. pumps, burettes), drug compatibility information, rate of administration, contraindications and side-effects, interactions,

unlicensed drugs and their use, anaphylaxis guidelines and drug administration guidelines.

- Signing and dating the drug charts to inform health professionals that a pharmacist has reviewed the specific prescription.
- Ensuring that the risks of medication errors are minimized throughout the process, from prescribing and dispensing to administration.
- Contributing towards the training of members of the healthcare team.
- Preparation of CIVAS (centralized intravenous additive service) for hazardous drugs, agents requiring specialist processes and clinical trials. In certain situations, the pharmacy department may be able to supply ready-made preparations.
- Advising on appropriate treatment for the management of adverse administration events such as extravasation or anaphylaxis.

Responsibilities of the nurse

The Nursing and Midwifery Council's *Code of Professional Conduct* (NMC 2004a) states that: 'As a registered nurse, midwife or health visitor, you are personally accountable for your practice'. The code emphasizes the need to act in a manner that promotes and safeguards the interests and well-being of patients by maintaining and improving professional knowledge and competence, acknowledging limitations in knowledge and expertise, and working towards achieving expertise in extended roles.

In addition to the *Code of Professional Conduct*, the NMC's *Guidelines for the Administration of Medicines* (NMC 2004b) establishes principles for safe practice in drug administration. It focuses on the requirement for a nurse practitioner to be satisfied with her or his competence and mindful of her or his personal accountability with respect to the administration of i.v. drugs.

In many NHS Trusts there is an 'approved list' of medicines that may be administered intravenously by nurses, midwives and allied health professionals who are competent in i.v. therapy. Many also have additional lists of 'specialist' drugs that may be administered intravenously by nurses working within certain specialist practice areas, e.g. coronary care units. Any drugs not included on the approved drugs list (or appropriate specialist list) should not be administered by nurses, but by the prescribing doctor. The drugs on the approved list are those whose action, method of administration and side-effects are well known and many hospitals supply additional information about these drugs in their i.v. drug administration policy.

Any nurse administering a drug that is not included in the approved or specialist list (where appropriate), may find the trust will not accept vicarious liability in the event of an incident (*See* Chapter 1). thus it is important to decline to administer drugs that are not on the list. Doctors should be advised that the approved list is constantly being updated as new drugs become available and others are no longer used. The procedure for including new drugs on the approved and specialist lists will vary from institution to institution but is usually relatively simple. When the drug has been approved, nurses may administer it intravenously and the trust will be vicariously liable as long as trust policies and procedures are followed.

Medicines may be administered by a single nurse who has demonstrated the necessary knowledge and competence; however, double-checks by a second nurse (or a doctor or pharmacist) will be employed in the case of controlled drugs, unlicensed medicines or clinical trial products, or when there are local restrictions, such as on specialist units (e.g. paediatrics and intensive care units) where infusions require complex calculations. Single-nurse administration applies to first-dose i.v. therapies as well as subsequent doses; nevertheless, if a nurse wishes to have her drug preparation checked (in any circumstances), then she/he is free to do so. O'Shea (1999) and Armitage and Knapman

(2003) note that previous studies suggest that single-nurse administration does not necessarily increase the risk of medication errors. Ross *et al.* (2000) demonstrated that most medication errors occurred despite checks being carried out by two practitioners. Nevertheless, the perception remains that double-checking provides a robust safeguard against medication errors (Armitage & Knapman 2003).

Nurses should refuse to administer an injection if they have not been present during its preparation in a clinical area, and the practice of preparing i.v. medication and storing it in the fridge for administration at a later date should be actively discouraged (Hyde 2002).

Record-keeping is an integral part of nursing practice. Good record-keeping protects the welfare of patients by promoting:

- high standards of clinical care
- continuity of care
- better communication and dissemination of information between members of the multidisciplinary healthcare team
- an accurate account of treatments and care planning and delivery
- the ability to detect problems such as a change in clinical condition at an early stage (NMC 2005).

Good practice in the administration of intravenous therapy

It is recommended that each hospital or community trust should have a local policy for i.v. therapy. Existing documents have usually been compiled by a multidisciplinary team overseen by the organization's Drugs and Therapeutics Committee which is ultimately responsible for policies and risk management related to the use of medicines. Such a document may focus on the importance of the recommendations of the independent professional bodies, as well as the principles stated within the specific local policy of a hospital/community trust (Clinical Research and Audit Groups 2002).

The following steps should be taken before authorization to allow administration of i.v. medicines.

- *Training.* Nurses must be satisfied that they demonstrate competence in intravenous medicine administration. Alternatively, training needs should be met by specific educational modules.
- *Policy.* Nurses must be aware of local policies produced by the Drugs and Therapeutics Committee and adhere to them.
- *Prescription chart.* The instructions given on the chart must be clear and concise in order to minimize the risk of errors occurring. Nurses must be satisfied that there is sufficient information detailing the dose, frequency, dilution, rate and method of administration, and the equipment necessary for use.

Conclusion

The administration of i.v. therapy is a complex and potentially hazardous process. To minimize the risk of errors occurring at any point during the process, a multidisciplinary team approach must be employed. Clinical considerations and the potential for adverse consequences to the patient require an understanding of the pharmacological aspects impacting on the administration of i.v. therapy. Figure 5.7 provides a summary of the pharmaceutical or medication-related issues that must be considered before, during and after the i.v. injection of medicines.

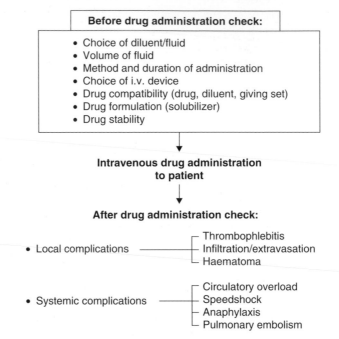

Intravenous drug administration
potential pharmaceutical problems

Before drug administration check:

- Choice of diluent/fluid
- Volume of fluid
- Method and duration of administration
- Choice of i.v. device
- Drug compatibility (drug, diluent, giving set)
- Drug formulation (solubilizer)
- Drug stability

**Intravenous drug administration
to patient**

After drug administration check:

- Local complications
  - Thrombophlebitis
  - Infiltration/extravasation
  - Haematoma

- Systemic complications
  - Circulatory overload
  - Speedshock
  - Anaphylaxis
  - Pulmonary embolism

Figure 5.7 Pharmaceutical issues to be considered before, during and after intravenous medicine administration.

References

Allwood M (1988) *Clinical Pharmacy Practice Guide – Drug Stability and Intravenous Administration*. United Kingdom Clinical Pharmacy Association, London.

Armitage G, Knapman H (2003) Adverse events in drug administration: a literature review. *Journal of Nursing Management* 11(2): 130–140.

Audit Commission (2001) *A Spoonful of Sugar; Medicines Management in NHS Hospitals* [www document]. www.audit-commission.gov.uk/

Beaney AM (2005) *Quality Assurance of Aseptic Preparation Services*, 4th edn. Pharmaceutical Press, London.

Bennett PN, Brown MJ (2003) General pharmacology. In: *Clinical Pharmacology*, 9th edn. Churchill Livingstone, London.

Campbell J (1996) Intravenous drug therapy. *Professional Nurse* 11(7): 437–42.

Cartensen JT, Rhodes CT (2000) *Drug Stability: Principles and Practices*. Marcel Dekker Inc, New York.

Clinical Research and Audit Groups (2002) *Good Practice Statement for the Preparation of Injections in Near-Patient Areas, Including Clinical and Home Environments*. NHS Scotland, Edinburgh.

Cooper A, Moore M (1999) IV fluid therapy. *Australian Nursing Journal* 7(6): 1–4.

Cousins D (1998) More must be done to cut errors. *Pharmacy Practice* 8: 342–6.

Cousins D *et al.* (2005) Medication errors in intravenous drug preparation and administration: a multicentre audit in the UK, Germany and France. *Quality and Safety in Health Care* 14: 190–5.

Crowley C *et al.* (2004) Describing the frequency of IV medication preparation and administration errors. *Hospital Pharmacist* 11: 330–336.

Department of Health and Social Security (1976) *Report of the Working Party on the Addition of Drugs to Intravenous Fluids* [HC (76) 9] (Breckenbridge report). HMSO, London.

Department of Health (1999) *Review of Prescribing, Supply and Administration of Medicines* [www document]. www.dh.gov.uk/assetRoot/04/07/71/53/04077153.pdf

Department of Health (2000) *An Organisation with a Memory: Report of an Expert Group on Learning from Adverse Events in the NHS*. TSO, London.

Department of Health (2004) *Building a Safer NHS for Patients: Improving Medication Safety.* TSO, London.
Department of Health (2005) *British Pharmacopoeia.* TSO, London.
Department of Health (2006) *Medicines Matters: A Guide to the Mechanisms for Prescribing, Supply and Administration of Medicines* [www document]. www.dh.gov.uk/assetRoot/04/13/77/24/04137724.pdf, accessed 24 September, 2007.
Dougherty L (2002) Delivery of intravenous therapy. *Nursing Standard* 16(16): 45–56.
Finlay T (2004) *IV Therapy.* Blackwell Publishing, Oxford.
Hand H (2001) The use of intravenous therapy. *Nursing Standard* 15(43): 47–55.
Henry JAH (2004) *The British Medical Association New Guide to Medicines and Drugs,* 6th edn. Dorling Kindersley Ltd, London.
Hepler CD, Strand LM (1990) Opportunities and responsibilities in pharmaceutical care. *American Journal of Hospital Pharmacy* 47(3): 533–543.
Horne MM, Heitz UE, Swearingen PL (1997) *Mosby's Pocket Guide to Electrolyte and Acid–Base Balance,* 3rd edn. Mosby, London.
Hyde L (2002) Legal and professional aspects of intravenous therapy. *Nursing Standard* 16(26): 39–42.
Ingram P, Lavery I (2005) Peripheral intravenous therapy: key risks and implications for practice. *Nursing Standard* 19(46): 55–64.
Jackson A (2003) Reflecting on the nursing contribution to vascular access. *British Journal of Nursing* 12(11): 657–65.
Katzung BG (2004) *Basic and Clinical Pharmacology,* 8th edn. Appleton and Lange, Connecticut.
Kayley J, Finlay T (2003) Vascular access devices for patients in the community. *Community Practitioner* 76(6): 228–231.
Lister S *et al.* (2004) Drug administration: general principles. In: Dougherty L, Lister S, eds, 184–227. *The Royal Marsden Hospital Manual of Clinical Nursing Procedures,* 6th edn. Blackwell Publishing, Oxford.
Maguire T (2001) More clarity, less dogma in our approach to pharmacy practice. *Pharmaceutical Journal* 266(7147): 651.
Mayne Pharma Ltd (2005) *Summary of Product Characteristics – Sodium Nitroprusside.* Electronic Medicines Compendium [www document]. http://emc.medicines.org.uk/, accessed 24 September, 2007.
McGavock H (2005) *How medicines work: Basic Pharmacology for Healthcare Professionals,* 2nd edn. Radcliffe Medical Press, Oxford.
Merck (1999) *The Merck Manual of Diagnosis and Therapy: Centennial Edition,* 17th edn. Merck Publishing, London.
Mosby CV (2005) *Mosby's Dictionary of Medicine, Nursing and Health Professions.* Mosby, Philadelphia.
MSD Ltd (2005) *Summary of product characteristics – Zocor (simvastatin).* Electronic Medicines Compendium [www document]. http://emc.medicines.org.uk/
NPC (2002) Medicines management services – why are they so important? *MeReC Bulletins* 12(6–21).
NPC (2003) *Supplementary Prescribing – A Resource to Help Healthcare Professionals to Understand the Framework and Opportunities* [www document]. www.npc.co.uk/publications/healthcare_resource.pdf, accessed 24 September, 2007.
NPSA (2007) *Promoting Safer Use of Injectable Medicines.* Patient Safety Alert 20, 28 March 2007.
Nursing and Midwifery Council (NMC) (2004a) *Code of professional conduct.* Nursing and Midwifery Council, London.
Nursing and Midwifery Council (2004b) *Guidelines for the Administration of Medicines.* Nursing and Midwifery Council, London.
Nursing and Midwifery Council (2005) *Guidelines for Records and Record Keeping.* Nursing and Midwifery Council, London.
Nursing and Midwifery Council (2006) *Standards of Proficiency for Nurse and Midwife Prescribers.* Nursing and Midwifery Council, London.
O'Shea E (1999) Factors contributing to medication errors: a literature review. *Journal of Clinical Nursing* 8(5): 496–504.
Pickstone M (1999) *A Pocketbook for Safer Administration of IV Therapy. Medical Technology and Risk Series.* Scitech Educational Ltd, Margate.
Ross LM, Wallace J, Paton JY, Stephenson T (2000) Medication errors in a paediatric teaching hospital in the UK: five years operational experience. *Archives of Disease in Childhood* 83: 492–7.
Royal College of Nursing (RCN) (2005) *Standards for Infusion Therapy.* Royal College of Nursing, London.
Schulman R *et al.* (1998) *UCL Hospitals Injectable Drug Administration Guide.* Blackwell Science Ltd, London.
Trissel LA (2005) *Handbook on Injectable Drugs.* American Society of Health Systems Pharmacy, Bethsheda.
Winter ME (2004) *Basic and Clinical Pharmacokinetics.* Lippincott Williams and Wilkins, Baltimore.

Section 1

Section 2
Practice

CHAPTER 6

Safe Administration and Management of Peripheral Intravenous Therapy

Teresa Finlay

Introduction

Most patients admitted to hospital have a venous access device (Dougherty 2000) and responsibility for administration and management of patients' intravenous (i.v.) therapy has shifted from doctors to nurses and midwives. In light of this, practitioners must have sound knowledge and understanding of the safe management of i.v. therapy. As with all aspects of healthcare, i.v. therapy management must be of the highest quality and based on available evidence. Most of the complications associated with peripheral i.v. therapy can be minimized or avoided by careful management; it is nurses' and midwives' responsibility to ensure i.v. therapy is managed with the requisite knowledge and skills to promote patients' health and recovery.

This chapter will address the following areas:

- care of the site of peripheral i.v. access devices
- preparation and management of i.v. infusions
- maintaining patency of peripheral i.v. cannulae
- the use of extension sets, three-way taps and other i.v. equipment with peripheral i.v. access devices
- safe i.v. drug administration
- removal of peripheral i.v. cannulae.

Care of the Peripheral Intravenous Site

Observation of the site

Peripheral cannula sites must be inspected *at least once a day*, and also when i.v. drugs are administered, infusion rates are altered, or infusion containers changed (DH 2005; RCN 2005a,b). They must be observed for the following.

1. *Phlebitis or thrombophlebitis (redness)* Phlebitis is inflammation of the intima (inner lining) of the vein and it should be assessed using a uniform scale to establish the severity of the inflammation. Jackson's venous inflammation phlebitis (VIP) scale provides a standard scale for assessment and action in the event of phlebitis (*See* Figure 6.1).
2. *Infection (heat)* Contamination of the cannula site will initially result in localized infection. The patient will experience pain, tenderness and inflammation at the site,

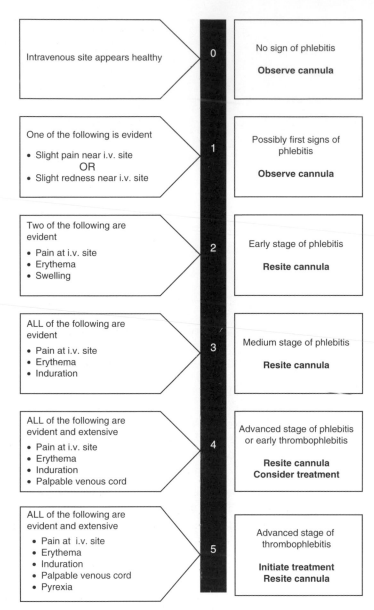

Figure 6.1   Vein infusion phlebitis. (Jackson 1998. Copyright Emap Public Sector Ltd 2007. Reproduced by permission of Nursing Times.)

and there may also be exudate. A fever and systemic infection may result if the device is not removed immediately. A swab should be sent for culture; findings and action must be documented. Patients who are immunocompromised are at particular risk (Finlay 2004). *See* Prevention of contamination below.

3. *Infiltration or extravasation (swelling around the site)* Infiltration is the unintentional infusion of a non-vesicant solution into the tissues surrounding a vein (INS 2006). Extravasation is the unintentional infusion of a vesicant solution into the tissues surrounding a vein (INS 2006). The latter may have severe consequences for the patient depending on the degree of tissue damage and necrosis incurred.

Grade	Clinical criteria
0	No symptoms
1	Skin blanched Oedema <2.5 cm in any direction Cool to touch With or without pain
2	Skin blanched Oedema 2.5–15 cm in any direction Cool to touch With or without pain
3	Skin blanched, translucent Gross oedema, >15 cm in any direction Cool to touch Possible numbness
4	Skin blanched, translucent Skin tight, leaking Skin discoloured, bruised, swollen Gross oedema >15 cm in any direction Deep pitting tissue oedema Circulatory impairment Moderate to severe pain Infiltration of any amount of blood product, irritant or vesicant

Figure 6.2   Infiltration Scale (INS 2006). Reprinted with permission of Lippincott Williams and Wilkins.

In either case, infusions or drug administration must be stopped immediately, the degree of infiltration/extravasation assessed and appropriate interventions implemented. The Infiltration Scale (INS 2006) gives a framework for assessment of infiltration (*See* Figure 6.2).

A cannula site should not be painful. There may be discomfort associated with the cannula and the patient may feel 'coolness' in the limb during rapid infusion or bolus drug administration, but it should not be painful between drug administrations or while an infusion is running. Some drugs may cause venous pain during administration but this should be minimized by slow administration and appropriate dilution (Weinstein 2007).

If the area around the cannula becomes painful or any of the signs listed above are present, i.v. therapy should be stopped, and the cannula removed and resited as indicated (INS 2006). In addition, the findings must be carefully documented in the patient's clinical record. Review of the need for continued i.v. access and the most appropriate type for the patient's needs should be made at the earliest opportunity (RCN 2005b). (*See* Chapter 7 for detail about complications of peripheral i.v. therapy.)

Prevention of contamination

Organisms implicated in contamination of peripheral cannulae are carried on the skin of both patients and the healthcare professionals handling their venous access devices and i.v. therapy. The most common of these organisms are staphylococci, and all are carried from one patient to another on the hands of the practitioners caring for them (Weinstein 2007). Thus the most important factor in prevention of contamination is hand hygiene. Hands must be washed and dried thoroughly before any manipulation of the cannula, i.v. fluid, administration set or i.v. site regardless of whether or not gloves are worn (DH 2003; RCN 2005a; INS 2006; Pratt *et al.* 2007). When changing the dressing, there is a risk of contact with blood and so gloves should be worn. Gloves should be well-fitting to allow dexterity and careful manipulation of the dressing and cannula. Non-touch techniques should be used when manipulating cannulae and infusion equipment to reduce extrinsic contamination (INS 2006). Asepsis is obligatory whenever:

- a device is inserted or removed
- the dressing is changed/site is exposed
- the continuity of the infusion system is 'broken' or disconnected at any point such as changing the infusion container or administration set, or administering a bolus injection.

Types of dressing

Peripheral cannulae need to be secured to prevent accidental removal, to promote the patient's comfort, and to prevent phlebitis due to movement of the cannula within the vein. In addition, securing the cannula will avoid contamination of the site due to entraining skin organisms should the cannula move in and out of the vein (Dougherty 2004; Weinstein 2007). The puncture site of a cannula constitutes a wound and must be treated as any other wound and a sterile dressing should be applied using aseptic technique. It must also be applied correctly, as per manufacturer's instructions (INS 2006). Nelson *et al.* (1996) reported an increase in the incidence of inflammation around the site when dressings were not applied appropriately. Poorly applied dressings may not secure the cannula adequately or may allow access to the cannula site by contaminating organisms where there are creases in the dressing material (Campbell & Carrington 1999). The choice of dressing is usually dictated by local infection control policy, availability and cost, but dressings for peripheral cannulae should:

- be sterile
- allow inspection of the site
- be able to secure the cannula but be easy to apply and remove
- keep the site free from exogenous infection
- be comfortable
- be cost-effective (Campbell & Carrington 1999).

Sterile gauze secured with clean tape provides a cheap dressing but does not enable immediate inspection and needs to be changed every time it is removed. Adhesive, transparent, semipermeable membrane (TSM) dressings meet the above criteria, although they are more expensive (Finlay 2004).

One manufacturer produces a dressing that combines sterile adhesive gauze and TSM and also incorporates a small gauze pad to sit under the wings of the cannula to increase patient comfort. The puncture site is covered by a small perforated aluminium pad which has bacteriostatic properties and encourages moisture absorption, leaving the surface in contact with the skin dry, and thus discouraging bacterial growth.

'Statlocks' are a specifically designed 'securement devices' that secure venous access devices (VADs) in place using a plastic mechanism that locks the cannula in place over an adhesive sterile pad. The device and pad are then covered with a TSM dressing. In a comparative review of studies comparing different approaches to securing VADs, Schears (2005) established that 'Statlocks' hold peripheral cannulae in place and reduce associated complications, thus prolonging the cannula dwell-times significantly more effectively than conventional tape and transparent film dressings. However, these devices are more often used for midline or central venous catheters and are a more costly option (Schears 2005).

Frequency of dressing change

If the dressing on a peripheral cannula is clean and secure and allows inspection of the cannula insertion site, it need only be changed when the cannula is removed/resited (INS 2006). As with any wound, there is a risk of introducing infection during dressing change and there is the additional risk of movement or even displacement of the cannula during the process (Vost & Longstaff 1997). However, if the dressing is wet or blood-stained or, in the case of the transparent type, there is fluid collecting around the site, the dressing must be changed (RCN 2005b; INS 2006).

If the site requires cleaning, 2% aqueous chlorhexidine or 70% alcohol chlorhexidine should be used and allowed to dry, without fanning or wiping, before the dressing is applied (Dougherty 2004; Pellowe *et al.* 2004; Weinstein 2007). Great care is required during removal of the old dressing to avoid displacement of the cannula. If the patient is confused or unable to cooperate by keeping still, help should be sought. Scissors should never be used to remove old tape or dressings because of the risk of accidentally cutting the cannula or injuring the patient (INS 2006).

Bandaging

Bandaging a peripheral i.v. access site should be undertaken only if the patient prefers it or circumstances indicate it will promote safety for the patient and their VAD. Using a bandage obscures the site from immediate view and means that the bandage must be removed every time the site is assessed and the VAD is used (INS 2006). If a transparent moisture-permeable dressing is used to secure the VAD, its permeability will be impaired if a bandage is placed over it, thus defeating the dressing's purpose (Dougherty 2004). Bandages may raise the skin temperature, encouraging growth of skin bacteria and increasing the risk of contamination of the i.v. access site (Finlay 2004).

However, some patients do prefer not to see their VAD and if they are confused, bandaging may be indicated to secure the device (Weinstein 2007). A study by Stonehouse found that 60% of patients complained that the port of their VAD frequently caught on nightwear and bed linen, causing them discomfort, and so they preferred to have the site bandaged (Stonehouse 1996).

If bandaging is deemed necessary, a light 'cling'-type bandage should be applied gently. Tight bandaging with crepe bandages or tubigrip should be avoided as these are designed to apply pressure which may constrict the flow of blood and the infusion through the vein, or cause damage to the skin under the cannula (Finlay 2004). The bandage must be removed at least once a day and every time a drug is administered to allow inspection of the site. The site should be inspected more frequently if the patient complains of pain or discomfort.

Use of splints

As with bandaging, use of splints should be considered carefully and indications for their use documented in the patient's record (RCN 2005b). Nerve damage may result from pressure of the splint during prolonged use, and contractures can result from joints being immobilized in non-functional positions (Weinstein 2007). Splints may be indicated in babies and young children, or in adults if the cannula is over a joint. In these circumstances a splint should be padded to promote comfort and be bandaged into

Section 2

place, firmly enough to immobilize the joint but not so as to constrict blood flow or cause skin damage. The bandage should be removed and re-applied at least once a day, the area inspected for redness or skin damage, and a range of movements of the affected joint(s) undertaken (INS 2006). Any complaints of pain or discomfort from the patient should be investigated without delay (RCN 2005a). Splints should be disposable (INS 2006).

Maintaining Patency of Peripheral Cannulae

Many peripheral i.v. cannulae do not have an infusion attached. They may be used for intermittent bolus administration of drugs or to provide i.v. access for the administration of drugs, infusions or transfusions should the patient's condition suddenly deteriorate. In order to maintain patency of these cannulae, regular flushing is necessary.

Flushing solution

A meta-analysis of the effects of heparin and 0.9% sodium chloride flushes for peripheral cannulae confirmed that 0.9% sodium chloride was as effective as heparin in maintaining patency of i.v. cannulae (Randolph *et al.* 1998). The use of 0.9% sodium chloride avoids the risk of side-effects of heparin, such as thrombocytopenia or iatrogenic haemorrhage, which have been reported despite the small doses involved (Goode *et al.* 1991; Dougherty 2004). It also eliminates the risk of heparin incompatibility with drugs such as gentamicin and other antibiotics (Goode *et al.* 1991), and is significantly cheaper. In many NHS trusts, 0.9% sodium chloride flushes do not require a doctor's specific prescription and are administered under a Patient Group Direction.

Amount

Twice the volume of the cannula plus any additional tubing is required to flush adequately; 5 mL of 0.9% sodium chloride is sufficient to flush a cannula that is not being used for drug administration (RCN 2005b). If drugs are being administered intermittently, 2 mL of 0.9% sodium chloride should be administered before the drug, and 3 mL after. If more than one drug is being administered, more will be needed so that the device can be flushed after each drug to prevent mixing in the cannula. If there is extension tubing on the cannula or an infusion is in progress and the injection port of the administration set is being used, a larger volume of solution will also be needed to ensure adequate flushing of the tubing as well as the cannula.

Frequency of flushing

Peripheral cannulae that are not in regular use require flushing at least once every 24 hours (Dougherty 2004). Those through which drugs are given intermittently should be flushed before, during and after drug administration as described above, to avoid mixing of incompatible solutions (NICE 2003).

Flushing technique

Flushing the cannula should be done using a pulsatile (push–stop–push) technique, and the syringe withdrawn from the cannula while positive pressure is still being exerted on the plunger; this is achieved by pushing on the plunger of the syringe with the thumb whilst the syringe is disconnected from the device. This avoids backflow of blood into the device and subsequent occlusion (Dougherty 2004; RCN 2005b) and is facilitated by the

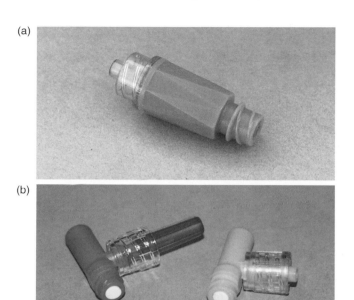

Figure 6.3 (a) Posiflow positive pressure injection cap. (b) CLC 2000 positive pressure injection caps (Dougherty 2006). Reprinted with permission of Blackwell Publishing.

device having an injectable, resealing port luer-locked onto its end (*See* Injectable caps on page 154). A more effective alternative is the use of a 'positive-pressure' injection cap on the end of the cannula. These have been manufactured to exert a positive pressure within the VAD as well as incorporating a closed, needle-free injection cap (*See* Figure 6.3) (Dougherty 2006).

If there is any sign of phlebitis, infection or infiltration before and during flushing, if the patient experiences pain, or if resistance is felt during flushing, the cannula should be removed. A review of the patient's ongoing need for peripheral i.v. access should be considered before resiting the cannula.

Preparation of the Intravenous Infusion

Inspection of infusion fluid

Most i.v. infusion fluids are manufactured in plastic infusion bags, although a few (e.g. human albumin solution) are provided in a glass bottle. The prescribed infusion fluid bags should be removed from their outer packaging and checked for leakage. The infusion fluid should be checked to ensure that the expiry date for use has not passed, the solution is clear and there are no particles present. Particles may indicate contamination of the fluid during the manufacturing process (although this is extremely rare), or precipitation of some component of the solution through improper storage. If particles are present, the solution must not be used and should be returned to the pharmacy so that the manufacturer can be alerted. If a solution containing particles is infused, it may cause particulate irritation of the venous endothelium, and blockage in the pulmonary or systemic circulation with potentially drastic effects (Weinstein 2007).

Section 2

Adding drugs to infusions

Many i.v. drugs are administered by continuous or intermittent infusion. Strict aseptic technique, preceded by hand-washing and disinfecting with alcohol hand-rub, must be used when adding drugs to an infusion bag or burette. When injecting into an infusion bag, it must be laid on a flat surface to avoid puncturing the bag when the injection is inserted (Lister 2004) and to facilitate mixing of the solution so that a bolus of the additive is not administered (Dougherty 2002). The injection port should be disinfected according to local policy, and the drug injected using a 23-G or 25-G needle. The injection membrane is designed to close completely after puncture and prevent the entry of microorganisms, provided a needle no bigger than 23-G or 25-G is used. The solution must then be mixed thoroughly to ensure even distribution.

A burette is useful for drug administration as the chamber allows mixing and dilution of the drug before administration. Care is required to ensure thorough mixing of the drug with the infusion fluid. Failure to mix thoroughly may result in a high concentration of the drug being administered over a short period of time.

A label must be affixed to the container or burette indicating:

- the name of the drug added
- the dose
- the date and time of its addition
- the signature(s) of the practitioner(s) who added/checked it (NPSA 2007).

Choosing the administration set

The nurse must choose an appropriate administration set, commonly referred to as a 'giving set'. A standard administration set is suitable for most i.v. infusions, with the exception of the following.

- *Blood and blood products.* A blood administration set, which has an integral filter chamber, must be used (*See* Chapter 13).
- *Platelets.* A special platelet administration set should be used (usually supplied with the platelet infusion) as filters in other sets will damage the platelets.
- *Neonates and paediatrics.* A burette should be used. This has a chamber into which a small amount of fluid from the bag is run before infusion to the patient. This prevents accidental overinfusion of large volumes of fluid. This may also be used for patients with heart failure to prevent accidental overload.

Different administration sets deliver different numbers of drops per millilitre (mL). This will need to be taken into consideration when calculating the drip rate of the infusion (*See* calculations on page 160). The different rates are:

- standard administration set: 20 drops/mL
- blood administration set: 15 drops/mL
- burette: 60 drops/mL.

Priming and connecting the administration set

Most administration sets have a date of sterilization on the packaging but may not have an expiry date by which they must be used. If the outer packaging is intact, has never been allowed to get wet and does not appear damaged in any way, the contents may be assumed to be sterile and usable. Both ends of the administration set are covered by protective caps to allow handling of the set without contamination of the part that will be inserted into the fluid bag or the end that will be attached to the VAD. All administration sets must be attached to the cannula using a luer-lock connection (INS 2006). *See* Boxes 6.1, 6.2 and 6.3.

BOX 6.1

Priming the administration set

- Close the flow control clamp before inserting the spike of the administration set into the fluid bag, as this prevents fluid running into the set before you are ready.
- Rest the bag of fluid on a flat surface to prevent accidental puncturing of the side of the bag when the spike is inserted.
- Remove the protective cover from the inlet port on the bag, and the protective cap from the spike of the administration set and push this firmly into the inlet port using a twisting movement to ensure it is fully inserted.
- Hang the bag on the infusion stand and squeeze the drip chamber several times until half full of fluid. Do not overfill it or you will be unable to see the drops forming.
- Expel all remaining air from the set by gradually opening the flow control clamp and allowing the fluid to flow slowly through the set.
- The protective cap on the end of the administration set should remain in place throughout to keep it sterile until use.
- If the infusion is in a glass bottle, an air inlet will be needed.

BOX 6.2

Connecting the administration set to the cannula

- The hands must be clean and gloves should be worn.
- If necessary, remove any bandaging and check the site for redness, swelling, heat or pain (*See* Chapter 7).
- Place a sterile gauze square under the end of the cannula when connecting the administration set to absorb any blood that leaks back from the cannula during connection (it must be sterile as it will come into contact with the exposed end of the cannula).
- With the exposed end of the administration set in your non-dominant hand and the sterile gauze in position underneath the end of the cannula, remove the cap or injectable cap on the end of the cannula.
- Alternatively, a needleless injection cap compatible with a luer-locked administration set connector may be used on the end of the cannula.
- Swiftly insert the end of the administration set and luer-lock into position.
- To reduce the flow of blood through the cannula as you connect the administration set, apply pressure to the vein just beyond the tip of the cannula.
- Discard the gauze in the clinical waste.

BOX 6.3

Changing an existing infusion

- If connecting a new bag to an existing infusion, inspect the infusion fluid as described in the text (*See* Inspection of infusion fluid, page 149).
- Close the roller clamp on the administration set. (Alternatively, bend the administration set back on itself and place the tubing in the clamp grippers at the back of the roller clamp. This will stop the flow of the infusion fluid. When the new infusion container has been connected, release the tubing from the clamp grippers and the infusion will continue at its preset rate.)
- Remove the old infusion from the stand and pull out the administration set, taking care not to contaminate the spike.
- Remove the protective cover from the inlet port of the new infusion bag, and whilst laying the bag flat (to prevent inadvertent puncture) insert the spike of the administration set, twisting until fully inserted.
- Replace the bag on the infusion stand and adjust the roller clamp to the prescribed flow rate or release the tubing from the clamp grippers as described above.

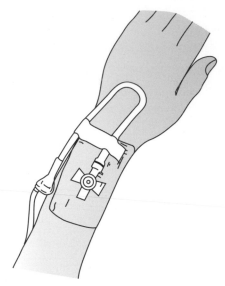

Figure 6.4   Fixing of tubing with tape.

Securing the administration set

Movement of the cannula in the vein causes mechanical phlebitis which damages the vein and reduces the flow of blood/infusate through the vein (Lister 2004). The tubing of an administration set can put traction on the cannula and cause phlebitis or dislodgement of the cannula. As cannula dressings are used to secure the device, so should administration set tubing be similarly secured to prevent it pulling on the cannula. This may be achieved by using a length of clean hypoallergenic tape; sterile tape is not required as it will have no contact with the insertion site wound. If required, loop the administration set tubing away from the patient's hand (Weinstein 2007) and place the tape completely around the circumference of the tubing and then on to the patient's skin away from the site dressing. Covering the site dressing with tape may prevent moisture loss through the dressing and increase the temperature at the site, thus encouraging bacterial growth (Finlay 2004). Ensure that the tubing between the tape and the cannula does not kink, is not pulling on the cannula and will not get caught and dislodge the cannula (*See* Figure 6.4).

Changing administration sets

Changing administration sets involves balancing the following:

- reducing the risk of contamination from the set (which increases with time and introduction of drugs)
- reducing manipulation of i.v. devices (which risks phlebitis and contamination)
- cost.

Administration sets for crystalloid infusions only need to be changed after 72 hours *in situ* (RCN 2005b; Pratt *et al.* 2007). This is congruent with recommendations by the United States Centers for Disease Control and Prevention (CDC 2002) whose guidance is supported by the results of a systematic review of studies researching optimum length of administration set use (Gillies *et al.* 2004). Administration sets used to infuse blood, blood products or lipid solutions need to be changed more frequently (CDC 2002; RCN 2005b; INS 2006; Pratt *et al.* 2007) (*See* Table 6.1).

Table 6.1   Changing administration sets.

Administration set type	Frequency of change
Continuous crystalloid infusion	72 hours Immediately if contaminated, when the set has been damaged in any way or when the i.v. access device is resited
Intermittent infusion, continuous drug infusions	24 hours when continuously connected to the i.v. access device Whenever administration set is disconnected if not continuously connected Immediately if contaminated or the set has been damaged in any way
Parenteral nutrition (PN)	Every 24 hours. This may be lengthened to 48 hours where a PN infusion runs continuously over that period and changing the set would disrupt the integrity of the infusion (Tait 2000) Immediately if contaminated or the set has been damaged in any way
Blood and blood products	12 hours When blood/blood product transfusion complete Immediately if contaminated or the set has been damaged in any way

(RCN 2005b; INS 2006; Pratt *et al*. 2007)

Administration sets must be changed using aseptic technique, following universal precautions and in line with the manufacturer's instructions. Using the procedures described in Boxes 6.1 and 6.2, administration set changes should coincide with commencement of a new infusion container to minimize the number of occasions that the closed infusion system is breached (INS 2006).

Administration sets should be labelled so that the change date or time is clearly visible, and a record kept in the patient's notes.

Three-Way Taps, Extension Sets and Other Equipment

Add-on devices for peripheral intravenous therapy include three-way taps, extension sets, injectable caps, needleless systems and in-line filters. Use of these devices should be kept to a minimum and they must only be used when indicated for the patient (DH 2003). They must be attached to the administration set and/or cannula using luer-locks in order to prevent disconnection (Dougherty 2004; INS 2006).

Three-way taps, ramping systems and extension sets

Three-way taps and ramping systems (also known as traffic lights) allow more than one infusion into a single vascular access device. For patients having short-term i.v. therapy this facilitates administering a continuous i.v. infusion with additional intermittent infusions or bolus drug administration, without disrupting the closed infusion system and risking contamination (Hindley 2004).

By virtue of their function, three-way taps and ramping systems require manipulation to alter the route of flow from different entry ports. This manipulation increases the risk of contamination and phlebitis considerably. The ports and turning mechanism on three-way taps are easily contaminated by both the patient's and the practitioners' skin flora; growing conditions for organisms are favourable and cleaning is difficult as their surface is uneven (Dougherty 2006). Repeated turning of the tap mechanism and flushing with infusion fluid makes colonization of the cannula more likely. Phlebitis results from

Section 2

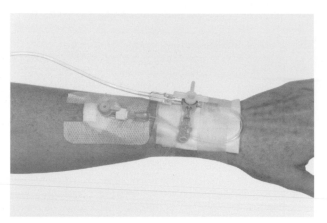

Figure 6.5   Using a three-way tap on a peripheral cannula (Finlay 2004). Reprinted with permission of Blackwell Publishing.

trauma to the lining of the vein caused by movement of the cannula whenever the three-way tap attached directly to the cannula is manipulated (Jackson 1998).

Any additional connection within an administration set increases the risk of infection (*See* Chapter 4). The use of three-way taps or ramping systems needs to be carefully considered in light of the benefits and risks. Where a device for multiple access is required on a peripheral cannula, it must always be used in conjunction with an extension set with all the connections luer-locked. Access ports on the three-way tap or ramping system must be capped off, preferably with needle-free injection caps to facilitate cleaning and subsequent drug administration or flushing (INS 2006; Weinstein 2007). A three-way tap should be secured to the patient's arm at a distance from the cannula, with a piece of sterile, low-linting gauze between it and the patient's skin. This will protect the tap from contamination, and the skin from pressure damage exerted by the plastic tap (*See* Figure 6.5). The extension set removes manipulations from proximity to the cannula, reducing the risk of contamination. Phlebitis is minimized as the flexibility of the extension set absorbs movement of the tap mechanism without dragging on the less flexible cannula (Finlay 2004). An extension set and three-way tap or ramping system should be changed with the same frequency as administration sets and at the same time as administration set(s) if used in conjunction with them (RCN 2005b).

Injectable caps

For intermittent bolus drug administration, an injectable cap that is either integral to an administration set or attached using a luer-lock on to the cannula (Figure 6.6) has several advantages. The injectable membrane is made of latex rubber that closes completely despite numerous punctures, provided a small needle is used; 23-g or 25-g is recommended (Lister 2004). This prevents the entry of microorganisms. The surface of the cap is easily disinfected and this should be done before each drug administration (NICE 2003). Using a needle with a small lumen means that the drug will be injected in a slow, controlled fashion. This allows the drug to be diluted by the blood flow in the vein, reducing chemical irritation to the vein wall. However, because a needle is used, there is some risk of needlestick injury (*See* Needleless systems on page 155).

Some cannulae are equipped with an integral injection port covered by a coloured protective cap. These are designed for drug administration by attaching the syringe hub directly onto the injection port, and as no needle is required, the risk of needlestick

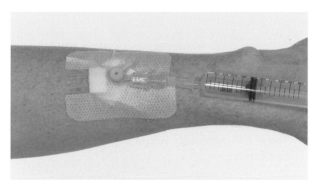

Figure 6.6   Ported cannula, dressed with transparent semi-permeable dressing with injectable cap attached (Finlay 2004). Reprinted with permission of Blackwell Publishing.

injury is reduced. However, as with three-way taps, there is a danger that the injection port will become contaminated, particularly as the protective cap frequently becomes loose, and the area is difficult to clean effectively (Clarke 1997). When the drug is administered, any microorganisms or debris present are flushed into the circulation.

Needleless systems

The risk of bloodborne infection from needlestick injury has been reduced significantly with the introduction of needleless systems. Provided they are used according to manufacturers' instructions, these appear to have all the advantages of injectable caps without the disadvantage of using a needle (Brown *et al.* 1997; Cookson *et al.* 1998; Mendelson *et al.* 1998). Their design involves a rubber membrane and valve mechanism that opens to admit a syringe tip, or plastic 'needle' but closes after their removal to provide a secure barrier against the entry of microorganisms. Most needleless systems also allow the attachment of an administration set so intermittent infusions may be attached without removing the cap and opening the system, which should also reduce the risk of infection (Weinstein 2007). In addition, some manufacturers provide administration sets with needle-free injection ports to enhance the safety of administration of drugs via the side-arm of the administration set.

US law has legislated that healthcare facilities must use safer devices including needleless systems, but there is no similar legislation in the UK at present. However, their use is recommended by both the RCN and NHS Employers (RCN 2005b; NHS Employers 2005). The decision to use needleless systems may be made locally and needs to weigh up the additional cost against the risk to practitioners of transmission of serious infection via needlestick injuries. The cost is significantly higher than an ordinary injectable cap and this is likely to influence a decision to use them in general clinical areas. However, their use should be considered with patients who are particularly vulnerable to infection and in areas where a needlestick injury would carry a high risk, such as areas where patients may have viral hepatitis or HIV. When selecting a needleless system, quality, ease of use, compatibility with other equipment, cost and perceived benefits to patients and staff need to be considered (Dougherty 2002).

In-line filters

Standard administration sets have integral filters of 15 microns (μm). Blood administration sets have filters of 170-μm width to prevent damage to the cells being transfused whilst filtering out particulate material or microaggregates (Finlay 2004). In-line filters of 0.2-μm width can be attached to the end of administration sets to prevent particulate matter, fungi, bacteria and endotoxins from entering the circulation. This reduces risks to the patient of contamination and reduces the frequency with which administration sets need to be changed (RCN 2005b; Weinstein 2007). However, studies have not been able to provide convincing evidence that they reduce bacterial contamination sufficiently to justify their universal use and the resulting cost (Johns 1996; Fennessy *et al.* 1999). Consequently the use of in-line filters is usually restricted to those who are immunodeficient or immunocompromised and those receiving multiple infusions with many additives.

Preparation for Intravenous Drug Administration

Checking procedures

Administration of drugs to patients is the final step in a series of actions involving a number of health professionals including pharmacists, doctors and/or non-medical prescribers, and nurses or midwives. Mutual trust and respect between these professional groups improves the safety of drug therapy for patients by facilitating questioning and clarification about treatment and prescribing decisions. Administering drugs to patients requires nurses to be familiar with the *Principles for the Administration of Medicines* (NMC 2004) (*See* Box 6.4).

BOX 6.4

***Principles for the Administration of Medicines* (NMC 2002)**

- 'know the therapeutic uses of the medicine to be administered, its normal dosage, side-effects, precautions and contraindications
- be certain of the identity of the patient to whom the medicine is to be administered
- be aware of the patient's care plan
- check that the prescription, or label on medicine dispensed by a pharmacist, is clearly written and unambiguous
- have considered the dosage, method of administration, route and timing of the administration in the context of the condition of the patient and coexisting therapies
- check the expiry date of the medicine to be administered
- check that the patient is not allergic to the medicine before administering it
- contact the prescriber or another authorized prescriber without delay where contraindications to the prescribed medicine are discovered, where the patient develops a reaction to the medicine, or where assessment of the patient indicates that the medicine is no longer suitable
- make a clear, accurate and immediate record of all medicine administered, intentionally withheld or refused by the patient, ensuring that any written entries and the signature are clear and legible...'

Meticulous checking of each element of preparing and administering a drug is essential to minimize drug errors and the associated potential harm to patients. With the exception of controlled drug administration, only one nurse need check drugs for administration in most areas. That nurse needs to be confident that all the principles for administering medicines have been addressed (NMC 2002). When these principles are adhered to, it follows that nurses will only administer intravenous drugs they have prepared themselves for immediate administration to an individual patient. Exceptions arise when drugs have been specially prepared for the patient in the pharmacy (such as cytotoxic drugs) and when nurses hand over the care of patients receiving intravenous drugs by an infusion that is still in progress. In both cases the infusions must be clearly labelled with the name of the drug, the dose, the time and date of preparation and the signature of the person who prepared the drug. A record of commencement of the infusion should be clearly made on the patient's drug chart (*See* Documentation and record keeping on page 163).

Ideally, preparation of drugs for i.v. administration should take place in a separate area where there are minimal distractions. This area should have hand-washing facilities and be stocked with the necessary equipment for safe preparation of drugs. This should aid concentration, reduce errors related to interruptions, and reduce contamination of the drugs being prepared or the individuals preparing them (Finlay 2004). Drugs for one patient should be prepared and then administered immediately (NPSA 2007). This reduces the risk of the drug(s) being given to the wrong patient. Also, some drugs may be stable for a short period only when reconstituted and so should be administered immediately (Dougherty 2002; NMC 2002; BMA/RPSGB 2007).

Individual nurses may wish to seek confirmation of their decision-making in drug administration by involving another nurse in the checking procedure. In such circumstances it is vital that both nurses check independently and come to an agreement about the elements of the process rather than one nurse relying on the other's decisions for perceived reasons of expertise, experience or hierarchy (Finlay 2004). In emergency situations, when drugs are prepared for administration by another practitioner, it is the responsibility of the individual administering the drug to be satisfied that the principles for administering medicines have been followed (NMC 2002).

A nurse administering a drug or caring for a patient receiving a drug infusion must be completely satisfied that the 'right drug' is being given to the 'right patient' in the 'right dose', at the 'right time' and by the 'right route'. The 'five rights' were proposed to provide a simple but thorough framework for checking that the elements of a drug administration procedure are correct (Clayton 1987).

The 'right patient'

The patient to whom the drug is to be given must have their identity checked to ensure the prescribed drug is given to the patient for whom it has been prescribed. The name and identifying information on the prescription must be the same as the patient's, and should be checked against the patient's identification band (NPSA 2006). In the absence of an identification band the patient should be asked their name and date of birth, and steps should be taken to fit the patient with an identification band as soon as possible. A study into drug errors found that in 79 drug incidents, 10 (12.7%) involved the incorrect patient (Gladstone 1995). The study found that giving a drug to the wrong patient is almost always linked to a failure to check the patient's identity, whether this is due to distractions or simply not following protocol. Anecdotal evidence suggests that patients sometimes answer to the wrong name, perhaps because they did not actually hear what was said or because they assume that the nurse knows who they really are and it was simply a 'slip of the tongue'.

Having confirmed that it is the right patient, it is important to ensure that a specific dose of the drug has not already been given to the patient. The patient should also be asked if they have any allergies relating to the drug about to be given, and if not already recorded, an entry must be made in the patient's notes and on the drug chart.

The 'right drug'

The patient's prescription (on the drug chart) must be checked for accuracy. It must be clearly written, dated and signed by the prescriber whose name and contact details must be stated. The drug must be correctly prescribed using its generic name (e.g. furosemide

Section 2

not Lasix) and must include the strength (where applicable), dose, route, frequency and timing of administration (Dougherty 2002). The drug to be used must also have its expiry date checked; it should be discarded with the rest of the batch if the expiry date has been exceeded.

It is also necessary to check the diluent for an i.v. drug in the same way. In addition, the compatibility of the drug with the diluent used, with other drugs being given and with any infusions that are running through the same i.v. access device must be established. Most i.v. drugs will be diluted with sterile water for injections to a volume of at least 10 mL (except in paediatrics). This is to reduce chemical irritation of the lining of the vein, which results in phlebitis (*See* Chapter 7). It also facilitates slower administration of the drug. Although there are some exceptions, most drugs should not be mixed with others before administration as this may cause chemical degradation of one or both agents, precipitation or unknown chemical reactions (Weinstein 2007). *See* Box 6.5.

If a number of drugs are being given as bolus injections, the cannula must be flushed between each drug to prevent mixing which can lead to precipitation or chemical reactions in the cannula (INS 2006); 0.9% sodium chloride is normally used for this (*See* Maintaining patency of peripheral cannulae on page 148) but a few drugs are incompatible with 0.9% sodium chloride (e.g. amphotericin) in which case 5% dextrose should be used instead. The *British National Formulary* (*BNF*) (BMA/RPSGB 2007) provides comprehensive information regarding the compatibility of various drugs with common infusion fluids. If in doubt, flush the cannula well before and after administration of the drug.

The 'right dose'

It is the nurse's responsibility to know the usual dose of the drug so that unusual prescriptions are queried with the prescriber or another authorized prescriber familiar with the patient's treatment plan (NMC 2002). A source of reference such as the hospital i.v. drug formulary or the *BNF* should be readily available to allow speedy checking. The dose should be clearly written using recognized abbreviations only. The abbreviations for milligrams (mg) and micrograms (µg) look very similar when handwritten and so micrograms should be written in full or the abbreviation 'mcg' should be used to avoid confusion. In addition, the nurse administering the drug must check that the prescribed dose is prepared and drawn up for administration. This may involve calculations and it is vital that nurses are competent at mathematical calculations so that the 'right dose' is administered (*See* Drug calculations below).

BOX 6.5

Knowledge a nurse must possess before administering intravenous drugs

- The action of the drug.
- The recommended dosage range.
- Possible side-effects.
- Any special precautions during and after administration (e.g. protection from light).
- The type of diluent to be used.
- The method of administration, (e.g. by slow i.v. bolus or intermittent infusion).
- Compatibility with other drug therapy and infusions.
- Any patient monitoring required before, during or after administration.

The 'right time'

One of the principal reasons for administering drugs intravenously is to establish and maintain adequate serum levels of the drug for optimum efficacy. With many treatment regimens, maintaining serum levels relies on accurate timing of administration of consecutive doses of the drug involved. Thus checking that the drug is due to be given (including the accurate time for administration) is important. If the prescription has not been signed as given, it is also important to check, if possible, whether or not the patient received the drug, to prevent double doses being administered.

The 'right route'

Nurses need to be familiar with drugs being administered intravenously in their practice area so that they can confirm the suitability of the intravenous route for administering individual drugs. The local hospital i.v. drug formulary or policy will indicate which drugs nurses competent in i.v. therapy may give; those not included will need to be given by the prescriber. In addition, nurses should also be familiar with the changes in dose required when this route is used for drug administration, and be able to question any discrepancies in prescriptions with the prescriber and/or a pharmacist.

Drugs suitable for i.v. administration should be labelled accordingly and the data sheet should include specific instructions for administration by this route (Scales 1996). Some intramuscular (IM) preparations may not be suitable for i.v. use and the appropriate dose may well vary. However, some drugs are being given intravenously before the manufacturer has obtained a product licence for that route. If a drug is prescribed for i.v. administration but the ampoule and data sheet state that it is for IM or subcutaneous (SC) use only, the nurse should check with the pharmacy before administration.

Drug errors made when drugs have been given by the wrong route can have serious consequences and even be fatal, usually because the i.v. dose is much smaller than that given IM, SC or orally. In addition, the nurse administering the drug intravenously must carefully check that the device through which the drug is about to be given is the appropriate, i.v. access device, rather than an alternative infusion device (e.g. an arterial or epidural catheter). Routinely checking the access site for phlebitis, inflammation or infiltration prior to administering i.v. drugs (*See* Observation of the site on page 143) should avoid this error, as the entire intravenous administration system is observed from insertion site back to administration set or injection cap.

Drug calculations

It is vital that the nurse is competent in accurate and reasonably speedy calculations relating to patients' i.v. therapy. Lower levels of numeracy have beennoted in students in higher education generally and among nursing students specifically (Sabin 2001). Many nurses find drug calculations challenging but given the critical nature of accuracy of calculations in intravenous therapy, it is crucial to develop numeracy skills. This can be achieved by seeking help and using numeracy education tools specifically developed for the purpose (*See* websites at the end of the chapter). Nurses are accountable for decisions they make in practice including checking the drugs they are giving and the volumes and rates they are administered in (Hutton 1998). Unlike oral tablets, the patient has no means of knowing whether the drug in the syringe is in fact correct: a syringe containing 250 mg of an antibiotic may look exactly the same as one containing 750 mg. Even totally different drugs may look exactly the same in the syringe.

There are three types of drug calculation that all nurses need to be able to perform competently for i.v. drug administration (Finlay 2004):

1. calculation of the volume of an injection (*See* below)
2. calculation of the number of drops per minute (drops/min) for gravity infusions and drip-regulating infusion devices
3. calculation of the number of millilitres per hour (mL/h) for volumetric infusion devices (*See* Chapter 8).

(*See* Chapter 15 on Calculations.)

Formulae

Knowing a few simple formulae will help the nurse perform drug calculations, provided the same SI units are used within each calculation (*See* Box 6.6).

BOX 6.6

Calculation of doses, concentrations and volumes

$$\frac{\text{What you want}}{\text{What you've got}} \times \text{volume available} = \text{volume required}$$

Example Gentamicin 120 mg has been prescribed. The stock ampoules are 80 mg in 2 mL. The calculation would be:

$$\frac{\text{Gentamicin } 120 \text{ mg}}{\text{Gentamicin } 80 \text{ mg}} \times 2 \text{ mL} = \frac{240}{80} = \textbf{3 mL}$$

Calculation of infusion rates

In millilitres per hour:

$$\frac{\text{Volume prescribed (mL)}}{\text{Hours of infusion time}} = \text{mL/hour}$$

In drops per minute:

$$\frac{\text{Volume prescribed (mL)}}{\text{Hours of infusion time}} \times \frac{\text{Drops per mL of giving set}}{60 \text{(minutes per hour)}}$$

Example An infusion of 500 mL of Hartmann's solution is prescribed to run over 6 hours. The calculation of infusion rate would be:

$$\frac{\text{Hartmann's solution } 500 \text{ mL}}{6 \text{ hours}} = \text{mL/hour} = \frac{500}{6} = \textbf{83.33 mL/hour}$$

Example An infusion of 500 mL of Hartmann's solution is prescribed to run over 6 hours. The calculation of drops per minute through a standard infusion set would be:

$$\frac{\text{Hartmann's solution } 500 \text{ ml}}{6 \text{ hours}} \times \frac{20}{60} = \text{drops per minute}$$

$$83.33 \times \frac{1}{3} = 83.33 \times 0.33 = 27.77 = \textbf{28 drops/minute}$$

Professional responsibility

Nurses' drug calculation errors and deviation from safe administration are known to be risk factors for medication errors, in particular in intravenous therapy (O'Shea 1999; Wirtz *et al.* 2003). Whilst the causes of drug administration errors are usually multifactorial, practitioners who prepare, administer and monitor the effects of drugs have a responsibility to patients to update and maintain their knowledge and skills in order to minimize their part in potential drug errors. The importance of being competent to accurately perform the calculations necessary for drug administration cannot be overemphasized. It is vital that nurses seek help if they have difficulty in this area, and pharmacists are usually willing to offer help and advice. Checking with another nurse may be advisable where calculations are involved (NMC 2002), but as stated earlier, the administering nurse must never rely on the second person to perform the calculation. Both nurses must perform the calculation and show the way the calculation achieved the answer, rather than simply exchanging answers. If there is any disagreement or uncertainty about the answer, help should be sought and the drug should not be given until the right dose, volume or rate is established.

Preparing the patient

Once sure that the prescribed drug is prepared for administration to the right patient, it is important to explain the procedure for drug administration and the aims of the treatment to the patient clearly. They need to be aware, as with any drug treatment, of the potential effects of the therapy (both desirable and undesirable), why they need to receive it, the frequency with which it will be administered and how it will be given. If additional monitoring of their condition is required in association with the i.v. drug therapy this must also be clarified (for example, regular monitoring of blood glucose level to titrate an insulin infusion). When appropriate, patients may be involved in monitoring the condition of their peripheral i.v. access site, to alert nurses to early signs of infiltration or phlebitis and to inform them of completion of an infusion. Providing comprehensive information and involving patients in their care according to their individual needs is likely to contribute to better outcomes and reduced anxiety (Wilson-Barnett & Batehup 1992; Drewett 2000).

Drug administration

Aseptic technique must be used in i.v. drug preparation and administration as in all other aspects of i.v. procedures, with thorough hand-washing and drying being undertaken at the beginning and end of the procedure (including immediately before the drug is administered). It is recommended that well-fitting gloves are worn to protect the nurse from absorption of the drug via their skin and contamination with the patient's microorganisms which may subsequently lead to cross-infection of other patients (DH 2001).

Before beginning administration of the drug(s), check the patient's identity, confirming it is the same as the prescription, confirm they are not allergic to the drug in question and inspect the peripheral i.v. access site to exclude phlebitis, infiltration or infection. Patency of the device must be checked by ensuring an existing fluid infusion is running freely, or flushing the cannula with 0.9% sodium chloride solution before administering any drugs. If there is any doubt about the patency of the device or health of the vein the drugs should not be administered and the cannula removed.

Peripheral cannulae are suitable for administration of drugs and fluid infusions that are isotonic, have an osmolality of less than 500 mOsm/L and a pH of between 5 and 9 when appropriately diluted (RCN 2005b; INS 2006).

Section 2

Drugs may be administered through a peripheral cannula in three ways:

1. by continuous infusion
2. by intermittent infusion
3. by intermittent injection (bolus injection).

Continuous infusion

A continuous infusion is used to administer a drug from either a syringe or a container at a constant rate over time. Pumps are often used to ensure a constant and accurate flow rate (Sarpal *et al.* 2004). Patients need to be made aware of what effects the infusion will have, and any side-effects it may have; these should be monitored in addition to checking the insertion site of the cannula for phlebitis or infiltration (Lister 2004).

The container or syringe needs to be clearly labelled with the name of the drug, the dose, the volume of the solution, the date and time of preparation and the signature of the person who prepared it (INS 2006). It is preferable that continuous drug infusions are administered via dedicated access rather than being administered in conjunction with another infusion. However, if this is not possible, a three-way tap and extension tube attached to the VAD may be used. Ensure that the tap and extension tube are primed with 0.9% sodium chloride solution before use (Finlay 2004).

Administration sets for drug infusions should be changed every 24 hours to avoid administering a less active solution of the drug, or a solution into which plasticizer has leached from the administration tubing (*See* Table 6.1).

Intermittent infusion

An intermittent infusion is one that is administered once only or at repeated intervals. It is usually given over 20 minutes to 2 hours and is indicated when peak levels of a drug are required (Rang *et al.* 2003). It may be given alone or in tandem with a compatible continuous infusion. As with continuous drug infusions, it is preferable that drug infusions have dedicated intravenous access via a single cannula. Where this is not possible, administration sets designed for additional access via a luer-locking side port or a three-way tap and extension tube may be used as described above. A similar procedure should be used in advising patients about the effects of the drug to be administered and in labelling the infusion. Between doses, the drug administration set may either be removed and discarded, or left *in situ*. If left *in situ*, the administration set must still be changed every 24 hours (*See* Table 6.1) (Dougherty 2004; Weinstein 2007).

Direct intermittent injection

Direct intermittent injections should be administered into the cannula using a 23-G or 25-G needle and syringe via an injectable cap, either attached to the end of the cannula, or incorporated into the fluid administration set. Needleless systems may be used by preference for administration into a cap directly attached onto the cannula or via the needleless injection port of an administration set (*See* Needleless systems on page 155). The drug should be administered at the rate specified by the manufacturer according to the drug's action and toxicity (Finlay 2004; Lister 2004). Where a compatible infusion is running, the drug may be injected into the administration set while the infusion is running to further dilute the drug and reduce the risk of chemical phlebitis (Dougherty 2002). If the infusion is not compatible, it must be turned off, the roller clamp moved down the tubing to the point just above the injection port, and the set flushed with 0.9% sodium chloride solution in sufficient volume to clear the tubing of residual fluid before the drug is administered.

After administration of the drug it must be flushed again to clear it of the drug solution. The fluid infusion may then be recommenced. The cannula (and administration set) must be flushed with 0.9% sodium chloride solution before drug administration, between each separate drug injection and when administration of drug therapy is complete, unless the drug concerned is incompatible with 0.9% sodium chloride solution in which case 5% dextrose may be used (Finlay 2004). (*See* Flushing technique on page 148.)

Documentation and record-keeping

Clear, timely record-keeping promotes patient care through written communication and is integral to professional practice (NMC 2005). All aspects of i.v. therapy should be documented according to local policy. This will usually include the following.

- Sites, insertion dates and types of i.v. access devices (DH 2003; INS 2006).
- Records of the condition of the insertion site including phlebitis scoring, suspected infection or infiltration scoring as indicated and the subsequent action taken.
- Flush regimen.
- The time an infusion started.
- The batch number of the fluid. This is recorded on the i.v. prescription chart so that in the event of an adverse reaction, the manufacturers will be able to trace the fluid back to the production stage.
- Most patients with an i.v. infusion will require fluid balance to be recorded. The new infusion and completion of the old should be written on a fluid balance chart.
- The signature of the practitioner(s) checking and administering i.v. infusions and drug therapy and the time of administration.

Infusion devices

Infusion devices, or pumps, are increasingly used to deliver i.v. infusions in most clinical areas and for many patients having intravenous therapy at home. The use of pumps aims to deliver fluids or drugs to the patient at a constant, set rate as part of the patient's treatment (Sarpal *et al.* 2004). Using a pump is indicated when overinfusion, underinfusion or irregular infusion rates are a risk, whether the patient's VAD is a peripheral or central device. The choice of pump is important and must be informed by the user's knowledge and competence in relation to appropriate device selection and use (INS 2006). *See* Chapter 8.

Removal of Peripheral Intravenous Cannulae

Peripheral cannulae should be removed when:

- the patient experiences pain, particularly when fluids are infused or on flushing the device
- there is any sign of phlebitis, thrombophlebitis or infection
- there is infiltration of infusate
- the cannula cannot be easily flushed
- therapy is no longer required.

When 72 hours have elapsed after insertion of a cannula, its removal and resiting should be considered if i.v. access is still required (CDC 2002). If the site shows no signs of the above complications and the device is patent, removal may be delayed (DH 2003; Dougherty 2004).

As with all other interventions with i.v. therapy devices, removing the cannula should be undertaken with an aseptic technique, gloves should be worn due to the likely contact with blood, and all the equipment required should have been assembled at the patient's side. Having stopped any infusion and lifted the cannula dressing from the skin, the device should be slowly and steadily withdrawn from the vein. Firm, continuous pressure should be applied to the site with a sterile gauze square immediately after complete withdrawal of the cannula (the patient may be able to do this). When bleeding has stopped, a small, sterile adhesive dressing may be applied. Relying only on gauze and tape to provide sufficient pressure to stop the bleeding should be avoided, as it is rarely successful and can result in extensive bruising (Godwin *et al.* 1992; INS 2006).

The cannula should be checked after removal to ensure that the complete device has been removed, and an appropriate record entered in the patient's notes. If it is suspected that the patient has bacteraemia or septicaemia, or there is a site infection, the cannula may be sent for culture and microscopy (INS 2006). Plastic cannulae may be disposed of in clinical waste bags whilst steel winged devices must be disposed of in sharps containers (MHRA 2004; Pratt *et al.* 2007).

Conclusion

Intravenous therapy has become a routine part of the nursing care of patients in hospital, and increasingly those in community settings as well (Kayley & Finlay 2003). The peripheral i.v. route clearly has several advantages, as well as risks. The nurse's role in the safe management of i.v. therapy is crucial. Through evidence-based practice, strict asepsis and thorough checking, many of the risks of i.v. therapy will be reduced, if not avoided altogether. Understanding the risks of phlebitis, infiltration and infection and taking appropriate steps to avoid them will result in a health-promoting, safe approach to managing patients' i.v. therapy (INS 2006).

References

British Medical Association/Royal Pharmaceutical Society of Great Britain (BMA/RPSGB) (2007) *British National Formulary*, 53. The Pharmaceutical Press, London.

Brown JD, Moss HA, Elliott TSJ (1997) The potential for catheter microbial contamination from a needleless connector. *Journal of Hospital Infection* 36(3): 181–189.

Campbell H, Carrington M (1999) Peripheral intravenous cannula dressings: advantages and disadvantages. *British Journal of Nursing* 8(21): 1420–1427.

Centers for Disease Control (CDC) (2002) Guidelines for the prevention of intravascular catheter-related infections. *Morbidity and Mortality Weekly Report* 51: RR10, 1–29.

Clarke A (1997) The nursing management of intravenous drug therapy. *British Journal of Nursing* 6(4): 201–206.

Clayton M (1987) The right way to prevent medicine errors. *Registered Nurse* June: 30–31.

Cookson S (1998) Increased bloodstream infection rates in surgical patients associated with variation from recommended use and care following implementation of a needleless device. *Infection Control Hospital Epidemiology* 19(1): 23–27.

Department of Health (DH) (2001) Guidelines for preventing infections associated with the insertion and maintenance of central venous catheters. *Journal of Hospital Infection* 47(Suppl): S47–S67.

Department of Health (2003) *Winning Ways: Working Together to Reduce Healthcare-Associated Infection in England*. Department of Health, London.

Department of Health (2005) *Saving Lives: a Delivery Programme to Reduce Healthcare-Associated Infection Including MRSA*. Department of Health, London.

Dougherty L (2000) Changing tack on therapy. *Nursing Standard* 14(30): 61.

Dougherty L (2002) Delivery of intravenous therapy. *Nursing Standard* 16(16): 45–52.

Dougherty L (2004) Vascular access devices: insertion and management. In: Dougherty L, Lister S, eds. *The Royal Marsden Hospital Manual of Clinical Nursing Procedures*, 6th edn, pp. 764–773. Blackwell Publishing, Oxford.

Dougherty L (2006) *Essential Clinical Skills for Nurses: Central Venous Access Devices: Care and Management*. Blackwell Publishing, Oxford.

Drewett S (2000) Complications of central venous catheters: nursing care. *British Journal of Nursing* 9(8): 466–477.

Fennessy P, Antonis P, Anderson J (1999) *What is the Efficacy of In-Line Filters in Reducing Microbiological Contamination of Intravenous Fluids?* Centre for Clinical Effectiveness, Monash Medical Centre, Southern Health Care Network, Victoria, Australia.

Finlay TMD (2004) *Essential Clinical Skills for Nurses: Intravenous Therapy*. Blackwell Publishing, Oxford.

Gillies D, O'Riordan L, Wallen M, Rankin K, Morrison A, Nagy S (2004) Timing of intravenous administration set changes: a systematic review. *Infection Control and Hospital Epidemiology* 25(3): 240–250.

Gladstone J (1995) Drug administration errors: a study into the factors underlying the occurrence and reporting of drug errors in a district general hospital. *Journal of Advanced Nursing* 22: 628–637.

Godwin PG, Cuthbert AC, Choyce A (1992) Reducing bruising after venepuncture. *Quality in Health Care* 1: 245–246.

Goode CJ, Titler M, Rakel B, Ones DS, Kleiber C, Small S, Triolo PK (1991) A meta-analysis of effects of heparin flush and saline flush: quality and cost implications. *Nursing Research* 40(6): 324–330.

Hindley G (2004) Infection control in peripheral cannulae. *Nursing Standard* 17(18): 37–40.

Hutton M (1998) Numeracy skills for intravenous calculations. *Nursing Standard* 12(34): 49–56.

Infusion Nurses Society (INS) (2006) Infusion nursing standards of practice. *Journal of Infusion Nursing* 29(1S) (Suppl) S1–S92.

Jackson A (1998) Infection control: a battle in vein infusion phlebitis. *Nursing Times* 94(4): 68–71.

Johns T (1996) Intravenous filters, panacea or placebo. *Journal of Clinical Nursing* 5: 3–6.

Kayley J, Finlay T (2003) Vascular access devices for patients in the community. *Community Practitioner* 76(6): 228–231.

Lister S (2004) Drug administration: general principles. In: Dougherty L, Lister S, eds. *The Royal Marsden Hospital Manual of Clinical Nursing Procedures*, 6th edn, pp. 184–227. Blackwell Publishing, Oxford.

Medicines and Healthcare Products Regulatory Agency (MRHA) (2004) *Reducing Needlestick and Sharps Injuries*. Medicines and Healthcare products Regulatory Agency, London.

Mendelson MH, Short LJ, Shechter CB *et al.* (1998) Study of a needleless intermittent intravenous access system for peripheral infusions: analysis of staff, patient and institutional outcomes. *Infection Control Hospital Epidemiology* 19(6): 401–406.

NHS Employers (2005) *The Management of Health, Safety and Welfare Issues for NHS Staff*. NHS Confederation (Employers) Company Limited [www document]. www.amicustheunion.org/pdf/NHSHandSBlueBook.pdf [accessed 25 January 2007]

Nelson RS, Tebbs SE, Richards N, Elliott TSJ (1996) An audit of peripheral catheter care in a teaching hospital. *Journal of Hospital Infection* 32(1): 65–69.

National Institute for Clinical Excellence (NICE) (2003) *Infection Control: Prevention of Healthcare-Associated Infection in Primary and Community Care*. National Institute for Health and Clinical Excellence, London.

National Patient Safety Agency (NPSA) (2006) Wristbands vital for matching care. *Safety Matters*, Spring, National Patient Safety Agency. http://www.npsa.nhs.uk/site/media/documents/1841_safetymatters_spring06_web.pdf [accessed 24 January 2007]

National Patient Safety Agency (2007) Promoting safer use of injectable medicines. *Patient Safety Alert* 20, 28 March.

Nursing and Midwifery Council (NMC) (2002) *Guidelines for the Administration of Medicines*. Nursing and Midwifery Council, London.

Nursing and Midwifery Council (2005) *Guidelines for Records and Record Keeping*. Nursing and Midwifery Council, London.

O'Shea E (1999) Factors contributing to medication errors: a literature review. *Journal of Clinical Nursing* 8(5): 496–504.

Pellowe CM, Pratt, RJ, Loveday HP *et al.* (2004) The *epic* project. Updating the evidence base for national evidence-based guidelines for preventing healthcare-associated infections in NHS hospitals in England: a report with recommendations. *British Journal of Infection Control* 5(6): 10–16.

Pratt RJ, Pellowe C, Wilson JA *et al.* (2007) epic 2: national evidence-based guidelines for preventing healthcare-associated infections in NHS hospitals in England. *Journal of Hospital Infection* 655 (Suppl): S1–S64.

Randolph AG, Cook DJ, Gonzales CA, Andrew M (1998) Benefit of heparin in peripheral venous and arterial catheters: systematic review and meta-analysis of randomized controlled trials. *British Medical Journal* 316(7136): 969–975.

Rang HP, Dale MM, Ritter JM, Moore PK (2003) *Pharmacology*, 5th edn. Churchill Livingstone, Edinburgh.

Royal College of Nursing (RCN) (2005a) *Good Practice in Infection Prevention and Control*. Royal College of Nursing, London.

Royal College of Nursing (2005b) *Standards for Infusion Therapy*. Royal College of Nursing, London.

Sabin M (2001) *Competence in Practice-Based Calculation: Issues for Nursing Education* [www document]. www.health.ltsn.ac.uk/publications/occasionalpaper/occasionalpaper03.pdf [accessed 24 January 2007]

Sarpal N, Dougherty L, Laverty D (2004) Drug administration: delivery (infusion devices). In: Dougherty L, Lister S, eds. *The Royal Marsden Hospital Manual of Clinical Nursing Procedures*, 6th edn, pp. 259–274. Blackwell Publishing, Oxford.

Scales K (1996) Legal and professional aspects of intravenous therapy. *Nursing Standard* 11(3): 41–46.

Schears GJ (2005) The benefits of a catheter securement device on reducing patient complications: a comprehensive review. *Managing Infection Control* 5(2): 14–26.

Stonehouse J (1996) Phlebitis associated with peripheral cannulae. *Professional Nurse* 12(1): 51–53.

Tait J (2000) Nursing management. In: Hamilton H, ed. *Total Parenteral Nutrition; a Guide for Nurses*. Churchill Livingstone, Edinburgh.

Vost J, Longstaff V (1997) Infection control and related issues in intravascular therapy. *British Journal of Nursing* 6(15): 846–857.

Weinstein SM, ed. (2007) *Plumer's Principles & Practice of Intravenous Therapy*, 8th edn. Lippincott Williams & Wilkins, Philadelphia.

Wilson-Barnett J, Batehup L (1992) *Patients' Problems: a Research Base for Nursing Care*. Scutari, London.

Wirtz V, Barber N, Taxis K (2003) An observational study of intravenous medication errors in the United Kingdom and in Germany. *Pharmacy World and Science* 25(3): 104–111.

Websites

http://newwww.nursing-standard.co.uk/archives/pn_pdfs/pnvol17n02/pncalculationskills.pdf
An RCN publication about drug calculations in paediatric nursing: contains sample calculations to do and useful information for all nurses.

http://www.dh.gov.uk
The Department of Health website: current guidance and policy, and links to other national healthcare agencies and resources.

http://www.mhra.gov.uk/home/idcplg?IdcService=SS_GET_PAGE&nodeId=5
The Medicines and Healthcare Products Regulatory Agency's website: publishes information about medical devices including those used in i.v. therapy.

http://www.nice.org.uk
The National Institute for Health and Clinical Excellence website: provides guidance on health promotion, ill-health prevention and treatments.

http://www.nmc-uk.org
The Nursing and Midwifery Council website: policy on nursing practice and conduct including medication administration, documentation and role development.

http://www.npsa.nhs.uk
The National Patient Safety Agency website: information on 'near misses' and incidents such as drug administration errors. Provides suggestions for future practice.

http://www.nursing-standard.co.uk/archives/ns/residentpdfs/quickrefPDFfiles/Quickref1.pdf
A short *Nursing Standard* publication on numeracy skills.

http://www.rcn.org.uk
The Royal College of Nursing website: information, publications, advice and guidance on practice issues and professional forums including the IV Therapy Forum.

CHAPTER 7

Local and Systemic Complications of Intravenous Therapy

Julie Lamb and Lisa Dougherty

Introduction

Patients who require intravenous (i.v.) therapy are likely to be those who, because of illness, are susceptible to infection. The insertion of a vascular access device that penetrates the body's skin defence mechanism will result in an additional potential hazard for these patients. It is now accepted that many patients receiving i.v. therapy will be exposed to associated risks and problems.

Peripheral venous cannulation is still a commonly performed procedure, with over 24 million cannulae (ported, non-ported, winged and straight) sold in the UK during 2004/2005 (PASA 2007). Whilst central venous catheterization is less common, the complications that can occur both during insertion and whilst *in situ* are more life-threatening. They include mechanical complications (5–19%), infection (2–26%) and thrombotic complications (2–28%) (McGee & Gould 2003). Complications increase hospital stays, duration of therapy, and nursing and medical responsibilities and can put the patient at risk of other medical problems. In addition, the patient experiences further discomfort and the organization's overall expenses are increased.

All nurses who are involved in the insertion and/or care of vascular access devices and i.v. therapy should have the knowledge and skills both to prevent complications and also to recognize and manage them appropriately (Ung *et al.* 2002; RCN 2005). Appropriate training, continuous support and the maintenance of i.v. skills are vital (RCN 2005). Practitioners who are expert in their skills, who know what to look for, who are aware of and understand the associated risks, and who are able to deal with them properly will significantly reduce i.v.-related problems and, as a consequence, improve patient care. It is recognized that the use of a skilled and dedicated i.v. team will significantly improve the quality of i.v. care provided. Studies have demonstrated that i.v. teams decrease the incidence of phlebitis (Mendez-Lang 1987; Scally *et al.* 1992); catheter-related bacteraemias (Maki *et al.* 1973; Miller *et al.* 1996; CDC 2002) and infiltration (Speechley 1984), as well as reducing the number of attempts and thus the anxiety and pain associated with insertion (Dougherty 1994, 1996; Hunter 2003).

This chapter will review the most common local and systemic complications of i.v. therapy, focusing on prevention and management.

Venous Spasm

A spasm is a sudden involuntary contraction of a vein (vasoconstriction) resulting in a temporary cessation of blood flow through a vessel. Stimulation by cold infusates or by mechanical or chemical irritation may produce spasms in veins (Perdue 2001; Macklin & Chernecky 2004; Phillips 2005; Weinstein 2007).

Clinical features

It is important to recognize the clinical features of spasms. Cramping or pain above an infusion site or a feeling of numbness is usually the first sensation the patient experiences (Perdue 2001), followed by slowing of the infusion (Phillips 2005).

Prevention

Venous spasm can be prevented or minimized by infusing medications or solutions known to be irritant at slower rates and by diluting them as much as possible (Perdue 2001; Phillips 2005; Weinstein 2007).

Blood warmers should be used for rapid infusions of potent cold agglutinins, exchange transfusions in neonates and treatment of patients with hypothermia. Fluid warmers may be used to warm i.v. solutions to prevent or reverse hypothermic conditions. All refrigerated medications and parenteral solutions should be allowed to reach room temperature before they are infused (Perdue 2001; Phillips 2005; Weinstein 2007).

Management

If a venous spasm occurs, discontinuation of the infusion is not necessary. The infusion rate should be decreased and if possible the medication or solution diluted further. If the spasm results from administration of a cold solution, warm compresses should be applied above the site; the heat provides vasodilation and increases the blood supply, thereby relieving the spasm and the pain (Perdue 2001; Phillips 2005; Weinstein 2007).

Ecchymosis and Haematoma

Ecchymosis is a term used to denote the infiltration of blood into the tissues, whereas haematoma usually refers to uncontrolled bleeding at the venepuncture site, leading to infiltration of blood in the tissues, creating a hard painful lump (Perdue 2001; Phillips 2005; Weinstein 2007).

Cause

Ecchymosis and haematomas are commonly associated with venepunctures that are performed by unskilled practitioners or on patients who have a tendency to bruise easily. Patients receiving anticoagulants and long-term steroid therapy are particularly susceptible to bleeding from vein trauma (Perdue 2001). Ecchymosis and haematomas often occur when multiple entries are made into a vein, or when attempts are made into hard-to-see veins or those that cannot be palpated (Perdue 2001; Macklin & Chernecky 2004). Haematomas may also result from extensive pressure being applied to a cannula site on removal (Perdue 2001).

The presence of ecchymosis and haematomas limit veins for future use and damages tissues. If a haematoma is severe, it may limit the use of an extremity (Perdue 2001; Weinstein 2007). The extremity should be monitored for circulatory, neurological and motor function (Perdue 2001).

Clinical features

These are discoloration of the skin, site swelling and discomfort, the inability to advance a cannula all the way into the vein and resistance to positive pressure (Phillips 2005).

Prevention

Ecchymosis cannot always be prevented. The best prevention for haematomas is to ensure that venepuncture and cannulation are performed by highly skilled practitioners (Perdue 2001). Inexperienced individuals should never perform venepuncture on patients with fragile veins or veins that are not visible or easily palpable (Perdue 2001). Use an indirect rather than a direct approach, apply the tourniquet just before venepuncture and use a blood pressure cuff on the elderly (Phillips 2005). Alcohol pads should not be used to apply pressure as alcohol inhibits clot formation (Perdue 2001; Macklin & Chernecky 2004). Elevating the extremity while continuing to apply pressure for 1 or 2 minutes helps stop the bleeding and prevents haematoma formation.

Additional prevention strategies should include the following.

1. Organizational guidelines regarding the prevention of haematomas.
2. Risk assessments to identify individuals who may be particularly susceptible to haematoma formation, including older people, those having anticoagulation therapy or on long-term steroids, patients with renal failure or diabetes mellitus, and children (Macklin & Chernecky 2004).
3. Use of strategies to minimize the risk of haematoma. Optimal pressure should be applied to the venepuncture site following a failed procedure or removal of a vascular access device, and the practitioner should have the appropriate level of expertise for insertion of the device.

Management

The practitioner should be competent to assess the access site and determine the need for treatment and/or intervention in the event of haematoma (RCN 2005). Should ecchymosis and haematoma occur during venepuncture, the cannula should be removed with light application of pressure over the insertion site. If too heavy pressure is applied, fragile veins may rupture and increase bleeding. A dry sterile dressing should be placed over the insertion site and the site monitored for breakthrough bleeding (Perdue 2001). The use of pharmacological methods such as hirudoid cream may be helpful (RCN 2005; BMA/RPSGB 2007).

The incidence of haematoma, together with the cause and its treatment, should be recorded in the patient's notes, so that possible steps for future prevention can be identified (RCN 2005). Statistics on the incidence, degree and cause of, and corrective action taken for haematomas should be maintained and readily retrievable (RCN 2005).

Phlebitis

Phlebitis is the inflammation of the intima of the vein and it is a commonly reported complication of i.v. therapy (Perdue 2001). Phlebitis rates are reported at between 7% and 70% of all peripherally inserted i.v. cannulae (Grune *et al.* 2004) and are associated with a relevant rate of cannula-associated infections as well as bloodstream infections with rates between 0.08% and 3% in hospital wards (Grune *et al.* 2004).

Clinical features

Inflammation occurs as a result of irritation to the endothelial cells of the vein intima creating a rough cell wall where platelets readily adhere. A variety of symptoms

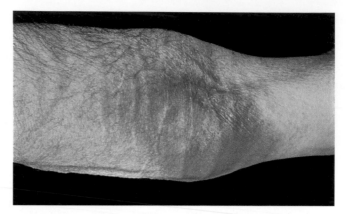

Figure 7.1 Phlebitis at the cannula site.

associated with phlebitis have been reported, including tenderness, pain, erythema, oedema, increased warmth, palpable cord and purulent discharge (Gallant & Schultz 2006). *See* Figure 7.1.

Incidence

Early studies found that 25–70% of all patients receiving peripheral i.v. therapy developed infusion-related phlebitis, although actual bacteraemia rates remain low at 0–0.2% (an acceptable incidence rate is usually placed at 5%) (Gallant & Schulz 2006; INS 2006). Infusion-related phlebitis may develop while the intravenous cannula is *in situ* and up to 96 hours after the i.v. cannula is removed (Gallant & Schultz 2004). This is defined as post-infusion phlebitis (Phillips 2005; Weinstein 2007). This can occur without any of the usual symptoms and there is no way to anticipate this type of phlebitis (Phillips 2005). Patients who do develop insertion site phlebitis may also have problems up to 5 months after the i.v. cannula is removed (Gallant & Schultz 2006).

Increased dwell time has been shown to increase phlebitis rates, with a phlebitis rate of between 12% and 34% after the first 24 hours, increasing to between 36% and 65% after 48 hours (Gallant & Schultz 2006). However, Gallant and Schultz (2006) reported that a recent systematic review of 13 studies with 4783 participants concluded that dwell times up to 96 hours did not increase the risk of bloodstream infections.

In 2002 the Centers for Disease Control and Prevention (CDC) recommended an increase in dwell time so that peripheral i.v. sites and administration sites were changed every 96 hours instead of every 72 hours, yet evidence from clinical practice shows that at least 25% of i.v. cannulae show no signs of phlebitis at 96 hours' dwell time. Research suggests that cannulae may safely be left indwelling for 5 days (120 hours) or even longer (Gallant & Schultz 2006).

The experience of the person inserting an i.v. cannula clearly influences the risk of phlebitis. In comparative trials, the availability of an i.v. therapy team of highly experienced nurses who insert i.v. cannulae and provide close surveillance of infusions resulted in a twofold lower rate of infusion-related phlebitis and an even greater reduction in catheter-related sepsis (Perdue 2001).

There are three types of phlebitis (Table 7.1):

1. bacterial
2. mechanical
3. chemical (Gallant & Schultz 2006).

Table 7.1 Types of phlebitis.

Type	Definition	Contributing factors
Bacterial (or septic)	An inflammation of the vein intima with a bacterial infection. It is the least common type of phlebitis and can be very serious as it predisposes the patient to the systemic complication of septicaemia. (Perdue 2001; Phillips 2005)	• Poor hand washing techniques • Failure to check equipment for compromised integrity • Poor aseptic technique in preparation of the site or system • Poor insertion technique • Poorly taped/secured cannula • Extended cannula dwell time • Infrequent site observation with failure to notice early signs of phlebitis (Perdue 2001)
Mechanical	Irritation of the vein by cannula movement (Perdue 2001). It can also be caused by certain cannula materials (Perdue 2001)	• Increased dwell time • Poor cannula placement i.e. areas of flexion • Poorly taped/secured cannula • Catheter material • Cannula gauge and length
Chemical	An inflammatory response that occurs by irritation when administering irritant or vesicant medications or the administration of hyperosmolar solutions such as dextrose 50% and additives (including some antibiotics and potassium chloride) (Gallant & Schulz 2004)	• Irritating medications or solutions • Medications improperly mixed or diluted • Medications or solutions administered at a rapid rate (Perdue 2001; Phillips 2005)

Phlebitis grading

Phlebitis should be rated according to a uniform scale (Perdue 2001). Measurement against this scale should be used in documenting phlebitis which should be graded according to the most severe presenting indicator (RCN 2005). (*See* Figure 6.1.)

Prevention

Each organization should have guidelines regarding the prevention of phlebitis. These should include appropriate device and vein selection, dilution of drugs and pharmacological methods, such as glyceryl trinitrate (GTN) patches (*See* Table 7.2). All vascular access sites should be routinely assessed for signs and symptoms of phlebitis and a phlebitis scale should be standardized and used in documenting phlebitis.

Management

All nurses should have knowledge of the management of phlebitis and when this occurs all interventions, treatments and corrective actions should be documented in the patient's nursing notes.

The infusion should be discontinued at the first signs of phlebitis (Grade I). Warm or cold compresses can be applied to the affected site. The patient should be referred to the doctor if the phlebitis rating is over 3. If bacterial phlebitis is suspected then the insertion site should be cultured and the cannula tip sent to microbiology (Macklin & Chernecky 2004; Phillips 2005). Any incident of phlebitis rating Grade I or higher should be investigated by an appropriate healthcare professional to identify cause and possible steps for future prevention. The acceptable phlebitis rate should be 5% or less in any given patient population. Each organization's policies and procedures should require calculation of phlebitis rates as a means of outcome assessment and performance improvement.

Table 7.2   Phlebitis prevention (Perdue 2001; Royer 2003; Gallant & Schulz 2006; Frey & Schears 2006).

Bacterial	Mechanical	Chemical
Thorough hand-washing techniques	Robust cannula securement	Use of filters
Checking all i.v. equipment for integrity	Frequent i.v. site observations and rotation of peripheral i.v. sites at regular intervals	Use of recommended solutions or diluents when mixing medications
Strict aseptic technique		Dilution of known irritant medications to the greatest possible extent
Competent insertion techniques		Administration of bolus medications through a port of compatible free flowing infusion
Robust cannula securement	Correct cannula placement avoiding areas of flexion	Administration of medication or solutions at the minimal rate recommended
Frequent i.v. site observations with cannula removal at recognition of early signs of phlebitis	Use of securement devices	Rotation of peripheral i.v. sites at recommended intervals
		Use of large veins for the administration of hypertonic or acidic solutions to provide greater haemodilution
		Use of the smallest gauge cannula that will adequately deliver prescribed therapy
		Use of heat pads
		Use of glyceryl trinitrate patches

The peripheral phlebitis incidence rate should be calculated according to a standard formula, e.g.

$$\frac{\text{Number of phlebitis incidents}}{\text{Total number of i.v. devices}} \times 100 = \% \text{ peripheral phlebitis}$$

Thrombophlebitis

This is the presence of vein inflammation and a blood clot on the vein wall (Macklin & Chernecky 2004) and is an extension of phlebitis.

Clinical features

Peripheral vein thrombophlebitis, the most frequent complication of i.v. infusion therapy, is characterized by pain, erythema, swelling and a palpable thrombosis of the cannulated vein (Tagalakis *et al.* 2002). The vein becomes hard and tortuous as it thromboses (Perdue 2001).
Causative factors include:

- duration of cannula dwell time
- cannula material
- type of infusate
- cannula site infections
- poor cannula/vein ratio
- cannula tip placed just below vein bifurcation (Tagalakis *et al.* 2002; Macklin & Chernecky 2004).

Dwell time is an important risk factor for i.v.-related complications, and a major discussion topic is whether elective replacement reduces the risk for thrombophlebitis (Maki & Ringer 1991; Lundgren *et al.* 1996; Bregenzer *et al.* 1998). Elective replacement has been suggested in the studies that used different catheters for the intervention. On the other hand, several observational studies have drawn the conclusion that elective replacement does not decrease the incidence of thrombophlebitis (Idvall & Gunningberg 2006).

These studies varied widely as regards samples, insertion routines, observational methods and the definition of thrombophlebitis. The number of peripheral cannulae varied from 60 to 2500 (Idvall & Gunningberg 2006).

Incidence

The incidence of thrombophlebitis as a peripheral i.v.-related complication has been reported to range from 5.3% to 77.5% (Idvall & Gunningberg 2006) which is well above the rate targeted by the Infusion Nurses Society (INS) standards of practice. Along with increased attention to cannula-specific risk factors, better characterization of biological factors will improve our understanding of the pathogens of i.v. thrombophlebitis and may allow the development of better management strategies (Tagalakis *et al.* 2002).

Tagalakis *et al.* (2002) reported that in a prospective study of 90 hospitalized patients with i.v. cannulae, 23 developed thrombophlebitis of which one third had complications that resulted in delay in i.v. therapy being administered and additional i.v. therapy needing to be prescribed due to complications, that led to an extended hospital stay.

Prevention

Thrombophlebitis can lead to serious systemic complications and measures should be taken to prevent their occurrence. These measures should include those outlined earlier under phlebitis as well as the following:

- venepuncture and cannulation should only be undertaken by a skilled practitioner
- avoid multiple venepuncture attempts
- use the smallest-gauge cannula possible for the solution to be adequately administered
- identify high-risk patients, e.g. those with poor circulation and venous stasis
- administer medications with compatible solutions only
- avoid the administration of medications with a high pH or tonicity whenever possible
- use filtration
- avoid cannulae constructed of thrombogenic materials (Perdue 2001).

Management

The i.v. site and vein should be observed at frequent intervals for signs and symptoms consistent with thrombophlebitis. The vein should be palpated for induration and tenderness; the patient should be questioned about pain at the site, along the vein and in the involved extremity (Perdue 2001). The patient should be observed for chills and fever and a full blood count evaluated for an elevated white cell count. If the thrombophlebitis goes untreated, it will render the vein unavailable for future use due to its sclerosed condition (Perdue 2001).

When thrombophlebitis occurs the infusion should be discontinued immediately and a doctor notified. If an infection is suspected the cannula should be cultured. The skin surrounding the cannula should be cleaned with alcohol and allowed to air dry before the cannula is removed for culture. When a purulent discharge is present, the culture of the discharge should be taken before the site is cleaned (Perdue 2001).

Cold compresses should be applied to the site initially to decrease the flow of blood and increase platelet adherence to the clot already formed. Then, warm compresses should be applied. The extremity should be elevated and the patient cautioned against rubbing or massaging the area as it may cause an embolus (Perdue 2001).

Repeated episodes of thrombophlebitis can lead to venous access difficulties and more invasive procedures such as central venous catheter (CVC) placement becoming

Section 2

necessary. As a result, administration of parenteral medications may be unnecessarily delayed and hospital stay lengthened (Tagalakis *et al.* 2002).

Infiltration

Infiltration is the inadvertent administration of a non-vesicant solution or drug into surrounding tissues as a result of dislodgement of a cannula or a vessel rupture (Fabian 2000; Perdue 2001; RCN 2005) and should not be viewed as a natural consequence of i.v. therapy (Fabian 2000). Royer (2003) found that of all the complications, 33.7% were as a result of infiltration.

Cause

Infiltration has a number of causes, from mechanical to inflammatory in origin (*See* Table 7.3). Complete infiltration occurs when a cannula moves out of the vein or is forced completely through the vessel wall on insertion (Figure 7.2). Partial infiltration occurs when only the tip of the cannula remains in the vein or the vessel wall does not seal around the cannula, allowing a slow leak into the subcutaneous tissues (Figure 7.3).

Clinical features

Fluid leaking into the tissue causes swelling which is the commonest sign of an infiltration. Infiltrated fluid is cooler than the surrounding body fluids, and as the skin temperature cools, the skin becomes blanched (Fabian 2000). Other clinical symptoms include leakage of fluid from the i.v. site, and if a large amount of fluid is trapped in the subcutaneous tissue, the skin may appear taut or stretched with the patient complaining of tightness and discomfort around the site (Fabian 2000). *See* Figure 7.4. The rate of the i.v. infusion will eventually diminish as the fluid accumulates in the subcutaneous tissue (Fabian 2000) but initially flow will continue until interstitial pressure overcomes gravity pressure.

Table 7.3 Why fluid infiltrates (adapted from Hadaway 2002).

Problem	Possible reasons
Mechanical	
Needle or cannula punctures vein wall	Traumatic insertion of cannula Inadequate securement of cannula Patient movement leads to device dislodgement
Needle dislodges from port	Inadequate securement of needle in port Poor selection of needle e.g. too short
Vascular access device becomes damaged or separated	Catheter separates from device—due to use of smaller syringes Pinch-off syndrome leads to catheter fracture Use of incorrect equipment on catheter resulting in damage
Obstructed blood flow resulting in back pressure and fluid leaking out of puncture site	Vasoconstriction due to irritants Thrombosis Pressure on veins from lymphoedema
Inflammatory reaction	Chemical irritation Physical trauma from cannulation or high-pressure injectors

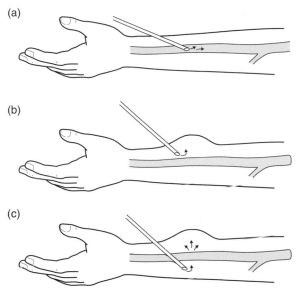

Figure 7.2 Complete infiltration. (a) The cannula is infusing solution into a patent vein. (b) The cannula tip has pulled out of the vein and is infusing into the surrounding subcutaneous tissue. (c) The cannula tip has passed through the vein wall and is infusing into surrounding subcutaneous tissue. (This occurs more commonly with steel needle winged devices.)

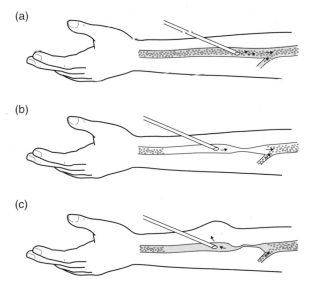

Figure 7.3 Partial infiltration. (a) The cannula is infusing into a patent vein with blood freely flowing through a side branch. (b) Constriction has occurred round cannula. Pressure has increased and resistance is apparent. The valve closes and dilution of the infusate with blood before the side branch ceases. (c) Complete occlusion. Due to the pressure around the cannula, its tip may increase the hole made on insertion, which will increase the likelihood of the infusate leaking into the surrounding tissues.

Section 2

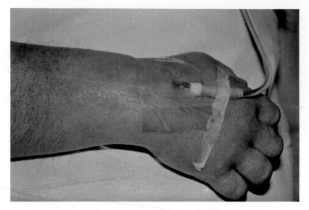

Figure 7.4   Infiltration of fluid into subcutaneous tissue around the cannula site.

This is why it is important not to rely on infusion pumps to detect early signs of infiltration (Marders 2005).

Prevention

To prevent infiltration it is essential that the cannula site is monitored regularly—the frequency will depend on the solution/medication being infused and the type of patient. Not all infiltrations can be avoided, but adhering to certain measures can aid in their prevention and minimize their severity. Flexion areas should be avoided and the site protected from excessive and unnecessary movement. Securement of the i.v. device is vital so that routine movement of the extremity will not cause excessive movement of the device (Fabian 2000; Schears 2005). Royer (2003) found that fixation devices reduced leaking at the site by 57% and infiltration by 100%.

Healthcare staff should be aware of infusion failures, and attempts to restart or encourage sluggish infusions by winding tubing around scissors or pens or by nipping the tubing should be discouraged as they increase the pressure within the vein; this in turn increases the risk of solutions or drugs leaking into the surrounding tissues (Dougherty 1992).

Patient education plays a key role in the prevention of infiltration, and the patient should be instructed in what signs and symptoms to recognize, how to reduce the risk and when to report any changes (Fabian 2000).

Management

The cannula should be removed immediately once an infiltration has been identified (Fabian 2000). An extensive assessment to determine the extent of the infiltration and volume of fluid infiltrated must be performed, using a scale such as the INS infiltration scale (INS 2006) (*See* Figure 6.2). The patient's range of motion and sensation of the extremity must be evaluated (any sensory deficit could be a sign of nerve damage or compartment syndrome) (Fabian 2000). The area of infiltration should be measured and the site monitored at regular intervals. Compresses should not be applied routinely until the type (cool or warm) and appropriateness is determined, which may be dependent on the type of infiltrated fluid (Fabian 2000).

Extravasation

Extravasation is the inadvertent administration of a vesicant or irritant solution into the surrounding tissues. A vesicant solution is one that causes the formation of blisters with

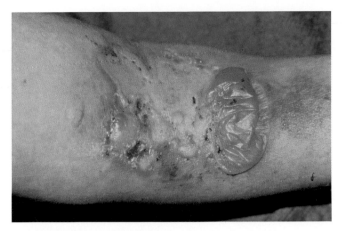

Figure 7.5   Extravasation of sodium bicarbonate.

> **BOX 7.1**
>
> **Drugs capable of causing severe tissue damage (non-cytotoxic)**
>
> Calcium chloride
> Calcium gluconate
> Phenytoin
> Hypertonic solutions of sodium bicarbonate (greater than 5%)
> Potassium chloride (> 40 mmol/L)
> Mannitol
> Aciclovir
> Amphotericin
> Cefotaxime
> Diazepam
> Ganciclovir

subsequent sloughing of tissues due to tissue necrosis (*See* Figure 7.5) (Perdue 2001; Polovich *et al.* 2004; RCN 2005; INS 2006). Drugs that contribute to extravasation necrosis are most often osmotically active or ischaemia-inducing, or cause direct cellular toxicity (Weinstein 2007) (Box 7.1). For details on cytotoxic drugs *See* Chapter 16.

Incidence

Peripheral   The incidence varies in the literature but has been documented as between 23 and 28% (Roth 2003).
Central   The actual number of central venous access device (CVAD) extravasations is unknown but a figure of 6% has been reported for port extravasations (due to needle dislodgement), and rates in non-randomized studies range from 3 to 50% (Lawson 2003; Masoorli 2003).

Cause

In peripheral devices the cause may be the practitioner (e.g. a poorly sited cannula or not checking for patency before administration) or the vein (e.g. in patients with thrombocytopenia or a vein that cannot withstand the volume or pressure of the administration)

(Dougherty 2004). In CVADs it may be a leaking or damaged catheter, fibrin sheath formation (Mayo 1998) or a port needle dislodgement (Schulmeister 1998).

Clinical features

Extravasation should be suspected if one or more of these are present.

1. The patient may complain of a burning, stinging pain or other acute change at the injection site (Hayden & Goodman 2005). This should be distinguished from venous spasm which may occur with some drugs; it can be caused by irritation and is usually accompanied by pain described as an achiness, a tightness or a feeling of cold (Hayden & Goodman 2005). Any change of sensation warrants further investigation (Goolsby & Lombardo 2006). It is important to note that pain is not always present.
2. Swelling is the most common symptom (Polovich *et al.* 2004) and may not always be immediately obvious if the cannula is sited in a deep vein or an area of deep subcutaneous fat, or if the leak is posterior (Dougherty 2006).
3. Blanching of the skin occurs (Springhouse Corporation 2002). Erythema can occur around the injection site but is not usually immediately present (Hayden & Goodman 2005).
4. Leakage may occur at the insertion site (Fabian 2000).
5. A resistance is felt on the plunger of the syringe if drugs are given by bolus (Vandergrift 2001; Stanley 2002).
6. The rate of the infusion may slow down or stop and this is not related to position (Vandergrift 2001; Stanley 2002).
7. Blood return is one of the most misleading of all signs, particularly in peripheral devices. If blood return is sluggish or absent in peripheral devices, this may indicate lack of patency or incorrect position of the device. However, if no other signs are apparent this should not be regarded as an indication of a non-patent vein, as a vein may not bleed back for a number of reasons and extravasation may occur even in the event of good blood return (Hayden & Goodman 2005). Any change in blood flow should be investigated (Hayden & Goodman 2005; Weinstein 2007). In CVADs there should always be blood return and if this is absent steps should be followed to verify correct tip or needle position or resolve a fibrin sheath.

Tissue sloughing is usually apparent within 1–4 weeks due to tissue necrosis (Perdue 2001). Necrosis can involve a small superficial area of tissue loss, which will granulate following debridement, if free of infection. It may also involve large areas and take in deep structures, including underlying connective tissues, muscles, tendons and bone, and may result in the need for wide surgical excision, debridement, grafting or even amputation to restore tissue integrity (Weinstein 2007).

Prevention (See Box 7.2)

Knowledge of the possible risk factors can help to prevent extravasation.

Patient risk factors

Extravasation injuries occur in seriously ill patients and may be more prevalent in children, elderly people and patients who require frequent venepunctures, such as those receiving chemotherapy. Patients who are unable to communicate pain include children, and anaesthetized or comatose patients (Dougherty 2006).

The status of the patient's venous access is an important contributory factor and the following factors are likely to increase the risk of extravasation:

- fragile veins
- elderly and debilitated patients with poor venous access

BOX 7.2

Prevention or minimization of the risks of extravasation

- Correct positioning of the cannula using the smallest gauge possible.
- Correct site placement—use the forearm; avoid sites near joints.
- Administer through a recently sited cannula.
- Consider a central venous catheter for slow infusions of high-risk drugs.
- Verify correct placement before vesicant administration.
- Administer by slow i.v. push into side-arm port of a fast-running i.v. infusion of compatible solution.
- Administer vesicant drugs first.
- Observe the site continuously.
- If in doubt, stop and resite cannula.
- Ask the patient to report any sensation of pain, burning or stinging.

In the event of an extravasation, treat promptly and document all the details in the patient's notes.

- patients with generalized vascular disease
- patients with obstructed venous drainage, following axillary surgery or radical mastectomy
- critically ill patients
- patients who are thrombocytopenic (which will inhibit the formation of a firm homeostatic plug at the cannula site and increase the risk of leakage)
- venous spasm as a result of changes in body temperature, raised blood pressure or psychological factors.

Device risk factors

Extravasation can occur as a result of inexperienced staff establishing venous access and administering drugs. If a vein is punctured repeatedly before a successful device is secured, drugs are more likely to leak into the surrounding tissues or cannula below a previous venepuncture site (Dougherty 2006). The type of device used can also affect the incidence of extravasation, as it has been shown that steel needles (e.g winged infusion devices) result in twice as many extravasations as those with plastic cannulae (Tully *et al.* 1981).

A peripheral device should not be sited over areas of flexion, and the hands should be avoided due to the close network of tendons and nerves that would be destroyed if an extravasation were to occur (Perdue 2001). If a cannula has been *in situ* for longer than 24 hours, it is prudent to consider replacing it, preferably on the opposite limb, before administration (Weinstein 2007).

Drug risk factors

The following features of drugs increase the risk of injury:

- ability to bind to DNA (e.g. doxorubicin)
- ability to cause direct cellular toxicity (e.g. vinca alkaloids)
- ability to cause local tissue ischaemia (e.g. vasopressors)
- formulations with high osmolality (e.g. glucose 20%)
- formulation pH outside the range 5–9 (e.g. phenytoin)
- formulations likely to precipitate (e.g. diazepam) (Roth 2003).

Monitoring of site

It is essential that an extravasation be identified early before a large volume of fluid leaks into the tissues. The intravenous site should be examined at regular intervals. As time progresses after extravasation, it becomes increasingly difficult to accurately palpate and measure the borders of induration, suggesting that surface assessments are most accurate when performed within a short period of extravasation (Yucha *et al.* 1993).

The i.v. site should always be checked for patency before, during and following administration. It is advisable to administer vesicant drugs via the side-arm of a fast-running infusion, as a free-flowing infusion will indicate a patent cannula and, should extravasation occur, the tissue damage may be reduced due to the concentration of the vesicant drug being diluted (Perdue 2001).

Policies and protocols

Most establishments have written protocols and procedures related to the management of such an event. Only trained staff knowledgeable in the administration of vesicant drugs should administer these agents. Knowledge of vesicant solutions and drugs and recognition of the clinical features of extravasation and preventative measures are imperative for the safe administration of these drugs. A major part of the prevention of such problems is the education of patients. Asking them to promptly report any sensation of pain or burning will assist in minimizing tissue damage (Dougherty 2004).

Management

If extravasation is suspected or confirmed, the injection or infusion must be stopped immediately and action must be taken (Polovich *et al.* 2004; INS 2006; Weinstein 2007).

Management can involve removal of the device, elevation of the limb, administration of compresses and/or antidotes and application of steroid cream.

For detailed guidelines on the management of extravasation *See* Chapter 16.

Occlusion

There are two types of occlusion.

1. Partial withdrawal occlusion (PWO): this is usually caused by fibrin sheath formation and identified by absent or sluggish blood return, although fluids can be infused. Fibrin sheaths can result in seeding of bacteria and drug extravasation (Mayo 2000, 2001).
2. Total occlusion: when there is an inability to withdraw blood or infuse fluids or medications.

Cause

Occlusion of a device is usually the result of:

- precipitate formation due to inadequate flushing between incompatible medications (Dougherty 2006)
- clot formation due to an administration set or electronic infusion device being turned off or ineffective or incorrect flushing of the device when not in use
- mechanical causes such as kinking or pinch-off syndrome which may also impair patency of the device (Dougherty 2004).

Prevention

The key to preventing an occlusion is:

- maintaining patency using the correct solution and method of flushing
- adequate flushing between medications.

Maintaining patency

Correct solutions   Two main types of solution are used to maintain patency in VADs: heparin inhibits the conversion of prothrombin to thrombin and fibrinogen to fibrin thus inhibiting coagulation and is therefore used to prevent the build-up of fibrin; and sodium chloride is used to clean the internal diameter of the device of blood and drugs (Camp-Sorrell 2004). The type of solution, strength and volume will depend on the type of device *in situ*. It is now well established that flushing daily with 0.9% sodium chloride can also adequately maintain the patency of the cannula (Goode *et al.* 1991), whilst weekly heparinized saline is still the accepted solution for maintaining the patency of open-ended CVCs for intermittent or infrequent use (RCN 2005; Pratt *et al.* 2007). All devices should be flushed with 10–20 mL 0.9% sodium chloride after blood withdrawal (RCN 2005; Dougherty 2006; INS 2006).

Method   Using the correct method to flush a VAD has been highlighted as one of the key issues in maintaining patency (Baranowski 1993; Goodwin & Carlson 1993). There are two stages in flushing.

1. Using a pulsated (push–pause) flush to create turbulent flow when administering the solution, regardless of type and volume. This removes debris from the internal catheter wall (Goodwin & Carlson 1993; Macklin & Chernecky 2004; Phillips 2005).
2. The procedure is completed using the positive pressure technique. This is accomplished by maintaining pressure on the plunger of the syringe while disconnecting the syringe from the injection cap, which prevents reflux of blood into the tip, reducing the risk of occlusion (Moureau 1999; Phillips 2005; INS 2006).

Manufacturers have now produced positive 'displacement' injection caps which achieve positive pressure without the practitioner being required to actively achieve the positive pressure (Weinstein 2007). These caps have been shown to significantly reduce the incidence of catheter occlusions (Berger 2000; Lenhart 2000; Mayo 2001; Rummel 2001).

Management

If a catheter becomes occluded the nurse should establish the cause of the clot—occlusion or precipitation (INS 2006). If precipitation occurs, then instillation of hydrochloric acid or ethyl chloride may be required (Holcombe 1992; LSC 2002).

Partial withdrawal occlusion can be resolved by the instillation of a thrombolytic agent such as urokinase or alteplase (Haire & Herbst 2000; Rinn 2001; Dougherty 2006; Weinstein 2007). A total occlusion can be resolved by instillation of a thrombolytic agent (Ponec *et al.* 2001; Deitcher *et al.* 2002; Timoney *et al.* 2002) or by use of an endoluminal brush (Archis *et al.* 2000; Weinstein 2007).

If a peripheral device is occluded then gentle pressure and aspiration may be sufficient to dislodge the clot. If not, then the device should be removed and resited.

Central venous access devices made of silicone can expand on pressure and allow fluid to flow around the clot, facilitating its dislodgement, but this should only be attempted using a 10-mL or larger syringe. Smaller syringes should never be used as they create a greater pressure (Conn 1993; Perdue 2001; Springhouse Corporation 2002; Camp-Sorrell 2004) which can result in rupture of the catheter, resulting in loss of catheter integrity, or dislodge the clot into the circulation (Perucca 2001). Instillation of thrombolytic agents should be performed using a three-way tap and negative pressure (Simcock 2001; Dougherty 2006). *See* Chapter 11.

Local Infection/Septicaemia

Any local i.v. site infection carries the risk of becoming a systemic infection. If the patient's health is already compromised, this complication can progress quickly and may prove fatal. Infection of the i.v. site can be caused by poor adherence to aseptic technique during procedures and manipulations; failure to maintain a clean site or closed delivery system; and failure to change administration sets and cannulae at regular intervals. Aseptic technique is the key preventative measure in reducing the likelihood of infection associated with i.v. therapy (CDC 2002; DH 2003; Hart 2004; RCN 2005). Hand-washing is the most basic, but often the most ignored, of all the techniques to minimize infection (DH 2001).

Patients are more at risk if they are malnourished, immunocompromised, less than 1 or more than 60 years of age, or if they already have an infection at another site (Weinstein 2007).

Septicaemia is a pathological state or pyrogenic reaction that is usually accompanied by systemic illness. It occurs when pathogenic bacteria invade the bloodstream. The presence of bacteria in blood is described as bacteraemia, and where bacteraemia is associated with symptoms of infection (e.g. rigors, fevers), this is termed septicaemia. Infection will depend upon the ability of the bacteria to survive and proliferate. The factors that influence their survival are:

- the specific organisms present
- the number of such organisms
- the resistance of the host
- environmental conditions.

(*See* Chapter 4)

Clinical features

The patient with septicaemia will usually present with chills, fever, malaise and headache, which occur when the pathogenic organisms first invade the circulation. As the fever increases, pulse rate increases and weakness occurs with accompanying symptoms of flushed face, backache, nausea, vomiting and hypotension. If the infection goes undetected or untreated, symptoms become more severe, and cyanosis, tachypnoea and hyperventilation can occur. As the offending organisms overcome the system, vascular collapse, shock and death can occur (Perdue 2001).

Prevention

Prevention strategies support the use of air-eliminating, bacteria-retentive filters, impregnated catheters, and use of correct antiseptic solutions (Pratt *et al.* 2007). Effective hand-washing techniques, cannula/catheter management protocols, and adherence to accepted standards of practice, administration set changes and proper cannula care will all assist in the prevention of septicaemia in the patient receiving i.v. therapy (RCN 2005; Dougherty 2006; Weinstein 2007).

Management

The course of action will often depend on patient factors, type of organism involved, need for CVAD and type of infection (Dougherty 2006). Local infection is usually treated with antibiotics given orally or intravenously (and sometimes topically). Systemic infection is often treated with intravenous antibiotics along with possible removal of the device (RCN 2005; Dougherty 2006).

Pulmonary Embolism

Pulmonary embolism occurs when a mass, usually a blood clot, becomes free floating and is carried by the venous circulation to the right side of the heart and into the pulmonary artery or the artery to the lobes, occluding arterial apertures at major bifurcations. If the pulmonary artery is obstructed, the patient will experience cardiac disturbances. If multiple emboli are passed into the pulmonary circulation, the patient will experience pulmonary hypertension and right-sided heart failure (Perdue 2001).

Clinical features

Clinical manifestations include dyspnoea, pleuritic pain or discomfort, apprehension, cough, unexplained haemoptysis, sweats, tachypnoea, cyanosis and low-grade fever (Weinstein 2007).

Prevention

Preventative measures include:

- use of a filter to remove particulates from solutions and drugs
- administration of blood through a microaggregate filter
- avoiding the use of lower extremities for cannulation in adult patients
- prevention of trauma to the vein intima, by ensuring that practitioners are skilled, by using the smallest and shortest cannulae appropriate for the prescribed therapy, by the use of large veins when irritating solutions are being administered, and by the use of correct fixation and securing techniques to prevent cannula movement
- use of good judgement when i.v. systems are being flushed—if, for example, there is any resistance within the device, undue force should not be employed as a blood clot may be released into the vascular system
- examining solution containers for particulates before use
- clipping of excessive hair and proper cleansing of the i.v. site to remove the potential for hair to be severed and carried into the circulation when the skin is breached (Perdue 2001).

Management

Medical and nursing intervention will include administration of oxygen to maintain correct blood gas levels, a lung scan and a prothrombin time before initiating anticoagulant therapy.

Air Embolism

Air embolism occurs when air enters a systemic vein and travels to the right ventricle via the vena cava. The bubble of air in the ventricle impedes its pumping ability, thus reducing the blood to the pulmonary vasculature (Dougherty 2006). The pulmonary arterioles then become occluded by tiny air bubbles pumped into them. As a result of the reduced output from the right ventricle, the venous pressure rises considerably. Further, the flow of blood from the left ventricle into the systemic circulation decreases and cyanosis occurs. Reduced blood flow to the brain causes syncope and the arterial blood pressure falls as a result of reduced cardiac output (Conrad 2002).

Cause

Air can enter into the venous system as a consequence of trauma or iatrogenic complications, especially CVC catheterization or pressurized i.v. infusion systems (Ostrow 1981). The frequency of clinically recognized air embolism following CVC is less than 2% (Conrad 2002). Symptomatic air embolism following CVC has a mortality rate as high as 30%. It can also occur following various surgical procedures and on removal of a CVC.

During insertion, large introducers are used (a 14-G needle allows air at 200mL/second into vein), and this enables air to be drawn into the central circulation in large amounts very rapidly. It is also more likely to occur if the patient is hypovolemic, and in vulnerable patients such as the critically ill and those gasping for air.

Air embolism can also occur during removal when air can enter the catheter tract between the catheter and sealing of the tract. The degree of risk is related to the length of time *in situ:* the longer in the vein, the longer the tract takes to seal (Ostrow 1981); although it can occur after a CVC has been in as little as 3 days. It may be delayed for 30 minutes or more.

Air drawn into the central system results in right ventricular dysfunction and pulmonary injury (Conrad 2002). Small amounts of air do not produce symptoms because air is removed from the circulation. Large boluses of air (3–8 mL/kg) can cause acute right ventricular outflow obstruction and result in cardiogenic shock and circulatory arrest. At 20 mL a patients will experience symptoms (Mennim 1992), so the small bubbles found in intravenous tubing are not usually a problem, but 70–105mL of air per second is usually fatal.

If a vented container is allowed to run dry, air enters the tubing and the fluid level drops to the proximity of the patient's chest. The pressure exerted by the blood on the walls of the veins controls the level to which the air drops in the tubing. A negative pressure occurs when the extremity receiving the infusion is elevated above the heart (Weinstein 2007).

Clinical features

These tend to develop immediately following embolization. The severity of the symptoms is related to degree of air entry and they include:

- dyspnoea
- chest pain
- tachycardia
- hypotension
- confusion
- anxiety
- lowered levels of consciousness
- neurological deficits
- circulatory shock or sudden death (Drewett 2000).

A loud continuous churning sound is often heard over the precordia. It is known as a Mill Wheel murmur and is produced by the presence of air and blood in the right ventricle. This classic murmur confirms the diagnosis, but it is not always present (Ostrow 1981).

Prevention

- Proper positioning of the patient during insertion and removal. The head should be tilted lower than the feet in the Trendelenberg position —this helps to engorge the veins and if air does enter it prevents it from travelling to the heart. If the patient performs the valsalva manoeuvre this can also reduce the volume of air that might enter.
- Whilst it would be ideal to have the patient rehydrated before CVC insertion, often the procedure is performed during emergency situations when the patient is bleeding and collapsed, and actually requires the catheter in order to receive the fluid and/or blood. However, wherever possible, ensure that the patient is not hypovolemic as this can also generate an increased sucking force.
- Use a closed CVC system and maintain vigilance during manipulation as air embolism can occur during accidental disconnection and dislodgement. It is therefore

recommended that only luer-lock connections should be used to reduce the risk of disconnection.

- The initial dressing after removal must be occlusive, and using valsalva during disconnection can also increase intrathoracic pressure as well as increasing the main pressure within the central vein (Ostrow 1981).
- The use of air-eliminating filters.
- Purging all i.v. administration sets before use.
- Changing solution containers before they empty completely. Infusion via CVCs poses a greater risk of air embolism when the solution container empties than an infusion via a peripheral vein. This is because the central venous pressure is lower than the peripheral venous pressure, and consequently there is a greater propensity towards negative pressure which could suck air into the circulation (Weinstein 2007).

Management

Staff should resist the temptation to sit a breathless patient upright in the case of a suspected air embolism. If air does enter the venous system, the patient should be turned onto the left side in a modified Trendelenburg position. This will decrease the flow of air into the vein during inspiration by decreasing intrathoracic pressure. The left lateral position allows the pulmonary artery to become inferior to the body of the right ventricle. The air bubble therefore rises into the right ventricle, relieving the obstruction to the pulmonary vasculature bed. Trendelenburg's position will then help to stop the flow of air into the vein and the left lateral position will improve the pumping ability of the right ventricle. 100% oxygen should be administered and the patient intubated if there are signs of respiratory distress. The patient's vital signs should be monitored and they should be reassured (Ostrow 1981). If air embolism is suspected during insertion of a CVC, the procedure should be terminated.

Catheter Damage

Catheter damage can occur at different points along the catheter.

1. The catheter hub.
2. The catheter near the hub or below a bifurcation.
3. Higher up the catheter or above a bifurcation.
4. Internal catheter fracture.

The site of damage will dictate whether the catheter can be repaired or needs to be removed (Dougherty 2004).

External catheter damage

For causes and management of external catheter damage *See* Table 7.4.

Internal catheter damage

There are a number of causes of catheter fracture and subsequent embolism.

- Separation of the catheter from the port—forceful flushing in the presence of distal obstruction, manufacturing defect or incorrect locking procedure.
- Catheter shear from needles/sutures or surgical instruments during insertion.
- On removal using traction or against excessive resistance.
- Catheter pinch-off syndrome (Ingle 1995; Andris & Krzywda 1997; Drewett 2000). This occurs when a CVC is inserted percutaneously via the subclavian vein and it

becomes compressed by the clavicle and the first rib (Andis & Krzywda 1997; Verhage & Van Bommel 1999). It results in:

- intermittent mechanical obstruction of the catheter
- complete or partial catheter transection
- possible catheter embolization into the central venous system (Ingle 1995).
- This syndrome is often unrecognized and underreported. The reported incidence is listed as between 0.1 and 1.12%. It is frequently identified retrospectively, after associated complications such as catheter fracture.

Clinical features

Pinch-off syndrome

- A positional catheter where there may be little, sluggish or no blood return or return only when the patient moves the arm to a right angle from his body during blood sampling or attempting to obtain blood return.
- During administration of drugs there is resistance on the plunger and poor flow during infusion, both which appear to be less problematic when the patient moves their arm.

Catheter fracture

- Infraclavicular pain and/or swelling on flushing or during an infusion.
- Palpitations.
- Chest pain.

Table 7.4 Causes and management of external catheter damage.

	Cause	Management
The catheter hub	'Overscrewing' of a cap onto the hub or applying the cap to the hub which has been cleaned with alcohol but not allowed to dry adequately (which effectively 'glues it on' causing difficulty when removing) can both result in cracking of the hub	This can be repaired easily by removing the damaged hub and replacing it, but does require the selection of the correct hub for the correct catheter. However, the ability to repair the hub will depend on the type of catheter as some have hubs which are integral to the catheter and cannot be repaired (Dougherty 2004)
Damage near the hub or below the bifurcation	This can occur if the wrong types of clamps are used. Silicone is a fragile material, prone to damage, and therefore only the clamps provided with the catheter or smooth-bladed forceps should be used. Artery or toothed forceps can cause small breaks in the wall of the catheter	Damage done to this section of catheter can be repaired by adding a small sleeve to the area of damage and gluing it into place. This should only be considered to be a temporary repair and the catheter should be replaced as early as possible due to the risk of contamination. In some cases such as PICCs the catheter can be shortened by cutting off the damaged portion and reapplying a new hub. This type of repair will affect the tip location as shortening the catheter will result in a new tip location and a chest X-ray must be performed to verify exact tip location (Ingle 1995; Dougherty 2004)
Damage higher up the catheter or above the bifurcation	This can occur on insertion and only be discovered once an infusion is commenced, but it more commonly occurs as a result of 'nicking ' the catheter when sutures are removed at the exit site or if small syringes are used to unblock a catheter and the pressure results in small holes or splits in the catheter	In the case of a skin-tunnelled catheter, when this occurs the only solution is removal of the catheter. Exchange over a guidewire may be carried out with non-tunnelled catheters or single-lumen PICCs. This is performed by cutting the end off the catheter, threading a guidewire along the catheter to a specified distance, removing the catheter and threading along a new catheter. This can only be performed if there are no signs of infection and requires the use of special guidewires, dilators and introducers (Dougherty 2004)

PICC, peripherally inserted central catheter.

When catheter tip embolizes patients may be asymptomatic—fewer than a third of patients have had associated symptoms.

Prevention

Damaged catheters result in removal of a working device, distress and discomfort for the patient and time delay in treatment as well as cost (Dougherty 2006). Prevention is the key, and the use of the correct equipment when manipulating the catheter, managing occluded catheters appropriately and taking care when handling the catheter all help to prevent damage (Ingle 1995; Andris & Krzywda 1997).

- Use clamps on clamping sleeves.
- Avoid using scissors or sharp objects around the catheter.
- Use short small-bore needles if accessing an injectable port.
- Check patency using 10-mL or larger syringes.
- Avoid using smaller syringes wherever possible.
- Administer medication without force.
- Monitor catheters for pinholes, cuts, leaks or tears.
- Check dressing for moisture or leaking at the insertion site during infusion and/or injection.
- Educate the patient for the signs and symptoms to look out for and when to report.

Management

It is important to ascertain that PWO is not due to another cause, such as fibrin sheath, tip against vein wall, clot/precipitate. Pinch-off syndrome can be diagnosed using the following method.

- Radiographic findings confirm pinch-off using fluoroscopy or i.v. contrast.
- The patient should be X-rayed with arms straight by sides and upright, not in the standard shoulder- raised and rolled-forward position (Ingle 1995; Andris & Krzywda 1997; Verhage & Van Bommel 1999).

The length of time is variable from when a catheter is placed until when it may fracture and embolize and the catheter fracture may be related to the degree of compression or frequency of catheter use or both. For any damage the immediate management would be to clamp the catheter and assess the degree of damage. Damaged catheters must be repaired or removed as any opening in the catheter can act as a potential entry for bacteria or air (Perdue 2001). Repair can only be performed in external catheters. Implanted ports have no external segment to repair and any fracture will require surgical replacement. Currently non-tunnelled catheters have no repair segments commercially available and so the best remedy is to exchange the catheter over a guidewire. Skin-tunnelled catheters and some peripherally inserted central catheters (PICCs) can be repaired, and this should be carried out in accordance with manufacturer's instructions (Reed & Philips 1996).

In the case of a catheter fracture, removal of the catheter and retrieval of the fragment can be successfully carried out using interventional radiology. In the case of a PICC fracture, in order to retrieve the fragment it may be necessary to perform a venous cutdown. If the fragment has migrated then percutaneous removal or a thoracotomy may be necessary (Ingle 1995).

Catheter Malposition

A catheter malposition is when the catheter tip is not in, or no longer in, the correct position. This will depend on where the tip was placed initially or where the tip placement was desired (e.g. in the superior vena cava, SVC). A catheter may become malpositioned during insertion or at any time whilst *in situ* (Perdue 2001; Dougherty 2006).

Incidence

Malposition can occur in 21–55% of insertions (Ingle 1995). Newer catheter materials predispose to greater frequency of looping, coiling or knotting in the vein.

Cause

During insertion

The catheter may have been inadvertently inserted into large tributaries of the SVC such as the jugular system, internal mammary, azygous, superior intercostal and pericardio-phrenic veins. It may be more common via the left brachiocephalic than the right (as this vein is more oblique and longer and has a larger number of tributaries). Placement via the basilic vein results in a greater chance of malposition into the internal jugular vein (Dougherty 2006).

Once *in situ*

Catheter migration out of the superior vena cava can occur from days to months following insertion or can occur spontaneously. Possible causes include vigorous upper extremity use, forceful flushing of catheter, change in intrathoracic pressure associated with coughing, sneezing, vomiting or constipation, congestive heart failure, or catheter foreshortening, due to repair (Dougherty 2006). Ports can become freely movable and migrate or flip over as a result of twiddler's syndrome. This syndrome is characterized by intentional or unintentional manipulation of a subcutaneous port or catheter and may lead to the catheter being 'removed' from the vein. The syndrome may be an indication of a patient's anxiety as they are often unaware of the manipulation (Ingle 1995; Dougherty 2006).

Clinical features

Malposition may be diagnosed if the catheter becomes longer at the exit site or the cuff is exposed (in a tunnelled catheter, especially following pulling of the catheter), more catheter is exposed at the insertion site of a PICC, or there is no blood return. Any of these would lead the practitioner to question tip placement (Dougherty 2006). Catheter malposition can be asymptomatic but there are a number of symptoms that can suggest malposition on insertion or when *in situ*:

1. resistance or discomfort during insertion
2. bending in guidewire when removed from catheter
3. 'ear gurgling' described by patients with catheter malpositioned in the internal jugular vein
4. arrhythmias (if tip too far into right atrium)
5. partial or complete catheter occlusion
6. headache, chest/shoulder or back pain with infusion
7. reduced infusion rate
8. signs of extravasation
9. ipsilateral extremity oedema
10. backflow of blood into external tubing unrelated to increased intrathoracic pressure (Perdue 2001; Camp-Sorrell 2004; Dougherty 2006; Weinstein 2007).

To obtain a definitive diagnosis the catheter must be X-rayed to verify tip location. This may necessitate a lateral as well as the standard PA view on chest X-ray. Venogram studies may also be performed (Perdue 2001).

Prevention

On insertion: correct positioning of the head to prevent jugular placement; a thorough assessment of the patient for any anatomical issues, history of previous difficulties inserting the catheter or fractured clavicles; accurate measurement to prevent placement in right atrium or ventricle.

Once *in situ* adequate securement of the device, both at the site and also of the extension sets, to prevent pulling at the exit site (Perdue 2001); education of the patient to ensure that it is not pulled, to report early if there are any changes to the length of external portion of the catheter and about what to do if it gets pulled out (Perdue 2001; Dougherty 2006).

Management

If malposition is suspected during insertion it can be rectified. Ultrasound of the jugular can indicate malposition in the vessel before sending patient for an unnecessary X-ray. If the wire is left in during PICC insertion or in a polyurethane catheter, the malposition may be rectified, or an over the guidewire exchange can take place. Other techniques for rectifying malposition include:

- positioning, such as sitting patient upright
- rapid flush during insertion (Perdue 2001; Camp-Sorrell 2004; Dougherty 2006).

Once *in situ* some cases of malpositioning may resolve spontaneously and return to the correct position. Difficult placements can be performed under X-ray guidance or may require repositioning using fluoroscopy (Ingle 1995). Guidance or assistance from an interventional radiologist may also correct coiled or malpositioned catheters. If the problem cannot be corrected removal may be necessary and is preferable if therapies include vesicant or hypertonic solutions or the patient reports pain (Dougherty 2006). If a catheter has been pulled or fallen out it should not be readvanced (RCN 2005).

Thrombosis

A thrombosis is a clot of blood that can be present at the tip of a catheter within the SVC (usually associated with fibrin sheath) or can surround the catheter; for example, a thrombosis in the upper arm caused by the presence of a PICC (Perdue 2001). Venous thrombi consist mainly of fibrin and tightly bound red blood cells. They are large with tapering tails that extend into larger veins and are attached to the venous intima, usually at a valve or bifurcation (Perdue 2001).

Incidence

The incidence of catheter-related thrombosis ranges from 3 to 79% (Moureau *et al.* 1999), with ultrasound studies showing an incidence of 33–67% after more than 1 week (Galloway & Bodenham 2004). However, clinical rates are low, particularly in long-term access, and asymptomatic subclavian vein thrombosis is more common than a symptomatic thrombosis, with only 1–5% demonstrating symptoms (Moureau *et al.* 1999).

Causes

The cause is usually multifactorial (Mayo 2000). Three factors are required for a thrombosis to develop (Mayo 2001; Perdue 2001). This is known as Virchow's triad:

1. stasis
2. endothelial damage and

Section 2

3. hypercoagulable state (caused by the following conditions: diabetes, malnutrition, dehydration, pregnancy, osteomyelitis, smoking, chronic renal failure, cirrhosis, cancer, obesity, sickle cell disease, surgery, congestive heart failure, oestrogen therapies; Mayo 2001; Perdue 2001).

There are certain conditions predisposing to thrombosis development (*See* Box 7.3).

BOX 7.3

Conditions predisposing to thrombosis (Perdue 2001; Dougherty 2006).

Malignancy—especially lung cancer and lymphoma
Venous compression by tumour metastases
Inflammatory bowel syndrome
Hypercoaguability
Infusion of sclerosing agents
Improper maintenance
Sepsis

Clinical features

Symptoms can be very acute or vague. The patient will usually complain of pain in the area such as the arm or the neck, oedema of neck, chest and upper extremity. There may be periorbital oedema, facial tenderness, tachycardia, shortness of breath and sometimes a cough, signs of a collateral circulation over the chest area, jugular venous distension and discoloration of the limb (Perdue 2001; Dougherty 2006).

Prevention

- Constant assessment of function while catheter is *in situ*.
- Early intervention with a thrombolytic agent.
- Meticulous flushing with a pulsatile positive pressure flush.
- Correct tip placement in the SVC.

Tip placement is associated with the incidence of thrombosis. It has been found that catheters whose tips lie in the axillary, subclavian or brachiocephalic veins have a greater incidence of thrombosis (Moureau *et al.* 1999; Vesely 2003). This is reduced by placing the tip into the lower third of the SVC or into the right atrium. The reason for this is that the blood flow is greater and the vessel larger and therefore there is less trauma and rubbing of the catheter against the vein wall.

Left-sided placement, particularly of PICCs, has also been associated with greater risk (Moureau *et al.* 1999; Perdue 2001). The skill of the practitioner may also have an impact; it has been noted that the rate of thrombosis is higher for those learning to insert PICCs, and this could be related to the amount of time taken for insertion and the additional trauma caused (Perdue 2001).

It has now been shown that the use of a low-dose anticoagulant such as warfarin whilst the catheter is *in situ* makes no difference to the incidence of thrombosis (Young 2005; Couban 2005).

Management

The patient should have a venogram and ultrasound to diagnose the thrombosis (Perdue 2001).

Pharmacological management of thrombosis includes anticoagulants and thrombolytics.

- Anticoagulants such as heparin (i.v.) act to impair blood coagulation by neutralizing several clotting factors. It does not assist in lysis of formed clots but reduces the occurrence. The main side-effect is haemorrhage. If the catheter is removed, patients will be prescribed i.v. heparin and then be changed on to an oral anticoagulant such as warfarin. This may continue for up to 3 months following removal of the catheter.
- Thrombolytics contain enzymes, which convert plasminogen into plasmin, resulting in lysis of the clot. Urokinase serum has a half-life of approximately 20 minutes (Moureau 1999; Perdue 2001).

Circulatory Overload/Pulmonary Oedema

Circulatory overload is precipitated by the presence of more fluid volume than the circulatory system can manage. When an excess of fluid volume occurs, there is an increase in venous pressure and the possibility of cardiac dilation (Perdue 2001). If the condition is allowed to persist, congestive cardiac failure and cardiac arrest can result. Circulatory overload is often precipitated by infusing too much fluid or increasing fluids too fast; this is particularly hazardous to elderly and paediatric patients as well as those with renal and cardiac problems (Perdue 2001; Macklin & Chernecky 2004).

Clinical features

Early signs include restlessness, slow increase in pulse rate, headache, shortness of breath, cough and possibly flushing (Perdue 2001; Macklin & Chernecky 2004).

As more fluid continues to build, the patient becomes hypertensive and dyspnoeic with gurgling respirations and starts to cough up frothy fluid. The patient should be assessed for venous dilation, indicated by engorged neck veins, pitted oedema in dependent areas, elevated pulmonary wedge pressure, and moist râles on auscultation. Some patients also experience puffy eyelids as fluids start to collect within the circulatory system (Perdue 2001).

Prevention

Preventative measures include the following.

1. Thorough patient assessment before commencing i.v. therapy. Take into account previous problems associated with i.v. therapy and any history of cardiac and respiratory problems. Assess present status related to the patient's ability to tolerate fluid volume.
2. Closely monitoring the patient receiving i.v. therapy for tolerance to the administration of medications or solutions.
3. Maintaining infusion rates as prescribed . Do not increase infusion rates for solutions that are behind schedule.
4. Slowing the infusion rate if signs and symptoms of circulatory overload are observed and asking the doctor to prescribe a decrease in the infusion rate.
5. Use of infusion devices when administering solutions or medications that require accurate measurement, and when administering solutions or medications to a neonatal, paediatric or elderly patient whose condition warrants critical management to prevent overload (Perdue 2001; Macklin & Chernecky 2004).

Management

If circulatory overload occurs the infusion must be slowed immediately to a rate that just keeps the vein patent and the patient placed in the high Fowler position (Perdue 2001): the position in which the head of the patient's bed is raised 90 cm with the knees elevated.

Section 2

The patient's vital signs and fluid balance should be monitored. The doctor should be notified and oxygen should be administered if required (Perdue 2001; Macklin & Chernecky 2004).

Medical intervention may include i.v. diuretics to produce rapid diuresis, an i.v. vasodilator to decrease afterload, morphine sulphate to decrease myocardial workload and venesection to relieve the heart's workload and reduce venous pressure (Perdue 2001)

Speedshock

Speedshock is a systemic reaction that occurs when a substance foreign to the body is rapidly introduced into the circulation (Perdue 2001; Weinstein 2007).

This phenomenon usually results from the administration of a bolus medication or an infusion containing a medication at a rapid rate. Speedshock should not be confused with circulatory overload as circulatory overload relates to volume whereas speedshock relates to the rapidity with which the medication is administered; it can occur even if a small volume of medication is given. Rapid injections enter the serum in toxic proportions and flood the heart and brain with medication (Perdue 2001; Phillips 2005).

Clinical features

When medications are administered the patient should be observed for dizziness, facial flushing, headache and medication-specific symptoms. It is important to recognize these symptoms early because progression is immediate, with the patient experiencing tightness in the chest, hypotension, irregular pulse and anaphylactic shock (Perdue 2001).

Prevention

Speedshock can be prevented. Practitioners should know the medication being administered and ensure that it is delivered at the manufacturer's recommended rate (Perdue 2001; Phillips 2005).

Gravity-flow administration sets, electronic flow control devices and volumetric chambers are available for use and the most suitable appliance should be used for those patients who are at risk of developing complications (Perdue 2001; Weinstein 2007).

Management

The administration of medicine and/or infusion should be performed over the specified time. The practitioner administering the medication and/or infusion should have the knowledge of the speed or rate over which to perform administration. S/he must be able to recognize the clinical features of speedshock and, should it occur be able to act accordingly, and notify the doctor (RCN 2005).

Nursing interventions should include immediate discontinuation of the infusion on recognition of the first symptom and maintaining the i.v. device for emergency treatment (Perdue 2001).

Allergic Reactions

An allergic reaction is a response to a medication or solution to which the patient is sensitive. Reactions may also occur from the passive transfer of sensitivity to the patient from a blood donor, or the patient may be sensitive to substances normally present in the blood, as is seen in blood transfusion reactions. Reactions may be immediate or delayed (Perdue 2001; Weinstein 2007).

> **BOX 7.4**
>
> **Medications commonly implicated in anaphylaxis (Scarlet 2006)**
>
> - Penicillin
> - Sulfa antibiotics
> - Allopurinol
> - Seizure and antiarrhythmia medications
> - Non-steroidal anti-inflammatory drugs (NSAIDs) such as asprin and ibuprofen
> - Muscle relaxants
> - Certain post-surgery fluids
> - Opioid analgesics
> - Vaccines
> - Radiocontrast media
> - Antihypertensives
> - Insulins
> - Blood products
> - Streptokinase

Clinical features

Patients receiving i.v. therapy should be monitored for symptoms of allergic reactions. The patient may experience chills and fever with or without urticaria, erythema and itching. Depending on the internal response to the allergen, the patient could experience shortness of breath with or without wheezing. The patient may also experience angioneurotic oedema (Perdue 2001). In severe cases anaphylactic shock may occur (Phillips 2005).

Incidence

In the United States approximately 550 000 serious allergic reactions to medications occur annually in hospitals. Incidences of drug-induced anaphylaxis from all drug types are reportedly increasing. This phenomenon may best be explained by the increased development and frequent use of new protein-based medications (Scarlet 2006) (*See* Box 7.4).

Prevention

Preventative measures include the following.

1. Patient assessment should be undertaken and the patient's previous drug allergies and sensitivities recorded. The patient's medical records should be flagged to alert all healthcare staff of any allergies; allergy alert bracelets should be used. Nurses should ensure that all appropriate checks are undertaken before administering any patient medication (Phillips 2005).
2. Adequate screening of donor and recipient blood can assist in the prevention of blood reactions. Policies and procedures should be in place for blood transfusion cross-matching, the cross-matching process, the identification process before blood administration and the interventions to be applied if a reaction occurs (Perdue 2001).

Management

In the event of an allergic reaction, the infusion should be stopped immediately, the tubing and the container changed and the vein kept patent to allow for treatment of possible anaphylactic shock. The doctor should be notified and interventions undertaken as prescribed (Perdue 2001).

Section 2

Antihistamines are usually administered; epinephrine or steroids are administered for more severe reactions. Sometimes antihistamines are used prophylactically when an allergic reaction is considered likely (Perdue 2001).

Conclusion

To optimize the potential for a patient receiving i.v. therapy to have a complication-free outcome, the provision of i.v. care must be considered within a multiprofessional framework. All parties need to be working in partnership towards the common goal of a successful intervention within the patient's treatment and therapy.

The nurse must consider her position from a legal and professional outlook. In relation to the Nursing and Midwifery Council Code of Practice (NMC 2004), nurses should embrace the expansion of their roles in the delivery of i.v. therapy only when they have the accompanying knowledge base and competence to ensure that they can deliver a service of excellence to their patients, of whom an estimated 80–90% will require i.v. therapy during their hospital stay (Perdue 2001).

Various investigators suggest that there is a degree of complacency surrounding the importance of asepsis, yet it is conclusively demonstrated that poor attention to asepsis in i.v. therapy is the cause of much morbidity and even mortality, particularly in the vulnerable patient groups (Perdue 2001; Gallant & Schulz 2006; Idvall & Gunninberg 2006).

It is evident that the longer i.v. therapy continues, the greater the risk of complications. A working knowledge and appreciation of correct standards of practice, knowing what to look for, being aware of the risks and dangers involved in therapy and being able to manage them effectively will help to reduce i.v.-related complications.

References

Andris DA, Krzywda EA (1997) Catheter pinch-off syndrome: recognition and management. *Journal of Intravenous Nursing* 20(5): 233–7.

Archis CA, Black J, Brown MA (2000) Does an endoluminal catheter brush improve flows or unblock haemodialysis catheters? *Nephrology* 5: 55–8.

Baranowski L (1993) Central venous access devices—current technologies, uses and management strategies. *Journal of Intravenous Nursing* 16(3): 167–194.

Berger L (2000) The effects of positive pressure devices on catheter occlusions. *Journal of Vascular Access Devices* 5(4): 31–3.

Bregenzer T, Conran D, Sakmann P, Widmer A (1998) Is routine replacement of peripheral intravenous catheters necessary? *Archives of Internal Medicine* 158(2): 151–156.

British Medical Association/Royal Pharmaceutical Society of Great Britain (BMA/RPSGB) (2007) *British National Formulary*, 53. The Pharmaceutical Press, London.

Camp-Sorrell D (2004) *Chemotherapy and Biotherapy Guidelines and Recommendations for Nursing Education and Practice.* Oncology Nursing Society, Pittsburgh.

Centers for Disease Control and Production (CDC) (2002) Guidelines for prevention of intravascular catheter-related infections. *Morbidity and Mortality Weekly Report* 51 (RR10): 1–26.

Conn C (1993) The importance of syringe size when using an implanted vascular access device. *Journal of Vascular Access Networks* 3(1): 11–18.

Conrad SA (2002) Venous Air embolism. *eMedicine Journal* 3: 4.

Couban S, Goodyear M, Burnell M, *et al.* (2005) Randomised placebo-controlled study of low-dose warfarin for the prevention of CVC-associated thrombosis in patients with cancer. *Journal of Clinical Oncology* 23(18): 4063–4069.

Deitcher SR, Tessen MR, Kiproff PM, *et al.* (2002) Safety and efficacy of alteplase for restoring function in occluded central venous catheters: results of the Cardiovascular Thrombolytic to Open Occluded Lines trial. *Journal of Clinical Oncology* 20(1): 317–24.

Department of Health (DH) (2001) Standard principles for preventing hospital-acquired infections. *Journal of Hospital Infection* 47 (Suppl): S21–S37.

Department of Health (2003) *Winning Ways. Working together to reduce Healthcare Associated Infection in England.* Department of Health Publications, London.

Dougherty L (1992) Intravenous therapy. *Surgical Nurse* 5(2): 10–13.

Dougherty L (1994) *A study to discover how cancer patients perceive the intravenous cannulation experience.* Unpublished MSc thesis, University of Surrey, Guildford.

Dougherty L (1996) The benefits of an IV team in hospital practice. *Professional Nurse* 11(11): 761–763.

Dougherty, L (2004) Vascular access devices. In: Dougherty, L & Lister S (eds) *The Royal Marsden NHS Trust Manual of Clinical Nursing Procedures*, 6th edn. Blackwell Publishing, Oxford.

Dougherty L (2006) *Central Venous Access Devices—Essential Skills Series.* Blackwell Publishing, Oxford.

Drewett S (2000) Central venous catheter removal: procedures and rationale. *British Journal of Nursing* 9(22): 2304–2315.

Fabian B (2000) IV complications: infiltration. *Journal of Intravenous Nursing* 23(4): 229–231.

Frey A, Schears GJ (2006) Why are we stuck on tape and suture. *Journal of Infusion Nursing* 29(1): 34–38.

Gallant P, Schultz AA (2006) Evaluation of a visual phlebitis scale for determining appropriate discontinuation of peripheral intravenous catheters. *Journal of Infusion Nursing* 29(6): 338–345.

Galloway, S, Bodenham A (2004) Long term central venous access. *British Journal of Anaesthesia* 92: 722–734.

Goode CJ, Titler M, Rakel B, *et al.* (1991) A meta analysis of effects of heparin flush and saline flush—quality and cost implications. *Nursing Research* 40(6): 324–30.

Goolsby TV, Lombardo FA (2006) Extravasation of chemotherapeutic agents: prevention and treatment. *Seminars in Oncology* 33: 139–143.

Goodwin M, Carlson I (1993) The peripherally inserted catheter: a retrospective look at 3 years of insertions. *Journal of Intravenous Nursing* 16(2): 92–103.

Grune F, Schrappe M, Basten J, Wenchal HM, Tual F, Stutzer H (2004) Phlebitis rate and time kinetics of short peripheral intravenous catheters. *Infection* 32: 1.

Hadaway L (2002) Why fluid escapes from the vein. *Nursing* 32(8): 36–43.

Haire WD, Herbst SF (2000) Use of alteplase. *Journal of Vascular Access Devices* 5(2): 28–36.

Hart S (2004) Aseptic technique. In: 30–2 Dougherty L, Lister S, eds. *The Royal Marsden Hospital Manual of Clinical Nursing Procedures*, 6th edn, pp. 50–63. Blackwell Publishing, Oxford.

Hayden BK, Goodman M (2005) Chemotherapy: principles of administration. In: Henke Yarbro C *et al.*, eds. *Cancer Nursing—Principles and Practice*, 6th edn, pp. 351–411. Jones and Bartlett, Massachusetts.

Holcombe B, *et al.* (1992) Restoring patency of long term central venous access devices. *Journal of Intravenous Nursing*, 15: 36–41.

Hunter MR (2003) Development of a vascular access team in an acute care setting. *Journal of Infusion Nursing* 26(2): 86–91.

Idvall E, Gunningberg L (2006) *Evidence for Elective Replacement of Peripheral Intravenous Catheter to Prevent Thrombophlebitis: a Systematic Review. The Authors Journal Compilation.* Blackwell Publishing, Oxford.

Infusion Nurses Society (INS) (2006) Infusion nursing standards of practice. *Journal of Infusion Nursing* 29(1) (Suppl).

Ingle RJ (1995) Rare complications of vascular access devices. *Seminars in Oncology Nursing* 11(3): 184–193.

Lawson T (2003) A legal perspective on CVC related extravasation. *Journal of Vascular Access Devices* 8(1): 25–28.

Lenhart C (2000) Prevention vs treatment of vascular access devices occlusions. *Journal of Vascular Access Devices* 5(4): 34–35.

LSC (2002) Standards of care; external central venous catheters in adults. London Standing Conference, London.

Lundgren A, Wahren LK, Ek AC (1996). Peripheral intravenous lines; time *in situ* related to complications. *Journal of Intravenous Nursing* 19(5): 229–238.

Macklin D, Chernecky C (2004) *IV Therapy.* Saunders, Missouri.

Maki DG, Goldmnan D, Rhame F (1973) Infection control in intravenous therapy. *Annals of Internal Medicine* 73: 867–887.

Maki DG, Ringer M (1991) Risk factor for infusion-related phlebitis with small peripheral venous catheters. *Annals of Internal Medicine* 114(10): 845–854.

Marders J (2005) Sounding the alarm for IV infiltration. *Nursing* 35(4): 18–20.

Masoorli S (2003) Extravasation injuries associated with the use of central vascular access devices. *Journal of Vascular Access Devices* Spring: 21–23.

Mayo DJ (1998) Fibrin sheath formation and chemotherapy extravasation: a case report. *Supportive Care in Cancer* 6: 51–56.

Mayo DJ (2000) Catheter-related thrombosis. *Journal of Vascular Access Devices* 5(2): 10–20.

Mayo DJ (2001) Catheter-related thrombosis. *Journal of Intravenous Nursing* 24 (Suppl 3): S13–S22.

McGee DC, Gould MK (2003) Preventing complications of CVC. *Medical Journals* 348(12): 1123–1133.

Mendez-Lang M (1987) Cost savings approach for justification of an IV team. *National Intravenous Therapy Association* September/October: 348–356.

Mennim P, Coyle CF, Taylor JD (1992) Venous air embolism associated with removal of central venous catheter. *British Medical Journal* 305: 171–172.

Miller J, Goetz A, Squier C, Muder R (1996) Reduction in nosocomial IV device-related bacteraemias after institution of an iv therapy team. *Journal of Intravenous Nursing* 19(2): 103–106.

Moureau N, Thompson McKinnon B, Douglas CM (1999) Multidisciplinary management of thrombotic catheter occlusions in VADs. *Journal of Vascular Access Devices* 4(2): 22–9.

Nursing and Midwifery Council (NMC) (2004). *Code of Professional Practice.* Nursing and Midwifery Council, London.

Ostrow L (1981) Air embolism and central venous lines. *American Journal of Nursing* November: 2036–2038.

PASA (2007) *Intravenous Cannula* [www document]. NHS Purchasing and Supply agency. www.pasa.doh.gov.uk/medical consumables/sharps/prod-ivc.stm [accessed 7 February 2007].

Perdue MB (2001) Intravenous complications. In: Hankin J *et al.*, eds. *Infusion Therapy in Clinical Practice*, 2nd edn, pp. 418–445. WB Saunders, Philadelphia.

Perucca R (2001) Obtaining vascular access. In: Hankin J *et al.*, eds. *Infusion Therapy in Clinical Practice*, 2nd edn, pp. 375–388. WB Saunders, Philadelphia.

Phillips L (2005) *Manual of IV therapeutics*, 4th edn. FA Davis, Philadelphia.

Polovich M, White JM, Kellher LO (2004) *Oncology Nursing Society Chemotherapy and Biotherapy Guidelines and Recommendations for Practice*, 2nd edn. Oncology Nursing Press, Pittsburgh.

Ponec D, Irwin D, Haire WD *et al.* (2001) Recombinant tissue plasminogen activator (alteplase) for restoration of flow in occluded central venous access devices: a double blind placebo controlled trial—the Cardiovascular Thrombolytic to Open Occluded Lines (COOL) efficacy trial. *Journal of Vascular Interventional Radiology* 12: 951–955.

Pratt RJ, Pellowe C, Wilson JA *et al.* (2007) Epic 2: national evidence-based guidelines for preventing healthcare-associated infections in NHS hospitals in England. *Journal of Hospital Infection* 655(Suppl): S1–S64.

Reed T, Philips S (1996) Management of central venous catheters occlusion and repairs. *Journal of Intravenous Nursing* 19: 289–294.

Rinn TL (2001) Fibrinolytic therapy in CVC occlusion. *Journal of Intravenous Nursing* 24 (Suppl 3): S9–S12.

Roth D (2003) Extravasation injuries of peripheral veins: a basis for litigation. *Journal of Vascular Access Devices* 8(1): 13–20.

Royal College of Nursing (RCN) (2005) *Standards for Infusion Therapy*. Royal College of Nursing, London.

Royer T (2001) "A case for posterior anterior and lateral CXR being performed following each PICC placement. *Journal of Vascular Access Devices* 6(4): 9–11.

Royer T (2003) Improving short peripheral outcomes: a clinical trial of two securemnt methods. *JAVA* 8(4): 45–49.

Rummel MA, Donnelly PJ, Fortenbaugh CC (2001) Clinical evaluation of a positive pressure device to prevent central venous catheter occlusion: results of a pilot study. *Clinical Journal of Oncology Nursing* 5(6): 261–265.

Scalley R, Van C, Cochran R (1992) The impact of an IV team on the related occurrence of intravenous related phlebitis. *Journal of Intravenous Nursing* 5(2): 100–109.

Scarlet C (2006) Anaphylaxis. *Journal of Infusion Nursing* 29(1): 39–44.

Schears GJ (2005) The benefits of a catheter securement device on reducing patient complications. *Managing Hospital Infection* 5(2): 14–20.

Schulmeister L (1998) A complication of vascular access device insertion. *Journal of Intravenous Nursing*, 21(4): 197–202.

Simcock L (2001) Managing occlusion in central venous catheters. *Nursing Times* 97(21): 36–38.

Speechley V (1984) The nurses role in intravenous management Nursing times 80(18): 31–32.

Springhouse Corporation (2002) *Intravenous Therapy Made Incredibly Easy*. Springhouse, Lippincott, Williams & Wilkins, Philadelphia.

Stanley A (2002) Managing complications of chemotherapy administration. In: Allwood M *et al.*, eds. *The Cytotoxic Handbook*, 4th edn, pp. 119–193. Radcliffe Medical Press, Oxford.

Tagalakis V, Khan S, Libman M, Blostein M (2002) The epidemiology of peripheral vein infusion thrombophlebitis: a critical review. *The American Journal of Medicine* 113:

Timoney JP, Malkin MG, Leone DM *et al.* (2002) Safe and effective use of alteplase for the clearance of occluded central venous access devices. *Journal of Clinical Oncology* 20(7): 1918–22.

Tully JL, Friedland GH, Baldrini LM, Goldmann DA (1981) Complications of intravenous therapy with steel needles and teflon catheters: a comparative study. *The American Journal of Medicine* 70: 702–706.

Ung L, Cook S, Edwards B *et al.* (2002) Peripheral intravenous cannulation in nursing. *Journal of Intravenous Nursing* 25(3): 189–195.

Vandergrift KV (2001) Oncologic therapy. In: Hankin J *et al.*, eds. *Infusion Therapy in Clinical Practice*, 2nd edn, pp. 248–275. WB Saunders, Philadelphia.

Verhage AH, Van Bommel EFH (1999) Catheter fracture: an under recognized and serious condition. *Journal of Vascular Access Devices* 4(2): 33–34.

Vesely TM (2003) Central venous catheter tip position: A continuing controversy. *Journal of Cardiovascular and Interventional Radiology* 14(5): 527–534.

Weinstein SM, ed. (2007) Plumer's Principles and Practice of Intravenous Therapy, 8th edn. JB Lippincott, Philadelphia.

Young AM, Begum G, Billingham LI *et al.* (2005) WARP: a Multi Centre Prospective Randomized Controlled Trial of Thrombosis Prophylaxis with Warfarin in Cancer Patients with Central Venous Catheters. *Journal of Clinical Oncology* 23: 16S Part I of II, June 1 Supplement, ASCO meeting proceedings, abstract 8004.

Yucha C, Hastings-Tolsma M, Szeverenyi N (1993) Differences among IV extravasation using four common solutions. *Journal of Intravenous Nursing* 16(5): 277–281.

CHAPTER 8

Intravenous Flow Control and Infusion Devices

Chris Quinn

Introduction

> Every year over 15 million infusions are carried out in the NHS. Infusion treatment is commonly used to deliver fluids and drugs via a drip into the veins of patients receiving re-hydration therapy or chemotherapy treatment.
>
> (NPSA 2004a)

The statement above is a conservative estimate of the number of intravenous (i.v.) infusions carried out in the UK every year. This estimate illustrates the scale of an increasingly high-risk practice area. The development of clinical procedures and treatments has prompted the ongoing technical development of infusion devices. The need for accurate flow control and other safety features to support the safe management of i.v. delivery has never been more apparent. Inevitably, this is a double-edged sword, because as infusion devices become more technically complex the risks associated with their use are also likely to increase (Quinn 1998).

This chapter will focus on infusion devices and related issues with an emphasis on risk management, national guidance, device management, functionality and use, patient perspectives and training.

Background to Infusion Risk

Infusion devices are used extensively across the NHS in both community and hospital care settings. They are used to accurately administer prescribed drugs or solutions through a designated vascular route over a set time. Infusion device technology has developed significantly over the past 20 years to support sophisticated procedures, techniques and risk management requirements. Infusion devices have moved from being tools that support clinical practice to being an integral requirement for treatment delivery. Without the use of infusion devices many procedures could not be carried out safely (Quinn 2000).

Such advances in medical technology have advantages and disadvantages. As devices such as large-volume infusion pumps and syringe pumps have technically improved it is inevitable that they will have become more complex. Consequently, appropriate training needs to be an integral part of infusion device practice (Quinn 1998; Amoore & Adamson 2003; NPSA 2004a).

The provision of infusion device training should be an integral part to any device management system; however, this may not be the case. In 2003 a report indicated that there were around 800 infusion device-related incidents reported to the Medicines and Healthcare products Regulatory Agency (MHRA) (MHRA 2003a). The actual number of infusion device-related incidents is probably significantly greater than this reported figure. This view is supported by one study (NPSA 2004b) that reviewed infusion device safety as part of a national project. The study identified 321 infusion device-related incidents in six NHS acute trusts. If these findings were extrapolated to the wider NHS (i.e. 189 acute NHS trusts in England and Wales at the time of the project); it is possible that there could be up to 10 000 infusion device incidents occurring yearly. If this were true it would reflect significant underreporting of infusion device-related incidents. It also supports the emerging views in the government report *Organisation With a Memory (OWAM)* which highlighted potentially high under reporting of adverse events (DH 2000).

In *OWAM*, research suggests that an estimated 850 000 adverse events occur in the NHS each year, with over 400 deaths per year where a medical device was implicated. This equates to approximately 1 in 10 patients (10.8%) admitted to hospital experiencing an adverse event. Another significant study, *A Spoonful of Sugar* (DH 2001b), goes on to state that of the adverse events experienced by 10.8% of admissions around one-third lead to greater morbidity and death; each event results in an average of 8.5 additional days in hospital; and 12% of all adverse events were related to medicines use. In a follow-up publication to *OWAM*, *Building a Safer NHS for Patients* (DH 2001a) it was recognized that over 400 people die or are seriously injured in adverse events involving medical devices every year. The problems associated with medication management are not just limited to the UK. The document *To Err is Human* (Kohn *et al.* 1999) in the United States was a major influence on the UK work *OWAM* with many similarities emerging during this work. What also emerged were similarities among incident rates from countries such as Denmark, Australia and New Zealand.

A report from the United States (Barker *et al.* 2002) recognized that medication errors are an increasing international healthcare problem and stated that typical hospital medication errors of one form or another occur in nearly one out of every five doses given to a patient. Another study (Kaushal *et al.* 2001) found that i.v. medications were involved in 54% of potential adverse drug events in the paediatric inpatient setting.

One study (Taxis & Barber 2003) found that in one London hospital, there was at least one error observed in 53% of observed i.v. drug administrations. In most cases the implications were negligible; however, in three instances the observer was required to intervene to prevent a potentially serious outcome.

The National Patient Safety Agency (NPSA)-sponsored national project that looked at infusion device safety found that the hospitals in its pilot study had, on average, over 30 different makes and models of infusion device available for use (NPSA 2004a; Quinn *et al.* 2004b). Apart from this situation being inefficient, it undoubtedly contributed to the occurrence of adverse drug events because of the potential confusion when clinicians are exposed to using many different devices.

The quality of training provision was also found to be extremely inconsistent, ranging from an unstructured 'ad hoc' approach (common) to less common comprehensive competency-based training. The best training observed was usually provided in conjunction with the infusion device manufacturers.

Finally, when adverse events do occur, an increasingly emerging risk that organizations and clinicians must consider is litigation. A recent study (Quinn & Upton 2006) reviewed 176 claims received by the NHS Litigation Authority (NHSLA) associated with infusion delivery. They found that:

- general wards were four times more likely to generate claims than any other area
- paediatric specialties generated three times as many claims as other specialties
- causes of most claims could be attributed to user error
- the nature of most claims related to extravasation leading to tissue damage and scarring
- the cost of claims was approximately £25 million.

It is therefore clear that greater awareness is required by users of infusion devices and associated equipment if patient safety is to be managed appropriately. The following sections provide insights into aspects of the infusion delivery system to assist the user to become a safer practitioner.

Infusion Systems: Selecting the Right Device

Before selecting an infusion device it is first necessary to understand what an infusion system is. The MHRA (MHRA 2003b) define this:

> as the process by which an infusion device and any associated disposables are used to deliver fluids or drugs in solution to the patient by the intravenous, subcutaneous, epidural, parenteral or enteral route.

This process, outlined in the MHRA document MHRA (2003b) comprises the following key stages:

- prescription of the drug or fluid
- preparation of the infusion solution
- selection of the appropriate infusion device
- calculation and setting of the rate of infusion
- administration of the fluid to the patient
- monitoring and recording the actual delivery
- disposal of equipment.

Infusion devices include the following.

- *Gravity controllers*, which employ a clamping mechanism to regulate the flow of fluid under the force of gravity.
- *Infusion devices*, which employ a positive pumping mechanism to deliver the fluid. These devices are powered items of equipment which together with an appropriate administration set provide an accurate flow of fluids over a prescribed period.
- *Syringe pumps*, which work by pushing the plunger of a syringe at a predetermined rate.

The type of infusion device required depends on factors including:

- the fluid or drug
- the volume and concentration of drug/solution
- the speed of the infusion required.

Other specialist infusion devices available to clinicians include the following.

- *Patient-controlled analgesia (PCA) pumps*, which allow the patient to have control of their infusion within accepted parameters.
- *Anaesthesia pumps*: syringe pumps specifically designed for anaesthesia or sedation administration and which should only be used for this purpose.

- *Ambulatory pumps*: small pumps designed to allow the patient independence either within hospital or at home.
- *Elastomeric devices*: disposable ambulatory devices that use an elastomeric reservoir from which a drug is delivered at a determined rate.

Flow Control

Flow control is an extremely important concept to understand, and can be defined as the delivery of i.v. fluids and medications at an appropriate rate and in a constant, accurate manner in order to achieve a therapeutic response and prevent complications such as over- or underinfusion (Millam 1990; MHRA 2003b; Emergency Care Research Institute (ECRI) 2004) *See* Box 8.1.

Gravity Flow

It is important to recognize that there are still many clinical situations where patients in the hospital or home-care setting will require minimal i.v. input, and where their therapy can be delivered with a simple administration set utilizing gravity flow. In many areas the cost of electronic infusion devices will be prohibitive or demand will overwhelm the hospital's supply, and it is therefore important that safe therapy can still be provided without these devices. *See* Box 8.2.

Indications for use

Indications for use of a gravity-type administration are as follows: (MHRA 2003b)

- delivery of fluids without additives
- administration of drugs or fluids where adverse effects are not anticipated if the infusion rate varies slightly
- where the patient's condition does not give any cause for concern and no complication is predicted.

When an infusion depends on gravity for its flow there will be a limitation to its rate and accuracy of delivery, and therefore for intensive or multimodality therapy, a flow control (infusion) device should be used (Hunt & Rapp 1996). A nurse may also be

---

BOX 8.1

Complications of inadequate flow control (MHRA 2003b; Finlay 2004; Gray & Illingworth 2004; RCN 2005)

Overinfusion
- Fluid overload with accompanying electrolyte imbalance
- Metabolic disturbances during parenteral nutrition
- Toxic concentration of medication which may result in 'speedshock'
- An increase in venous complications caused by reduced dilution of irritant substances
- Air embolism if containers run dry earlier than anticipated

Underinfusion
- Dehydration
- Metabolic disturbances
- A delayed response to medications or subtherapeutic dose
- Occlusion of i.v. device due to slow cessation of flow

BOX 8.2

Advantages and disadvantages of gravity flow (MHRA 2003b; Gray & Illingworth 2004; RCN 2005)

Advantages
- Low cost
- Familiar to all staff
- Easy to set up
- Infusion of air is less likely
- Minimizes risk of excessive extravascular infusion

Disadvantages
- Variability of drop size
- Delivery not accurate
- Infusion rates limited
- Risk of free flow
- Requires frequent observation and adjustment

---

required to calculate the rate of administration. Numerous reports have highlighted the need for calculation skills (Hutton 1998; Elliott 2005; Emergency Nurse 2005; Wilson 2006) and recommend a range of standard formulae to achieve delivery requirements.

To calculate drops per minute the following formula can be used:

$$\frac{Quantity\ to\ be\ infused\ (mL) \times no.\ of\ drops/mL}{No.\ of\ hours\ over\ which\ infusion\ to\ be\ delivered \times 60\ min} = no.\ of\ drops/min$$

(Gatford 1990)

It should be noted that the number of drops per millilitre (drops/mL) is dependent on the administration set and the viscosity of the fluid. An increased viscosity, such as blood or plasma, will cause a larger drop size. Crystalloid fluid being administered by gravity flow is delivered at the rate of 20 drops/mL, whereas red blood cells given via a blood set are delivered at 15 drops/mL (Atterbury & Wilkinson 2000; Finlay 2004; Gray & Illingworth 2004). If greater safety is required, a burette administration set can be used, particularly if large bolus volumes could be harmful, such as in children or patients with cardiac failure. A burette has a discrete 150–200-mL chamber which can be filled from the infusion bag each hour. This allows the nurse to ensure that the patient receives no more than the prescribed hourly rate.

There are many factors that will affect the rate of flow of gravity flow infusions (*See* Box 8.3).

Fluid and container

The type and viscosity of the infusion fluid, as well as the temperature at which it is delivered, may influence flow rates (Phelps & Cochran 1989; Quinn 2000; Cornelius *et al.* 2003), as cold or irritating solutions may cause venous spasm, impeding the rate of flow (Finlay 2004). A warm pack placed on the vein proximal to the device will offset this reaction (Finlay 2004).

For gravity flow to be effective, the infusion will need to be suspended at an adequate height above the patient. The amount of fluid within the container exerts a pressure and any change in gravity by elevating or lowering the container will affect the flow rate (Morling 1998; Weiss *et al.* 2000; Kern *et al.* 2001). Generally, the faster the infusion rate required, the higher the infusion will need to be placed; thus, increasing the distance

> **BOX 8.3**
>
> **Factors that affect flow control (MHRA 2003b; Finlay 2004; Sarpal 2004)**
>
> - Condition and size of vein
> - Gauge size and length of device
> - Type and location of device
> - Partial or total occlusion and kinking of the device
> - Administration set
> - In-line devices: antisiphon valves, in-line filters, antireflux valves
> - Type and viscosity of fluid
> - Temperature of fluid
> - Height of container
> - Roller clamp control
> - The patient
> - Other in-line devices, e.g. filters
> - Venous access device
> - Occlusion of the device caused by clot formation or fibrin sheath. This can occur as a result of restricted venous circulation, e.g. blood pressure cuff on the infusion arm, restraints on or above device, the patient lying on the arm receiving the infusion, blood backtracking down the device due to an empty infusion bag, or container lowered preventing gravity flow
> - The position of the device within the vein, e.g. if the bevel of the device is against the inner wall of the vein, flow will be slow

between the bag/bottle and the patient will increase the rate (MHRA 2003b). The optimum height of the container above the patient is 1.5 m (MHRA 2003b), which is the reason that gravity infusions sometimes slow down when the patient's position is changed (e.g. sitting up, lying down, in ambulant patients or during transportation).

Roller clamp control

The roller clamp used to control flow may become loose and slip, or even distort the administration set tubing, and this results in a phenomenon known as 'free flow' (Finlay 2004). This risk has prompted recommendations that emphasize the need to prevent free flow (MHRA 2003b; ECRI 2002, 2004).

The patient

Patients may occasionally tamper with the roller clamp control or inadvertently adjust the height of the infusion container or other equipment without realizing the effect it will have on flow rate (Meadows 2003; Quinn 2003; Richardson 2004).

Flow Control Devices

Certain patient groups are more at risk of complications associated with flow control, and it is in these circumstances that a flow control infusion device must be used. There are also a number of other factors to consider when selecting the appropriate infusion system for a particular situation, such as risks to the patient, delivery parameters and environmental features. *See* Boxes 8.4 and 8.5.

MHRA classification

In order to aid the selection of an infusion device, the MHRA of the Department of Health, in collaboration with users, manufacturers and technical and clinical specialists, has produced guidance to assist users when identifying a suitable device for use.

BOX 8.4

Groups at risk of complications associated with flow control (Sarpal 2004)

- Infants, young children and the elderly
- Patients with compromised cardiovascular status, impairment/failure of organs or major sepsis
- Postoperative or post-trauma patients
- Patients suffering from shock
- Stressed patients
- Patients receiving multiple medications, whose clinical status may be changing rapidly

---

BOX 8.5

Factors to consider when selecting an appropriate infusion system (MHRA 2003b; Finlay 2004)

Risk to patient of:
- Over or under infusion
- Uneven flow
- Inadvertent bolus
- High delivery pressure
- Extra vascular infusion

Delivery parameters
- Infusion rates and volume required
- Degree of short and long-term accuracy required
- Alarms required
- Ability to infuse into chosen site (venous, arterial, subcutaneous)
- Suitability of infusing the type of drug (half-life, viscosity)

Environmental features
- Ease of operation
- Frequency of observation and adjustment
- Type of patient (child, very sick)
- Mobility of patient

The MHRA state that:

> 'Pumps (infusion devices) are designed for a variety of clinical applications and their performance characteristics will vary. The same level of technical performance of pumps is not necessary for every clinical therapy. We have divided therapies into three major categories according to the potential infusion risks to help purchasers and user(s) select the pump (infusion device) most appropriate for their needs.
>
> These categories are shown in Table 4a with a list of performance parameters critical to each, and the important safety features are given in Table 4b. These have been selected on the principle that, in general, the greater the potential risks associated with therapies, the higher the performance needed and the more important are the safety features.'

See Table 8.1.

Because of the complexity and functionality of new infusion devices, all offering a range of features to choose from, it can be confusing for the clinician when choosing which device(s) to purchase. The MHRA have listed a number of features in order of importance that need to be considered when purchasing an infusion device (*See* Box 8.6).

One significant safety feature relatively new to the infusion device market is the development of medication safety software. This software solution prevents the inappropriate programming of dangerously incorrect doses. The 'dose-limiting' software alerts the user to a potential problem with the device programming and can prevent the infusion

Table 8.1   MHRA DB2003(02) *Infusion Devices* (MHRA 2003b. Reproduced with permission).

Therapy category	Therapy description	Patient group	Critical performance parameters
A	Drugs with narrow therapeutic margin	Any	Good long-term accuracy
			Good short-term accuracy (see below)
	Drugs with short half-life[1]	Any	Rapid alarm after occlusion
			Small occlusion bolus
	Any infusion given to neonates	Neonates	Able to detect very small air embolus (volumetric pumps only)
			Small flow rate increments
			Good bolus accuracy
			Rapid start-up time (syringe pumps only)
B	Drugs, other than those with a short half-life[1]	Any except neonates	Good long-term accuracy
			Alarm after occlusion
	TPN	Volume sensitive except neonates	Small occlusion bolus
	Fluid maintenance		Able to detect small air embolus (volumetric pumps only)
	Transfusions		Small flow rate increments
	Diamorphine[2]	Any except neonates	Bolus accuracy
C[3]	Fluid maintenance	Any except volume sensitive or neonates	Long-term accuracy
	Transfusions		Alarm after occlusion
			Small occlusion bolus
			Able to detect air embolus (volumetric pumps only)
			Incremental flow rates

[1] The half-life of a drug cannot usually be specified precisely, and may vary from patient to patient. As a rough guide, drugs with half-lives of the order of 5 minutes or less might be regarded as 'short' half-life drugs.
[2] Diamorphine is a special case. The injected agent (diamorphine) has a short half-life, whilst the active agent (the metabolite) has a very long half-life. It is safe to use a device with performance specifications appropriate to the half-life of the metabolite.
[3] Not all infusions require a pump. Some category C infusions can appropriately be given by gravity.

BOX 8.6

The MHRA infusion device safety features in descending order of importance (MHRA 2003b)

- Anti-free-flow device in administration set
- Free-flow clamp in pump when door is opened
- Provision against accidental modification of settings
- Two distinct actions to change rate
- Two distinct and/or simultaneous actions to initiate a bolus
- Syringe barrel clamp alarm, door open alarm or equivalent
- Syringe plunger disengagement alarm or equivalent
- Patient history log
- Volume infused display
- Technical history back-up
- Battery back-up

---

from proceeding. One international safety organization recommends that only infusion devices fitted with this software should be purchased (ECRI 2002). The MHRA have carried out evaluations on a number of devices which use dose-limiting infusion software and are worth reviewing (MHRA 2004). *See* Box 8.7.

> **BOX 8.7**
>
> **Types of equipment available (MHRA 2003b)**
>
> **Using a syringe**
> - Syringe infusion pumps
> - Syringe drivers
> - Anaesthetic pumps
> - Patient-controlled analgesia (PCA) pumps
>
> **Gravity controllers**
> - Drip rate controllers
> - Volumetric controllers
>
> **Infusion pumps**
> - Drip rate pumps
> - Volumetric pumps
> - PCA pumps
>
> **Ambulatory pumps**
> - Continuous infusion
> - Multimodality pumps
> - PCA pumps

(a)

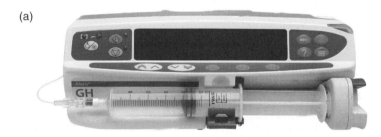

(b)

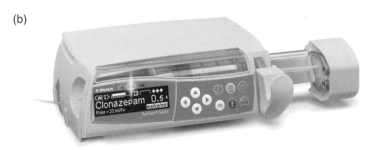

Figure 8.1   Two syringe pumps of differing designs. Both can carry out similar functions despite having a different user interface. (a) The Alaris GH (reproduced by permission of Alaris). (b)The B. Braun Space (reproduced by permission of B. Braun).

Infusion Devices That Use a Syringe (Figure 8.1)

Syringe infusion pumps

These are devices in which a syringe containing fluid or a drug in solution is fitted into the pump and the plunger of the syringe is driven forwards at a predetermined rate. These pumps are usually set to run at millilitres per hour (MHRA 2003b).

Section 2

Application

Syringe infusion pumps are designed for the accurate delivery of fluids at low flow rates and are recommended where a prescribed drug flow rate is prescribed at less than 5 mL/h (MHRA 2003b). This is because historically the mechanisms used in large-volume infusion pumps (discussed later) have not been as accurate at lower flow rates (MHRA 2003b). Syringe pumps are therefore ideally selected for the safe infusion of fluids and drugs to neonates or children and drugs to adults (MHRA 2003b).

Features

When using syringe infusion pumps for drugs with a short half-life (less than 5 minutes) it is essential that the infusion device meets the delivery recommendations as set out in the MHRA device bulletin (MHRA 2003b).

- Good long-term accuracy.
- Good short-term accuracy.
- Rapid alarm after occlusion.
- Small occlusion bolus.
- Able to detect very small air embolus.
- Small flow rate increments.
- Good bolus accuracy.
- Rapid start-up time.
- Internal rechargeable battery that will provide power (if the mains power fails) without interruption and without losing memory of set parameters or patient data.
- The syringe barrel and plunger must be located securely in order to ensure accurate function. If the syringe is incorrectly inserted, there should be activation of an alarm and automatic disablement of the pump so that the infusion cannot continue.
- Although not essential, it is recommended that the pump has the ability to record and recall its service or technical history.
- Comprehensive alarm and tamper prevention features are also important considerations.

Safety issues

- Use the smallest syringe that the device will accept and that is able to hold the required volume of drug. A smaller syringe ensures improved consistency of flow and occlusion response times are decreased (MHRA 2003b).
- If using several pumps simultaneously with one patient in a high-dependency or critical care setting, ensure that the pumps can be mounted horizontally as this makes checking of the rate easier and thus minimizes the potential for errors (Quinn 2000; Powell & Carnevale 2004). It also enables more pumps to be attached to one intravenous stand.

Anaesthesia pumps (Figure 8.2)

The early anaesthetic pumps appeared similar to all other syringe pumps with the exception that they were designed to allow rapid changes in flow rate and bolus to be made while the pump is infusing, where other pumps require the user to stop the pump first before adjusting the rate (MHRA 2003b).

There are also new-generation anaesthetic pumps called total intravenous anaesthesia (TIVA) pumps and target-controlled infusion (TCI) pumps that can deliver i.v. anaesthetic drugs using a pharmacokinetic software delivery model. These highly specialized devices control the induction, maintenance and reversal phases of drug delivery and require close supervision by the anaesthetist (Absalom & Struys 2006).

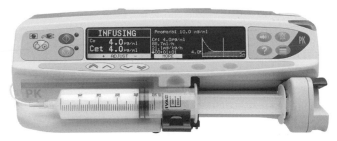

Figure 8.2 Anaesthesia pump. Although they look like any other syringe pump they have markedly different software algorithms which allow accurate delivery of the anaesthetic agent in relation to the weight and age of the patient. These pumps must only be used in those areas where anaesthesia is delivered.

Application

These pumps are only to be used in areas where anaesthesia may be administered, such as operating departments and critical care areas. They are designed to provide induction of anaesthesia or sedation and therefore have to be able to provide much greater flow rates and larger boluses than other devices (e.g. several hundred mL/h). The benefits of this type of i.v. anaesthesia are that it minimizes the risk of postoperative nausea and vomiting (PONV) and shortens recovery time (Guarracino *et al.* 2005; Absalom & Struys 2006). There is also evidence that i.v. anesthesia is not only efficient but cost effective (Fombeur *et al.* 2002).

Special features

These pumps often have a range of special features:

- built-in drug information systems
- software that can automatically calibrate the pump for the drug being delivered
- programming for the individual patient's body weight and the drug concentration being used
- computer interface for control and for connection to the patient monitoring system; some pumps have the ability to change drug rates depending on changes in the patient's haemodynamic status (Absalom & Struys 2006).

Safety issues

Because these pumps can give large boluses, run at high rates and deliver specific anaesthetic drug algorithms, it is essential that they are only used in critical care areas under close supervision. Measures must be instituted to ensure that these pumps never follow the patient out of these areas to a general ward (MHRA 2003b).

Patient-controlled analgesia (PCA) pumps (Figure 8.3)

Background

The literature demonstrates that in the late 20th century, patients who had undergone surgery reported that they experienced severe unrelieved pain (Kuhn *et al.* 1990). Kuhn *et al.*'s work showed that 40% of postoperative patients (*n* = 33) reported that the 'postoperative period had been very painful'. The authors postulated several reasons for the inadequacy of analgesia, the most likely being that clinicians were still concerned about the possibility of opiate dependency and therefore chose minimal dosages. This research and several other studies led to a report being produced by the Royal College of Anaesthetists and the Royal College of Surgeons (RCS & RCA 1990). This report

(a)

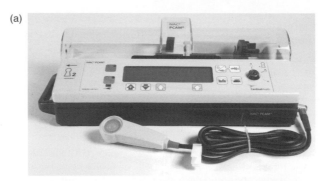

(b)

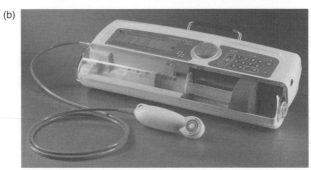

Figure 8.3   Patient-controlled analgesia (PCA) syringe pumps allow the patient to press a button to self-administer a predetermined dose within set limits. (a) The Alaris PCA pump used generally in acute hospital settings (reproduced by permission of Alaris). (b) The Graseby CADD Legacy PCA pump which is ideal for home settings (reproduced by permission of Graseby).

recommended that patients should have access to pain teams and that one of the pain control methods which should be available for patients was patient-controlled analgesia.

Although often regarded as a recent advance, the concept of patient-managed or -controlled analgesia has its roots in the 1960s both in the USA and in the UK. In the USA in the late 1960s, Dr Sechzer devised an experimental approach to measuring pain experienced by postoperative patients. He taught patients to press a button when they felt pain and a nurse observer would then administer a bolus of i.v. analgesia. Meanwhile in the UK, in the late 1960s, Scott (Levy & Williams 1992) was experimenting with a hand-held spring-loaded clamp which controlled an i.v. bottle containing a solution of glucose 5% with 300 mg of pethidine. His patients were taught to grip the clamp each time they experienced pain. The clamp would then close automatically and prevent further analgesia doses if the patient fell asleep.

One of the advantages of the PCA system is that the patient can deliver the dose when they choose. For this reason it is sometimes known as 'demand analgesia'. It is recognized that there are many factors that influence the intensity of the pain experience and it therefore seems wise to individualize the approach to a patient's pain relief (Brown 2004; Gara 2004; Rourke 2004; Godfrey 2005; Hsu *et al.* 2005).

It is important to recognize that PCA is not a universal panacea for all postoperative pain and is not successful in some patients. Indeed, recent research has indicated that there are a multitude of factors that need to be considered before treating pain appropriately (Tyrer & Davis 2005).

An important factor in the success of PCA is patient education and compliance, both of which will be influenced positively by a well-designed device (MHRA 2003b).

There are now several varieties of PCA pump, which deliver the analgesia via a syringe, a reservoir bag or a disposable elastane (elastomeric) balloon (the reservoir and disposable devices will be discussed later in this chapter).

Application

PCA is most commonly used in the postoperative setting, but it has proved useful in other areas of acute and chronic pain, such as the pain resulting from osteoarthritis (Taylor 2000) or pain management in rehabilitation (Dawkins 2003; Tyrer & Davis 2005).

PCA can be used in virtually any clinical care setting where the need arises.

Features

These devices are similar to the syringe infusion pumps described previously, but they have the following special features (MHRA 2003b):

- a hand-held button or switch which allows the patient to deliver a preset bolus
- a preset lock-out time between boluses
- the ability (some models) to deliver a continuous background or basal infusion, providing a continuous low rate of analgesia
- a loading dose to be delivered on setting up the pump
- a memory log which can be accessed by the clinician to ascertain the number and frequency of boluses used, and the total volume of opiate used in a given time.

Safety issues

The general safety issues described previously for syringe infusion pumps apply, but the following apply particularly to the PCA pump.

The concept of PCA is that the patient takes an active role in their therapy. In many instances of i.v. therapy this may not be the case (Quinn 2003; Richardson 2004). In order to promote an active role, the patient must firstly receive an explanation of PCA and then, if they consent to this type of therapy, they should be trained in its use (MHRA 2003b). It is therefore essential that the pump is easy to use. The following safety design features are therefore recommended:

- simple-to-follow steps for accessing a bolus
- easily depressed or gripped device (some patients may have peripheral sensory problems).

All PCA pumps must have the facility to 'lock out' the programming device from the patient. If there is any concern that the patient's respiratory function or conscious level could be altered then it may be safer to select a bolus-only setting. This means that there will be *no* background infusion and the patient can only receive a bolus dose when they push the button.

It is also imperative that nursing and medical staff receive training and understand the specific functions of the PCA pump.

Syringe Drivers

Syringe drivers are sometimes known as miniature syringe pumps because they are light and easily portable.

Applications

Syringe drivers are used in the following situations:

- when the patient is mobile in hospital or receiving treatment at home and in the community for delivering cytotoxic chemotherapy where a small volume is delivered over several days or weeks

- when the ambulant patient requires continuous pain relief via the subcutaneous, i.v. or epidural route.

Safety issues

Syringe drivers are designed to be set over hours or a day (24 h). When using the hourly driver, the rate is set in 'mm/h'; the 24-h driver, however, should be set to 'mm/24 h'. Manufacturers have endeavoured to clearly label the devices, but care should still be taken when setting up the driver (MHRA 1995). Because of their design, older types of these devices are prone to programming errors. This is especially problematic where both device models are available for use. Standardization is recommended wherever possible (NPSA 2004a,b; Quinn *et al.* 2004b).

These types of syringe drivers are not suitable for neonatal infusions because of their scant alarm function. They should not be used for any category A infusions as discussed earlier in the section on MHRA classifications and in Table 8.1 (MHRA 2003b).

Gravity Controllers

These are seldom seen in hospitals as they are old technology. The first infusion pumps were controller devices and worked by constricting the administration set. These controllers relied solely on the height of the fluid bag above the patient as the device has no pumping action.

The rate of the infusion was monitored by a sensor (drop counter) attached to the drip chamber of the administration set. The sensor ensures that there was no overinfusion of fluid, but if there is any resistance to flow, i.e. occlusion in access device or administration set, there may be underinfusion of fluid. If the device had not delivered the prescribed volume of fluid the controller would alarm. Some models of controller had a 'flow status' system which then allowed the clinician to view whether there was any resistance to flow (MHRA 2003b). There were two main types of gravity controllers: the drip rate controller and the volumetric controller.

Drip rate controllers

These controllers have no pumping action, as described above, and are powered by mains or battery. They tend to have few controls and are therefore very easy to operate.

Application

These controllers were suitable for most of the lower-risk infusions such as simple fluid infusions (e.g. sodium chloride or dextrose).

Safety issues

The accuracy of a drip rate controller is dependent upon the sensor counting drops. However, several factors can influence the volume of fluid in each drop (Finlay 2004; MHRA 2003b; RCN 2005):

- the shape, condition and size of the hole in the administration set from which the drop falls
- the drip rate that has been set
- the type of fluid, its osmolality, temperature and surface tension.
- As therapy and drug treatment have developed and the need for more accurate infusion devices increased, these devices are virtually obsolete and are not recommended for use (MHRA 2003b).

Volumetric controllers

These devices are rarely used now, if at all, having been surpassed by newer, more technically competent infusion devices (discussed below). They could be set in 'mL/h'. They had a drop sensor and needed a dedicated administration set or a disposable 'add-on' rate clip. Volumetric controllers had more settings and alarms than the drip rate controllers, but although they could compensate for the drop size, their flow rate accuracy was only ± 10%, and as for the controller above, they are no longer recommended for use (MHRA 2003b).

Gravity flow control devices

These devices incorporate a mechanism/dial into the infusion set to regulate the rate and flow of the infusion, with gravity providing the driving pressure. The accuracy of this type of system ranges widely, and because of the many high-risk drugs now administered, and the associated requirement for accuracy, these are not used widely in the UK. They have been used mainly for the delivery of low-risk, large-volume infusions such as crystalloids.

Infusion Pumps (Figure 8.4)

These devices pump fluid from an infusion reservoir such as a bag, bottle or infuser via an administration set.

Volumetric pumps

These are the preferred option for larger flow rates and a wide range of large-volume infusion devices are available in the UK healthcare market. This range of pumps ensures

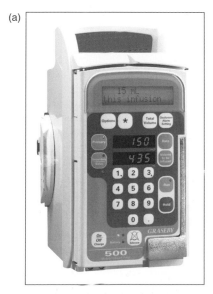
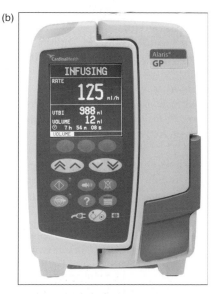

Figure 8.4 These pumps are preferred for the accurate delivery of large-volume infusions. The Graseby 500 (a) and the Alaris GP (b) are examples of commonly available pumps. (a) Reproduced by permission of Graseby; (b) reproduced by permission of Alaris.

that there is a volumetric pump available to meet the delivery requirements of all patient groups, including neonates.

They usually weigh between 3 and 5 kg and are designed to be 'stationary', i.e. attached to an i.v. drip stand or a bed rail (MHRA 2003b).

Volumetric pumps should have the facility to work on either mains or battery but should always be used 'plugged in' to a mains supply. Most of these pumps use batteries designed to last for at least 3 hours when fully charged. The user manual provided by the manufacturer of the device should always be checked to determine how long any specific pump will function on battery. The pump manual will usually indicate the battery life in specific terms (e.g. 'the pump will work for 5 hours at 5 mL per hour').

The infusion rate is set using mL/h. Most devices can be programmed to between 1 and 1000 mL/h, but at rates below 5 mL/h, accuracy will decrease (MHRA 2003b). Most pumps use a linear peristaltic pumping action, although there are other mechanisms with devices using a cassette or other dedicated administration set (MHRA 2003b).

Application

Modern volumetric pumps have a comprehensive range of safety and alarm features and can be recommended for use in a range of care settings. *See* Box 8.8.

Features

Some pumps have a drop sensor which is used for safety monitoring and alarms (e.g. 'empty infusion bag'), but unlike the drip rate pumps this sensor is not integral to the rate mechanism.

In most volumetric pumps the infusion pressure can be configured so that the pump will alarm and stop above a certain preset pressure level. Some of these pumps can set pressure occlusion limits in single units, whilst others set 'levels' of pressure. The advantage of

---

BOX 8.8

Infusion pump use by common care settings (Markman 2000; Finlay 2004; Absalom & Struys 2006)

Acute care settings
- Fluids—both crystalloid and colloid solutions
- Antimicrobials
- Blood and blood products
- Cardiac and vasoactive drugs—inotropes and antiarrhythmic
- Total parenteral nutrition (TPN), electrolyte infusions such as magnesium, calcium, phosphate
- Dialysate used in haemodialysis or more commonly in the continuous filtration methods, such as continuous venovenous haemodiofiltration (CVVHD)
- Rapid fluid resuscitation

General wards
- Fluid management
- Blood transfusions—particularly in the elderly or those with a degree of cardiac failure
- Prehydration regimens before regimens such as anticancer chemotherapy
- TPN and electrolyte infusions (as 'acute care')
- Infusion antimicrobials

Home-care setting
- Fluids
- Antimicrobials
- Anticancer chemotherapy
- Pain control
- Peritoneal dialysis fluid
- TPN, electrolyte infusions

single-unit setting is that it can be set just above the pumping pressure, whereas the stepped pressure level increments in levels of 50 or 100 mmHg. Single-unit settings allow an earlier alarm alert, minimizing the risk of potential harm to the patient following extravasation. Anecdotally, whilst pressure occlusion may not prevent extravasation, it can certainly minimize the risk of complications from extravasation, and in many neonatal and paediatric units where 'single-unit' variable pressure pump settings are used, extravasation problems are usually uncomplicated. This may be the consequence of being able to programme low pressure occlusion settings, combined with frequent monitoring by staff.

One study (Quinn & Upton 2006) identified extravasation as the most common area for negligence claims in i.v. therapy in the UK. Extravasation accounted for over 50% of all claims, at an average cost of around £45 000 per claim. It would appear that a greater focus on and understanding of pressure management is still required by clinicians to minimize the risk and impact of extravasation and its associated complications and costs. Whilst it is clear that having the capability to set low occlusion pressures shortens the time for the pump alarm following occlusion, it does not prevent extravasation from occurring. However, having shortened times to alarm increases the chance of preventing the development of complications from extravasation (Quinn & Upton 2006).

Safety issues

It is estimated that there are over 15 million intravenous infusions taking place in the UK every year with many using an infusion pump to control delivery (NPSA 2004a). These pumps generally have a good safety record; however, because of their increased sophistication mistakes do still happen with their use (DH 2001b; ECRI 1998, 2002, 2003; MHRA 2003b). As these pumps can deliver rates of up to a 1000 mL/h, care must be taken to ensure that the pump rate is set correctly (e.g. taking particular care to set 10 mL/h rather than 100 mL/h). This is especially important in the paediatric setting (Hutton 1998; Emergency Nurse 2005).

In the acute care setting, care must also be taken to ensure that pumps that are not in use are left plugged into the electrical supply. This can become extremely important if a critically ill patient needs to be moved and cannot manage without supportive drug therapy. The pumps need to be fully charged so that they can be powered by their battery (MHRA 2003b; NPSA 2004a).

Ambulatory Pumps (Figure 8.5)

These pumps are small portable devices that will fit easily into a pocket, a handbag or a waist belt. They can use either a small syringe or a reservoir bag of 100–250 mL that can be housed in a plastic 'wallet' that clips onto the pump. Most of these pumps are preprogrammable. They are therefore an ideal choice for the patient who can be taught a few basic care rules whilst in hospital and can then receive a preset dose of drug over several days or weeks. These pumps are powered by a small battery and so patients are advised to have a spare battery available.

Application

Like ambulatory syringe pumps, these devices are best suited to small volumes of solution. Depending on the reservoir size, a dose regimen can be set up for weeks or months.

Ambulatory pumps are therefore well suited for anticancer chemotherapy, long-term antibiotic therapy, anticoagulant therapy and pain control (Cabrera & Arias 2001; Coyte *et al.* 2001; New *et al.* 1991). Increasingly, manufacturers are providing a variety of ambulatory pumps which may include a PCA function.

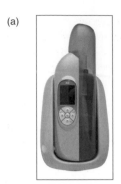
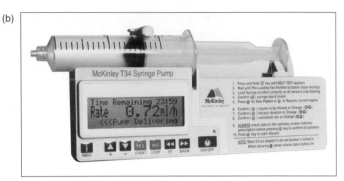

Figure 8.5   Two examples of an ambulatory infusion device: (a) the Alaris AD;
(b) the McKinley T34. Different designs but both are light and easy to carry.
(a) Reproduced by permission of Alaris; (b) reproduced by permission of McKinley Medical UK
Limited.

Features

These pumps have the same safety features as listed in the section on PCA syringe pumps.

As it may be necessary for patients and/or their carers to access any of the controls (e.g. to change a dose), the settings should be 'user-friendly' with buttons or a soft pad large enough to be visualized and activated easily.

Safety issues

As these pumps are predominantly used in the home and community setting, it is essential that they are reliable and require the minimum maintenance. In recent times, manufacturers have greatly improved the reliability and durability of their designs (MHRA 2003b).

Implanted Pumps

In recent years, as biotechnology has advanced, so has the manufacture of dedicated devices. Implanted pumps have been developed for ambulatory patients who need long-term, low-volume therapy (Dionigi *et al.* 1995; Buchwald & Rohde 1997; Tono & Monden 2000; Gin *et al.* 2001; Nielsen & Sinkjaer 2004).

Application

These pumps were designed to target chemotherapy or biological behaviour modifiers directly to a site of cancer (Markman 2000). Regional anticancer chemotherapy is used at the following sites:

- *intra-arterial chemotherapy*: hepatoma, metastatic colorectal cancer, osteosarcoma, glioblastoma, astrocytoma and tumours of the head and neck
- *intraperitoneal chemotherapy*: localized ovarian cancer (although more recently, combination systemic regimens have become more popular)
- *intrathecal or intraventricular chemotherapy*: acute lymphocytic leukaemia, brain tumours and palliation for metastatic disease in the brain.

More recently, implanted pumps have been successfully developed to be used in long-term anticoagulant and pain management therapy.

Features

There are several devices available, all working on the principle of a periodically 'topped-up' port. In some pumps, the device is powered by the vaporization of a 'charging' fluid in a reservoir adjacent to the drug reservoir. The pressure of this vapour exerts a pressure on some bellows which, in turn, force the drug out through a filter and flow restrictor to the dedicated implanted catheter. In another device, a septum port is periodically filled and then programmed telemetrically.

Safety issues

In dealing with implanted devices, access to the device will be solely through repeated filling of reservoirs. Therefore, although there is less for the patient and carer to learn about the device, education concerning aseptic technique is essential (RCN 2005).

Patients must also be trained to recognize any alteration in the appearance of the site of the implanted pump (e.g. signs of infection) or any signs that the pump has become dislodged or that it is no longer working, and told of the necessity for quick reporting to their relevant referral team.

Disposable Pumps

Compared to infusion devices these pumps are relatively new. These non-electronic devices have several advantages for the patient in that they are generally very lightweight and small so that they can be easily worn or carried even whilst performing physical exercise. They are usually very 'user-friendly', requiring the minimum of input from the patient. They do not require a battery, so they are less expensive and the patient does not have to remember to carry a spare battery. Finally they can be purchased prefilled, thus minimizing patients' and carers' exposure to needles and ampoules.

Application

These lightweight pumps have been used predominantly in the ambulatory and home-care setting, but because of their predictable small-volume, low-rate capacity, they have also been used in acute care settings. The following are the most common uses:

- anticancer chemotherapy
- anticoagulant therapy
- pain control, particularly when coupled with a disposable PCA device such as the 'wristwatch' attachment (Sheldon & Bender 1994).

Features

The disposable pumps work on the principle of an elastomeric balloon which is situated inside a plastic cylinder. When the balloon is filled, the resulting hydrostatic pressure inside the balloon is enough to power the infusion. The drug is then infused through a small-bore administration set which usually has a rate restrictor at the patient end. The size of this bore determines the flow rate of the drug or solution.

Cost implications

The disposable pumps are intended to be filled only once, the usual reservoir size being 50–70 mL; the infusor is then discarded following use. These devices can also be purchased prefilled by private pharmaceutical companies or hospital pharmacies. Another cost advantage of the disposable non-electronic pump is that there are no maintenance or servicing costs (Kelly & Brull 1995).

Management of Infusion Devices

Any technical medical equipment will only function optimally if it is cared for in an appropriate manner and all such devices are supplied with recommendations from the

Section 2

manufacturer as to servicing and maintenance. Whichever department is concerned with the technical management of these devices, it is imperative that clinicians have a direct input into this area.

Indeed, clinical practitioners are bound by their professional codes to recognize their individual responsibility and accountability for practice. For nurses in the UK, the NMC code of professional conduct: standards for conduct, performance and ethics (NMC 2004) section 6 states that:

- You must keep your knowledge and skills up-to-date throughout your working life. In particular, you should take part regularly in learning activities that develop your competence and performance.
- To practise competently, you must possess the knowledge, skills and abilities required for lawful, safe and effective practice without direct supervision. You must acknowledge the limits of your professional competence and only undertake practice and accept responsibilities for those activities in which you are competent.
- If an aspect of practice is beyond your level of competence or outside your area of registration, you must obtain help and supervision from a competent practitioner until you and your employer consider that you have acquired the requisite knowledge and skill.

A nurse, whether working clinically with patients or as a manager responsible for a care environment, must recognize that it is unacceptable to use any device that:

- is not suitable for an application
- has not been maintained
- is partly broken
- is unknown to the user (Cuthrell 1996; ECRI 2002; MHRA 2003b).

Every year government agencies such as the MHRA receive many reports of adverse incidents or errors involving infusion devices.

Recognition of the need for clinical staff to be closely involved with the monitoring of device management has led to increasing nurse involvement in 'focus' groups concerned with product design (Haslar 1996). As a consequence of reports received by the MHRA involving infusion device-related adverse incidents, the UK National Patient Safety Agency (NPSA) sponsored a project in 2002 which looked to establish the root causes of infusion device-related incidents and develop solutions to prevent and minimize their recurrence. The *Infusion Device Project* produced guidance (NPSA 2004a,b; Quinn *et al.* 2004b) for the NHS that promotes the need for trusts to *'Buy Right, Manage Right, Use Right'* infusion devices. It made four key recommendations that will support good practice and safety with infusion device use.

1. Standardization of infusion device stock as a key action for hospitals to improve safety.
2. Evaluation of infusion devices before purchase to ensure good usability.
3. Centralization of infusion (and other) devices (e.g. equipment libraries).
4. The need for users to be competent in the use of infusion devices.

Nurses especially are encouraged to become more involved in purchasing these devices by influencing procurement decisions. All too often decisions to purchase infusion devices are made in isolation by those staff whose primary concern is financial; this often leads to a false economy. If the cheapest available infusion device is purchased and that device is difficult to operate or maintain, then the initial cost saving will be lost due to error and repair costs. The development of the competency-based training required to improve patient safety is discussed later.

Selection and procurement

Care should be taken to involve all relevant personnel in the initial planning and selection stage, including:

- clinical representatives—it is essential that there is some representation from those directly involved with patient care and using the device
- supplies or administrative personnel who are familiar with the process of ordering, supply and delivery
- an accountant or financial adviser
- a biomedical/clinical engineer or staff involved with the maintenance and servicing of equipment
- the directorate manager or staff with a link to the manager with responsibility for the relevant budget
- a risk manager, who can provide information on adverse events that would inform the specification requirement for a potential infusion device model.
(NPSA 2004a; Quinn *et al.* 2004b)

Clinical representative

It is essential that there is involvement from staff that have been working in the clinical environment where new equipment is required. The representative should have experience in the specific needs of the area but also have knowledge of the relevant literature on devices; in some areas a nurse with this degree of experience may be the clinical nurse specialist or the senior sister.

Medical staff, particularly anaesthetists or intensivists, may also wish to be involved. However, it is the nurses at the bedside who frequently set up and change rates on devices, as well as discovering faults and sending the devices for repair. For these reasons it is recommended that nurse membership be included in such groups. In hospitals where they exist, an important addition to this group would be a member of the i.v. team whose experience will be a valuable resource in the selection and the management of devices (Dougherty 1996).

Before a meeting of the above personnel, the clinical staff should discuss the clinical application for which an infusion device is to be used and devise a written specification which should include the following (MHRA 2003b):

- the reason for choosing the equipment and the benefits to be gained from a particular device
- the problems that might occur
- whether it is user-friendly
- type of patient—neonate, child, adult
- type of infusion category infusion device is required to infuse—Category A, B or C as discussed earlier (MHRA 2003b)
- environment—home care, ambulatory, general ward use, theatres and anaesthetics, acute care
- portability
- budget limit for capital purchase and ongoing expenditure on disposables
- standardization of devices (where possible) to facilitate training and minimize the risk of user error (NPSA 2004a).

Supplies or administrative personnel

It is important to include staff experienced in liaison with manufacturers and in the arrangement of purchasing deals that may include standing orders for disposables. Such staff will also have experience and knowledge of the reliability of different manufacturers concerning delivery of disposables, and also customer care and after-care, especially with technical and staff training support (PASA 2004).

Accountant or financial adviser

It is imperative that an accountant or financial adviser is involved in the initial stages when contracts are being discussed. They may also be very helpful in the negotiation of any trial periods or discounts on bulk purchasing. They can advise on high cost, which may have to follow a specific process as part of the tender process. As of 1 January 2006 high-cost tenders (over £93 000) need to be advertised throughout the European Union (EU) as part of this mandatory process (PASA 2004).

Biomedical/clinical engineer

Although clinical staff will be aware of clinical needs, it is important that any device should also be considered from a mechanical and scientific viewpoint. Technical reports such as those produced by the MHRA can be helpful, but local expert technical help and experience are also vital. Most large biomedical engineering departments build up a library of devices which have been evaluated and they can therefore offer valuable advice on how a device will perform over time.

Trust/directorate managers

It is advisable that wherever possible the purchasing of equipment be standardized through-out a trust (NPSA 2004a,b). Devices are often moved with patients or are loaned through various wards and departments. Standardization and centralization of equipment will help to minimize user error and ensure ease of training of personnel (NPSA 2004a,b).

A trust or directorate manager may be able to influence or liaise with other directo-rates to ensure that there is a more streamlined approach to the selection and purchasing of devices. In some areas of the UK, several trusts have joined together to form groups or consortiums to develop greater purchasing power for device selection and purchasing (PASA 2004).

Staff development and competency training

Historically in the NHS, the delivery of training has been inconsistent and in many hospitals extremely limited. A national e-learning qualification for infusion device use was launched in February 2006 at the NPSA Risk Conference. The *Certificate in the Safe Use of Infusion Devices* (C&G 2006) is accredited through City & Guilds and the Open College Network, and incorporates a process that takes the learner through e-learning modules (knowledge) as well as practical training (skills), both elements requiring assess-ment. This learning was designed to get trusts to use the training skills of manufacturers as part of the process.

The qualification aims to:

- provide an overview of the key concepts underpinning the use of infusion devices
- take the learner through the process of setting up, monitoring and closing down an infusion, drawing your attention to critical issues at each stage
- provide an overview of generic practical issues related to the use of infusion devices
- train the learner in the practical use of one model of syringe pump and one model of volumetric pump
- provide an awareness of the associated risks
- review and practise drug calculation skills.

The need for staff to receive training is reflected in national recommendations includ-ing NPSA (NPSA 2004a,b), MHRA (MHRA 2003b) and the NHS Litigation Authority Clinical Negligence Scheme for Trusts (CNST) standards (CNST 2006).

Storage of devices and tracking strategies

Care should be taken to comply with the manufacturer's instructions regarding storage of supplied equipment. The following general rules apply.

- Any device that has a battery back-up facility needs to be plugged in continuously even when not in use; therefore storage areas need enough electrical sockets.
- Pumps powered by small removable batteries (such as ambulatory pumps) should be stored without their batteries.
- All devices should be stored clean and ready for use.
- If possible, devices should be stored in a central collection area such as an equipment library (NPSA 2004a) where they can be logged in and out and their use monitored. This system can help to prevent devices being stored in inappropriate places such as in cupboards or on window sills, and it also ensures that pumps are available.

All devices will at some time need repairing or updating and it is therefore essential that device use is logged. If a tracking system is used it should be possible to identify a particular device that has malfunctioned more times than expected or to be able to check that all the department's devices are returned.

Another use for a tracking or logging system is to ensure that all devices are routinely maintained and serviced at least as often as the manufacturer recommends.

Routine tracking of all medical devices is becoming commonplace in many areas and although it requires some resource allocation, this can be justified as part of the institution's risk management programme (Quinn *et al.* 2004b). As medical litigation becomes more common (Quinn & Upton 2006), patients and their families are becoming more aware of their right to be cared for in an institution that has an optimum safety network.

Maintenance and servicing

All devices need to be maintained and serviced as directed by the manufacturer. Once infusion devices are out of warranty, usually 1–3 years, they will often need an annual service. Most of these devices are easily portable and in the hospital setting they could be difficult to locate. Therefore, to enable the pumps to be easily located, a tracking record system is essential.

Each institution or department should have guidelines which ensure the following:

- careful cleaning and decontamination of pumps before handling by service and maintenance personnel
- immediate withdrawal of a device from the clinical area if it has been dropped or subjected to other damage
- documentation of all service and maintenance checks and of any repair work carried out for each individual pump—using a bar code or the manufacturer's code number can be useful.

It is important to rigorously discourage any repair of devices by clinical staff or carers in the hospital or community setting. Modern devices are complex machines and should only be attended to by designated biomedical engineers or the manufacturer. If a device malfunctions and causes a patient incident, its service history will be checked. If a non-designated person has carried out any work on the device, the manufacturer may have a case in law to place the responsibility onto the institution (MHRA 2000).

Most countries have a system of reporting whether a device has been involved in a patient incident. In the UK, if a device is involved in an incident it is recommended that it is reported to the MHRA. There are strict guidelines for reporting such an incident, including the retention for examination of any related disposable such as the syringe/reservoir or administration set that was used (MHRA 2003b).

It is vitally important that such patient incidents are reported to a central body, because it is this reporting that can provide the necessary large database to recall a device from general sale and thus help to protect future patients.

Reporting errors with devices

The continuous infusion of i.v. drugs is increasing as technological advances in equipment and pharmacological improvements in drugs are introduced into clinical practice. Such technology, however, can also introduce potential new complications (Department of Health & Design Council 2003). As discussed earlier, the MHRA receives many reports of adverse patient incidents where an infusion device has been used. Some of these incidents are due to the malfunctioning of equipment, but many reflect user error. In 53% of all reports received by MHRA no cause was established, with the infusion device found to be working to specification (Quinn *et al.* 2004a). User error in infusion device incidents was almost three times that of any other medical device. This could imply that in the 53% of incidents where no cause was established, user error is a probable explanation (NPSA 2004a; Quinn *et al.* 2004b).

Anecdotal evidence suggests that the majority of clinicians, nursing staff and pharmacists have little or no knowledge or understanding of the types and suitability of pumps for intravenous infusions (Pickstone *et al.* 1994). Inadequate understanding of equipment makes it difficult to interpret information correctly and diagnose false alarms (McConnell 1998). Nurses who do not understand the purpose, capabilities, limitations and functioning of a device may be unable to point out malfunctions, which will increase liability and the risk of harm to the patient.

Whilst it is difficult in the absence of good reporting systems to establish the precise numbers of deaths attributable to infusion devices, one study (*See* Box 8.9) illustrates the nature of reported deaths.

A number of reviews (Hutton 1998; McConnell 1998; Amoore & Adamson 2003; Meadows 2003; Quinn 2003) found that training and education were a major problem for machine use in direct patient care for a variety of reasons.

- New equipment frequently arrived on the unit for almost immediate use.
- Nurses had difficulty in getting time off to attend training courses.
- Device use education was, in some instances, limited to on-the-job training from partially knowledgeable colleagues or learned from an equipment supplier's manual.
- There was inadequate time to learn from suppliers' demonstrations which may be narrow in scope and skewed to favour the device.

BOX 8.9

Device-related deaths (Richardson 1995)

- A patient died when diamorphine was infused via a clockwork pump which was not accurate enough for the purpose.
- A patient died when a drug was infused at nearly 50 times the required rate; the pump had been returned from the serving department and set at a high rate which was not reset by nursing staff before use.
- A patient died because a pump designed for use with a dedicated administration set was used with a standard set.
- A patient died when no drug was infused because an in-line tap was closed. The pump drive mechanism was badly worn and slippage meant that the alarm was not activated.
- A patient died when the roller clamp on the administration set was not closed; when the pump was opened it caused a massive overinfusion of drug.

As a result nurses generally felt that their device education was inadequate (NPSA 2004a,b; Quinn *et al.* 2004b).

Nurses caring for patients with electromechanical devices need to fulfil their professional responsibility to protect their charges and should therefore possess comprehensive device knowledge, which includes a conceptual understanding of the technology involved. It will only be when the nurse is fully conversant, competent and proficient in the use of mechanical devices in direct patient care that the potential for error will be at its minimum. However, there are also some additional management tools that can be used to ensure safety.

- A network for near-miss reporting (Kohn *et al.* 1999; DH 2001a) is recommended by national governments. These reports from the UK and USA address the need to learn from mistakes and near-misses and avoid a 'blame' culture which has been so prevalent in recent times. The premise is that clinicians are more likely to report incidents and near-misses when they know that blame will not be apportioned.
- A compassionate and professional attitude to incident reporting—this may encourage reporting.
- A computerized database of all incidents—to allow for the recognition of repeated similar errors to be collated and management action to be taken.
- Regular updates for clinical staff on errors reported and the management action taken.
- Awareness of the NPSA and MHRA reporting system as noted above.

As technological advances make further inroads into device development, more pumps can now incorporate a failure/error log, which may be useful for local data collection.

Following the Clothier report requested by the Department of Health in the UK (Medical Devices Agency 1995), many manufacturers have developed devices that require 'specific button push combinations' to prevent or minimize tampering. Manufacturers have now developed 'dose-limiting' software incorporated within the infusion device. This helps prevent inadvertent programming errors and potential overdoses. A number of these dose-limiting systems have been evaluated by the MHRA (MHRA 2004).

Disposal of devices

It is imperative that all obsolete or failed infusion devices are removed from the clinical area immediately (MHRA 2003b). Each trust will need written documentation for the procedure to be followed when a device is condemned and to document this removal from the hospital database.

The practice of sending out-of-date medical equipment to developing countries is *not* recommended as all safety issues will be further compounded in countries and regions that have no technical back-up facilities (MHRA 2000).

Audit of practice

As hospital inspections are carried out, for example by the Healthcare Commission and NHS Litigation Authority (CNST), the need to produce good evidence across a range of identified areas is imperative. This is especially so in the area of i.v. medication administration (CNST 2006; DH 2001b). Trusts are required to demonstrate how they are identifying and addressing problems with the overall aim of improving patient safety (DH 2001b).

This could take the following form:

- a review of documentation
- a review of data collection: incident reports, device failure/repairs, maintenance issues

- interviews with all levels of the multidisciplinary clinical team
- spot checks of clinical practice to determine policy compliance.

Conclusion

There has been an emphasis on safety and the prevention of error throughout this chapter. However, this is with due recognition to the huge contribution that infusion devices make to clinical care. Indeed, many aspects of therapeutic care that we perform today would not be possible without the aid of these devices.

It is also known from experience and the literature that patients are increasingly keen to learn about the devices used in their treatment, and they are sometimes now being involved in the development or selection of devices (Richardson 2004). It should therefore be our aim to ensure continuous education for all staff, patients and their families in this area, as in other clinical areas.

Finally, it is through becoming more knowledgeable, and therefore more confident, that healthcare professionals will be able to enter the debate with manufacturers and work together to ensure the highest standards of clinical excellence for patients.

References

Absalom A, Struys M (2006) *An Overview of TCI & TIVA*, 1st edn. Academia Press, Belgium.

Amoore J, Adamson L (2003) Infusion devices: characteristics, limitations and risk management. *Nursing Standard* 17(28): 45–52.

Atterbury C, Wilkinson J (2000) Blood transfusion. *Nursing Standard* 14(34): 47–52.

Barker KN, Flynn E, Pepper G *et al.* (2002) Medication errors observed in 39 health care facilities: Implications for prevention. *Archives of Internal Medicine* 162(16): 1897–1903.

Brown D (2004) A literature review exploring how healthcare professionals contribute to the assessment and control of postoperative pain in older people. *Journal of Clinical Nursing* 13(6): 74–90.

Buchwald H, Rohde TD (1997) International study group for implantable infusion devices 1996. The world's only implantable infusion pump society. *American Society for Artificial Internal Organs Journal* 43(3): 132–136.

Cabrera FJ, Arias HM (2001) Continuous ambulatory chemotherapy with elastomer pump. *Revista de Enfermeria* 24(9): 76–78.

City & Guilds:(C&G) (2006) *Certificate in the Safe Use of Infusion Devices*. City & Guilds, London.

Clinical Negligence Scheme for Trusts (CNST) (2006) *Clinical Negligence Scheme for Trusts; Standard 5*. CNST Standards, London.

Cornelius A, Frey B, Neff TA, Gerber AC, Weiss M (2003) Warming of infusion syringes caused by electronic syringe pumps. *Acta Anaesthesiologica Scandinavica* 47(5): 549–553.

Coyte PC, Dobrow MJ, Broadfield L (2001) Incremental cost analysis of ambulatory clinic and home-based intravenous therapy for patients with multiple myeloma. *Pharmacoeconomics* 19(8): 845–854.

Cuthrell P (1996) Managing equipment failures: nursing practice requirements for meeting the challenge of the Safe Medical Devices Act. *Journal of Intravenous Nursing* 19(5): 264–268.

Dawkins S (2003) Patient-controlled analgesia after coronary artery bypass grafting. *Nursing Times* 99(47): 30–31.

Department of Health (DH) (2000) *An Organisation with a Memory*. The Stationery Office, London.

Department of Health (2001a) *Building a Safer NHS: Implementing OWAM*. The Stationery Office, London.

Department of Health (2001b) *A Spoonful of Sugar: Medicines Management in the NHS*. The Stationery Office, London.

Department of Health & Design Council (2003) *Design for Patient Safety*. Department of Health Publications, London.

Dionigi P, Cebrelli T, Jemos V, Minoli L, Gobbi P, Dimitrov G (1995) Use of subcutaneous implantable infusion systems in neoplastic and AIDS patients requiring long-term venous access. *European Journal of Surgery* 161(2): 137–142.

Dougherty L (1996) The benefits of an IV team in hospital practice. *Professional Nurse* 11(11): 761–763.

Emergency Care Research Institute (ECRI) (1998) Infusion pump inspection frequencies. How often is inspection really needed? *Health Devices* 27(4–5): 148–150.

Emergency Care Research Institute (2002) Evaluation: health devices. *Health Devices* 31(10): 352–387.

Emergency Care Research Institute (2003) Infusion devices. Inspection and preventive maintenance procedure. *Health Devices* 32(5): 197–202.

Emergency Care Research Institute (2004) JCAHOs national patient safety goal for infusion pump free-flow protection. ECRI's assessment of the protection offered by general-purpose, PCA, and ambulatory pumps. *Health Devices* 33(12): 430–435.

Elliott M (2005) Mapping drug calculation skills in an undergraduate nursing curriculum. *Nurse Education in Practice* 5(4): 225–229.

Emergency Nurse (2005) Calculation skills: paediatric dosages. *Emergency Nurse* 13(6): 1–17.

Finlay T (2004) *Intravenous Therapy.* Blackwell Publishing, Oxford.

Fombeur PO, Tilleul PR, Beaussier MJ, Lorente C, Yazid L, Lienhart AH (2002) Cost-effectiveness of propofol anesthesia using target-controlled infusion compared with a standard regimen using desflurane. *American Journal of Health-System Pharmacy* 59(14): 1344–1350.

Gara D (2004) Acute pain management choices. *World of Irish Nursing* 12(10): 35–37.

Gatford JO (1990) Nursing calculations. Churchill Livingstone, Edinburgh. 3rd edition.

Gin H, Melki V, Guerci B, Catargi B (2001) Clinical evaluation of a newly designed compliant side port catheter for an insulin implantable pump: the EVADIAC experience. Evaluation dans le diabete du traitement par implants actifs. *Diabetes Care* 24(1): 175.

Godfrey H (2005) Pain management. Understanding pain, part 2: pain management. *British Journal of Nursing* 14(17): 904–909.

Gray A, Illingworth J (2004) *RCN: Right Blood, Right Patient, Right Time: RCN guidance for Improving Infusion Practice.* Royal College of Nursing, London.

Guarracino F, Lapolla F, Cariello C *et al.* (2005) Target controlled infusion: TCI. *Minerva Anestesiologica* 71(6): 335–337.

Haslar R (1996) Human Factors Design: what is it and how can it affect you? *Journal of Intravenous Nursing* 19(3): S5–S8.

Hsu Y, Somma J, Hung Y, Tsai P, Yang C, Chen C (2005) Predicting postoperative pain by preoperative pressure pain assessment. *Anesthesiology* 103(3): 613–618.

Hunt M, Rapp R (1996) Intravenous medication errors. *Journal of Intravenous Nursing* 19(3): 9–15.

Hutton M (1998) RCN continuing education. Numeracy skills for intravenous calculations, *Nursing Standard* 12(43): 49–52.

Kaushal R, Bates D, Landrigan C (2001) Medication errors and adverse drug events in pediatric inpatients. *Journal of the American Medical Association* 285: 2114–2120.

Kelly D, Brull S (1995) The cost of modern technology. *Journal of Clinical Anaesthesia* 7: 80–81.

Kern H, Kuring A, Redlich U *et al.* (2001) Downward movement of syringe pumps reduces syringe output. *British Journal of Anaesthesia* 86(6): 828–831.

Kohn L, Corrigan C, Donaldson M (1999) *To Err is Human: Building a Safer Health Care System.* Archives of Internal Medicine, Washington DC, USA.

Kuhn S, Cook K, Collins M, Jones J, Mucklow J (1990) Perceptions of pain relief after surgery. *British Medical Journal* 300: 1687–1689.

Levy D, Williams C (1992) Recent developments in the management of post-operative pain. *The Pharmaceutical Journal* September: 12–15.

Markman M (2000) Regional delivery of anticancer drugs: current applications. *Cleveland Clinic Journal of Medicine* 67(8): 584–586.

McConnell EA (1998) Infusion devices require educated users. *Nursing Management* 29(11): 55–58.

Meadows M (2003) Strategies to reduce medication errors. *FDA Consumer* 37(3): 20–27.

Medical Devices Agency (1995) *Clothier Report: The Report of the Expert Working Group on Alarms on Clinical Monitors in Response to Recommendation 2: Allitt Enquiry.* Department of Health, London.

Medicines and Healthcare products Regulatory Agency (MHRA) (1995) *MDA HN9506 (Graseby MS 16 & 26 ambulatory syringe pumps).* Medicines and Healthcare products Regulatory Agency, London.

MHRA (2000) *Equipped to Care: The Safe Use of Medical Devices in the 21st Century.* Medicines and Healthcare Products Regulatory Agency, London.

MHRA (2003a) *Adverse Incident Reports: 2002: DB 2003(01).* Medicines and Healthcare Products Regulatory Agency, London.

MHRA (2003b) *Infusion Devices: Device Bulletin (DB 2003(02)).* Medicines and Healthcare Products Regulatory Agency, London.

MHRA (2004) *Dose Limiting Software For Infusion Devices: Evaluation 04097. Evaluation Bulletin.* Medicines and Healthcare Products Regulatory Agency, London.

Millam DA (1990) Controlling the flow. Electronic infusion devices. *Nursing* 20(8): 65–68.

Morling S (1998) Infusion devices: risks and user responsibilities. *British Journal of Nursing* 7(1): 13–6, 18, 20.

National Patient Safety Agency (NPSA) (2004a) *Safer Practice Notice (01): Infusion Devices.* National Patient Safety Agency, London.

National Patient Safety Agency (2004b) *Standardising and Centralising Infusion Devices—A Project to Develop Safety Solutions for NHS Trusts.* National Patient Safety Agency, London.

New PB, Swanson GF, Bulich RG, Taplin GC (1991) Ambulatory antibiotic infusion devices: extending the spectrum of outpatient therapies. *American Journal of Medicine* 91(5): 455–461.

Nielsen JF, Sinkjaer T (2004) Guided intrathecal baclofen administration by using soleus stretch reflex in moderate-severe spastic multiple sclerosis patients with implanted pump. *Multiple Sclerosis* 10(5): 521–525.

Nursing and Midwifery Council (NMC) (2004) *The NMC Code for Professional Conduct. Standards for Conduct, Performance and Ethics.* Nursing and Midwifery Council, London.

Phelps SJ, Cochran EB (1989) Effect of the continuous administration of fat emulsion on the infiltration of intravenous lines in infants receiving peripheral parenteral nutrition solutions. *JPEN Journal of Parenteral and Enteral Nutrition* 13(6): 628–632.

Pickstone M, Jacklin A, Langfied B, Wooton R (1994) Intravenous infusion of drugs; measuring and minimising the risks. *British Journal of Intensive Care* 5(Suppl): 338–343.

Powell ML, Carnevale FA (2004) A comparison between single and double-pump syringe changes of intravenous inotropic medications in children. *Dynamics* 15(4): 10–14.

Purchasing and Supply Agency (PASA) (2004) *Safe use of infusion device*. UK Purchasing & Supply Agency, NHS. www.pasa. nhs.uk/infusiondevices

Quinn C (1998) Infusion devices: a bleeding vein of clinical negligence? *Journal of Nursing Management* 6(4): 209–214.

Quinn C (2000) Infusion devices: risks, functions and management. *Nursing Standard* 14(26): 35–41.

Quinn C (2003) Infusion devices: understanding the patient perspective to avoid errors. *Professional Nurse* 19(2): 79–83.

Quinn C, Upton D (2006) A review of claims against the NHS relating to IV therapy. *Health Care Risk Report* 12(14): 15–18.

Quinn C, Boult M, Cotteril R(2004a) An infusion of safety. *Health Care Risk Report* 10(2): 12–15.

Quinn C, Stephenson E, Glenister H (2004b) NPSA infusion device toolkit: A cost saving way to improve patient safety. *Clinical Governance* 9(3): 195–199.

Royal College of Nursing (RCN) (2005) *Standards for Infusion Therapy*. Royal College of Nursing, London.

Royal Colleges of Surgeons and Anaesthetists (RCS & RCA) (1990) *Working Party of the Commission on the Provision of Surgical Services. Pain after Surgery*. Royal Colleges of Surgeons and Anaesthetists, London.

Richardson N (1995) A review of drug infusion incidents: the situation from the national perspective. *British Journal of Intensive Care* 8(9): Suppl.

Richardson A (2004) Infusion devices: the views of patients. *Health Care Risk Report* 10(2): 16.

Rourke D (2004) The measurement of pain in infants, children, and adolescents: from policy to practice. *Physical Therapy* 84(6): 560–570.

Sarpal N (2004) Drug administration infusion devices. In: Dougherty L, Lister S, eds. *The Royal Marsden Hospital Manual of Clinical Nursing Procedures*, 6th edn, pp. 260–274. Blackwell Publishing, Oxford.

Sheldon P, Bender M (1994) High-technology in home care. *Nursing Clinics of North America* 29: 507–519.

Taxis K, Barber N (2003) Ethnographic study of incidence and severity of intravenous drug errors. *British Medical Journal* 326(7391): 684.

Taylor L (2000) *The Assessment and Management of Chronic Pain: a Case Study of a Patient with Osteoarthritis, St Vincent's Hospital, New South Wales, Australia* [www. document]. www.ciap.health.nsw.gov.au/hospolic/stvincents/2000/chronic_pain.html

Tono T, Monden T (2000) [The role of prophylactic hepatic arterial infusion chemotherapy after potentially curative resection of hepatic metastases from colorectal cancer]. *Nippon Geka Gakkai Zasshi* 101(8): 568–573.

Tyrer S, Davis E (2005) Central pain states: etiology and management in rehabilitation. *Critical Reviews in Physical and Rehabilitation Medicine* 17(2): 131–162.

Weiss M, Fischer J, Neff T, Baenziger O (2000) The effects of syringe plunger design on drug delivery during vertical displacement of syringe pumps. *Anaesthesia* 55(11): 1094–1098.

Wilson A (2006) Nurses' Maths: Researching a practical approach. *Nursing Standard* 17(47): 33–36.

CHAPTER 9
Obtaining Peripheral Venous Access
Lisa Dougherty

Introduction

Venepuncture and cannulation are the most commonly performed invasive procedures in the UK. Neither of these procedures is based simply on technical skill, each requiring adequate knowledge of the relevant anatomy and physiology, the impact that such a procedure can have on a patient and the expected outcomes of therapy. The ability to assess the patient and make an informed choice on the selection of the vein and the device to be inserted is based on observation, nursing judgement, the use of clinical and nursing notes and the ability to problem-solve. The aim should be to provide the patient with a functional, comfortable peripheral vascular access device (Perucca 2001).

The procedures are defined as follows:

- venepuncture—the insertion of a needle into a vein for the withdrawal of a blood specimen (Weller 2005)
- cannulation—the process of introducing a hollow tube made of plastic into a peripheral blood vessel to enable the administration of drugs or fluids, which can remain in situ for variable periods of time (Philips 2005).

Psychological Effect on Patient

Venepuncture and cannulation have become routine procedures for both doctors and nurses to perform, but for a patient who is unfamiliar with the procedure, it may be a frightening experience (Weinstein 2007). It is important to never underestimate the anxiety provoked by having a blood test or a cannula inserted, which can be caused by previous bad experience, a degree of needle phobia or dislike of needle procedures (Lavery & Ingram 2005).

Fears and phobias

Agras *et al.* (1969) performed a study on a population of a medium-sized city to discover the incidence and predict the prevalence of common fears and phobias. The results showed that the bulk of the population was affected by common fears such as visiting the dentist and the sight of blood. This is also supported by Marks (1988). Mild phobias affect a significant but lesser portion of the population, and severe disabling phobias are much less common. Interestingly, Agras *et al.* (1969) discovered that 57 out of 1000 individuals had sought advice from a physician about a severe fear or phobia related to a medical procedure, such as blood tests and injections, in order to minimize their fearful response.

Humans have a natural tendency to be squeamish at the sight of blood, and discomfort, faintness and nausea are triggered by cues involving blood such as blood sampling (Marks 1988). This natural, mild human fear usually causes no difficulty in normal life and is only termed a phobia if it becomes severe and causes a marked or even life-threatening disability. For many patients, it is the fear and anticipation of fainting that brings on anxiety, and so they avoid anything that could result in fainting such as contact with blood or any injury. Blood phobia is defined as a fear and avoidance of situations involving direct and indirect exposure to blood or injuries and is common and potentially life-threatening. It is estimated that blood phobias occur (in varying degrees of severity) with a 3.5–4% lifetime prevalence (Koppel 1999; Patel *et al.* 2005).

Those with blood phobias usually also have injection phobia (Ost 1992). Injection phobia is the fear and avoidance of receiving various types of injection and having a blood sample drawn through venepuncture (Ost 1992).

Early work in the field of injection fear was performed on dental patients, who tend to have high levels of anxiety and rank their common fears as pain, blood and needles (Berggren 1992). However, Ost (1992) discovered that it was often fear of the pain rather than the fear of the injection that led to phobic reactions, highlighting the anticipatory effect of fear and anxiety on the perception of pain. It is considered that developmental learning has a role to play through direct conditioning, vicarious conditioning (observing another person's fear) or the transmission of information or instruction (Rogers & Gournay 2001).

Fears of blood and injection tend to start in childhood and this may be as a result of modelling. Parents who exhibit fear of a particular situation may pass this onto their children through vicarious conditioning (Marks 1988, Ost 1992). Some parents may pass fears more directly to their children by warning them against specific situations. However, these fears tend to disappear in adulthood because of repeated exposure to the feared situation (Mavissakalian & Barlow 1981). But if the exposures are traumatic, the memory of the experience may induce a conditioned response. Auerbach *et al.* (1976) found that anxiety states in dental patients were related to previous dental contacts of an aversive nature.

In a study performed by Ost (1991) more than half the patients (53.5%) ascribed the origin of their phobia to direct experiences of the conditioning type. Condition theory seems to accommodate the way in which the majority of both injection (57%) and blood (49%) phobics acquired their phobias (Ost 1991). Steel *et al.* (1986) also recognized that diabetic injection phobias were usually acquired as a conditioned response.

Problems can result from blood and injection phobic conditions, and serious consequences can arise for the patient whose survival depends on injections and blood tests, such as diabetics (Steel *et al.* 1986) (*See* Box 9.1). It has been found that phobias in adults rarely disappear spontaneously without treatment (Agras *et al.* 1972), but once the cause of the phobia is ascertained there are various types of therapies to manage the phobia such as referral to nurse therapists and self-help groups (e.g. triumph over phobias—TOPS), systemic desensitization/exposure therapy (Koppel 1999; Rogers & Gournay 2001), cognitive behavioural therapy or medication (Rogers & Gournay 2001).

Effects of anxiety and pain

In 1983 Coates *et al.* carried out a study of cancer patients to discover what caused the most distress during chemotherapy. At the time 'having a needle' was ranked as sixth most distressing. This study was repeated in 1993 (Griffin *et al.* 1996), when fear of a

---

BOX 9.1

'Jab-fear woman is saved from herself' (Morris 1996)

Doctors were forced to carry out a life-saving caesarean operation on a woman too terrified of needles to agree to an anaesthetic injection … the women had agreed in principle to a caesarean but because of her needle phobia insisted on gas rather than an injection … the judge decided that L's extreme needle phobia rendered her incapable of weighing relevant treatment information.

'The fear that condemned a man to die in agony from rabies' (Verity 1993)

Mark Sell enjoyed the reputation as an action man. He was fearless in his high-risk job … only one thing frightened him—needles. And when he was bitten by a friend's dog in Thailand 2 months ago, he refused to have an anti-rabies injection that might have saved his life … 'He couldn't stand to even look at a syringe, it was that bad,' his father Terry said yesterday. 'He was a brave man … but he was terrified of injections.'

---

needle was ranked in the top five most severe side-effects by more women and this finding was statistically significant.

Age certainly appears to play a role in the amount of pain and distress associated with needles. Agras *et al.* (1969) showed that the incidence of injection fear in the general population rises sharply from 0 to 15 years and then there is a steep decline ending at 30 years of age, suggesting that the fear is short-lived. However, both Wilson Barnett (1976) and Coates *et al.* (1983) found that hospitalized patients under 40 years of age responded more negatively to injections than those aged 40 and over. Age has also been correlated to the level of distress associated with routine venepuncture and this could account for the variability in degree of distress and pain reported (Bennett-Humphrey & Boon 1992).

Gender does not appear relevant in children and adolescents, but in adults it appears that women (particularly those under the age of 45) are more anxious about needles than men (Coates *et al.* 1983). Van den Berg and Abeysekera (1993) found that more female patients had greater pain scores and more responses during the cannulation procedure, suggesting that female patients may need more care and attention during the procedure. However, it must be remembered that men tend to have been socialized to appear brave and not express pain (Levine & De Simone 1991). Miaskowski (1997) found that studies indicate that women exhibit lower pain thresholds than men and also exhibit less tolerance to noxious stimuli than men. This is supported by Berkley (1997) but both report that studies are small and exist only for certain forms of stimulus and are affected by situational variables such as disease. Results may also be explained by hormonal status as well as being compounded by the gender of the experimenter. Men have reported less pain in front of female than male experimenters, although this did not influence responses in females. Other studies have shown that gender does not affect the results (Miaskowski 1997). Berkley (1997) also reported on a study where views relating to anticipation of pain of an impending venepuncture differed between male and female children but there were no differences in rates of the pain actually produced. What is key is that attitudes towards pain can affect coping mechanisms and response to treatment. Kelley *et al.* (1997) compared pain and distress in women undergoing urethral catheterization with women undergoing peripheral venous cannulation. Distress levels were the same for both procedures but cannulation caused more pain.

Coates *et al.* (1983) found that anxiety was often related more to the fear of having a needle inserted than the pain of the needle itself, and this is supported by Bennett-Humphrey and Boon (1992) and reflected in patients' own accounts of venepuncture and cannulation. Buckalew (1982) described how she became anxious before and after chemotherapy and identified one of the sources of her anxiety as the pain of having intravenous (i.v.) infusions started. One bad experience of an infiltrated i.v. infusion had led to feelings of extreme anxiety before venepuncture and cannulation. She listed fear, anticipation of pain and severe anxiety as being more painful than the pain of the procedure itself.

Inducing pain during a procedure can provoke feelings of incompetence and frustration in the nurse, and lack of confidence, apprehension, distress and even hostility in the patient (Millam 1995). Investigations into the pain associated with venepuncture and cannulation in both adults and children have concentrated on influencing variables such as age, sex, device and vein site, as well as the relief of physical pain caused by the insertion of needles.

A study by Van den Berg and Abeysekera (1993) investigating venous cannulation in a large sample of patients (1422) considered a range of influencing factors during the insertion of a cannula. These included arm used, vein site, cannula size and pain on cannulation. Pain was assessed by a verbal analogue scale and observation of patients' responses. Use of the cephalic vein and a larger gauge (16-G) cannula produced more responses, but reported pain was reduced when lignocaine was used.

Cannula design has also been implicated in the degree of reported pain, with thin-walled cannulae appearing to cause less pain than thick-walled cannulae (Ahrens *et al.* 1991). This evidence reinforces the necessity for careful selection of vein, device design and size. Hecker *et al.* (1983) performed a study using glyceryl trinitrate (GTN) ointment to increase vasodilation and facilitate easier venous access. They recommended its use to reduce patient trauma and save time.

Vasovagal reactions

The ill patient is susceptible to fears, which become exaggerated, triggering an undesirable autonomic nervous system response known as a vasovagal reaction. Such a reaction may present as syncope. Sympathetic reaction may follow and result in vasoconstriction. This limits available veins, complicates the procedure and makes therapy more difficult (Weinstein 2007). It has been well established that fainting or vasovagal syncope is a common feature of venepuncture and cannulation (Kaloupek *et al.* 1985; Pavlin *et al.* 1993). Although typically benign and self-limited, these episodes may cause traumatic injury if unanticipated and are considered stressful and embarrassing by patients. Symptoms include feeling faint, light-headed, sweaty, hot, cold or nauseated (Pavlin *et al.* 1993), followed by vasovagal bradycardia and a drop in blood pressure, ending in fainting (Stark & Brener 2000; Rogers & Gournay 2001).

Pavlin *et al.*'s (1993) study investigated how to identify subjects who are at greatest risk of vasovagal reaction and provided direction for future methods of prevention or treatment. They found that patients responded to various aspects, including psychological stress, pain, anticipated pain, the sight of blood and the act of donating of blood. Only the age of the patient, the duration of cannulation and prior history of fainting were identified as independent predictors of vasovagal reaction (Kaloupek *et al.* 1985, Pavlin *et al.* 1993).

The number of attempts at venepuncture and the duration of cannulation had equally strong associations with developing symptoms but were not independent of each other. The incidence of reaction was 16.6% in patients aged 40 or less; those with a history of fainting (33.3%) reacted 50% of the time; and 12% of female patients reacted compared with 9% of males. Pavlin *et al.* (1993) strongly recommended the use of a reclining chair to prevent the mechanical trauma that may occur during syncope; it also allows rapid change from the upright to the horizontal. However, the study did not show that selecting the horizontal position before venepuncture would alter the incidence of vasovagal reaction.

Methods to Help Reduce Anxiety and Pain

Information/education of the patient

Provision of clear and comprehensive information on the procedure should reduce the patient's anxiety and pain (Lucker *et al.* 2003). Patients should be approached in a calm and reassuring manner, and encouraging the patient to ask questions provides information that helps to alleviate fear and anxiety. The nurse should be honest and forthright, convey self-assurance and appear confident (Alexander *et al.* 2001). The nurse must provide a careful explanation of the procedures which will do much to alleviate the fear and ensure patient compliance (Weinstein 2007). Many patients will be apprehensive and this anxiety may cause vasoconstriction—making venepuncture or cannulation more difficult for patient and practitioner and more painful for the patient. Careful patient teaching and a confident understanding attitude will help patients relax and cooperate (Springhouse 2002). Information is helpful, reduces anxiety and can ensure a positive experience. To reduce patient anxiety, and as good practice, patients should be asked if they have had venepuncture or cannulation performed previously. Attention should be paid to any adverse outcomes or experiences and the patient should be reassured (Lavery & Ingram 2005).

The skilled practitioner

> Only a skilled clinician should perform a venipuncture on an anxious patient who has limited access and difficult veins. (Weinstein 2007, page 243)

The skill of the practitioner appears to be relevant to the feelings attached to the procedure of venepuncture and cannulation and is recounted in patients' experiences. Kaplan (1983) described his major fear as having the novice intern taking bloods and being poked, prodded and probed time after time. Cohn (1982) described how staff would not listen to his warnings about his veins and what would or would not work.

Both Buckalew (1982) and Kaplan (1983) stressed that patients should not have to endure unnecessary assaults because of inexperienced practitioners. It appears that patients feel less anxious when the procedure is performed by a skilled practitioner, and they also equate the skill of giving injections with caring behaviour. Larson (1984) and Mayer (1987) found that cancer patients identified 'knows how to give an i.v. and manage equipment' as the most important caring behaviour.

Pain relief

There are a number of methods for reducing pain in invasive procedures, both pharmacological and non-pharmacological.

Non pharmacological methods of reducing pain

1. *Distraction.* The effectiveness of the cough trick as a method of pain relief during venepuncture was tested by Usichenko *et al.* (2004). It appeared to reduce the intensity of the pain during venepuncture and whilst they concluded that it seemed effective, the mechanism remains unclear.
2. *Massage.* Wendler (2003) studied the use of gentle physical touch, called the Tellington Touch technique. The study reviewed heart rate, blood pressure, anxiety and procedural pain before venepuncture. There was a significant decrease in blood pressure and heart rate in the touch group, but no other significant differences. It was also noted that there were many limitations in the study including the gender and type of subjects, and the authors concluded that the technique needed further study.

Section 2

3. *Transcutaneous electrical nerve stimulation (TENS).* Coyne *et al.* (1995) investigated whether the application of TENS decreased the pain and unpleasantness of i.v. needle insertion. Their double-blind randomized study placed patients in one of three groups—placebo, TENS or control. The use of modified brief intense TENS did not produce a reduction in pain (sensory or affective) associated with cannulation. However, the use of TENS has been shown to reduce procedural pain in both children (Lander & Fowler-Kerry 1992) and adults (Webster *et al.* 1992). The benefits are the lack of long-term side-effects or complications.

Pharmacological methods of reducing pain

Use of local anaesthetics   Local anaesthetics (LA) can work in two ways: (a) to reduce the pain of venepuncture or cannulation and (b) to lessen the anxiety associated with procedures involving a needle (Scales 2005). They are widely used in paediatrics and also for anxious adults (*See* Table 9.1).

Table 9.1   Local anaesthetic agents. (From Weinsten 2007.)

	EMLA cream	Ametop gel	Lidocaine
Time to effectiveness	It takes 1 hour to be maximally effective (Lavery & Ingram 2005) although some state it should be left on up to 90 minutes	It is recommended that it is left on for 30–45 minutes and no longer than 60 minutes	Immediate
Side effects	Associated with blanching and vasoconstriction and this in turn can result in difficult cannulations (Browne *et al.* 1999)	Side effects include erythema (in one-third of subjects) oedema and pruritis (Lavery & Ingram 2005). All topical LA agents should be removed before venepuncture or cannulation as prolonged skin contact has been associated with skin damage (Hewitt & Scales 1998). Repeated exposure to Ametop has been shown to cause possible red raised areas and blistering in children and the site should be observed every 10 minutes (Lavery & Ingram 2005)	Hypersensitivity
Contraindications	The application is not recommended for patients under 3 months, for anyone with known hypersensitivity or for use on open areas of skin (Macklin & Chernecky 2004)		
Application	The product comes as a 5 g tube and the recommended application is 2.5 g or half a tube over a small area of skin.	The contents of any topical LA should be left in a small mound and covered with a bio-occlusive dressing. It is not required to spread it as it will spread itself.	Use small needle e.g. 25 g. Ensure LA is at room temperature Use only a small amount of LA e.g. 0.1–0.3mL Buffering the lidocaine with bicarbonate can reduce the stinging (Macklin & Chernecky 2004)

LA, local anaesthetic.

Topical local anaesthetic

EMLA   Eutectic mixture of local anaesthetics (EMLA) is a cream mixture of lidocaine 2.5% and prilocaine 2.5%. These are emulsified in water and thickened into a cream that becomes oily at room temperature or when applied to the skin (Macklin & Chernecky 2004). The release of the local anaesthetic into the epidermal and dermal layers of the skin provides anaesthesia (Weinstein 2007). Absorption of EMLA is site specific, being more effective on thin epidermal areas than on thick epidermal layers. It is capable of anaesthesia to the maximal depth of 5–6 mm below the skin (Macklin & Chernecky 2004).

Ametop   Ametop is a topical anaesthetic gel containing amethocaine 4%. It is usual practice to apply it to more than one potential site in case the first application fails (Macklin & Chernecky 2004; Lavery & Ingram 2005). Browne *et al.* (1999) compared Ametop with EMLA and found that cannulation was less painful using Ametop, and it also caused less vasoconstriction and facilitated easier cannulation.

Intradermal

This technique is suitable for situations that will not allow the prolonged application time required for creams. It refers to the injection or infiltration of medication around the potential site of the venepuncture or cannulation (*See* Figure 9.1). The basic goal is to carry out this procedure in order to reduce the level of discomfort of the second (cannulation). However, if done incorrectly the injection can be as painful as inserting a smaller-gauge cannula without local anaesthetic (Macklin & Chernecky 2004). The benefits are that it provides an effective, economical and rapid anaesthesia and can be administered immediately prior to the procedure.

However, the Infusion Nurses Society (INS)(2006) advocates monitoring the use of local anaesthetic due to the disadvantages such as increased risk of allergic reaction, anaphylaxis and possible inadvertent injection of the drug into the vascular system as well as obliteration of the vein (Weinstein 2007). They state an alternative is to administer an intradermal injection of 0.8% sodium chloride to the side of the vein which provides an

Administering a local anaesthetic

A local anaesthetic may be prescribed when starting peripheral i.v. therapy. To administer a local anaesthetic, follow the steps below.

1. Using a U-100 insulin syringe with a 25g needle draw 0.1 mL of lidocaine 1%.

2. Clean the venepuncture site.

3. Insert the needle next to the vein, introducing about one-third of it into the skin at a 30° angle. The side approach carries less risk of accidental vein puncture (indicated by blood appearing in the syringe). If the vein is deep, however, inject the lidocaine over the top of it. To be sure you don't inject lidocaine into the vein—thus allowing it to circulate systemically—aspirate to check for a blood return. If this occurs, withdraw the needle and begin the procedure again.

4. Hold your thumb on the plunger of the syringe during insertion to avoid unnecessary movement once the needle is under the skin.

5. Without aspirating, quickly inject the lidocaine until a small wheal appears (as shown). You may not have to administer the entire amount in the syringe.

6. Quickly withdraw the syringe and massage the wheal with an alcohol swab. This will make the wheal disappear so the vein won't be hidden—although you'll see a small pinprick of blood. The skin numbness will last about 30 minutes.

7. Insert the venepuncture device into the vein.

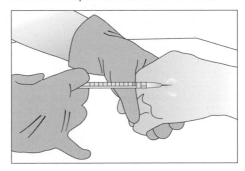

Figure 9.1   Administering a local anaesthetic. (After Springhouse 2002. Reproduced with permission of Lippincott Williams and Wilkins.)

Section 2

anaesthetic effect but does not increase the patient's risk. All types of injectable local anaesthetics can be administered, but lidocaine is the most common and comes in different concentrations (0.5, 1 or 2%). Research has shown that the pain of cannulation using 22-G or larger cannulae is reduced significantly by prior subcutaneous infiltration with 1% lignocaine when compared with cannulation without infiltration. Moreover, there was no increased difficulty associated with cannulation (Harrison *et al.* 1992; Dennis *et al.* 1995).

Iontophoresis   This technique provides analgesia by use of a handheld device with two electrodes using a mild electric current to deliver charged ions of lidocaine 25 and epinephrine 1 : 100 000 solution into the skin. It is effective in 10–20 minutes, has a penetration depth of 10 mm, and causes minimal discomfort without distorting the tissues, making it an excellent choice for numbing a site in children (Galinkin *et al.* 2002; Springhouse 2002).

Improving Venous Access

Difficult peripheral access is traumatic for the patient. Application of a tourniquet, tapping and stroking of veins, vigorous swabbing, clenching the hand to pump up veins, hanging the forearm downwards and application of local warmth are all commonly used aids for cannulation (Perucca 2001; Witt 2004).

Application of a tourniquet promotes venous distension. The tourniquet should be tight enough to impede venous return while not affecting arterial flow (Perucca 2001; Witt 2004; RCN 2005). It should be applied around the upper forearm about 6–8 inches above the venepuncture site (Phillips 2005) to promote dilation of the veins, and time should be allowed for the veins to fill. A blood pressure cuff may also be used, with the cuff being inflated to a pressure just below the diastolic pressure (Phillips 2005). A tourniquet can be applied over a thin layer of clothing if there is a chance that it could cause injury or bruising of the skin (Witt 2004). This is particularly the case for elderly patients, those with extremely fragile veins and thrombocytopenic patients, making it necessary to release the tourniquet as soon as the vein is entered. It should not pinch the patient's skin once it is tightened and should not be left on for longer than 1 minute before venepuncture as it may result in haemoconcentration or pooling of blood leading to inaccurate blood results (Ernst & Ernst 2001). If left on for extended periods of time it may also result in ecchymosis (RCN 2005). If venous access is difficult, it may be necessary to release the tourniquet and allow refilling; then, once it is tightened, the search for the vein may continue (Perucca 2001).

There are several types of tourniquets available (*See* Figure 9.2). The most effective is a good-quality single-hand, quick-release tourniquet but the choice will depend on the practitioner and availability (Witt 2004; RCN 2005). Consideration should be given to the ability to decontaminate the tourniquet or the use of a single-use tourniquet where there is the potential for cross-infection (Golder 2000; RCN 2005).

Other methods used to improve venous distension include lowering the extremity below the level of the heart, and opening and closing the fist (the action of the muscles forces blood into the veins, causing them to distend) (Phillips 2005). This action may affect certain blood results, e.g. potassium (Ernst & Ernst 2001; Garza & Becan McBride 2002). Light tapping of the vein may be useful as this releases histamines beneath the skin and causes dilation (Phillips 2005), but it can be painful and may result in the formation of a haematoma; again, elderly patients and those with fragile veins are most at risk (Witt 2004).

When these methods fail, applying a warm compress in the form of a heat pack or electric heating blanket or immersing the limb in a bowl of warm water for 10–15

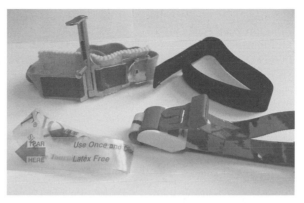

Figure 9.2   Types of tourniquets.

minutes helps to increase vasodilation and promote venous filling (Dougherty 1996; Perucca 2001; Lenhardt *et al.* 2002; Weinstein 2007). Ointments or patches containing small amounts of GTN have been used to improve vasodilation (Gunwardene & Davenport 1990); this also reduces the incidence of chemical phlebitis and increases site survival time (Hecker 1988).

Finally, new technologies such as transillumination (Venoscope) to illuminate or ultrasound can be used to locate veins that the practitioner is unable to palpate (Phillips 2005).

Site Preparation

Asepsis is vital when performing venepuncture or cannulation, as the skin is breached and a foreign object is introduced into a sterile circulating system. The two main sources of microbial contamination are:

- cross-infection from practitioner to patient
- skin flora of the patient (Maki 1991).

It is therefore essential that the nurse employs good hand-washing and drying techniques (Hart 2004). In order to adequately clean the skin and remove the risk presented by the skin flora, most transient skin flora can be removed with soap and water using mechanical friction (Carlson *et al.* 2001). Firm and prolonged rubbing with an antiseptic solution such as chlorhexidine in 70% alcohol or 2% aqueous solution is then recommended (Maki 1991; Ryder 2001; DH 2004; RCN 2005).

The prepared area should be 2–3 inches in diameter and the solution applied with friction from the insertion site outward (Perucca 2001). It is imperative during the skin cleansing procedure not only to use the most effective antiseptic, but also to clean the skin for a long enough period of time—at least 30 seconds to a minute for peripheral cannulation (Dougherty 2004; Weinstein 2007). For the antimicrobial solution to be effective and ensure coagulation of the organisms, and to prevent stinging as the needle pierces the skin, the area should be allowed to air dry for a minimum of 30 seconds. Fanning, blowing and blotting of the prepared area are contraindicated (Perucca 2001; Dougherty 2004; RCN 2005).

Skin cleansing is a controversial subject and it is acknowledged that a cursory wipe with an alcohol swab fails to reduce bacterial counts prior to peripheral cannulation (Dougherty 2004). The skin must not be touched or repalpated once it has been cleaned. If it is necessary to repalpate, then the same cleaning regimen should be repeated (Dougherty 2004).

Section 2

There is no evidence demonstrating the need to shave the site prior to cannulation. It has been suggested that shaving might cause microabrasions and therefore encourage microbial growth (Carlson 2001; RCN 2005). Depilatories are not recommended because of allergic reactions that could cause skin eruptions (Perucca 2001). Electric razors or scissors are therefore recommended for clipping and removing excess hair, but must be cleaned between patients to prevent cross-infection or have disposable heads for single-patient use (RCN 2005).

Selecting an Appropriate Environment

It is important that the patient is provided with privacy, but it may be that the patient wishes to have a friend or relative with them during the procedure for support or distraction (Dougherty 1994). Adequate lighting of the environment is essential for performing accurate venous assessment and achieving successful venepuncture or cannulation. It may be necessary to use a bedside light or to increase the lighting if it is not sufficient (Perucca 2001).

The next step is to ensure that the patient is in a comfortable position. It is helpful to place a pillow or a rolled towel under the extended arm for support and to provide a firm, flat surface. It is also vital that the nurse is in a comfortable position and it may be necessary to adjust the height or position of the bed or chair to prevent unnecessary bending or twisting (Perucca 2001).

The temperature of the environment is also a consideration. The room should be warm enough to encourage vasodilation, but if it is too warm, the patient may feel faint. If the room is too cold then the patient's venous access will be more difficult to assess. As Sagar and Bomar (1982) stated:

> a sufficiently warm room not only provides a feeling of comfort to the patients but by promoting dilation and filling of the veins will facilitate selection and entry of the vein.

Approach to the Patient

How the practitioner approaches the patient may have a direct bearing on that person's response to the venepuncture or cannulation procedure (Weinstein 2007). An efficient, unhurried approach will reinforce the impression of the nurse's competence. A nurse who feels unsure of her abilities will transmit that feeling to the patient (Sagar & Bomar 1982). The practitioner should ensure that all the equipment is prepared in advance and is on hand at the patient's bedside (Sommer *et al.* 2002).

Once the environment has been prepared, the practitioner must discover whether the patient has ever undergone such a procedure before; if not, an explanation should be given and the patient encouraged to ask questions. In order to eliminate fear of the unknown, it may be useful to show the patient what the equipment looks like, as well as providing information about the general aspects of i.v. therapy, drugs, etc. and being honest about the discomfort that may be experienced.

Patients may previously have had a bad experience of venepuncture or cannulation, and as a result may feel anxious before insertion. The practitioner should listen to what the patient says about previous experiences and, in order to gain trust and encourage compliance, the patient should be involved in the decision-making. Being offered a choice of where the device is to be sited is important to patients (Dougherty 1994). Even being asked to point out areas to be avoided, such as previous painful sites or areas of poor venous access, represents a degree of choice and patients may feel more in control of their i.v. therapy if they are encouraged to become active participants (Hudek 1986).

Mills and Krantz (1979) found that patients given a choice of arm for blood donation showed reduced self-rated discomfort and pain relative to no choice. However, some patients may feel that they are happy to make the choice of which arm to use, but that any more detail should be left to the experts (Dougherty 1994). The final step is encouraging the patients to use individual coping skills, as well as employing interventions such as distraction or relaxation techniques. Only once the patient is fully informed can consent be obtained. It is usual to accept a verbal consent (Lavery 2003; Lavery & Ingram 2005).

Choice of Vein

> The selection of vein may be a deciding factor in the success of the infusion and the preservation of veins for subsequent treatment. The most prominent vein is not necessarily the most suitable. (Weinstein 2007, page 245)

It is important to make a full assessment of the patient and their veins before the vein and device are chosen. The main factors which should be considered are the clinical status of the patient, the location and condition of the vein, and the purpose and duration of the therapy.

The clinical status of the patient

Injury or disease may prevent the use of a limb for venepuncture or cannulation for a variety of reasons. There may be a reduction in the venous access due to amputation, fracture or a cerebrovascular accident. Surgery often dictates which arm can be used. Veins should be avoided in the affected arm of an axillary node dissection such as a mastectomy, as the circulation may be impaired. This can lead to impaired lymphatic drainage, which can influence venous flow regardless of whether there is any obvious lymphoedema (Rowland 1991). If it is necessary to cannulate the affected arm, permission should be sought from the doctor and the patient's arm should be closely monitored for any signs of an increase in swelling. An oedematous limb should be avoided as there is danger of stasis of lymph predisposing to complications such as phlebitis and cellulitis (Rowland 1991; Millam 1992).

Positioning of the patient may dictate the site of choice, for example if a patient is to be turned on one side during an operation. The lower portion of the arm is preferred for an i.v. infusion, as the increased venous pressure in the lower arm may interfere with the free flow of the solution (Weinstein 2007). The placement of a cannula into the affected limb of a patient who has had a cerebrovascular accident is contraindicated. This is due to the reduced or absent neurological sensation in the limb, which prevents the patient from detecting pain as a result of an infiltration or developing phlebitis. There is also often limited venous access because of reduced mobility (Perucca 2001).

An extremity where an arteriofistula or graft is situated should not be used for routine peripheral cannulation. It is usually inserted only for dialysis and requires special consideration when selecting the site. Patients who are in shock or dehydrated will have reduced peripheral circulation, making venous access difficult. Not only do the veins not dilate sufficiently, but they may also collapse more quickly. Patients who are obese tend to have veins located deep in the subcutaneous tissue and fat, making the veins much more difficult to palpate. A hand vein may be the only easily accessible vein (Millam 1992). Malnourished patients may have more obvious venous access; however, there is a lack of subcutaneous support, and the veins may be mobile and more friable (Macklin & Chernecky 2004).

In the elderly, there is a thinning of elastin fibres in the skin and a loss of subcutaneous supporting tissue. In addition, the skin undergoes a generalized loss of water and loose skin folds appear. There is also a loss of fat on the dorsal aspects of the hands and arms.

Veins and bones of the hand become prominent (Whitson 1996) but tend to be tortuous and fragile, have narrow lumens and may be thrombosed.

The type of medication currently being taken by patients may influence the condition of the vein. Those taking anticoagulants or on long-term steroid therapy may present with fragile, friable veins and thin, dry parchment skin, and have the potential to bruise (Dougherty 2004). Another problem may be restriction of a patient's mobility, especially if the best veins for cannulation lead to a patient being unable to use a crutch or other lifting/mobilizing aids (Dougherty 2004; Macklin & Chernecky 2004). Therefore, it is important to consider which is the dominant arm and if more appropriate, then use the non-dominant arm.

Type of treatment

The purpose of the therapy and the type of solution/medications to be infused or administered dictate the rate of flow required. If large quantities are to be administered or the solution has a high viscosity, such as packed cells, then a large vein with adequate blood flow will be required. It is also useful to select a large vein when using hypertonic or irritant solutions. These types of solution cause trauma to smaller vessels, leading to phlebitis, as the supply of blood is not sufficient to dilute the drugs (Weinstein 2007). If vesicant drugs are to be administered, small veins or those over joints should be avoided due to the local damage and tissue necrosis that may occur in the event of an extravasation.

Length of therapy

The length of therapy often dictates the choice of vein. It is recommended that the most distal site should be selected for cannulation or venepuncture. If a prolonged course of therapy is required, sites can be maintained for longer by starting distally and moving more proximally with subsequent insertions. However, patient comfort and cooperation are required and, if infusions or therapy are to be administered over an extended period of time, areas of joint flexion, for example, should be avoided (Weinstein 2007).

Patient preference

Patients have reported anxiety and pain associated with the location of the cannula (Dougherty 1994). Allowing patients to choose the site may help to reduce anxiety and improve compliance (Hudek 1986). It is important to position the cannula away from a joint and, where possible, in the non-dominant arm to allow the patient maximum use of the arm (Macklin & Chernecky 2004). Patients have also identified that the veins in the wrist and the back of the hand are often the most painful and awkward places to have a cannula sited, causing discomfort and restricted movement. Overall, patients prefer the veins of the forearm—they are more convenient, cannulation appears to be less painful, the cannula remains *in situ* for longer and allows flexion and movement, enabling the performance of normal daily activities (Dougherty 1994). This is supported by Marsigliese (2001) who studied comfort levels related to location of peripheral cannulae. She defined comfort as freedom from physical pain, degree of inconvenience and ability to perform certain self-care activities. She found that regardless of dominance, the forearm was more comfortable and was associated with less complications than the hand, and that the devices remained *in situ* longer. She concluded that the decision to select a site for insertion of a peripheral cannula should be based on what benefits the patient rather than a site that is easy to locate, suggesting that experienced staff such as i.v. teams are best suited to providing cannulation for patients.

Location of the vein

The superficial veins of the lower portion of the arm are used for venepuncture and cannulation because they are located just beneath the skin in the superficial fascia ~~...~~ page 37) Cannulation of the lower extremities is usually avoided due ~~...~~ ~~...~~ pulmonary embolism (which ~~...~~ 05). Stagnant blood in vari- ~~...~~ ons when a toxic concentra- ~~...~~ nula is inserted into a lower ~~...~~ priate site can be found. It is ~~...~~ used in preference to lower ~~...~~ se veins are used, the dorsum ~~...~~ of choice (Millam 1992). ~~...~~ cubital fossa are available for ~~...~~ or a variety of reasons.

~~...~~ veins in the antecubital fossa ~~...~~ municates with the basilic by ~~...~~ and superficial location makes ~~...~~ ular and connective tissue. They ~~...~~ providing copious and repeated ~~...~~ a good technique is used (Witt ~~...~~ r a number of reasons.

~~...~~ t any motion could dislodge the ~~...~~ , extravasation of the drug or ~~...~~ ernecky 2004; Weinstein 2007). ~~...~~ y are large and will enable large ~~...~~ to be rapidly diluted and circu- ~~...~~ illam 1992).

~~...~~ ke movement of a device over the ~~...~~ rom the skin into the circulation, ~~...~~ feeling is to avoid the use of the ~~...~~ by, as one infusion of a long dura- ~~...~~ s that most readily provide ample

~~...~~ nerves (the median cephalic vein ~~...~~ aken to prevent accidental arterial

The size and position of the cep... xcellent vein for transfusion administration. It readily accommodates a large-gauge cannula (Hadaway 2001). However, its position at a joint may increase complications such as mechanical phlebitis and even general discomfort and patient compliance. The presence of tendons controlling the thumb can lead to these obscuring the vein during insertion of a device (Hadaway 2001), and care must be taken not to hit the radial nerve.

The basilic vein

This is a large vein, which is often overlooked due to its inconspicuous position on the ulnar border of the hand and forearm. It is found on palpation when the patient's arm is placed across the chest, with the practitioner opposite the patient (Hadaway 2001).

Venepuncture access can be awkward due to its position and it can be difficult to observe. There is also a tendency for this vein to have many valves, which can hinder the advancement of the cannula. It tends to roll easily and a haematoma may readily occur if the patient flexes their arm, which results in the blood being squeezed from the engorged vein into the tissues.

The dorsal venous network

The dorsal venous network of the hand allows for successive sites in proximal locations. The veins can usually be visualized and palpated easily. The digital veins are small and may be prominent enough to accommodate a small-gauge needle as a last resort for fluid administration, but may be of more use for venepuncture. With adequate taping, the fingers can be immobilized, thus preventing the cannula from piercing the posterior wall of the vein and leading to bruising or infiltration (Hadaway 2001).

The metacarpal veins

The metacarpal veins are accessible, easily visualized and easily palpated, and are well suited for i.v. use as they allow for successive sites in a proximal location (Hadaway 2001). They tend to be smaller veins than those of the forearm and may prove difficult to use in infants because of excessive subcutaneous fat. Use of these veins are contraindicated in the elderly as there is diminished skin turgor and loss of subcutaneous tissue, making the vein difficult to stabilize, they often take longer to fill (venous distension takes longer due to slower venous return and reduced competence of venous valves), and they are difficult to secure (Whitson 1996; Powers 1999; Hadaway 2001; Walther 2001; Springhouse 2002). Insertion may be more painful due to increased nerve endings and they are more likely to become phlebitic (Weinstein 2007). These veins are a better option for short-term or outpatient i.v. therapy. In the wrist the veins may appear to be suitable for venepuncture, but they are usually situated between two branches of the median nerve, which results in extremely painful venepuncture. The veins are thin-walled and small and are associated with bruising, phlebitis and infiltration (Hadaway 2001). Although these tend to be easy to stabilize and accessible (Hadaway 2001), they should only be used if absolutely necessary.

Condition of the vein

Assessment should start with the visual inspection of both upper limbs, followed by palpation of the veins likely to be used. Visual inspection will enable the practitioner to avoid:

- areas of phlebitis
- areas of infection
- areas of oedema
- bruised or inflamed veins
- any veins which have undergone multiple punctures.

If previous phlebitic or infiltrated areas are used for cannulation, accurate site assessments cannot be performed. Also if damaged veins are used, greater injury to the skin and vein will occur (Perucca 2001).

Palpation of the vein is an important assessment tool. It helps to determine whether the vein is located in the superficial fascia or deep tissue. Stroking the vein downward and observing the venous refill are helpful in determining the condition of the vein. This procedure also enables the practitioner to differentiate veins from arteries and to locate valves (Dougherty 1996; Weinstein 2007). Palpation should be performed before every venepuncture or cannulation, even if the vein appears large and easy to cannulate. To palpate a vein, place one or two fingers over it and press lightly; then release pressure to assess the vein's elasticity and rebound filling (Millam 1992). Always use the same finger(s) to palpate veins, in order to develop sensitivity for assessing them. Usually the index finger and the third forefinger of the non-dominant hand have the most sensitivity (Perucca 2001); the thumb should not be used as it is not as sensitive and a pulse may be detected which could be confused with an aberrant artery (Perucca 2001; Weinstein 2007).

An ideal vein feels soft and bouncy as it is palpated. It should refill quickly once it has been depressed and should be straight, visible and well supported (Dougherty 1996). Using veins that are tender, sclerosed, thrombosed, fibrosed or hard is unacceptable, and can result in pain, repeated attempts and undue stress (Weinstein 2007). A thrombosed vein may be detected by its lack of resilience, its hard cord-like feeling, and its tendency to roll easily (Weinstein 2007).

Arteries tend to be placed much deeper than veins and have thicker, tougher walls. Veins do not pulsate—arteries do! Aberrant arteries pulsate and are located superficially in an unusual location. It is estimated that 1 in 10 people have an aberrant artery in the antecubital fossa, and they can also frequently occur in the hand or wrist (more commonly in a thin emaciated person) (Perucca 2001). Aberrant arteries should not be used for peripheral cannulation, because if drugs are administered, spasm will result, followed by contraction, necrosis and gangrene. If an artery is cannulated, the patient may complain of severe pain in the hand or arm and bright red blood will be observed, although this is not always a clear indicator (Weinstein 2007).

Valves are folds of epithelium present in larger vessels to prevent backflow of blood into the extremity (*See* Figure 2.6). They can be detected by a small visible bulge in the vein, and on palpation they will feel like a small lump. There is little or no documentation about the specific location of valves, probably due to the great variation among individuals (Hadaway 2001). They tend to occur at points of branching and junctions. Applying a tourniquet impedes venous flow so that when suction is applied (as in blood withdrawal), the valves compress and close the lumen of the vein; this prevents the backward flow of blood and interferes with the process of venepuncture. In palpating the vein and locating the valves, the practitioner can resolve the difficulty by slightly readjusting the needle to facilitate blood withdrawal (Weinstein 2007). When cannulating, valves can also prevent the advancement of the cannula and, if forced, can cause pain and rupture of the vessel.

Device Selection

The practitioner must always select the device to be used only after assessing the condition and accessibility of the individual patient's vein. The selection should be based on:

- the needs of the patient
- the number of samples required (venepuncture)
- the use and location of the device (cannulation)
- the type of fluid/drug to be administered (cannulation) (Perucca 2001).

In general, the smallest-gauge needle or cannula possible should be used to prevent damage to the intima of the vein (Perucca 2001; Macklin & Chernecky 2004). The measurement used for needles and cannulae is standard wire gauge (swg), which measures the internal diameter—the smaller the gauge size, the larger the diameter. Standard wire gauge measurement is determined by how many cannulae fit into a tube with an inner diameter of 1″ (1 inch = 25.4 mm) and uses consecutive numbers from 13 to 24 (Witt 2004). Needles tend to be odd-numbered, e.g. 19 g, 21 g, etc., whilst cannulae are even-numbered, e.g. 18 g, 20 g, etc. Most manufacturers simply refer to the gauge or the Charrière, commonly known as 'French', which relates directly to catheter size, i.e. 1 Ch = 0.33 mm.

Venepuncture

The device most commonly used to perform venepuncture for blood sampling is a straight steel needle or a steel winged infusion device (*See* Box 9.2). Either of these can then be attached to a vacuum system or a standard syringe.

Steel needle

The steel needle is commonly used for blood sampling either on a syringe or as part of a vacuum system. Consideration should be given to the length of the bevel, gauge and length of the needle (Weinstein 2007). The optimum gauge for blood sampling is 21 g which enables blood to be withdrawn at a reasonable speed without undue discomfort

---

BOX 9.2

Procedure for venepuncture (using a winged infusion device)

- Explain the procedure to the patient and give them the opportunity to voice any concerns, express any preferences or ask any questions. Ensure the patient gives their consent; this is usually implied when the patient rolls up their sleeve and places their arm in a position ready for the procedure to be performed. However, the practitioner should also get the patient to verbally consent to the procedure.
- Check the patient's identity by asking for name and date of birth. These must be checked against the information on the request forms. It is vital that the practitioner ensures that the correct samples are taken from the correct patient.
- Gather all the equipment that will be required.
- Wash hands with an appropriate bactericidal solution.
- Position yourself and the patient, ensuring there is adequate lighting and ventilation.
- Apply the tourniquet and use methods to encourage venous access.
- Assess and select the vein, and release the tourniquet.
- Select the device based on the vein size, location, etc.
- Reapply the tourniquet.
- Apply the cleaning solution to the selected vein for a minimum of 30 seconds and allow to air dry. Do not repalpate the vein or touch the skin.
- Apply a pair of clean gloves.
- Remove the device from the packaging and inspect it for any faults.
- Stabilize the vein by applying manual traction on the skin.
- Hold the wings firmly and insert the needle (bevel up) through the skin at the selected angle and observe for backflow of blood into the tubing.
- Level off the needle (by decreasing the angle of the needle to the skin) and advance slightly in order to stabilize the needle within the vein.
- Gently release the skin tension and, if necessary, tape one wing to stabilize the device.
- Attach syringes or vacuumed bottles and withdraw the required volume of blood.
- During filling of the last bottle/syringe, release the tourniquet to decrease the pressure within the vein.
- Place a sterile swab over the insertion site, remove the needle and apply pressure.
- Discard the needle and holder into a designated sharps container.
- Apply firm digital pressure directly over the puncture site until bleeding has ceased.
- Cover with a clean dressing and/or an adhesive plaster to prevent leakage or introduction of bacteria, and advise the patient to keep it in place until healing is complete.
- Transfer blood into bottles where necessary and label all bottles with relevant details.
- Remove gloves.
- Discard waste appropriately.

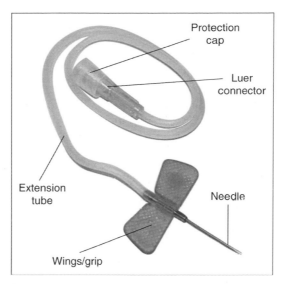

Figure 9.3   BD winged needle set. (Reproduced by permission of BD.)

to the patient or possible damage to the blood cells (Witt 2004). A short bevel reduces the risk of trauma to the endothelial wall and haematoma formation (Weinstein 2007).

Winged infusion devices (Figure 9.3)

The steel winged infusion device, commonly referred to as a 'butterfly', is used for venepuncture and short-term intravenous therapy, as well as single-dose medications. The device comprises a steel needle with a pair of flexible wings and plastic tubing (Perucca 2001). The wings enable the device to be easily grasped during insertion, and once placed in the vein, the wings are flattened and provide an anchor for stabilization. The device is available in a variety of gauge sizes, although the usual size for venepuncture is a 21 or 23 g. The steel needle is inflexible and so greatly increases the risk of vein damage, infiltration and extravasation (Perucca 2001). Tully *et al.* (1981) found, when steel needles were compared with plastic cannulae, that they were significantly associated with infiltrations but that the risk of phlebitis was much lower. Therefore, this device is recommended for non-vesicant therapies only.

Whilst the choice of whether to use a needle or a winged infusion device is dependent on the patient's venous access and the experience of the practitioner at handling the equipment, it has been shown that using a winged infusion device significantly reduces patient discomfort (Hefler *et al.* 2004).

The advantages and disadvantages of each system are outlined in Table 9.2.

Vacuum systems

Using a syringe has many inherent problems. The correct syringe size needs to be selected according to the volume of blood required, and if a large volume is required, e.g. 40–50 mL, the syringe may become cumbersome and difficult to manipulate, especially if attached to a straight steel needle. It also leaves the practitioner with the need to decant the blood into bottles, which can increase the risk of spill and contamination by blood.

The vacuum system is a safer system and has increased the efficiency of blood sampling. It consists of a plastic holder which contains or is attached to a sterile disposable double-ended needle or an adaptor (Figure 9.4). Once the needle is in the vein, the rubber-topped tube is pushed onto the needle and the rubber sheath covering the shaft of the needle is forced back, allowing the blood to flow into the tube. Samples may be

Table 9.2   Choice of venepuncture device. (From Dougherty & Lister 2004.)

Device	g	Advantages	Disadvantages	Use
Needle	21	Cheaper than winged infusion devices. Easy to use with large veins	Rigid. Difficult to manipulate with smaller veins in less conventional sites. May cause more discomfort Venous access only confirmed when sample tube attached	Large, accessible veins in the antecubital fossa. When small quantities of blood are to be drawn
Winged infusion device with or without safety shield	21	Flexible due to small needle shaft. Easy to manipulate and insert at any site. Causes less discomfort Usually shows a 'flashback' of blood to indicate a successful venepuncture	More expensive than steel needles The 12–30 cm length of tubing on the device may be caught and dislodge the needle	Veins in sites other than the antecubital fossa. When quantities of blood greater than 20 mL are required from any site
	23	Flexible due to small needle shaft. Easy to manipulate and insert at any site. Causes less discomfort. Smaller gauge and therefore useful with fragile veins	More expensive than steel needles, plus there can be damage to cells which can cause inaccurate measurements in certain blood samples, e.g. potassium	Small veins in more painful sites, e.g. inner aspect of the wrist, especially if measurements are related to plasma and not cellular components

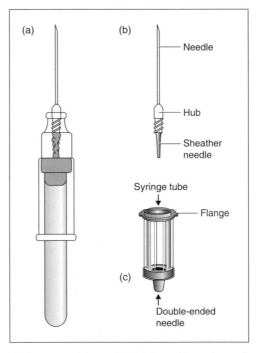

Figure 9.4   The evacuated tube system (a), consisting of a multisample needle (b) attached to a needle adapter (c). (Sommer *et al.* 2002. Reproduced with permission of Saunders.)

obtained one after another by removing the filled tube and replacing it with another. As the tube is removed the rubber sheath slips back over the needle, preventing blood from leaking into the holder and contaminating the practitioner (Sommer *et al.* 2002). This makes it a closed system, reducing the risk to the practitioner of contamination during the venepuncture and removes the need to decant the blood. The tube is vacuumed in order to obtain the exact volume of blood required for the test, and the filling ceases once that occurs (McCall & Tankersley 2003).

The disadvantage of this system is that it is more expensive. If the bottles are not vacuumed properly they have to be discarded and the suction in the tubes can sometimes cause collapse of smaller veins, making blood withdrawal more difficult (Weinstein 2007). It is important always to remove the last tube from the holder before removing the needle, as it can cause backflow of blood out of the needle, leading to possible contamination of the practitioner (Phillips 2005).

Cannulation (Box 9.3)

A cannula is defined as a hollow plastic tube used for accessing the vascular system (Weller 2005). The first plastic cannula was introduced in 1945. The over-the-needle type of cannula is the most commonly used device for peripheral venous access and is available in various gauge sizes, lengths, composition and design features. The cannula is mounted on the needle and once the device is pushed off the needle into the vein, the needle is removed. Nightingale and Bradshaw (1982) listed some of the desirable properties for a peripheral venous cannula (*See* Box 9.4).

BOX 9.3

Suggested procedure for cannulation (using the one-handed technique)

- Explain the procedure to the patient and give them the opportunity to voice any concerns, express any preferences or ask any questions. Ensure the patient gives their consent.
- Gather all the equipment that will be required.
- Wash hands with an appropriate bactericidal solution.
- Position yourself and the patient, ensuring there is adequate lighting and ventilation.
- Apply the tourniquet and use methods to encourage venous access.
- Assess and select the vein, and release the tourniquet.
- Select the device based on the vein size, location, etc.
- Open a pack and place a sterile towel under the patient's arm.
- Reapply the tourniquet.
- Apply the cleaning solution to the selected vein for a minimum of 30 seconds and allow to air dry. Do not repalpate the vein or touch the skin.
- Apply a pair of clean gloves.
- Remove the device from the packaging and inspect it for any faults.
- Stabilize the vein by applying manual traction on the skin.
- Ensure the cannula is in the bevel up position and, placing the device directly over the vein, insert the cannula through the skin at the selected angle according to the depth of the vein.
- Wait for the first flashback of blood into the flashback chamber of the stylet.
- Level the device by decreasing the angle between the cannula and the skin and advance the cannula slightly to ensure entry into the lumen of the vein.
- Withdraw the stylet slightly and a second flashback of blood will be seen along the shaft of the cannula.
- Maintaining skin traction with the non-dominant hand, slowly advance the cannula off the stylet and into the vein with the dominant hand.
- Release the tourniquet and apply pressure to the vein above the cannula tip and remove the stylet.
- Dispose of the stylet into an appropriate sharps container.
- Attach an injection cap, extension set or administration set.
- Flush with 0.9% sodium chloride to check patency, observing the site for signs of swelling or leakage, and ask the patient if any discomfort or pain is felt.
- Secure and dress with an appropriate dressing.
- Remove gloves.
- Discard waste appropriately.

BOX 9.4

Properties of a cannula

- Sterility
- Sharp-tipped introducing needle
- Non-toxic/non-irritant material
- Thin walls
- Good flow rates
- Wide range of gauge sizes and lengths
- Easily secured
- Strong, firm components
- Comfortable grip
- Radio-opaque
- Kink recovery
- Non-tapering shaft
- Smooth insertion
- Quick and easily observable flashback

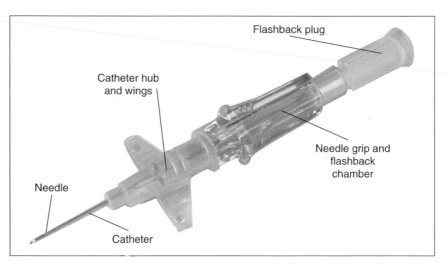

Figure 9.5 BD Insyte-NTM. (Reproduced by permission of BD.)

Components of a cannula

See Figure 9.5.

Cannula size and length

Cannulae are available in a range of gauge sizes (14–26 g) and lengths (¾″–2 inches (19–50 mm). It has been shown that the incidence of vascular complications increases as the ratio of cannula external diameter to vessel lumen increases. Therefore, most of the literature recommends the use of the smallest, shortest-gauge cannula suitable for any given situation (Perucca 2001; Dougherty 2004; RCN 2005).

When selecting a cannula the practitioner should not only determine the gauge size required but also consider the flow rates, which may vary among different manufacturers (*See* Table 9.3). Flow rate through a cannula is related to its internal diameter and is inversely proportional to its length. The principle is that as you double the length the flow rate will be halved, so long cannulae have slower rates than short cannulae (Macklin & Chernecky 2004). Also, as the length of the cannula increases, so does the

Table 9.3   Gauge sizes and average flow rates (using water).

Gauge	Flow rate (mL/min)	General uses
14 g	350	Used in theatres or emergency for rapid transfusion of blood or viscous fluids
16 g	215	As 14 g
18 g	104	Blood transfusions, parenteral nutrition, stem cell harvesting and cell separation, large volumes of fluids
20 g	62	Blood transfusions, large volumes of fluids
22 g	35	Blood transfusions, most medications and fluids
24 g	24	Medications, short-term infusions, fragile veins, children

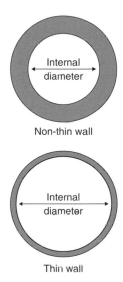

Figure 9.6   Same-gauge catheter. (Macklin & Chernecky 2004. Reprinted with permission from Elsevier.)

likelihood of vascular complications. A large, long device will fill the vessel, preventing adequate blood flow around it, causing mechanical trauma to the vessel; both factors would contribute to the development of phlebitis (Tagalakis *et al.* 2002).

The internal diameter is the distance from one inside edge of the cannula lumen to the opposite side. Catheter wall thickness determines the internal diameter of the device and cannulae can be thin or thick walled (Figure 9.6). Ideally, the walls of the device should be thin to provide a large internal diameter, so that maximum flow rates may be achieved whilst reducing complications such as phlebitis. They are also smoother on insertion as they have a more tapered fit to the inner stylet (Perucca 2001; Macklin & Chernecky 2004).

Needle/cannula design (*See* Figure 9.5)

A sharp-tipped needle or stylet facilitates penetration into the vein and the type of graduation from the cannula to the needle can affect the degree of trauma to the vessel and the cannula tip, allowing negligible resistance to tissue penetration. A thin, smooth-walled cannula tapering to a scalloped end causes less damage than one which is abruptly cut off (Perucca 2001).

If the distance from the bevel of the introducing needle to the tip of the cannula is short (less than 1.0 mm), it will minimize the risk of flashback of blood with the needle tip in the vessel lumen and the cannula tip still outside it. A short bevel reduces the risk of trauma to the endothelial wall of the vein, which could lead to infiltration from a puncture to the posterior wall. When a needle with a long bevel is inserted into the vein, blood may leak into the tissue before the entire bevel is within the lumen of the vein (Weinstein 2007), resulting in haematoma or extravasation.

The cannula should have a non-tapering shaft in order to reduce the overall size. The incidence of complications such as thrombophlebitis is higher when the tapering portion is inside the lumen of the vein (Nightingale & Bradshaw 1982, Peters *et al.* 1984). Turbulent flow is also decreased with parallel-sided cannulae, which improves flow rates.

Material

The ideal material is one that is non-irritant and does not predispose to thrombus formation (Payne-James *et al.* 1991). Ideally it should be radio-opaque or contain radio-opaque material for radiographic visualization in the event of catheter embolus (Fuller & Winn 1999; Perucca 2001; Weinstein 2007). Materials include polyvinylchloride, teflon and polyurethane. There are certain properties of materials that increase the risk of thrombogenicity and bacterial colonization.

Surface irregularities These are created during manufacturing and consist of pits, ridges and grooves. They are usually revealed by scanning with an electron microscope. These defects act as ideal sites for bacterial colonization and may cause turbulent flow. This in turn enhances platelet adhesion, platelet disintegration and thrombogenesis, leading to thrombophlebitis (Goodison 1990).

Chemical composition It appears that bacteria have affinities for certain materials, in particular certain types of synthetic polymer; this affinity is lowest in steel. This was demonstrated by Maki (1976) who found that the incidence of bacteraemia was lowest when steel needles were used (0.2%), while rates for plastic cannulae ranged from 0 to 8%. Crow (1987) also suggested that some plastic catheters actually appeared to promote the growth of organisms such as *Staphylococcus epidermidis*.

Flexibility There may be enhancement of the flexibility of a material in fluids at body temperature. Absorption of water by the cannula material enhances its plasticity and therefore makes it less likely to cause mechanical trauma (McKee *et al.* 1989; Weinstein 2007). Softer devices are also more kink resistant (Scales 2005).

Studies have compared polyurethane and teflon to ascertain which material has the lowest potential risk for phlebitis. Gaukroger *et al.* (1988) found that vialon (a type of polyurethane) was superior to teflon, although the phlebitis scores for both types of device increased with the duration of infusion. This result has been supported by other studies (McKee *et al.* 1989; Kerrison & Woodhull 1994; Keradag & Gorgulu 2000). By contrast, Payne-James *et al.* (1991) found that, although vialon was theoretically superior as a cannula material, under controlled conditions there appeared to be little difference in the capacity of both materials to cause thrombophlebitis. It must be noted that studies comparing catheter materials often use different phlebitis scales and calculations for creating a total score for each device. Other variables to consider are the differences in catheter size, skin preparation, the use of dressings, the type of solution being infused and the skill of the practitioner inserting the device (Dougherty 2004).

Sterility and packaging

All cannulae are single-use items (MDA 2000) and all products should be CE marked (MHRA 2005a). All packaging should be inspected for integrity before use, and when opened, should enable the practitioner to maintain sterility prior to insertion. The device itself should also be inspected to ensure that it is complete, there are no barbs and the needle is not defective in any way. Some manufacturers suggest that the stylet is twisted to release the cannula and make advancement off the needle into the vein easier. All components and connections should be checked to ensure they are firmly connected before insertion.

Flashback chamber (*See* Figure 9.5)

The flashback chamber is a small space at the hub of the stylet. When the stylet punctures the vein, the increased pressure in the vein forces the flow of blood into the flashback chamber. The chamber is closed with a small plug to allow air to escape and prevent blood spill (Perucca 2001). It is an important aspect of the cannula as it enables immediate visual indication to the practitioner that the cannula has entered the vein (Scales 2005).

Grip (*See* Figure 9.5)

The practitioner should be able to perform the cannulation smoothly and comfortably, so the design of the cannula for grip is also important. Some devices have a fingerguard to help stabilize the device, which also helps with the advancement of the device into the vein.

Other features (Figure 9.7a,b)

Winged cannulae can provide more control when the device is being manipulated, which also enables the cannula to be easily secured to the skin (Perucca 2001; Dougherty 2004).

(a)

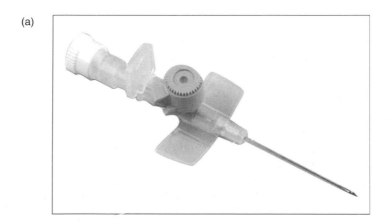

(b)

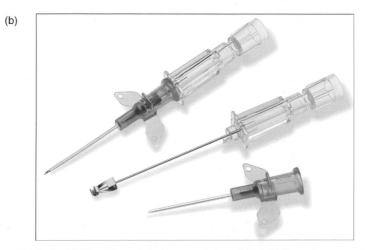

Figure 9.7   (a) BD VenflonTMPro. (Reproduced by permission of BD.) (b) Braun introcan safety cannula. (Reproduced with permission of Braun Medical Ltd.)

Section 2

Other devices have ports for intermittent injections. There has always been controversy attached to ported devices and they are used only in Europe, not in the USA. The main advantage is the ability to administer drugs without interfering with continuous infusion. Opinion remains divided as to the risk of infection associated with ported devices (Cheeseborough & Finch 1984), and it has been recommended that ports, if used, should be equipped with a bacterial filter (Brismar *et al.* 1984) or should have a needle-free injection cap attached to ensure a closed system which can be adequately cleaned.

Safety cannulae are now available. The main feature is to provide the practitioner with a safer stylet and prevent needlestick injury—some have self-sheathing stylets which recess into a rigid chamber or a soft plastic casing. Some have the ability to blunt the stylet and make it safe to dispose. Most are active devices, in that the practitioner has to activate the safety device to make it safe. The RCN (2005) recommend that ideally all peripheral devices should be equipped with a safety device, and risk assessments should be undertaken concerning their use.

Midline catheters

A midline catheter is defined as a catheter which is inserted into an antecubital vein and advanced until the tip is in an upper arm vein but does not extend past the axilla (Perucca 2001; Dougherty 2004; RCN 2005). It offers an alternative to peripheral and central venous access and can stay *in situ* for weeks, making it suitable for therapies of 1–4 weeks (Carlson 1999). Midline catheters provide venous accessibility, along with an easy and hazard-free insertion. As the catheter is in a larger vein, it is useful for patients who:

- require frequent resites of their peripheral cannula or
- have exhausted their lower arm peripheral veins or
- present with poor venous access, but who do not require a central venous catheter.

Benefits to patients include less frequent resiting of the device and a reduction in associated venous trauma (Perucca 2001). The main problem associated with these devices is the risk of mechanical phlebitis, which usually occurs within the first week following insertion. This can be resolved by close observation, resting the limb and the use of heat. However, if it does not resolve, it will become necessary to remove the catheter and resite it in another vein, preferably in the opposite arm if possible. X-ray verification of the tip is not required (Carlson 1999; Dougherty 2004; Camp-Sorrell 2005) and it is because of this that some institutions do not recommend that vesicant drugs, parenteral nutrition or solutions/medications with pH less than 5 or greater than 9 are administered via this type of catheter (Banton & Leahy-Gross 1998; Hadaway 2000; Frey 2001; Dougherty 2004). This is because of the risk of extravasation, which would not be easily detected.

Most catheters are made of silicone or polyurethane (Kupensky 1998; Hadaway 2000) and are available as single- and dual-lumen catheters in gauges of 4 and 5 Fr, with lengths of up to 20 cm. The catheter is then cut to the desired length following measurement of the arm (Frey 2001; Dougherty 2004). The main vein of choice is the basilic vein due to its larger size and straighter course for advancement (Weinstein 2007). Insertion should be performed by an experienced nurse and requires a sterile approach (*See* Box 9.5). The optimal dwell time for a midline is not known (RCN 2005), although the INS (2006) recommend a maximal dwell time of 2–4 weeks. Longer dwell times should be evaluated based on site assessment and patient condition (Kupensky 1998). Removal requires gentle firm traction, and pressure should be applied for 3–4 minutes (Dougherty 2004). The catheter integrity should be checked and its length measured to ensure an intact device has been removed (RCN 2005).

BOX 9.5

Midline catheter insertion

- Explain the procedure to the patient and give them the opportunity to voice any concerns, express any preferences or ask any questions. Ensure the patient gives their consent.
- Gather all the equipment that will be required.
- Wash hands with an appropriate bactericidal solution.
- Position the patient.
- Apply the tourniquet and use methods to encourage venous access.
- Assess and select the vein. The vein site should be two to three fingerbreadths above or one fingerbreadth below the bend of the elbow (antecubital fossa). The basilic is better as it tends to be straighter and larger. Release the tourniquet.
- Measure from the selected insertion site to the axilla.
- Select the gauge size based on the vein size, location, etc.
- Open a sterile pack and place a sterile towel under the patient's arm.
- Apply sterile gloves.
- Cut the catheter to the desired length.
- Apply the cleaning solution to the selected vein, working outwards to an area of 4–5″ in diameter for 1 minute and allow to air dry. Do not repalpate the vein or touch the skin.
- Reapply the tourniquet.
- Remove and discard gloves.
- Don a second pair of sterile gloves.
- Drape the arm with a fenestrated drape.
- Stabilize the vein—the veins above the antecubital fossa tend to be deeper and more mobile.
- Insert introducer needle and, once flashback is observed, advance into the vein until stabilized.
- Release the tourniquet.
- Apply digital pressure on the vein above the tip of the introducer needle and remove the stylet.
- Insert the catheter and advance slowly through the introducer until it reaches the desired length.
- Do not force the catheter; if any resistance is encountered, reposition the patient's arm at a different angle, rotate the wrist or get the patient to open and close their fist.
- Remove the guidewire and attach flushing solution.
- Flush the catheter with sodium chloride 0.9% and check for patency, discomfort and swelling.
- Gently retract the introducer and remove according to manufacturer's instructions.
- Secure the device and apply a dressing.

Techniques Used During Insertion

Stabilizing the vein

Vein stabilization is one of the most important elements for successful venepuncture or cannulation (Perucca 2001; Dougherty 2004). Superficial veins tend to roll, and to prevent this, the vein must be anchored in a taut, distended and stable position. The wrist and hands are flexible and so hand veins are often easier to immobilize than veins in the forearm (Millam 1993).

Veins are stabilized by applying traction to the side of the insertion site or below it using the non-dominant hand. This will also provide countertension, which will facilitate a smoother needle entry. Where and how traction is applied will depend on the vein and the preference of the practitioner.

Various methods can be used. The thumb can be used to stretch the skin downwards or the hand of the practitioner can be placed under the patient's arm and traction applied with the thumb and forefinger on either side, creating an even traction (Springhouse 2002; Dougherty 2004; *See* Figure 9.8). A vein can be stretched between forefinger and thumb, but this can cause problems for the trainee. Draping the patient's hand over a pillow will create a degree of tension in the skin and help to stabilize hand veins. Problems arise

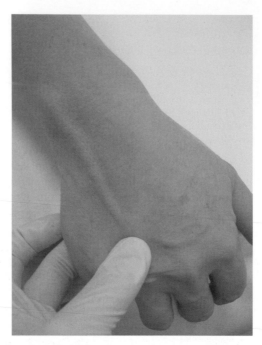

Figure 9.8 Anchoring the vein with the thumb.

when the practitioner's thumb is too close to the venepuncture site, preventing the correct angle of approach. Sometimes, once the skin has been pulled taut, the position of the vein alters slightly, so that the practitioner enters to the side of the vessel, necessitating realignment of the needle.

Stabilization of the vein must be maintained throughout the procedure until the needle or cannula is successfully sited. If the tension is released halfway through the procedure, it can result in the needle penetrating the opposite wall of the vein, causing a haematoma (Dougherty 2004).

Device placement

It is important that the needle enters the skin with the bevel up. This is to aid a smooth venepuncture, as the sharpest part of the needle will penetrate the skin first and will produce less trauma to the skin and vein. It also reduces the risk of piercing the vein's posterior wall (Weinstein 2007). The method of inserting the needle bevel down to prevent extravasation in small veins is described by Weinstein (2007), but this is not a commonly used or recommended technique and is more associated with subcutaneous infusions.

The angle of the needle varies with the type of device used and the depth of the vein in the subcutaneous tissue. The literature recommends a range of 10–45° (Perucca 2001; Weinstein 2007; Springhouse 2002). A vein located superficially, such as a hand vein, certainly requires a smaller angle of approach, whilst a large or deeply placed vein will require a greater angle. Once the device is in the vein, the angle will always be reduced in order to prevent puncturing the posterior wall of the vein (Perucca 2001).

The vein can be approached using either the direct or indirect method. The direct method is when the device enters the skin directly above the vein. The advantage is that the vein is entered immediately. However, with small, fragile veins, this method may lead to the vein bruising more easily or puncturing of the posterior wall (Dougherty 2004). For these types of vein, the indirect method may be preferable. To achieve this, the device is inserted through the skin, then the vein is relocated and the device advanced into the vein. It is a form of tunnelling and may be useful in veins which are palpable and visible for only a short section. This method enables a more gentle entry and thus reduces trauma to the vein (Hadaway 2000; Perucca 2001; Dougherty 2004).

Flashback into the tubing of a winged infusion device or into the flashback chamber of a cannula is an indication that initial entry into the vein has been successful (Scales 2005). This may be accompanied by a popping or 'giving way' sensation felt by the practitioner (and sometimes the patient). This is felt when there is resistance from the vein wall as the device enters the lumen of the vein. It tends to be more obvious when inserting devices into large, strong-walled veins and more difficult to discern in thin-walled veins with a small blood volume (Perucca 2001; Springhouse 2002). If the device punctures the posterior wall, the flashback will stop. However, it must be remembered that with small-gauge cannulae or in hypotensive patients the flashback may be slow (Perucca 2001)

Advancing the device

During venepuncture, once the needle has successfully entered the vein, it needs only to be advanced slightly in order to stabilize it and prevent dislodgement during blood sampling. The distance it should be advanced will depend on the length of the needle and the size and position of the vein.

There are several methods of advancing the cannula into the vein. It should be advanced gently and smoothly, and the technique used will often depend on how the practitioner was taught. However, students may need to try several approaches in order to find the most suitable (Dougherty 2004).

- *The one-handed technique.* This is more difficult to learn but it is attributed with a greater success rate (*See* Box 9.3). The hand used to perform cannulation also withdraws the stylet and advances the cannula into the vein. This allows skin traction to be maintained while the device is advanced and, if the patient is uncooperative, enables the practitioner to stabilize the patient's arm (Hadaway 2000; Perucca 2001; Dougherty 2004).
- *The one-step technique.* In this case, when the cannula has entered the vein, the practitioner slides it off the stylet in one movement. The disadvantage with this method is that the stylet must remain completely still in order to prevent damage to the vein. It is best accomplished on a straight vein and is more helpful if the cannula has a small finger guard which can be used to 'push' the cannula off the needle into the vein.
- *'Floating'.* Floating the cannula into the vein is useful if the device comes up against a valve, which usually prevents advancement. If enough of the cannula is within the vein, the stylet can be removed and a syringe or an infusion of sodium chloride 0.9% can be attached; as the fluid opens the valve, the device can then be advanced and 'floated' into the vein.
- *The two-handed technique.* This is when the practitioner uses one hand to perform the cannulation and then releases skin traction to use the other hand to hold and withdraw the stylet, while the dominant hand advances the cannula off the stylet. Millam (1992) suggested that this method prevents blood spill, but it requires the release of skin traction which can often lead to the puncturing of the posterior vein wall, particularly in mobile or fragile veins. It may be an easier technique to learn but is not recommended unless the vein is straight, large and well supported by subcutaneous tissue (Dougherty 2004).

Once the cannula is advanced into the vein, the tourniquet should be released. Then, using a finger just above the location of the tip of the cannula, apply pressure (to prevent blood spillage) and remove the stylet completely. An injection cap, extension set or administration set can then be attached.

If the cannulation is unsuccessful, the stylet should never be reintroduced into the cannula. This could result in shearing or puncturing of the cannula wall, which could lead to pieces of cannula breaking off and causing an embolism (Perucca 2001; RCN 2000).

Section 2

A new device should be used for each venepuncture or cannulation. All devices are single use (MDA 2000).

A practitioner should only have two attempts, as multiple attempts cause unnecessary trauma to the patient and limit vascular access (Phillips 2005).

If bruising occurs during the procedure, the tourniquet should be released immediately, the device removed and pressure applied to prevent haematoma formation. If the tourniquet is reapplied to the same arm too soon after a venepuncture, a haematoma will form (Weinstein 2007).

Securing the Device

On completion of a successful cannulation it is important to secure the device to prevent mechanical phlebitis and accidental dislodgement. Clean tape may be used, providing it does not come into contact with the insertion site as this may contaminate and obscure the site, making observations for early signs of phlebitis difficult (Figure 9.9a and b). Moureau and Iannucci (2003) found that using an adhesive pad with an integrated retainer designed to hold a cannula in place offered more security than tape. They reviewed

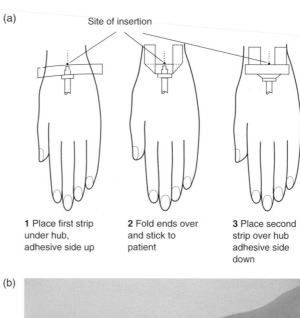

(a)   Site of insertion

1 Place first strip under hub, adhesive side up

2 Fold ends over and stick to patient

3 Place second strip over hub adhesive side down

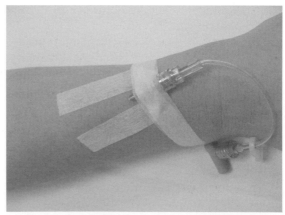

(b)

Figure 9.9   (a) Taping a peripheral cannula (Dougherty 2004). Reprinted with permission of Blackwell Publishing. (b) Cannula secured by tape.

a number of studies and found that compared to tape, securing devices such as a Statlock, reduced device dislodgement (in 67%), complications (in 50%) and unscheduled restarts (in 78%), for both peripheral and CVADs (such as PICCs). Dwell times were also increased (Smith 2006; Frey & Schears 2006). The cannula may then be dressed using a recognized dressing such as dry sterile gauze or a transparent dressing (Maki & Ringer 1987). Any tubing should also be taped to prevent pulling on the cannula. A light bandage can be applied over gauze but should not be applied to a transparent dressing as this defeats the object of the transparent dressing (Dougherty 2004). If the device is located over a joint, or in an uncooperative or confused patient or child, the joint should be splinted to prevent movement and possible dislodgement. The use of the correct type of splint is important. The choice will depend on the type of joint being splinted, e.g. elbow or wrist. Complications such as contracture, particularly in patients with oedema and muscle weakness, can arise if hands are not correctly immobilized on a splint in order to ensure a functional position (Weinstein 2007).

Care of the Device

Once sited and dressed, an injection cap (preferably needle free) (MHRA 2005b; RCN 2005) can be attached directly to the cannula or via an extension set and the cannula should be flushed with a solution of sodium chloride 0.9%. Flushing should be performed before and after each use and if a cannula is not in use then it should be flushed every 24 hours (Kamimoto & Olson 1996; Campbell *et al.* 2005). The recommended technique is to use turbulent flow (brisk flush), achieved by a push–pause method, and to complete with a positive pressure (achieved by maintaining pressure with the thumb on the plunger of the syringe whilst removing the syringe from the injection cap) (Perucca 2001; Dougherty 2004). This is effective but if not performed correctly can still result in occlusion (Dougherty 2006). For this reason, manufacturers have developed a needle-free positive displacement injection cap, which is attached to the end of the device or extension set and provides the benefits of a closed needle-free system, but also creates the positive pressure required to maintain patency (Figure 9.10). Berger (2000) found that using positive pressure devices resulted in a significant decrease in the incidence of occlusion. Finally, details regarding the insertion (date, time, vein used, device size and signature of the practitioner) should be documented in the patient's notes or care plan (DH 2003; RCN 2005).

Resiting of Cannula

It has been recommended that peripheral cannulae should be resited every 48–72 hours to reduce the risk of phlebitis (DH 2003; Barker *et al.* 2004; RCN 2005). However, this may be difficult to achieve in certain groups, such as oncology or paediatric patients. In these cases, it may be preferable to ensure careful monitoring of the site, and to remove and resite the cannula at the first indications of tenderness, infiltration or phlebitis (Grune *et al.* 2004). The sites should be alternated whenever possible to allow time for cannula sites to rest and recover, and for any local complications (e.g. phlebitis or infiltration) to resolve.

Removal of Needle/Cannula

On completion of venepuncture, pressure should not be applied until the needle has been fully removed or it will cause the needle to be dragged out of the vein, causing pain and

Section 2

(a)

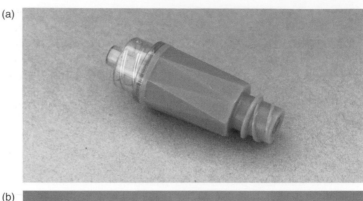

(b)

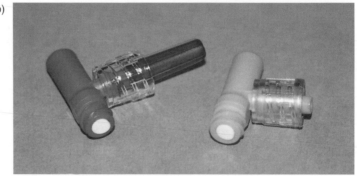

Figure 9.10   CLC 2000. An example of a positive displacement cap.

venous damage. The device should be removed carefully, using slow, steady movement and keeping the hub parallel to the skin, in order to prevent damage to the vein. On removal of a cannula, the integrity and length of the device should be checked, to ensure that the entire device has been removed (RCN 2005).

Once a needle or cannula has been removed, firm digital pressure should be applied over the puncture site and the arm kept straight. It is not recommended to apply pressure whilst flexing the arm (McCall & Tankersley 2003; Dougherty 2004; Weinstein 2007). Dyson and Bogod (1987) concluded that the practice of flexing the elbow after venepuncture was not an efficient way of preventing bruising in the antecubital fossa. It has also been suggested that the practitioner should apply the pressure, rather than the patient, as this also reduces the incidence of bruising (Godwin *et al.* 1992). Applying pressure prevents leakage and haematoma formation. In some patients, it may take longer for bleeding to cease, especially if they are on medication that interferes with clotting mechanisms (e.g. warfarin or heparin), or their disease predisposes them to bleeding (e.g. thrombocytopenia or haemophilia) (Dougherty 2004). Weinstein (2007) instructs patients to elevate the arm, which causes a negative pressure in the vein, collapsing it and facilitating clotting, although it is not recommended in cardiac patients. The nurse should remain with the patient until bleeding has stopped and only then should a dressing be applied.

The date, time and reason for removal of the cannula must be documented in the patient's notes (DH 2003; RCN 2005).

Safety of the Practitioner

Manual dexterity is required for venepuncture or cannulation, both of which are invasive and potentially hazardous procedures, so the practitioner should select well-fitting gloves (ICNA 2003; RCN 2005). Gloves will protect practitioners against unexpected spill or contamination, and also the wiping effect on the needle by the glove may reduce the volume of blood to which the practitioner is exposed, thereby reducing the risk of infection (Mitchell Higgs 2002; NAO 2003; ICNA 2003). However, gloves will not prevent a needlestick injury and so it is vital that safe technique and practice are used at all times. Used needles should not be resheathed, and any sharp should be disposed of immediately into a non-permeable, puncture-resistant, tamperproof container (ICNA 2003; NICE 2003; NHS Employees 2005; RCN 2005).

Systems are now available that reduce the risk of accidental needlestick injury, such as vacuum collection systems, needleless injection caps and sharps injury protection devices, and these should be used wherever possible (ICNA 2003; NHS Employees 2005; RCN 2005).

If a needlestick injury does occur, the area should be made to bleed and washed under running water. Usual steps following such an injury include testing both patient and practitioner for hepatitis B, documentation of the accident and reporting the incident to the occupational health department. HIV anaphylaxis may also be necessary. Practitioners should have knowledge of and refer to their organization's policy.

Problem-Solving Techniques

Anxious patient

Some patients may be anxious before venepuncture or cannulation because of:

- previous traumatic experiences
- fear of needles or blood
- ignorance about what the procedure involves.

Prevention

- Approach the patient in a calm and confident manner.
- Explain what the procedure involves and show them the equipment if appropriate.
- Offer the patient the opportunity to lie down or recline during the procedure.
- Use all methods of improving venous dilation to ensure success on the first attempt.
- Listen to the patient's previous experiences and involve them in site selection.
- Offer a local anaesthetic (by gel or injection).

Action

- Refer the patient for psychological support if anxiety and fear are of phobic proportions.

Difficulty in locating a suitable vein

Some patients may have limited venous access due to:

- excessive previous use
- shock or dehydration
- anxiety
- fragile, thready veins (e.g. the elderly or patients on anticoagulant therapy)
- thrombosed veins as a result of treatment (e.g. cytotoxic therapy).

Prevention

- Alternate sites wherever possible to avoid overuse of certain veins.
- Use the methods described above to reduce anxiety.

Action

- Reassure the patient.
- Use all methods of improving venous access before attempting the procedure; for example, use warm water/GTN to encourage venous dilation.
- Do not attempt the procedure unless experienced.

Spurt of blood on entry

When the bevel enters a large or superficial vein, before the entire bevel is under the skin it may result in a small spurt of blood onto the patient's skin and cause a small blood blister.

Prevention

- Select a less superficial vein where possible.
- Enter the vein smoothly and without hesitation.

Action

- Reassure the patient that there is nothing to be concerned about, and wipe away any blood after removal of the needle.

Missing the vein on insertion of the needle

The needle fails to be inserted directly into the vein because of:

- inadequate anchoring
- collapse of the vein
- incorrect position of practitioner or patient
- inadequate palpation
- poor vein choice
- lack of concentration
- failure to penetrate the vein properly due to incorrect insertion angle.

Prevention

- Ensure good position and lighting.
- Improve preparation and concentration.
- Use good technique and accurate vein selection.

Action

- Withdraw the needle and manoeuvre gently to realign it and correct the angle of insertion.
- Check during manoeuvring that the patient is not feeling any pain.
- If the patient complains of pain, remove the needle.
- If unsuccessful then remove the needle.
- Where necessary, pass to a colleague with more experience.

Blood stops flowing through the device

In this case, blood flashback is seen and then the blood stops flowing because of:

- venospasm
- bevel of needle up against a valve
- penetration of the posterior vein wall by the device
- possible vein collapse.

Prevention

- Try to locate valves before insertion and insert the device just above the valve.
- Carefully level off once in the vein to prevent penetration of posterior wall.
- Use a good angle of approach to the vein to prevent through-puncture.
- Check expiry date of bottle as vacuum reduces when out-of-date bottle is used to obtain blood sample.

Action

- Massage the veins above the needle tip to pull blood into the vein.
- Release and tighten the tourniquet.
- Gently stroke the vein above the needle to relieve venous spasm.
- Withdraw the needle slightly to move the bevel away from the valve.
- If the vein wall is penetrated, remove the device.

Difficulty in advancing

The practitioner may have difficulty advancing the needle/cannula, which could be due to:

- removing the stylet too far so that the cannula is now no longer rigid enough to be advanced
- encountering a valve
- not releasing the cannula from the needle before insertion
- poor anchoring or stretching of the skin
- releasing the tourniquet too soon, causing the vein to collapse.

Prevention

- Ensure the tourniquet remains sufficiently tight until insertion is completed.
- Ensure the cannula is released from the stylet before insertion, to allow for smooth advancement.
- Ensure that a sufficient length of the cannula is inserted into the vein before stylet withdrawal.
- Use good technique.
- Assess the vein accurately, observing for valves, and avoid where possible.

Action

- In the event of early stylet removal or encountering a valve, connect a syringe of sodium chloride 0.9%, flush the cannula and advance at the same time in an effort to 'float' the device into the vein.
- Tighten the tourniquet and wait for the vein to refill.

Difficulty in flushing once the cannula is *in situ*

Sometimes the cannula has been successfully inserted, but on checking patency by flushing, the practitioner has difficulty because:

- the cannula tip is up against the valve
- the cannula has pierced the posterior wall of the vein
- the cannula tip is resting on the wall of the vein
- there is an occlusion.

Prevention

- Avoid areas along the vein where there may be valves.
- Ensure careful insertion to prevent puncturing the posterior wall of the vein.

Action

- Withdraw the cannula slightly to move it away from the vein wall or valve and attempt to flush.
- If the vein wall is pierced, remove the cannula.
- Attempt to withdraw the clot and clear the occlusion.

Complications

Pain

Pain can be caused by any of the following:

- tentative stop–start insertion (often a problem with hesitant or new practitioners)
- hitting an artery, nerve or valve
- poor technique—inadequate anchoring causes skin to gather as the needle is inserted
- alcohol is not allowed to dry adequately before insertion, resulting in stinging pain
- using a frequently punctured, recently used or bruised vein
- anxious patient with low pain threshold
- use of large-gauge device
- use of veins in sensitive areas.

Prevention

- Use methods to relax and relieve anxiety.
- Avoid use of bruised, used or sensitive areas.
- Use local anaesthetic creams or injections.
- Ensure good technique is employed.

Action

- Reassure the patient and explain, especially in the case of nerve pain, that it may last for a few hours.
- Depending on the cause (e.g. nerve or artery), it may be necessary to remove the device immediately.
- Document the incident.

Haematoma

This is a swelling of blood under the skin which occurs during the insertion procedure or after removal. It can be caused by:

- failure to remove the tourniquet promptly or before removing needle
- penetration of the posterior vein wall
- incorrect choice of needle for vein size
- fragile veins
- anticoagulant therapy
- spontaneous rupture of the vessel on application of the tourniquet or cleaning of the skin
- inadequate pressure on venepuncture site following removal of the needle.

Prevention

- Remove the tourniquet before removing the needle.
- Use good vein and device selection.
- Employ careful technique.
- Be aware of patients with fragile veins or those on anticoagulant therapy.

- Apply adequate pressure on removal of the needle/device.
- Do not apply the tourniquet to a limb where recent venepuncture has occurred.
- Do not leave the tourniquet for any longer than necessary.

Action

- Remove the needle immediately.
- Apply pressure to the site for a few minutes.
- Elevate the extremity if appropriate.
- Reassure the patient and explain the reason for the bruise.
- Apply a pressure dressing if required.
- Apply an ice pack if bruising is extensive.
- Apply hirudoid or arnica ointment.
- Do not reapply the tourniquet to the affected limb.
- Document the incident.
- Give the patient an information sheet with advice about whom to contact and when if the haematoma gets worse or they develop numbness.

Syncope/vasovagal reaction

Patients may feel faint, light-headed, sweaty, hot, cold or nauseated (Pavlin *et al.* 1993), or go on to a vasovagal reaction characterized by bradycardia and hypotension (Kaloupek *et al.* 1985). It can be caused by:

- fear of needles or blood
- a hot stuffy environment
- feeling very hungry
- being pregnant
- feeling unwell.

Prevention

- The practitioner should have a confident reassuring manner and approach.
- A facility for the patient to lie down during the procedure should be available.
- Spend time before the procedure discussing fears and anxieties with the patient.
- Be aware of which patients are more vulnerable.

Action

- A patient who feels faint should be encouraged to put their head between their legs; but this may be difficult, especially if the patient has the device in the vein.
- Try to get the patient to lie down.
- If the patient faints then the vein will collapse; if possible, it may be useful to secure the device in case the patient requires any medication as a result of the reaction and so that it can be used once the patient has recovered.
- It may be necessary to remove the device and resite it once the patient has recovered.
- Document the incident.

Hitting an artery

Accidental puncture of an artery is characterized by pain and bright-red blood.

Prevention

- Adequate assessment and recognition of arteries before performing the procedure will help to prevent this occurring.

Action

- Remove the device immediately and apply pressure to the puncture site for up to 5 minutes.
- Reassure the patient.
- Do not reapply the tourniquet to the affected limb.
- Document the incident.
- Give the patient an information sheet with advice about whom to contact and when if they develop numbness or tingling in the limb.

Hitting a nerve

If a nerve is accidentally hit on insertion of the needle into the vein, this will result in severe shooting pain (Yuan & Cohan 1987).

Prevention

- Ensure that the location of superficial nerves is known. For example, a common place to hit a nerve is the cephalic vein and this can be avoided by placing three fingers at the wrist and inserting the needle above this (the nerve runs deeper at that point and therefore the practitioner will be less likely to touch it) (Boeson *et al*. 2000; Masoorli 2002).

Action

- The needle should be removed immediately.
- Reassure the patient and explain that the pain may last for a few hours and the area may feel numb. Explain that the pain can sometimes last for a few days and that if it continues or gets worse, medical advice should be sought.
- Give the patient an information sheet with advice about whom to contact and when.
- Document the incident.

Blood Tests

Blood tests are routinely performed to:

- indicate relatively common disorders
- enable diagnosis
- follow the course of a disease
- regulate therapy (Weinstein 2007).

Each blood test requires a different type of tube containing a specific additive to enable the serum or plasma to be analysed or the blood to be collected in an anticoagulated form or as a clotted sample (*See* glossary of terms in Box 9.6). Immediately following collection of blood, it is important that the specimen tubes are gently inverted 6–8 times to mix the blood with the additives (Sommer *et al*. 2002). However, excessive shaking of the sample can cause cells to become agitated, resulting in haemolysis (Sommer *et al*. 2002). Haemolysis results from the destruction of red blood cells and the liberation of haemoglobin into the fluid portion of the specimen. This affects certain tests and a haemolysed specimen as a result of procedural error is usually not analysed and discarded (Garza & Becan McBride 2002).

General sources of variability

Increased capillary hydrostatic pressure can cause water to shift from the intravascular to the interstitial space. This increases the concentration of the constituents of blood, a process called haemoconcentration. It can result from a systemic increase in capillary pressure such as that seen with prolonged standing and from local effects such as

> **BOX 9.6**
>
> **Glossary of terms used in blood sample analysis**
>
> - *Anticoagulated blood*—sample of blood collected in a tube containing an anticoagulant such as EDTA or lithium heparin, which prevents the blood from clotting.
> - *Clotted blood*—sample of blood collected in a plain glass or plastic tube and allowed to clot.
> - *Blood serum*—extracellular fluid of clotted blood, i.e. the fluid that remains when the cellular elements of clotted blood have been removed.
> - *Blood plasma*—extracellular fluid of anticoagulated blood, i.e. the fluid that remains when the cellular elements of anticoagulated blood have been removed.
> - *Haemolysis*—the rupture of red cell membranes causing release of haemoglobin, which can occur if blood is withdrawn through a very small gauge needle or if withdrawal is very slow and prolonged.

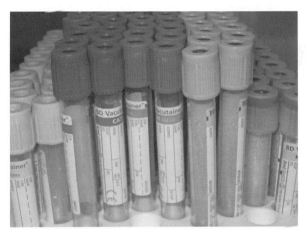

Figure 9.11   Types of blood bottles.

prolonged application of the tourniquet during venepuncture (Sommer *et al.* 2002). Therefore, standing time before venepuncture and length of tourniquet application should both be kept to a minimum. The recommendation for tourniquet application is not more than 1 minute before venepuncture and not more than 2–3 minutes for the entire procedure (Ernst & Ernst 2001; Garza & Becan McBride 2002; Weinstein 2007).

Rapid flow of blood through small-bore needles, especially if exposed to large negative pressures, leads to haemolysis. This can be minimized by the use, where possible, of large-bore needles, moderate flow rates and moderate negative pressures. Blood samples may become contaminated with infusion fluid and therefore blood should not be taken from a site above an infusion, but where feasible should be obtained from a site in the opposite arm or below the infusion site (Sommer *et al.* 2002; Weinstein 2007). Some authors advise that the infusion should be switched off for a certain period of time (less than 2 minutes) before taking blood from the arm with an infusion (Sommer *et al.* 2002). Others state that samples should never be taken above an infusion even it is has been discontinued (Ernst & Ernst 2001). There is also the risk of the device becoming occluded if not flushed properly to maintain patency.

Equipment

The vacuumed tubes often used for collecting samples of venous blood come in various sizes appropriate to the age of the patient and the type of laboratory analysis. The colour of the top or stopper usually indicates the presence and type of additive (*See* Figure 9.11

BOX 9.7

Example of Order of Draw (Check with Manufacturer's Instructions)

1. Blood cultures
2. Light-blue top
3. Red or pink top
4. Green gold
5. Lavender
6. Pink

and Box 9.7). Care must be taken to ensure that the correct tube is used for the test to be performed, that they are used in the correct order (*See* Box 9.7 for order of draw) and that the tube is used before its expiration date (Sommer *et al.* 2002; McCall & Tankersley 2003; Philips 2005).

If a needle and syringe are used, when blood is decanted into the sample tube, it should be allowed to flow gently down the inside of the tube. If using vacuumed bottles, where possible a 21-G needle should be used to prevent haemolysis (McCall & Tankersley 2003).

Haematology tests

Full blood count—lavender top tube

The full blood count is the most commonly requested and performed blood test. It is not one but rather a group of tests, including the following:

- a count of the cellular elements of blood—red blood cells, white blood cells and platelets
- the measurement of haemoglobin concentration in the blood
- assessment of size and appearance of the cells.

It is generally used to investigate anaemia, but in the oncology setting is used extensively to assess leucopenia and thrombocytopenia (Higgins 1995a).

Method of collection   Blood for a full blood count is usually collected in a tube which contains K2 EDTA. Blood must be mixed immediately after collection to prevent clumping and microclot formation (McCall & Tankersley 2003).

Coagulation studies—light-blue top tube

Screening for haemostasis and thrombosis, as well as anticoagulant control, is carried out using a tube containing sodium citrate. There is a critical 9:1 ratio of blood to anticoagulant so it is important to fill tubes to the stated capacity. Underfilled tubes will not be accepted for testing (McCall & Tankersley 2003).

Electrolytes, and liver and kidney function tests

Electrolytes—green or gold top tube

Electrolyte imbalances are serious complications in the critically ill patient and must be recognized and corrected immediately. Levels of potassium, sodium, calcium, chlorides and phosphorus are all measured, and their accuracy is largely dependent on the proper collection and handling of the samples.

Method of collection   Potassium alterations can occur due to any of the following.

- A tourniquet left on for an extended length of time will affect potassium levels. The longer it is on the greater the amount of potassium leaks from the tissues into the blood (Garza & Becan McBride 2002).

- Haemolysis should be prevented as this releases potassium from blood cells into serum and causes an elevation in serum potassium levels (Weinstein 2007).
- Leucocytes and platelets are rich in potassium and, at high levels, can release potassium during the clotting process.

Calcium variations in sample collection technique can also affect the results. Acid–base changes can occur from prolonged tourniquet application and variations in the amount of heparin in the collecting tube can alter the measured calcium ions.

Liver function tests—green or gold top tube

These tests may be useful in diagnosing kidney and liver disease or in determining the effectiveness of treatment; they include albumin, globulin and total protein. Bilirubin tests differentiate between impairment of the liver by obstruction and haemolysis.

Kidney function tests

Creatinine and blood urea nitrogen are both used to measure kidney function.

Blood sugar tests—grey top tube

The test for blood sugar is used to detect any disorders of glucose metabolism; for example, raised levels may indicate diabetes or chronic liver disorder, and low levels may indicate insulin overdose, tumours of the pancreas or insufficiency of the endocrine glands (Weinstein 2007).

Fasting blood sugar usually requires the patient to fast for 8 hours before the blood is taken. It must be remembered that results will be elevated above baseline if the patient is receiving parenteral glucose, regardless of the site from which the sample is withdrawn.

Glucose tolerance tests involve a fasting blood sugar, followed by the patient drinking a quantity of glucose; blood and urine samples are then taken at 30, 60, 90, 120 and 180 minutes after ingestion of the glucose.

Acid–base balance and enzymes

When deviations occur in the normal acid–base ratio, a change in pH results and is accompanied by a change in bicarbonate concentration.

Method of collection

Carbon dioxide measurement is performed by collecting the blood in either a heparinized syringe which is put immediately on ice, a heparinized tube, or a dry tube without any anticoagulant. The containers should always be filled to the top with blood and it is important that the patient avoids clenching the fist. This is because muscular activity in the arm raises carbon dioxide levels in the blood (Weinstein 2007).

Acidity (pH) is measured once blood has been collected in a heparinized 2-mL syringe which is capped off or in a vacuumed bottle containing heparin. It should not be agitated and should be packed in ice after collection.

Enzymes Tests such as amylase, acid and alkaline phosphatase, aspartate aminotransferase (AST) and alanine aminotransferase (ALT) will be inaccurate if the sample is haemolysed.

Blood typing—red or pink top tube

Blood typing is a common test required to be carried out on all blood donors and all patients who may require a blood transfusion. The ABO system denotes four main groups—A, B, AB and O, and the antigens such as D, E, C, etc. belong to the Rhesus system. Other tests include direct or indirect Coombs' tests (Weinstein 2007).

Section 2

Identification of the patient and clear and correct labelling of the sample bottle and request form are essential. The patient must give his or her full name and date of birth, and the sample and form must be signed by the practitioner collecting the blood.

Method of collection

Venous blood is collected and allowed to clot. Usually one bottle is enough, but occasionally the laboratory may request two or three samples to be collected.

Antibiotic assays

Some antibiotics, e.g. vancomycin and aminoglycosides, are potentially nephrotoxic and ototoxic. Therefore, patients receiving these drugs should have serum sent regularly for antimicrobial assay. The purpose is to avoid toxic accumulation and to check that therapeutic levels are being achieved (Verity 2004).

Method of collection

Levels should be sent every 2–3 days or daily in the presence of marked renal failure. Pre-dose levels are taken just before administration of the antibiotic. Post-dose levels are usually taken 1 hour after bolus injection or the end of an infusion. It is important that the samples are taken at standardized times so that the results can be interpreted accurately and the dosage adjusted accordingly (Verity 2004).

Serum samples of blood should be collected in a plain tube, usually 10 mL directly from a vein. Neither pre- nor post-dose levels should be taken from a cannula or catheter because the device may have been contaminated by previous administration of antibiotic; if it is necessary, then it should be documented on the microbiology request card (Verity 2004).

Blood culture

This test is usually performed during febrile illnesses and when a patient is having chills with a spiking fever (Sommer *et al.* 2002). The number of bacteria in the blood of an infected individual is too low for visual confirmation of bacteraemia, so a blood culture sample may be taken in order to culture the bacteria in a nutrient solution (which rapidly increases the number of any bacteria present) to enable identification of microorganisms (Higgins 1995b; Weinstein 2007).

Most laboratories provide two bottles for blood cultures. One is for culturing aerobic bacteria and has oxygen in the headspace above the liquid media. The second has a gas mixture and no oxygen, for culture of anaerobic species (Sommer *et al.* 2002).

Method of collection

Blood for cultures must be taken from a peripheral vein and not from an indwelling cannula or catheter, which might itself be contaminated. The only exception is when it is the cannula or catheter which is suspected of being the cause of infection (Verity 2004). This would necessitate obtaining two sets of cultures: one from the catheter/cannula and one from a peripheral vein. Both sets should be clearly marked with the site from which they were taken. It is also important to sample blood before administration of antibiotics, otherwise the bacteraemia is suppressed, making isolation difficult (Verity 2004).

Aseptic collection technique is critical to obtain meaningful results (Sommer *et al.* 2002; Ernst 2005; Hoetke 2006; DH 2007). It is important to collect blood samples without introducing any contaminating bacteria from the skin or the environment which could lead to a false-positive result (Sommer *et al.* 2002). It has been suggested by some institutions that the practitioner should wear sterile gloves; however, it is more important that the site of the venepuncture should be cleaned thoroughly with 2% chlorhexidine (DH 2007). The blood should then be collected and injected via the rubber septum (cleaned with an antiseptic swab) into the blood culture bottles.

Drawing the correct volume is also critical because the ratio of blood to culture media depends on the system used. The volume is usually between 5 and 10 mL per bottle (Sommer *et al.* 2002). It is recommended that vacuumed bottles or a separate syringe and needle be used to decant blood into each bottle. Some laboratories recommend taking a second sample not less than an hour later (Sommer *et al.* 2002). The bottles should be clearly labelled and transported immediately to the laboratory or placed in an incubator maintained at 37°C (Higgins 1995b).

General considerations

High-risk samples

These samples should be clearly labelled and identified as high risk. They are usually double-bagged, with the request form separated from the sample to prevent accidental contamination. Staff asked to take blood from high-risk patients should be informed of the risk and ensure universal precautions are practised when sampling.

Special preparation

The practitioner must be aware of the activities or habits that may influence the results of blood tests, and ensure that the patient is aware of any activities that will need to be restricted before venepuncture (Box 9.8). If a patient is to have bloods taken that require a dietary restriction, such as a special diet, fasting or omitting medications, the practitioner must ensure that the patient understands what is required and the reasons for it. Verbal instruction should be reinforced with written information to ensure that patients' and practitioners' time is not wasted. Herbal remedies such as St John's wort can affect clinical laboratory testing (Weinstein 2007).

Sampling from a peripheral cannula or a central venous catheter

When taking blood samples from any venous access device, consideration should be given to the type of sample to be obtained, and the effect of the catheter size/material and the pressure on the ability to obtain the blood samples (Frey 2001). A peripheral cannula should not be used for routine blood sampling unless it has been placed specifically for that reason (e.g. pharmacokinetics) (RCN 2005). The presence of a central venous catheter makes obtaining frequent blood samples easier; however, it requires some method

Section 2

BOX 9.8

Activities or conditions that may need to be managed before venepuncture

- Vigorous exercise
- Ingestion of alcohol
- Intramuscular injections
- Certain surgical procedures
- Smoking
- Previous blood transfusions
- Immunizations
- Traumatic venepunctures (especially for haematology tests)
- Anxiety
- Pain
- Dehydration
- Herbal remedies

of removing the contents of the lumen such as the drugs recently administered, saline or heparinized saline (Frey 2002). This is in order to prevent inaccurate laboratory values which have been reported when blood specimens are obtained via this route. Samples can be taken with a vacuum systems with the aid of an adaptor or a syringe (RCN 2005).

The proximal lumen of a multilumen catheter is the preferred site from which to obtain the sample. The largest lumen should also be reserved for blood sampling (Dougherty 2004). It may also be necessary to discontinue infusions for a short period before the catheter sample is obtained. There are also a number of methods of withdrawing the sample to reduce the risk of inaccurate results, although the most appropriate method has not yet been established by research (Keller 1994). There are currently three main methods used: discard, reinfusion and mixing.

Discard   This is when the first sample is withdrawn (usually 5–10 mL of blood) and then discarded (Cosca *et al.* 1998; Holmes 1998; Sommer *et al.* 2002). This ensures that any residual drug is removed, but may result in excessive blood removal in small children or those requiring multiple samples.

Mixing   This method involves flushing the catheter with sodium chloride 0.9%, withdrawing 6 mL of blood in a syringe and then injecting it back and forth several times without removing the syringe. This removes any residual solution, reduces exposure to blood and there is no blood wastage (Holmes 1998; Perucca 2001). Problems include difficulty in obtaining enough blood and the chance of haemolysis caused by agitation of the blood (Frey 2002).

Reinfusion   This method is performed by taking the first 6 mL of blood, capping off the syringe, taking the samples and then reinfusing the blood first taken (Keller 1994). It does not result in depleted blood volume but does expose the practitioner to blood contamination and may introduce clots into the system (Cosca *et al.* 1998; Dougherty 2004).

An important aspect of care once the sample has been withdrawn is to ensure adequate flushing of the device in order to clear the device of all residual blood to reduce the risk of clot formation and subsequent infection (RCN 2005).

Conclusion

Following the reduction in junior doctors' hours, one of the responsibilities actively taken on by nurses has been the practice of venepuncture and cannulation. The nurse is both accountable and responsible for maintaining the technical expertise and high level of skill necessary for performing these procedures (NMC 2004). The practitioner must ensure that s/he has knowledge of the anatomy and physiology of the venous system, how to choose the appropriate vein and equipment, as well as the associated complications, in order to meet the physical, social and psychological needs of the patient undergoing venepuncture and cannulation.

References

Agras S, Sylvester D, Olivean D (1969) The epidemiology of common fears and phobias. *Comprehensive Psychiatry* 10(2): 151–157.

Agras WS, Chapkin HN, Olivean DC (1972) The natural history of phobia. *Archives of General Psychiatry* 26: 315–317.

Ahrens T, Wiersma L, Weilitz PB (1991) Differences in pain perception associated with intravenous catheter insertion. *Journal of Intravenous Nursing* 14(2): 85–89.

Alexander MC, Webster HK (2001) Legal aspects of intravenous nursing. In: Hankin *et al.*, eds. *Intravenous Therapy in Clinical Practice*, 2nd edn, pp. 50–64. WB Saunders, Philadelphia.

Auerbach SM, Kendall PC, Cutter HF, Levitt NR (1976) Anxiety, locus of control, type of preparatory information and adjustment to dental surgery. *Journal of Consulting and Clinical Psychology* 44(5): 809–818.

Banton J, Leahy-Gross K (1998) Assessing catheter performance – 4 years of tracking patient outcomes of midline, mid-clavicular and PICC line program. *Journal of Vascular Access Devices* 3(3): 19–25.

Barker P, Anderson ADG, MacFie J (2004) Randomised clinical trial of elective re-siting intravenous cannulae. *Annals of the Royal College of Surgeons of England* 86: 281–293.

Bennett-Humphrey G, Boon CMJ (1992) The occurrence of high levels of acute behavioural distress in children and adolescents undergoing routine venepuncture. *Paediatrics* 90(1): 87–91.

Berger L (2000). The effects of positive pressure devices on catheter occlusions. *Journal of Vascular Access Devices* 5(4): 31–33.

Berggren U (1992) General and specific fears in referred and self-referred adult patients with extreme dental anxiety. *Behavioural Research Therapy* 30(4): 395–401.

Berkley KJ (1997) Sex differences in pain. *Behavioural and Brain Sciences* 20: 371–380.

Boeson MB, Hranchook A, Stoller J (2000) Peripheral nerve injury from intravenous cannulation: a case report. *AANA Journal* 68(1): 53–57.

Brismar B, Malmborg AS, Nystrom B, Strandberg A (1984) Bacterial contamination of intravenous cannula injection ports and stopcocks. *Clinical Nutrition* 3: 23–26.

Browne J, Awad I, Plant R, McAdoo J, Shorten G (1999) Topical amethocaine (Ametop) is superior to EMLA for intravenous cannulation. *Canadian Journal of Anesthesia* 46(11): 1014–1018.

Buckalew PG (1982) On the opposite side of the bed: a nurse clinician's experience of anxiety during chemotherapy. *Cancer Nursing* 5(6): 435–439.

Campbell SG, Trojanowski J, Ackroyd-Stolarz SA (2005) How often should peripheral intravenous catheters in ambulatory patients be flushed? *Journal of Infusion Nursing* 28(6): 399–404.

Camp-Sorrell D((2005) *Oncology Nursing Society Access Device Guidelines; Recommendations for Nursing Practice and Education*. Oncology Nursing Society, Pittsburgh, Pennsylvania.

Carlson K, Perdue MB, Hankins J (2001) Infection control. In: Hankin J *et al.*, eds. *Infusion Therapy in Clinical Practice*, 2nd edn, pp. 126–40. WB Saunders, Philadelphia.

Cheeseborough JS, Finch R (1984) Side ports—an infection hazard? *British Journal of Parenteral Therapy* 5(4): 155–157.

Coates A, Abraham S, Kaye SB, Sowerbutts T, Frewin C, Fox RM, Tattersall MHN (1983) On the receiving end—patient perception of the side effects of cancer chemotherapy. *European Journal of Cancer Clinical Oncology* 19(2): 203–208.

Cohn KH (1982) Chemotherapy from an insider's perspective. *Lancet* 1: 1006–1009.

Cosca PA, Smith S, Chatfield S *et al.* (1998). Reinfusion of discard blood from venous access devices. *Oncology Nursing Forum* 25(6): 1073–1076.

Coyne PJ, MacMurren M, Izzo T, Kramer T (1995) Transcutaneous electrical nerve stimulator for procedural pain associated with intravenous needlesticks. *Journal of Intravenous Nursing* 18(5): 263–267.

Crow S (1987) Infection risks in intravenous therapy. *Journal of the National Intravenous Therapy Association* 10: 101–105.

Dennis AR, Leeson-Payne CG, Langham BT, Aikenhead AR (1995) Local *anaesthesia* for cannulation—has practice changed? *Anaesthesia* 50: 400–402.

DH (2003) *Winning Ways: Working Togther to Reduce Healthcare Associated Infection in England*. Department of Health, London.

DH (2004) *Saving Lives; A Delivery Programme to Reduce Healthcare Associated Infection (HCAI) including MRSA*. Department of Health, London.

DH (2007) *Saving Lives: a delivery programme to reduce healthcare associated infection including MRSA: Taking blood cultures – a strategy for NHS Trusts, a summary of best practice*. Department of Health, London.

Dougherty L (1994) *A study to discover how cancer patients perceive the intravenous cannulation experience*. Unpublished MSc thesis, University of Surrey, Guildford.

Dougherty L (1996) Intravenous cannulation. *Nursing Standard* 11(2): 47–51.

Dougherty L (2004) Vascular access devices. In: Dougherty L, Lister S, eds. *The Royal Marsden NHS Trust Manual of Clinical Nursing Procedures*, 6th edn, pp. 724–773. Blackwell Publishing, Oxford.

Dougherty L (2006) *Central Venous Access Devices*. In: *Essential Skills Series*. Blackwell Publishing, Oxford.

Dyson A, Bogod D (1987) Minimising bruising in the antecubital fossa after venepuncture. *British Medical Journal* 294: 1659.

Ernst DJ (2005) *Applied Phlebotomy*. Lippincott Williams & Wilkins, Philadelphia.

Ernst DJ, Ernst C (2001) *Phlebotomy for Nurses and Nursing Personnel*. Healthstar Press, USA.

Frey AM (2001) IV therapy in children. In: Hankin J *et al.*, eds. *Infusion Therapy in Clinical Practice*, 2nd edn, pp. 561–591. WB Saunders, Philadelphia.

Frey AM (2002) *Drawing Labs From Venous Access Devices*. Presentation at NAVAN 15th Annual Conference, Virginia.

Frey AM, Schears GJ (2006) Why are we stuck on tape and suture. *Journal of Infusion Nursing* 29(1): 34–38.

Fuller A, Winn C (1999) Selecting equipment for peripheral inravenous cannulation. *Professional Nurse* 14(4): 233–6.

Galinkin JL, Rose JB, Harns K *et al.* (2002) Lidocaine iontophoresis versus eutectic mixture of local anaesthetics (EMLA) for IV placement in children. *Anesthesia and Analgesia* 94(6): 1484–8.

Garza D, Becan-McBride K (2002) *Phlebotomy Handbook: Blood Collection Essentials*. Pearson Education Inc, New Jersey.

Gaukroger PB, Roberts JG, Manners TA (1988) Infusion thrombophlebitis: a prospective comparison of 645 Vialon and Teflon cannulae in anaesthetic and postoperative use. *Anaesthesia and Intensive Care* 16(3): 265–271.

Section 2

Godwin PGR, Cuthbert AC, Choyce A (1992) Reducing bruising after venepuncture. *Quality in Health Care* 1: 245–246.

Golder M (2000) Potential risk of cross contamination during peripheral venous access by contamination of tourniquets. *Lancet* 355: 44.

Goodison SM (1990) The risks of IV therapy. *Professional Nurse* 5(5): 235–238.

Griffin AM, Butow PN, Coates AS *et al.* (1996) On the receiving end V: Patient perceptions of the side effects of cancer chemotherapy in 1993. *Annals of Oncology* 7: 189–195.

Grune F, Schrappe M, Basten J *et al.* (2004) Phlebitis rate and time kinetics of short peripheral intravenous catheters. *Infection* 32: 30–32.

Gunwardene RD, Davenport HT (1990) Local application of EMLA and glyceryl trinitrate ointment before venepuncture. *Anaesthesia* 45: 52–54.

Hadaway L((2000) Peripheral IV therapy in adults. In: *Self Study Workbook*. Hadaway Associates, Georgia.

Hadaway L (2001) Anatomy and physiology related to intravenous therapy. In: Hankin J *et al.*, eds. *Infusion Therapy in Clinical Practice*, 2nd edn, pp. 65–97. WB Saunders, Philadelphia.

Harrison N, Langham BT, Bogod DG (1992) Appropriate use of local anaesthesia for venous cannulation. *Anaesthesia* 47: 210–212.

Hart, S (2004) Aseptic technique. In: Dougherty L, Lister S, eds. *The Royal Marsden NHS Trust Manual of Clinical Nursing Procedures*, 6th edn, pp. 50–63. Blackwell Publishing, Oxford.

Hecker J (1988) Improved techniques in IV therapy. *Nursing Times* 84(34): 28–33.

Hecker JF, Lewis BH, Stanley H (1983) Nitroglycerine ointment as an aid to venepuncture. *Lancet* 1: 202–206.

Hefler L, Grimm C, Leodolter S, Tempfer C (2004) To butterfly or to needle: the pilot phase. *Annals of Internal Medicine* 140(11): 935–6.

Hewitt T, Scales K (1998) Prolonged contact with topical anaesthetic cream: a case report. *Paediatric Nursing* 10(21): 22–23.

Higgins C (1995a) Haematology testing. *Nursing Times* 91(7): 38–40.

Higgins C (1995b) Measuring renal function with urea and creatinine tests. *Nursing Times* 90(51): 35–36.

Hoetke LB (2006) *The Complete Textbook of Phlebotomy*, 3rd edn. Thomson Delmar Learning, Canada.

Holmes K (1998) Comparison of push pull versus discard method from central venous catheters for blood testing. *Journal of Intravenous Nursing* 21(5): 282–285.

Hudek K (1986) Compliance in intravenous therapy. *Journal of the Canadian Intravenous Nursing Association* 2(3): 7–8.

Infection Control Nurses Association (ICNA) (2003) *Reducing Sharps Injury—Prevention and Risk Management*. Infection Control Nurses Association, London.

Infusion Nurses Society (INS) (2006) Infusion nursing standards of practice. *Journal of Infusion Nursing* 29 (1S).

Kaloupek DG, Scott JR, Khatami V (1985) Assessment of coping strategies associated with syncope in blood donors. *Journal of Psychosomatic Research* 29(2): 207–214.

Kamimota V, Olson K (1996) Using normal saline to lock peripheral intravenous catheters in ambulatory cancer patients. *Journal of Intravenous Nursing* 19(2): 75–78.

Kaplan M (1983) Viewpoint: the cancer patient. *Cancer Nursing* 6(2): 103–107.

Keller CA (1994) Method of drawing blood samples through central venous catheters in paediatric patients undergoing bone marrow transplant. *Oncology Nursing Forum* 21: 879–884.

Kelley L, Sklar DP, Johnson DR, Tandberg D (1997) Women's perceptions of pain and distress during intravenous catheterization and urethral mini-catheterization. *American Journal of Emergency Medicine* 15: 570–572.

Keradag A, Gorgulu S (2000) Vialon better than teflon. *Journal of Intravenous Nursing* 23(3): 158–66.

Kerrison T, Woodhull J (1994) Reducing the risk of thrombophlebitis—comparison of teflon and vialon cannulae. *Professional Nurse* 9(10): 662–666.

Koppel S (1999) Treating needle phobia. *Practice Nursing* 10(7): 12–13.

Kupensky DT (1998) Applying current research to influence clinical practice—utilization of midline catheters. *Journal of Intravenous Nursing* 21(5): 271–4.

Lander J, Fowler-Kerry S (1992) TENS for children's procedural pain. *Pain* 52: 209–216.

Larson PJ (1984) Important nurse caring behaviours perceived by patients with cancer. *Oncology Nursing Forum* 11(6): 46–50.

Lavery I (2003) Peripheral cannulation and gaining consent. *Nursing Standard* 17(28): 40–42.

Lavery I, Ingram P (2005) Venepuncture: best practice. *Nursing Standard* 19(49): 55–65.

Lenhardt R, Seybold T, Kimberger O *et al.* (2002) Local warming and insertion of peripheral venous cannulae: single blinded prospective randomised controlled trial and single blinded randomised crossover trial. *British Medical Journal* 325: 409.

Levine FM, De Simone LL (1991) The effects of experimenter gender on pain report in male and female subjects. *Pain* 44: 69–72.

Lucker P, Stahlheber-Dilg B (2003) Pain related to optiva 2, biovalve and Venflon 2 intravenous catheters. *British Journal of Nursing* 12(22): 1345–1351.

McCall RE, Tankersley CM (2003) *Phlebotomy Essentials*, 3rd edn. Lippincott Williams & Wilkins, Philadelphia.

McKee JM, Shell JA, Warren TA, Campbell VP (1989) Complications of intravenous therapy: a randomised prospective study–Vialon vs teflon. *Journal of Intravenous Nursing* 12(5): 288–295.

Macklin D, Chernecky C (2004) *IV Therapy*. Saunders, Missouri.

Maki DG (1976) Preventing infection in IV therapy. *Hospital Practice* 11(4): 95–104.

Maki DG (1991) *Improving Catheter Site Care*. Royal Society of Medicine Services Ltd, London.

Maki DG, Ringer M (1987) Evaluation of dressing regimes for prevention of infection with peripheral IV catheters. *Journal of the American Medical Association* 258(17): 2396–2403.

Marks I (1988) Blood injury phobia: a review. *American Journal of Psychiatry* 145(10): 1207–1213.

Marsigliese AM (2001)Evaluation of comfort level and complication rates as determined by peripheral intravenous catheter sites. *CINA Journal* 26–39.

Masoorli S (2002) Catheter related nerve injury: inherent risk or avoidable outcome. *Journal of Vascular Access Devices* 7(4): 49.

Mavissakalian M, Barlow DH (1981) *Phobia, Psychological and Pharmacological Treatment*. The Guildford Press, New York.

Mayer DK (1987) Oncology nurses' versus cancer patients' perceptions of nurse caring behaviours: a replication study. *Oncology Nursing Forum* 14(3): 48–52.

Medical Devices Agency (MDA) (2000) Single-use medical devices: implications and consequences of reuse. In: *Device Bulletin 2000*, 04. Department of Health, London.

Medicines and Healthcare products Regulatory Agency (MHRA) (2005a) *Alert MDA 2005/01 and Device Bulletin DB 2005(01). Reporting Adverse Incidents and Disseminating Medical Device Alerts*. Medicines and Healthcare products Regulatory Agency, London.

Medicine and Healthcare products Regulatory Agency (2005b) *Medical Device Alert on all Brands of Needle Free Intravascular Connectors*, MDA/2005/030, issued 17 May 2005. Medicines and Healthcare products Regulatory Agency, London.

Miaskowski C (1997) Women and pain. *Critical Care Nursing Clinics of North America* 9(4): 453–458.

Middleton J (1985) Don't needle the patient. *Nursing Mirror* 161(4): 22–24.

Millam D (1992) Starting IVs—how to develop your venipuncture skills. *Nursing* 92: 33–46.

Millam D (1993) How to teach good venipuncture technique. *American Journal of Nursing* 93(7): 38–41.

Millam D (1995) The use of anaesthesia in IV therapy. *Journal of Vascular Access Devices* 1(1): 22–29.

Mills RT, Krantz DS (1979) Information, choice and reactions to stress. A field experiment in a blood bank with laboratory analogue. *Journal of Personality and Social Psychology* 3(4): 608–620.

Mitchell Higgs N (2002) *Personal protective equipment—improving compliance*. All points conference. Safer Needles Network, London.

Morris S (1996) Jab-fear woman is saved from herself. *Mail on Sunday.*

Moureau N, Iannucci AL (2003) Catheter securement: trends in performance and complications associated with the use of either traditional methods or adhesive anchor devices; *Journal of Vascular Access Devices* Spring: 29–33.

National Audit Office (NAO) (2003) *A Safer Place To Work—Management of Health and Safety Risks in Trusts*. National Audit Office, London.

NHS Employers (2005) *The Management of Health, Safety and Welfare Issues for NHS Staff*. NHS Confederation (Employers) Company Ltd, London.

National Institute for Clinical Excellence (NICE)((2003) *Infection Control—Prevention of Healthcare Associated Infection in Primary and Community Care*. Clinical Guideline 2. National Institute for Health and Clinical Excellence, London.

Nightingale KW, Bradshaw EG (1982) A review of peripheral cannulae. *British Journal of Intravenous Therapy* 3(4): 14–23. *of Clinical Lab Studies*. Williams and Wilkins, Baltimore, pp. 870–873.

Nursing and Midwifery Council (NMC) (2004) *The NMC Code of Professional Conduct: Standards for Conduct Performance and Ethics*. Nursing and Midwifery Council, London.

Ost LG (1991) Acquisition of blood and injection phobia and anxiety response patterns in clinical patients. *Behavioural Research and Therapy* 29(4): 323–332.

Ost LG (1992) Blood and injection phobia: background and cognitive psychological and behavioural variables. *Journal of Abnormal Psychology* 101(1): 68–74.

Patel MX, Baker D, Nosarti C (2005) Injection phobia: A systematic review of psychological treatments. *Behavioural and Cognitive Psychotherapy* 33: 343–349.

Pavlin DJ, Links S, Rapp SE, Neesley ML, Keyes HJ (1993) Vasovagal reactions in ambulatory surgery centre. *Anesthesia and Analgesia* 76: 931–935.

Payne-James JJ, Rogers J, Bray MJ, Rana SK, McSwiggon D, Silk DB (1991) Development of thrombophlebitis in peripheral veins with Vialon and PTFE-teflon cannulas: a double blind randomised controlled trial. *Annals of the Royal College of Surgeons of England* 73: 322–325.

Perucca R (2001) Obtaining vascular access. In: Hankin J *et al.*, eds. *Intravenous therapy: in clinical practice*, 2nd edn, pp. 375–388. WB Saunders, Philadelphia.

Peters JL, Frame JD, Dawson SM (1984) Peripheral venous cannulation: reducing the risks. *British Journal of Parenteral Therapy* 5: 56–58.

Phillips L (2005) *Manual of IV therapeutics*, 4th edn. FA Davis, Philadelphia.

Powers FA (1999) Can you keep her safe? *Nursing* 99: 54–5.

Rogers P, Gournay K (2001) Phobias: nature, assessment and treatment. *Nursing Standard* 15(30): 37–43.

Rowland R (1991) Making sense of venepuncture. *Nursing Times* 87(32): 41–43.

Section 2

Royal College of Nursing (RCN) (2005) *Standards for Infusion Therapy*. Royal College of Nursing, London.

Ryder M (2001) The role of biofilm in vascular catheter related infections. *New Developments in Vascular Disease* 2(2): 15–25.

Sagar DP, Bomar SK (1982) *Intravenous Medications*. JB Lippincott, Philadelphia, pp. 12–21.

Scales K (2005) Vascular access: a guide to peripheral venous cannulation. *Nursing Standard* 19(49): 48–52.

Smith B (2006) Peripheral intravenous catheter dwell times. *Journal of Infusion Nursing* 29(1): 14–17.

Sommer SR, Warekois RS, Robinson R (2002) *Phlebotomy Workbook and Procedures Manual*. WB Saunders, Philadelphia.

Springhouse (2002) *IV Therapy Made Incredibly Easy*, 2nd edn. Lippincott Williams & Wilkins, Philadelphia.

Stark MM, Brener N (2000) Needle phobia. *Journal of Clinical Forensic Medicine* 7: 35–38.

Steel J, Taylor R, Lloyd G (1986) Behaviour therapy for phobia of venepuncture. *Diabetic Medicine* 3: 481.

Tagalakis V, Kahn SR, Libman M, Blostein M (2002) The epidemiology of peripheral vein infusion thrombophlebitis: a critical review. *The American Journal of Medicine* 113: 146–151.

Tully JL, Friedland GH, Baldrini LM, Goldmann DA (1981) Complications of intravenous therapy with steel needles and teflon catheters: a comparative study. *The American Journal of Medicine* 70: 702–706.

Usichenko TI, Pavlovic D, Foellner S, Wendt M (2004) Reducing venipuncture pain by a cough trick: a randomized crossover volunteer study. *Anesthesia and Analgesia* 98: 343–345.

Van den Berg AA, Abeysekera RM (1993) Rationalising venous cannulation: patient factors and lignocaine efficacy. *Anaesthesia* 48(1): 84.

Verity E (1993) The fear that condemned a man to die in agony. *Daily Mail*, 1 July 1993.

Verity R (2004) Specimen collection. In: Dougherty L, Lister S, eds. *The Royal Marsden NHS Trust Manual of Clinical Nursing Procedures*, 6th edn, pp. 663–676. Blackwell Publishing, Oxford.

Walther K (2001) Intravenous therapy in the older adult In: Hankin J *et al.*, eds. *Intravenous Therapy in Clinical Practice*, 2nd edn, pp. 592–603. WB Saunders, Philadelphia.

Webster D, Pellegrini L, Duffy K (1992) Use of transcutaneous electrical neural stimulation for fingertip analgesia: a pilot study. *Annals of Emergency Medicine* 21: 1472–1475.

Weinstein SM (2007) *Plumer's Principles and Practice of Intravenous Therapy*, 8th edn. JB Lippincott, Philadelphia.

Weller BF (2005) *Baillières Nurses Dictionary*, 24th edn. Elsevier, Edinburgh.

Wendler MC (2003) Effects of Tellington Touch in healthy adults awaiting venipuncture. *Research in Nursing and Health* 26: 40–52.

Whitson M (1996) Intravenous therapy in the older adult: special need and considerations. *Journal of Intravenous Nursing* 19(5): 251–255.

Wilson Barnett J (1976) Patients' emotional reactions to hospitalisation: an exploratory study. *Journal of Advanced Nursing* 1: 351–358.

Witt B (2004) Venepuncture. In: Dougherty L, Lister S, eds. *The Royal Marsden NHS Trust Manual of Clinical Nursing Procedures*, 6th edn, pp. 774–785. Blackwell Publishing, Oxford.

Yuan RTW, Cohan MD (1987) Lateral antebrachial cutaneous nerve injury as a complication of phlebotomy. *Journal of Canadian Intravenous Nurses Association* 3(3): 16–17.

CHAPTER 10

Vascular Access in the Acute Care Setting

Katie Scales

Introduction

Intravenous (i.v.) access is necessary for the reliable and predictable administration of medications and fluids when the traditional oral route is no longer appropriate or possible. The selection of the vascular access device (VAD) will be dependent upon the nature and duration of treatment as well as the severity of illness and the potential for adverse change in the condition of the patient.

In acute care, access may be required for the administration of fluids and electrolytes, blood products, medications, parenteral nutrition and dialysis. In critical care environments access may also be required for haemodynamic monitoring, haemofiltration, transvenous pacing or biopsy procedures. These procedures require central venous access. Central venous access is the route of choice when administering vasoactive medications such as inotropes and vasodilators. These drugs are administered centrally in conjunction with arterial monitoring in order to provide real-time haemodynamic information which will allow titration of the medications within agreed haemodynamic parameters. Central venous access is also the route of choice if the drugs or fluids to be administered are irritant to peripheral veins due to extremes of pH or osmolarity and have the potential to cause tissue necrosis should extravasation occur. The local concentration of a drug often determines the degree of irritation to the vessel. High concentrations of drugs entering a small, low-flow vessel will cause a high intravascular concentration and can result in local inflammation (phlebitis); the same drug further diluted or delivered into a high-flow vessel will result in a lower intravascular concentration and less inflammation (Soni 1989). The ability to further dilute drugs will depend largely on the clinical condition of the patient (e.g. their ventricular or renal function) and the stability of the drug in a more dilute solution.

Once seen as a last resort, the use of central venous access is now commonplace for an increasing number of patients in the acute hospital setting. Despite this trend, the use of more traditional access routes should not be forgotten as the use of central venous access is not without risk. Muhm (2002) estimates the risk of major and minor complications to be as high as 10% and healthcare workers must evaluate the relative advantages and disadvantages when selecting the most appropriate route for intravenous therapy. Unfortunately, vascular access devices carry a significant and often underestimated risk of iatrogenic disease, most commonly bloodstream infections associated with infection of the device or contamination of the solutions infused through the device (Maki & Crnich 2003).

Because of the significant morbidity and mortality associated with central venous catheters a risk–benefit analysis must be undertaken to ensure that their use is reserved for patients for whom the benefits outweigh the risks.

Peripheral Venous Access

Peripheral access should not be excluded from the management of acute-care patients. Peripheral venous access is associated with fewer complications than central venous access, but there are also limitations to its use.

There are many sites of potential peripheral venous access, and some are more advantageous than others. Arm veins have the benefit of easy access but the disadvantage of flexure points and close proximity to arterial structures. Leg veins can hamper mobility and are associated with an increased risk of venous thrombosis.

The choice of site and the size of cannula will be determined by the indication for its placement (Soni 1989). For example, patients who require fluid resuscitation need a large cannula in a large vein which can be accessed at the first attempt. By contrast, patients who require elective low-risk drug administration need a smaller cannula with more attention paid to patient convenience and comfort.

In acute settings such as the emergency department or the anaesthetic room, large-gauge cannulae are often selected to facilitate large-volume fluid replacement in patients who are considered to be at high risk of haemorrhage or circulatory collapse. A 14- or 16-gauge cannula is usually selected. A 45-mm, 16-gauge peripheral cannula is capable of infusing on average 14 litres of crystalloid per hour (Scales 2005), twice as quickly as a 20-cm 16-gauge central venous catheter.

In the conscious patient, large peripheral cannulae can be associated with significant pain and can contribute to the development of cannulation-related anxiety. Research demonstrates that the pain associated with insertion, the residual pain of the *in situ* cannula and the anxiety associated with cannulation can all be reduced by the use of local anaesthetic creams before cannulation (Spiers *et al.* 2001). Dennis *et al.* (1995) demonstrated that, despite the publication of conclusive research into the use of local anaesthesia for peripheral cannulation, 46% of the anaesthetists surveyed were unaware of it. They also concluded that junior anaesthetists were less likely to use local anaesthesia than their more experienced colleagues.

Traditionally it has been recommended that peripheral cannulae be replaced every 48–72 hours because of the infection risks associated with their use (Collin *et al.* 1975; Maki & Ringer 1987; Soni 1989). However, since these early papers were written, cannula design has improved significantly and most modern peripheral cannulae are made from polyurethane rather than Teflon or polyvinyl chloride (PVC). Polyurethane catheters are associated with reduced phlebitis as the material softens after insertion and causes less wear and tear to the tunica intima of the peripheral vein (Gaukroger *et al.* 1988; Jensen 2001). Modern polyurethane catheters can remain *in situ* for 72–96 hours but cannulae made from more rigid materials should still not remain *in situ* for longer than 48–72 hours (RCN 2005). Peripheral cannulae that have been inserted in an emergency, where aseptic technique may have been compromised, should be replaced within 24 hours (RCN 2005).

In the shocked patient whose peripheral circulation is shut down, the palpation of peripheral vessels may be impossible. It is relatively commonplace to attempt central venous access in the absence of peripheral veins; however, in patients with trauma to the trunk and abdomen, central venous access may prove equally difficult and potentially hazardous.

> **BOX 10.1**
>
> **A technique for venous cut-down of the saphenous vein at the ankle**
>
> - Locate the vein—2 cm above and anterior to the medial malleolus.
> - Make a transverse incision in the skin over the vein.
> - Locate the vein using blunt dissection with forceps or scissors.
> - Place ties around the vein, a lower one tying off the vessel, and another one higher up.
> - Incise the vein, taking care not to cut through it, and introduce the cannula into the vessel.
> - Flush the cannula to check patency.
> - Use the upper tie to secure the cannula.

Cut-Down Venous Access

This once common technique has become largely redundant since the establishment of central venous access as a routine method of drug and fluid administration in the critically ill patient.

In the event that cut-down access is required, a large vein which is not prone to anatomical inconsistency is usually selected (Soni 1989). It is important to have an understanding of the related anatomy if complications are to be avoided. For example, when cutting down to a vein in the antecubital fossa, it is important to know that the area also contains the brachial artery and the median nerve. The most common sites for cut-down access are the veins of the antecubital fossa and the saphenous vein at the ankle (Soni 1989). This procedure is usually restricted to medical personnel with appropriate skills as it requires a surgical technique to locate and access the vein. The development of what is now referred to as the 'Seldinger technique' for insertion of central venous catheters and improvements in technology have all but eliminated the need for surgical cut-down in order to gain access to the venous circulation. Cut-downs should no longer be performed routinely (RCN 2005).

A technique for venous cut-down of the saphenous vein at the ankle, as recommended by Soni (1989), is given in Box 10.1.

Central Venous Access

The actual number of central venous catheters (CVCs) inserted annually in the UK is unknown. In 1993 Elliot estimated the number to be 200 000 annually and this number is certain to have risen. In 2001 it was reported that the USA purchased more than 150 million VADs annually and that of these approximately 5 million were CVCs (Mermel *et al.* 2001).

Central veins are usually considered to be veins that lie within the thorax and which are in direct continuity with the right atrium (*See* Figure 10.1). Access to the central veins can be achieved from several approaches: internal or external jugular, subclavian, femoral or peripheral veins. Each site has its relative indications and most appropriate technique.

Site Selection

The cubital fossa

This is an established route into the central venous system and has the advantage of a low incidence of mechanical complications (Mermel *et al.* 2001). It is also advantageous

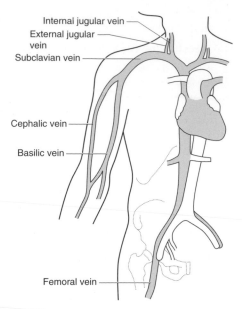

Internal jugular vein

External jugular vein

Subclavian vein

Cephalic vein

Basilic vein

Femoral vein

Figure 10.1　The central veins.

for the patient who cannot tolerate the supine position traditionally required for CVC insertion. The cubital fossa allows percutaneous cannulation of the basilic, cephalic and median cubital veins (RCN 2005) or cut-down cannulation of the brachial vein (Seneff 1987a). The introduction of ultrasound guidance has all but eliminated the need to cut down to the brachial vein to obtain access via the antecubital fossa.

The first report of a peripherally inserted central catheter (PICC) was in 1929 when Forssman, a German physician, passed a 4-FG ureteric catheter up to his heart via a wide-bore needle in his cubital fossa (Abi-Nader 1993). The use of the basilic or saphenous vein catheter was reported by Hughes and Magovern (1959) for the assessment of central venous pressure.

In these early years, the catheter materials were relatively rigid and resulted in a high incidence of thrombosis, malposition, sepsis and phlebitis (Abi-Nader 1993). In 1962, the first silicone elastomer (silastic) catheter was introduced, but there was no method of advancing this soft, malleable catheter into the central circulation. In the 1970s a spring stylet was introduced which produced enough rigidity for the catheter to be threaded into the central circulation (Abi-Nader 1993). A range of PICC devices are now available.

Complications as a result of PICC insertion are in general more minor when compared to traditional central venous access routes; however, PICC placement is not without complication. In a study of 332 consecutively placed PICCs Loughran and Borzatta (1995) reported a 9.7% incidence of catheter fracture. Lowenthal *et al.* (2002) reported the most common complications to be phlebitis, malposition and tip migration. Controversy exists about the dwell time for PICCs—early studies from the 1960s (utilizing older catheter materials, e.g. polyethylene) suggested that a PICC inserted via the cubital fossa should not be left *in situ* in excess of 72 hours. More modern catheter materials, such as elastomeric polyurethane or silicone, which are considered to be more flexible and biocompatible, are designed for more prolonged use. In a study by Cardella *et al.* (1993) the average dwell time was 72.7 days (range 2–307 days). However, in the intensive care setting, PICCs carry a similar risk of infection to that seen in non-cuffed multilumen CVCs (Maki & Crnich 2003) and cannot be recommended for long-term use.

The incidence of complications associated with the use of PICCs is reported to have been reduced by the introduction of novel securement devices that do not involve sutures (Maki & Crnich 2002).

The femoral vein

The femoral vein is a well-established access route with relatively consistent anatomy. The femoral artery lies lateral to the femoral vein in the region of the inguinal ligament, and the femoral nerve lies lateral to the artery. This is usually a relatively easy access site for the inexperienced operator, and should the femoral artery be punctured, pressure is easy to apply.

Some medical personnel shy away from the femoral vein as a routine access route because of the potential risk of infection. This concern is supported by the recent critical analysis of the evidence undertaken by Pellowe *et al.* (2004) who state that

> femoral catheters have been demonstrated to have relatively high colonization rates when used in adults and should be avoided.

Timsit *et al.* (1999) suggest tunnelling non-cuffed acute-care femoral CVCs in order to reduce the incidence of bacterial colonization in the critically ill, and demonstrated a fourfold reduction in the incidence of septic complications. The use of a tunnel to reduce infective complications was supported by Nahum *et al.* (2002) in a study of critically ill children.

Merrer *et al.* (2001) demonstrated a statistically significant increase in the incidence of infective and thrombotic complications when femoral venous access was compared with the subclavian site in critically ill adults. Whilst the evidence may support the use of one specific route over another, in practice we are rarely dealing with the ideal situation. Long-term critical illness will require site rotation of VADs and specific clinical conditions may make the recommended routes impossible. As in all aspects of medicine a risk–benefit analysis will be required and the best vascular access route for the given situation will be selected.

There has also been concern over the incidence of false aneurysm in the femoral artery. In practical terms this is exceptionally rare, far less common than a pneumothorax following subclavian vein cannulation. Seneff (1987a) pointed out that during resuscitation, the femoral vein can provide central access without the need to stop chest compressions.

A retrospective case-matched controlled study by Gutierrez *et al.* (2003) found that children with diabetic ketoacidosis (DKA) had an increased incidence of deep vein thrombosis (DVT) associated with the placement of femoral CVCs. This finding was supported by Worly *et al.* (2004); both studies demonstrated a 50% incidence of DVT when femoral CVCs were used in children with DKA. It is therefore recommended that femoral CVCs are avoided for children with DKA (Worly *et al.* 2004).

The more rare complications of femoral vein cannulation include massive scrotal haemorrhage (Sung *et al.* 1981) and arteriovenous fistula formation (Fuller *et al.* 1976).

The external jugular

The external jugular vein can be used for central vascular access, although its high incidence of anomalous anatomy and its severe angle with the subclavian vein make it an unpopular choice. In its favour is the relatively low risk of pneumothorax and the fact that it is part of the surface anatomy of the neck and therefore easily located. Soni (1989) suggested that its superficial nature may make it more susceptible to sepsis and therefore less suitable as a long-term access route.

The major disadvantage of this access site is the difficulty in threading a catheter into the central circulation. The tight angle with the subclavian can be difficult to negotiate, even

Section 2

with the help of a 'J' wire. Soni (1989) emphasized the need for radiographic placement of catheters inserted via the external jugular site in view of the cannulation difficulties.

When this vein is selected, it is not uncommon to find that the operator has used a peripheral cannula to access it, rather than the traditionally longer central catheter. It is important to establish whether this is the case as minimal cannula dislodgement could lead to extravasation, with the associated hazard of haemorrhage, infiltration and loss of systemic effects of the drug being infused.

In an unusual study that sought to use the size of the external jugular vein as a predictor of the size of the internal jugular vein, Stickle and McFarlane (1997) used ultrasound to assess the diameter of the internal jugular whilst visualizing the external jugular vein. They found that there was an inverse relationship between the size of the vessels: a large external jugular vein was an accurate predictor of a small internal jugular vein. No other patient dimension (height, weight, BMI, neck circumference) predicted internal jugular vein diameter. The results suggest that a large external jugular vein of 7 mm or greater is a predictor of a small internal jugular vein (Stickle & McFarlane 1997).

Complication from external jugular catheterization is rare, but Ghani and Berry (1983) reported four cases of hydrothorax 24–48 hours after external jugular vein cannulation. It was presumed that the catheter tip had rested transversely across the wall of the superior vena cava (SVC) and that this had led to erosion and subsequent infusion of fluids directly into the pleural space.

The internal jugular

The internal jugular vein is probably the most common site for central venous access. Seneff (1987b) stated that its high success rate and low incidence of complications make it an extremely good site for central venous catheterization. He believes the main complications of this approach to be carotid artery puncture and laceration of local neck structures from needle probing. Soni (1989) suggested the main contraindication to the internal jugular approach to be coagulopathy, as this is a relatively blind technique which punctures a deeply situated vein in close proximity to the carotid artery. These concerns may be reduced by the use of two-dimensional (2-D) ultrasound guidance. This has been recommended as the preferred method of insertion of CVCs into the internal jugular vein in adults and children in elective situations since guidance was issued by the National Institute for Health and Clinical Excellence (NICE) in 2002. NICE (2002) also recommend that 2-D ultrasound be considered in most clinical circumstances, whether elective or emergency. A confidential postal survey of consultant paediatric anaesthetists in the UK revealed that despite the NICE guidance only 39% of the anaesthetists who responded to the survey used 2-D ultrasound routinely for the insertion of internal jugular vein CVCs (Bosman & Kavanagh 2006) though 75% of responders believed that there should be training on the use of 2-D ultrasound and that it should be available if required.

Anatomically the neck is highly innervated and both the insertion procedure and the residual cannula can cause extreme tenderness to the patient. The vagus nerve lies in a posterior position between the internal jugular vein and the carotid artery, and the sympathetic trunk lies behind the vagus. The phrenic nerve lies lateral and posterior to the internal jugular vein (Woodburne & Burkel 1994). Damage to the sympathetic chain by either needle puncture or infiltration with local anaesthetic can lead to Horner's syndrome (Soni 1989; Doğan *et al.* 2005), which is the term given to a collection of symptoms arising from damage to sympathetic nerves in the cervical region. The syndrome includes a constricted pupil, ptosis and an absence of sweat gland activity over the affected side of the face.

In practice, catheters in the internal jugular vein can provide a nursing challenge. Beard growth in men, diaphoresis in the febrile patient and poor control of oral secretions in the patient with altered consciousness or swallowing difficulties can all lead to problems with fixation of the catheter and the need for repeated dressing of the site. Invariably the catheter or its associated administration sets and connections are in close proximity to the patient's hair.

Inadequate fixation of the catheter can lead to increased mobility and subsequent mechanical thrombophlebitis. Soni (1989) suggested that head movement may contribute to catheter movement and subsequent contamination of the site. Regular observation of the site for signs of inflammation or infection is required.

The subclavian

In adult patients the subclavian site is the preferred site from the perspective of infection control (Pellowe *et al.* 2004), but the use of this site is not without clinical risk (Soni 1989).

The technique of subclavian vein catheterization was first described by Aubaniac (1952) and there continues to be debate over the advantages of using this site.

Before the introduction of modern, high-specification catheterization kits, this was often considered as a last-resort access route and was approached with a great deal of respect. The literature reports a range of complications—some fatal—and by the late 1960s there were calls for this route to be abandoned (Shapira & Stern 1967). There has been a revival in the popularity of the site, perhaps due to the increased amount of long-term access or perhaps because of the realization that no site is perfect. Soni (1989) suggested that, with the recent increase in use of this site, there has also been an increase in the complacency with which the venepuncture is performed. He postulated that the operator who has never experienced a complication from this site has either not performed very many or has been exceptionally lucky. Gopal *et al.* (2006) also demonstrated in a prospective study that a nurse-led subclavian CVC service was both safe and effective.

Soni (1989) cited coagulopathy as one of the most significant contraindications to the selection of this access route. The subclavian vein is located in close proximity to the artery, and in view of the relatively 'blind' nature of the technique, arterial puncture is a significant complication. Once arterial puncture has occurred, it may be impossible to arrest the bleeding as there is no point at which pressure can be applied to the artery. A surgical repair via thoracotomy may be the only solution though the literature does report the use of an endovascular stent to repair iatrogenic injuries to the subclavian artery (Bartorelli *et al.* 2001).

The subclavian is probably the most popular and convenient site for long-term venous access. It is easy to secure the catheter to the chest wall, and as a result there are fewer incidents of mechanically induced thrombophlebitis and infection.

The commonly acknowledged complications of this route reflect the structures that are in close proximity to the subclavian vein. Soni (1989) noted that the pleura, subclavian artery, phrenic nerve and even the trachea are all within easy reach of 'a misguided needle'. He also noted that a guidewire that has been forced can end up in the mediastinum, as can a catheter.

Pneumothorax is usually considered to be the most common complication of subclavian vein catheterization; however, in a meta-analysis of the literature Ruesch *et al.* (2002) identified catheter tip malposition as the most commonly occurring complication. The incidence of catheter tip malposition from internal jugular and subclavian CVCs was 5.3% and 9.3% respectively. In the prospective nurse-led study by Gopal *et al.* (2006) involving a total of 348 catheter insertions the incidence of pneumothorax was 1%. The presentation of the pneumothorax may be immediate or delayed. Even if a 'check X-ray' has been performed, it is not uncommon to discover a small pneumothorax a couple of days after the insertion of the catheter (Soni 1989). The incidence of pneumothorax can increase significantly if the patient is undergoing positive pressure ventilation and may present as a tension pneumothorax.

Section 2

Subclavian artery puncture is reported to be as frequent a complication as pneumothorax but the literature comes mainly from the 1970s, before the introduction of modern catheterization kits. Soni (1989) believes the incidence to be lower than for pneumothorax. Seneff (1987b) suggested that a platelet count of less than 50 000 or a partial thromboplastine time (PTT) ratio greater than 3 predisposes the patient to haemorrhage. Fatal subclavian artery haemorrhage as a complication of subclavian vein catheterization is reported in the literature as recently as 1995 (Mercer-Jones *et al.* 1995). In a meta-analysis of the literature Ruesch *et al.* (2002) concluded that the incidence of arterial puncture was greater using the internal jugular approach (3%) than it was using the subclavian approach (0.5%). Gopal *et al.* (2006) reported a 4% incidence of arterial puncture.

Another acknowledged complication is subclavian vein thrombosis. There is much in the literature to support the existence of thrombosis (Hansen & Christensen 1983; Maurer *et al.* 1984; Weiner *et al.* 1984), but the reports are inconsistent because of the range of criteria used to diagnose the condition. Seneff (1987b) considered this complication to be underdiagnosed. De Cicco *et al.* (1997) reported a high incidence of subclavian vein thrombosis associated with the use of silastic catheters in cancer patients. The work of De Cicco *et al.* suggests that the thrombosis risk is highest in the first few days after insertion and that the left subclavian vein is associated with a greater incidence of thrombosis than the right subclavian vein.

The literature is more consistent in reporting the thrombogenic nature of the subclavian vein when used for large-bore, double-lumen renal catheters (Barton *et al.* 1983; Vanherweghem 1986; Brady *et al.* 1989; Cimochowski *et al.* 1990). In a retrospective study by Trerotola *et al.* (2000) 774 dialysis catheters placed under radiological guidance in either the internal jugular or the subclavian vein were evaluated. Trerotola and colleagues demonstrated an increased incidence of thrombosis in the subclavian group (13% versus 3%) and the mean time to thrombosis was 36 days for the subclavian catheters compared to 142 days for the internal jugular catheters. Evidence suggests that the internal jugular vein is the optimal access route for short-term non-tunnelled and longer-term tunnelled dialysis catheters (National Kidney Foundation 1997; Trerotola *et al.* 2000).

Seneff (1987b) suggested that the incidence of thrombosis is proportional to the length of time that the catheter remains *in situ*. However, he acknowledged that the mechanism is inconclusive as there are reports of subclavian thrombosis after unsuccessful attempts at subclavian cannulation (Weiner *et al.* 1984).

In the early 1980s there were many reports of subclavian vein thrombosis associated with the use of parenteral nutrition (PN) (Padberg *et al.* 1981; Fabri *et al.* 1982; Ross *et al.* 1982). However, it is difficult to find specific evidence of this in current literature. Whether this reflects changes in clinical management as PN is used far less frequently in critically ill patients now than it was 20 years ago, or whether this reflects improvement in catheter design is unknown. Seneff (1987b) postulated that the hyperosmolar nature of PN could be a contributive factor to the development of thrombosis.

Seneff (1987a) suggested that there are no absolute contraindications to CVC placement in patients who require it, although there may be absolute contraindications to specific approaches. For example, subclavian access should be avoided in patients whose baseline respiratory function would not tolerate a pneumothorax.

Catheter Selection

The ideal catheter should fulfil several important criteria. It should:

- carry a low risk of infection
- be non-thrombogenic
- be hypoallergenic

- be atraumatic to the intimal lining of the blood vessel
- have a smooth surface to prevent the attraction of cells and microorganisms
- be easy to insert
- be comfortable for the patient
- have an inherent tensile strength to withstand normal wear and tear, thus preventing catheter embolism
- be radio-opaque.

Given the known complications of CVCs, it is essential that modern catheters are routinely manufactured with luer-lock fittings and, where possible, in-line clamps. Elliot *et al.* (1994) advocated that catheters should have graduated markings to facilitate placement and monitoring of their position, and recommended that they be kink resistant and have a means of securing them to the skin.

There is an enormous range of CVCs on the market. Modern catheters are biocompatible and many utilize novel technology to reduce the risk of catheter-related bloodstream infection (CRBSI). When choosing a catheter for central access, it is important to consider the intended use and duration of placement in order that the correct catheter is selected.

Even in the short term, if the therapy to be delivered is damaging to blood vessels (e.g. PN, chemotherapy or concentrated inotropes) then central access will be required to facilitate haemodilution and safe administration of the products. In general, if the pH of the product to be administered is less than 5 or greater than 9, or if the osmolarity of the final solution is greater than 500 mOsm/L, a CVC will be required (Bard 2006).

Short-term therapies usually justify the placement of non-tunnelled, percutaneous CVCs, though it is acknowledged that this VAD carries the highest incidence of CRBSI (Maki & Crnich 2003). Several weeks or months of therapy may indicate the need for a PICC or other longer-term catheter, while long-term therapies will require the placement of long-term tunnelled catheters or implantable devices (Gabriel *et al.* 2005).

The selection of a multilumen device will depend on the range of therapies required, the compatibility of the therapies and the need for sampling or monitoring access. Multilumen catheters may have two, three, four or five lumens. Complex catheters such as cardiac output (CO) catheters may have five or more lumens. In general, the greater the number of lumens the greater the diameter of the catheter.

Other considerations for device selection include the general medical history of the patient, their activity level, an evaluation of their peripheral veins and the landmarks for locating central veins, their psychological needs and the duration of the intended therapy. The medical team should not be solely responsible for the selection of the device; where appropriate, the patient or their carer should be involved in the decision-making process. This is more of an issue for longer term therapy than for the emergency setting (Gabriel 2000).

Catheter materials

Early catheters were made of rigid materials such as polyethylene, polyvinyl chloride and Teflon. The rigidity of these materials meant that insertion was easy, even over long distances. These materials have largely been superseded as they had a tendency to damage the intimal lining of the vessel, causing platelet aggregation and thrombus formation (Hadaway 2001). The more modern polyurethane catheters show less thrombogenicity than their predecessors, are rigid enough to facilitate insertion, but then become more pliable as they attain body temperature. Baranowski (1993) noted the superior tensile strength of the polyurethane catheter and that this allows the manufacture of thinner-walled catheters, which subsequently reduces the degree of vessel obstruction caused by the catheter. Some catheter manufacturers have further enhanced the biocompatibility of the polyurethane catheter by constructing the tip out of a silicone elastomer (silastic) material, thus reducing the likelihood of intimal damage to the blood vessel.

Silastic is a lightweight material which floats within the blood vessel, and is therefore less likely to cause damage to the vessel wall (Baranowski 1993). Some short-term catheters are made of this material, but they require specialized insertion techniques and it is more common to see polyurethane catheters for short-term acute-care use. The majority of longer-term access catheters are designed using this type of material.

Topography

The topography of the catheter surface is of importance. Catheter surfaces that are uneven or pitted can promote the adherence of platelets and microorganisms. It is thought that a catheter's relative thrombogenicity predisposes the patient to an increased risk of bacterial colonization and subsequent septicaemia (Elliott 1988; Lopez-Lopez *et al.* 1991). A number of bacteria (in particular coagulase-negative staphylococci) excrete a carbohydrate-based 'slime' which coats intravascular catheters and helps microorganisms to bond to them. This substance is known as a microbial biofilm. The organisms embed themselves in the biofilm which provides a degree of protection from antibiotics and subsequently reduces the effectiveness of antibiotic therapy (Kamal *et al.* 1991). Much work has been done over the last decade to improve our understanding of the biofilms that are now known to be associated with CVCs (Costerton *et al.* 1999; Murga *et al.* 2001; Ryder 2001; Wilcox *et al.* 2001).

Another concern is the development of a fibrin sheath along the length of the catheter. Within seconds of insertion, intravascular catheters are coated with plasma proteins and subsequently with platelets (Kristinsson 1989). Some catheter materials are more predisposed to platelet attraction than others (Borow & Crowley 1985). Within 5–7 days, this coating will have developed into a fibrin sheath (Baranowski 1993). Organisms such as coagulase negative staphylococci, *Staphylococcus aureus* and *Candida albicans* all bind well with the fibrin sheath, enhancing the correlation between thrombogenesis and infection.

In an attempt to address the problems of biofilm and fibrin sheath development on CVCs, manufacturers now produce catheters which are coated or bonded with substances thought to reduce the incidence of these problems.

Bonded catheters

Polyurethane catheters bonded with antiseptic substances were developed in the late 1980s and marketed in the early 1990s. The first available product was impregnated with silver sulphadiazine and chlorhexidine. Maki *et al.* (1991) performed a randomized prospective study on this product in a surgical intensive care unit. Their findings were encouraging, with a 50% reduction in catheter colonization and a 75% reduction in catheter-related septicaemia. The catheter was designed to sustain the release of the antiseptic agents over a 15-day period, although small amounts (> 1%) continued to be released after this period (Farber 1993). There have now been 15 randomized controlled trials of this catheter. Most have shown a reduction in CVC colonization, but only two studies have demonstrated a significant reduction in CRBSI (Maki & Crnich 2003). While no resistance to or adverse effects from this product have been found in the USA (Maki & Crnich 2003), 12 cases of anaphylactoid reactions have been reported in Japan (Oda *et al.* 1997) and 1 case in the UK (Stephens *et al.* 2001).

Further developments were seen with the introduction of a minocycline and rifampin-coated catheter. Raad *et al.* (1997) undertook a randomized double-blind clinical trial involving nearly 300 short-term CVCs and demonstrated an important reduction in the incidence of catheter colonization rates and CRBSIs.

In 1999 Darouiche and colleagues (Darouiche *et al.* 1999) compared the silver sulphadiazine and chlorhexidine-impregnated catheter with the minocycline and rifampin-coated catheter and found that the antibiotic-coated catheter was less likely to be colonized and that overall rates of bloodstream infection were lower. Maki and Crnich (2003) postulate that the superiority of the minocycline–rifampin catheter is due to both the internal and external surfaces of the catheter being coated, whereas only the external surface of the silver sulphadiazine and chlorhexidine catheter was coated. Maki and Crnich (2003) also note that the minocycline and rifampin catheter retains surface antimicrobial activity for longer than the silver sulphadiazine and chlorhexidine catheter and that its activity against staphylococci is far superior. In response, Arrow International have launched a new antiseptic CVC with a higher level of chlorhexidine–silver sulphadiazine in the catheter material; the internal and external surfaces of the catheter have been coated as well as the catheter hub. Trials of this new catheter are under way (Maki & Crnich 2003). The Centers for Disease Control and Prevention (CDC) only recommend the use of antimicrobial or antiseptic-impregnated catheters in adults when the CVC has an anticipated dwell time of more than 5 days and when the individual institution's rate of CRBSI is above their target despite the implementation of a comprehensive strategy to reduce CRBSI (O'Grady *et al.* 2002). This view was supported in the 2004 EPIC guidelines update (Pellowe *et al.* 2004).

Heparin-bonded catheters were launched in the early 1980s to reduce the thrombogenicity of the catheter and to improve their biocompatibility (Hoar *et al.* 1981). Heparin is commonly bonded to the surface of pulmonary artery catheters using benzalkonium chloride, which fortuitously has antimicrobial activity (Crnich & Maki 2002a). One prospective study has demonstrated a reduction in CRBSI associated with heparin-bonded pulmonary artery catheters (Mermel *et al.* 1993); however, this has not been born out in trials relating to short-term CVCs (Moss *et al.* 2000).

Cuffs

The 1980s also saw the development of an attachable cuff made of biodegradable collagen and impregnated with silver ions (Hadaway 2001). The cuff is placed subcutaneously around the CVC at the time of insertion. The collagen promotes tissue growth, which provides a physical barrier to bacteria that may try to migrate from the skin surface along the catheter and into the circulation. The silver ions produce a chemical barrier against microbial colonization. Despite initial enthusiasm for this product subsequent clinical trials have proved inconclusive and there is currently no evidence base to support their use (Cicalini *et al.* 2004). In particular, the attachable cuff failed to reduce the incidence of CRBSIs in catheters that remained *in situ* for more than 20 days (Groeger *et al.* 1993; Dahlberg *et al.* 1995). The biodegradable nature of the collagen and the release of the silver ions over the initial 3–7-day period are suggested as possible causes of this failure (Cicalini 2004). Pellowe *et al.* (2004) concluded that the silver-impregnated collagen cuff failed to demonstrate an effect in both short- and long-term use.

Dacron cuffs have been available on long-term skin tunnelled catheters for many years. Long-term CVCs such as the Hickman catheter incorporate a Dacron cuff on the section of the catheter that will lie in a subcutaneous skin tunnel distal to the vein. There was a time when tunnelled catheters were only considered for use within oncology but their use is increasing in acute-care areas. Whether this is always the most appropriate device is questionable in acute care, but at least clinicians are beginning to consider alternative forms of access rather than restricting themselves to peripheral or acute-care CVCs.

Section 2

Catheter design

Most modern central venous catheters are constructed with in-built extensions, which facilitate the manipulation of connections with minimal disturbance of the entry site. The advantage of this is the reduction in the incidence of mechanical thrombophlebitis from movement of the catheter within the vessel. These extensions usually have in-built clamps to reduce the likelihood of air embolism during tubing changes or any other procedure that opens the CVC to the atmosphere. Some catheter materials are easily damaged by in-line clamps, e.g. silastic catheters, and these are usually manufactured with a reinforced area where it is safe to clamp.

Multilumen catheters have an advantage in the acute care setting where patients require continuous infusions of incompatible products. Multilumen catheters for short-term access usually have lumens which exit at different points along the length of the catheter; those for long-term access often have lumens which open at the same place at the tip of the catheter.

Considering that one advantage of a multilumen catheter is the ability to simultaneously infuse incompatible products through the same access site, this would appear to be a design fault of some long-term catheters.

Collins and Lutz (1991) undertook an *in vitro* study of simultaneous infusion of incompatible drugs in multilumen catheters. They highlighted the lack of data on the subject and sought to use an *in vitro* model to investigate the administration of PN and phenytoin, known to be incompatible, via multilumen catheters. The catheters compared were a triple-lumen catheter with staggered openings (the type typically used in the UK for short-term acute access) and a double-lumen catheter with adjacent openings at the tip of the catheter (the type usually associated with long-term catheters or implantable ports). Their findings concluded that the catheter with adjacent openings was inferior to that with staggered openings, as it resulted in drug precipitation.

Concern has been raised over the possible increased infection risk associated with multilumen catheters (Kovacevich *et al.* 1988; Powell *et al.* 1988; Gil *et al.* 1989; Horowitz *et al.* 1990). It is difficult, however, to draw conclusions from these studies as the populations vary, their samples sizes are relatively small and the criteria for determining catheter-related sepsis are not the established ones suggested by authors such as Maki *et al.* (1977). In contrast, Gianino *et al.* (1992) were able to demonstrate a low incidence of infection amongst multilumen catheters when a specialist team is involved in the management of the venous access.

The study by Dezfulian *et al.* (2003) concluded that multilumen CVCs may be associated with a slightly higher risk of infection when compared with single-lumen CVCs; however, this is likely to be offset by an increase in convenience which may justify their use.

Catheter Insertion

There are three methods of central venous catheter placement:

- over a needle
- through a cannula
- over a guidewire.

Placement over a wire and through a cannula both allow for the introduction of a multilumen catheter if required. (It is important when inserting multilumen catheters that all of the lumens are flushed with sodium chloride 0.9% before insertion, which both ensures patency and prevents air embolism.)

Each insertion method has advantages and disadvantages which need to be considered when selecting the method of choice.

Over a needle

This technique usually involves the use of an extra-long cannula, which is inserted in the same way as a standard cannula. This is most commonly associated with the placement of cannulae in the internal jugular vein (Soni 1989). This technique is often favoured by anaesthetists who are placing short-term or emergency cannulae, e.g. at the scene of a cardiac arrest.

As for all central cannulation, the patient is laid flat and, where possible, placed in a head-down position (Trendelenburg). This assists with the filling of the neck veins to facilitate palpation and cannulation (Figure 10.2).

The head is usually turned away from the insertion site and the vessel is punctured. A flashback is seen when the vessel is entered, and the cannula is advanced and the trochar withdrawn in the same manner as for peripheral cannulation. The cannula is aspirated to ensure free flow of blood, which implies that the cannula has not left the vessel, that it is well positioned within the vessel and that it is not kinked.

The advantages of this technique are speed of access, minimal handling and low cost. The disadvantages include the length of the trochar which can cause significant trauma if the operator is inexperienced (Soni 1989), the limitation of a single-lumen catheter and the reduced range of catheter material available for this insertion method. Soni also suggests that this minimal handling technique can result in a tendency to 'skimp on aseptic technique'. This technique is usually restricted to the jugular approach in the emergency situation.

Through a cannula

This is an established technique whereby a small, wide-bore cannula is inserted into a central vein, in a very similar manner to peripheral cannulation. Having established a

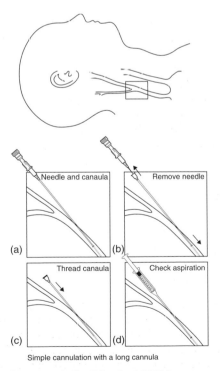

Simple cannulation with a long cannula

Figure 10.2 Placing a cannula over a needle. (After Soni 1989.)

Section 2

flashback, the trochar is withdrawn. It is important to avoid introducing air into the venous system when the trochar is removed, so it is common practice for the operator to occlude the end of the cannula using a sterile gloved finger. A flexible catheter is then threaded through the cannula. The catheter is aspirated to confirm placement and patency. It is usual practice to flush the catheter with sodium chloride 0.9% or heparinized saline to prevent obstruction from clot formation. This method can be used to place short or long catheters.

The introducing cannula is often removed, although this will depend on the construction of the catheter that has been passed and the risk of bleeding, as the introducer cannula is inevitably of a larger diameter than the catheter that has been passed through it.

This method is employed for the placement of temporary transvenous pacing wires, for the placement of pulmonary artery or CO catheters and to facilitate transvenous biopsies (e.g. myocardial or hepatic biopsy). For these procedures a percutaneous introducer sheath with a side arm and self-sealing diaphragm is usually selected. The self-sealing diaphragm allows the therapeutic device (pacing wire, CO catheter etc.) to be fed through the diaphragm and into the circulation without the risk of air embolism that would occur if there were a gap between the device and the lumen of the introducer. There are two main types of percutaneous introducer sheaths: a composite device and a two-part device. These devices are intended to facilitate the use of another therapeutic device; they are not intended for routine vascular access (Darovic 2002). The wide bore of the introducer carries a high risk of air embolism should the two-part device become disconnected. The self-sealing diaphragm is designed to create a seal once the pacing wire or other therapeutic device has been removed. To ensure that there is no risk of air embolism the manufacturer provides an obturator which is intended to be placed in the self-sealing diaphragm when the therapeutic device is removed (Darovic 2002). MacGregor *et al.* (1998) tested the self-sealing diaphragm without the obturator in place and concluded that although the obturator would improve safety it was unlikely that any patient would generate intrathoracic pressure of a magnitude great enough to induce an air embolism.

Over a guidewire

This method of placement is known as the Seldinger technique. It was first described by Dr Seldinger in 1953 and has continued to gain in popularity ever since (Seldinger 1953). Commercially produced kits for CVC insertion continue to evolve, with many labour-saving and hazard-reducing features built into their design.

The basic Seldinger kit comprises a wide-bore hollow needle, a flexible guidewire which will fit through the needle, and a catheter to be threaded over the guidewire. More elaborate kits include smaller needles and wires with a series of dilators which are used to prepare the vessel for the cannula placement. The use of dilators means that flexible, large catheters can be passed into the vein.

The vein is punctured using a needle (or a cannula and trochar depending upon the type of kit selected) and the needle is aspirated to ensure placement in the vein. Avoiding the introduction of air, the syringe is removed and a guidewire is passed down the needle into the vein (*See* Figure 10.3). The needle is withdrawn, leaving the wire in the vein. A catheter is now threaded over the wire and fed into the vein. As the catheter is advanced the wire is removed. More advanced catheter kits use a system which enhances continuity of action for the operator. The syringe which is used to aspirate the needle has a central bore down which the wire is passed. This reduces the risk of either air embolism or operator contamination with blood.

If a kit with a dilator is selected, it will be easy to pass the catheter through the skin and into the vessel because the skin hole will have been enlarged by the dilator.

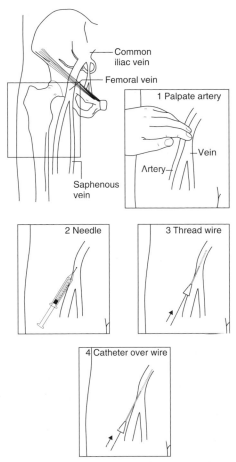

Femoral vein cannulation using Seldinger technique

Figure 10.3   Placing a catheter over a wire. (After Soni 1989.)

If a dilator kit is not selected, it may be necessary to nick the skin with a blade to facilitate passage of a malleable catheter through the barrier of the skin. Blood is aspirated from the catheter in the usual way to ensure correct placement in the vein. The catheter is then flushed with sodium chloride 0.9%.

Care must be taken not to lose the guidewire as it has been known for operators to push both the catheter and the wire into the circulation.

There are a variety of guidewires on the market, some with different coatings, some with different-shaped ends. The 'J' wire has evolved to help placement of catheters which are difficult to thread into the vein. The difficulty in threading a jugular vein can be due to the relative right angle with which the internal jugular enters the subclavian vein, and the 'J' shape to the end of the wire facilitates its passage around such a corner. Most wires, whether 'J' or standard, are usually manufactured with a flexible end and a rigid end. It is important that it is the flexible end which is inserted into the vein. Most modern seldinger CVC kits contain a 'J'-tipped wire.

An advantage of the Seldinger technique is the small needle puncture, allowing the vessel to be dilated up to an exact fit with the cannula size. This reduces the risk of bleeding and the likelihood of air entrainment around the catheter. The use of a dilator removes the need for a surgical nick in the skin and reduces the size of the skin hole.

Patient Considerations

Irrespective of insertion method, it is essential to explain the intended procedure to the patient and to obtain their informed consent to the procedure. Where this is not possible, it is important to explain to a family member the intended actions of the practitioner and the objectives of the treatment. Although consent of one adult for another has no basis in law, keeping family members up to date with treatment is of benefit to promote good relations with the public and to prevent misunderstandings (Medical Defence Union 1996).

During the insertion procedure, it is important that the patient is offered psychological support. The positioning of the patient may be uncomfortable, particularly for those who experience shortness of breath. Cannulation of the neck veins usually requires the placement of sterile towels over the head and face, which can be particularly traumatic for claustrophobic patients.

Despite infiltration of the skin and subcutaneous tissues with local anaesthetic, central vein cannulation can still be an uncomfortable procedure. A significant amount of pressure is usually experienced by the patient as the operator locates, cannulates and dilates the vessel. These experiences are compounded when the operator is inexperienced or when the vessels prove to be difficult to cannulate. It is not uncommon during a prolonged procedure for the local anaesthetic to have worn off by the time the operator is ready to suture the cannula to the skin. It is debatable which is more uncomfortable, repeated infiltration with local anaesthetic or two transient needle pricks to suture the cannula in place.

If the patient is troubled by lying flat, it may be possible to elevate the head of the bed as soon as the catheter is in place. Securing the catheter and applying the dressing can be done with the patient in an upright position.

Management of Central Venous Access

Aseptic technique

A strict aseptic technique is required for the placement of CVC, irrespective of the method chosen. Despite the wealth of research into the infective complications of CVCs, aseptic precautions vary between centres and operators. Stringent aseptic technique is considered mandatory for short- or long-term central catheter placement and its importance should not be underestimated.

Elliott *et al.* (1994) recommended that staff should prepare themselves as for theatre: sterile gown and gloves, mask and hat and a full surgical scrub technique performed prior to gowning. Maki and Crnich (2003) confirm the importance of barrier precautions and state that:

> long-sleeved sterile surgical gowns, mask, cap and a large sterile drape, as well as sterile gloves, significantly reduces the risk of CVC-related bloodstream infection and has further been shown to be highly cost-effective.

It has often been assumed that catheters inserted in the operating theatre pose a lower risk of infection than those inserted in a ward environment. The results of two prospective studies did not support this view and in fact demonstrated that it is the amount of barrier precaution utilized during the insertion process, rather than the environment, which influences the incidence of infection in CVCs (Mermel *et al.* 1991; Raad *et al.* 1994). Pearson (1995) demonstrated that operators who only use sterile gloves and a small fenestrated drape produced a higher incidence of infection than those who use maximal barrier precautions. Pellowe *et al.* (2004) confirm that maximal sterile barrier precautions remain key to the reduction of CRBSIs.

Skin preparation and site care

The intended insertion site should be clean (INS 2006). If there is gross contamination of the skin, Elliott *et al.* (1994) recommended that it be cleaned with soap and water prior to routine disinfection of the site. What form that disinfection should take has been the subject of much research and debate.

For many years, the use of an alcohol-based iodine solution to clean the insertion site was recommended. This has now been superseded by the work of Maki *et al.* (1991), who demonstrated the efficacy of aqueous chlorhexidine for the management of central access sites. Alcohol-based iodine products are most efficacious when they are applied, and as they dry they lose their activity (Hibbard 2005). By contrast, aqueous chlorhexidine 2% has been shown to remain active on the skin surface for 6 hours after application. Pellowe *et al.* (2004) in their review of the evidence, accepted the Healthcare Infection Control Practice Advisory Committee (HICPAC) recommendation for the use of an alcoholic solution of chlorhexidine gluconate 2% for skin antisepsis prior to catheter insertion and for site care unless contraindicated by the manufacturer of the vascular access device. This has been confirmed by the epic2 project (Pratt *et al.* 2007).

Just as important as the selection of the cleansing solution are the method and duration of the cleansing process. Elliott *et al.* (1994) emphasized the need to clean beyond the intended site of insertion. As an example, they suggested that for jugular or subclavian access, the skin preparation should include the neck and top of the trunk of the patient. They also recommended that the insertion site be cleaned again after correct placement of the catheter. It is important, when doing this, to avoid further contamination of the site. The recommended agent of choice for skin antisepsis is 2% chlorhexidine gluconate and 70% isopropyl alcohol (Pratt *et al.* 2007) and the first licenced product, ChloraPrep®, has now been approved for use in the UK. To prepare a dry insertion site such as the arm or abdomen the manufacturer recommends a side-to-side motion for approximately 30 seconds, ensuring that the intended site is completely wet. This skin should then be allowed to air dry for 30 seconds. If, however, a moist insertion site is selected, for example the femoral site, the intended insertion site should be cleaned for 2 minutes and allowed to dry for 1 minute (ChloraPrep 2007). In the event of allergy, povidone iodine in alcohol may be used and should remain on the skin for at least 2 minutes, or longer if not yet dry (O'Grady *et al.* 2002).

The use of antimicrobial ointments to prevent local colonization of CVC sites is controversial. Maki and Band (1981) were unable to demonstrate any effectiveness of antibiotic- or iodine-based ointments in the prevention of catheter-related sepsis. Concern has been raised that antibiotic ointments may disrupt normal skin flora and promote the growth of yeasts such as *Candida* (Pearson 1995). The use of mupirocin, an antistaphylococcal agent, in conjunction with tincture of iodine before catheter insertion, has been shown to reduce the incidence of internal jugular colonization in cardiac surgical patients (Hill *et al.* 1990). One randomized study of dialysis catheters demonstrated a reduction in the incidence of exit site infections, catheter tip colonization and bloodstream infections with the routine use of povidone iodine ointment (Levin *et al.* 1991). Mupirocin resistance has been reported, and concern has been raised that mupirocin may affect the integrity of polyurethane catheters. O'Grady *et al.* (2002) did on balance recommend the use of an iodine-based ointment at dialysis catheter exit sites only, and with the proviso that it should not harm the specific catheter *in situ*.

Dressings

The type of dressing to use on vascular access sites provokes perhaps the greatest discussion of all. Gauze and tape or transparent dressings are the most common methods employed in the literature.

Section 2

Transparent self-adhesive dressings have the obvious benefit of facilitating observation of the entry site without disturbance. The earlier transparent dressings were occlusive in nature, the type now considered appropriate for wound management. The concern with these dressings was the build-up of moisture beneath the dressing and the infection hazard that this might cause. Craven *et al.* (1985) and Conly *et al.* (1989) reported an increased incidence of *Candida* growth with the introduction of the early transparent dressings; however, other studies were unable to confirm this finding (Ricard *et al.* 1985; Hoffman *et al.* 1988). Maki and Ringer (1987) investigated the use of transparent dressings on peripheral devices and could establish no clinical significance between the use of gauze and the transparent moisture-permeable dressing. The authors advocated that the transparent dressing placed on the cannula at the time of insertion be left *in situ* until the cannula was removed, providing that the cannula was routinely replaced 48–72 hours post insertion.

Modern transparent dressings for intravascular catheters are described as moisture permeable and are reported to produce less moisture build-up at the entry site. Manufacturers usually provide the statistics on the 'moisture vapour transmission rate' (MVTR) of their product. Moisture-permeable transparent dressings usually have a MVTR of 400–900 $g/m^2/24$ h (Jones 2004). The two most common products marketed in the UK are IV3000 by Smith & Nephew and Tegaderm by 3M; both have markedly different MVTR statistics. IV3000 claims an MVTR of 11 000 $g/m^2/24$ h, while Tegaderm reports an MVTR of 735 $g/m^2/24$ h (Jones 2004). The study by Reynolds *et al.* (1997) was unable to identify any statistically significant difference between the two dressings when accumulation of fluid, skin colonization, local infection and systemic infection were compared in 100 critically ill liver patients with a CVC.

O'Grady *et al.* (2002) recommend that the user selects the most appropriate dressing for the situation as they could not determine any difference in the incidence of infection when gauze and semipermeable transparent dressings were compared. They comment that if a CVC site is bleeding or if the patient is diaphoretic, it may be more appropriate to select a gauze dressing because of its absorbency. Transparent semipermeable dressings are recommended to be changed weekly or if they are visibly loose or soiled (O'Grady 2002). The epic2 guidelines (Pratt *et al.* 2007) concluded that a sterile, transparent semipermeable dressing should be used to cover a CVC entry site however, they also noted that a gauze and tape dressing was more appropriate in the presence of profuse sweating or if the entry site was bleeding. They recommend that a gauze dressing be changed when it becomes damp, loose or soiled or if visual inspection is needed and that it is converted to a transparent dressing as soon as possible (Pratt *et al.* 2007).

Most of the literature surrounding CVC dressings relates to short-term, non-tunnelled catheters. Less is written about long-term, tunnelled catheters; however, O'Grady and colleagues were able to conclude that a well-healed tunnelled CVC may not require a dressing.

The development of the Biopatch® dressing has been an interesting new development in the prevention of CRBSI. The Biopatch® by Johnson & Johnson is a synthetic foam disc impregnated with chlorhexidine gluconate and available in a range of sizes to accommodate the range of vascular devices available. The dressing is applied around the catheter entry site and changed when the entry site dressing is changed. The Biopatch® has been shown to reduce the incidence of CRBSI and no adverse reactions have been reported in association with its use (Banton & Banning 2002; Maki & Crnich 2003; Crawford *et al.* 2004).

Securing the catheter

That the catheter should be secured is undisputed: a mobile catheter is not only prone to mechanical phlebitis but may also become dislodged. Long-term catheters are usually immobilized by their Dacron cuffs, whereas short-term CVCs have traditionally been sutured.

The development of the 'Statlock', a novel sutureless device to stabilize and anchor CVCs, has challenged the traditional management of CVCs and the use of sutures has become increasingly controversial.

Sutureless devices have been shown to reduce the incidence of PICC-related bloodstream infection in both adults and children as well as reducing the incidence of PICC-associated thrombosis and catheter loss in children (Maki & Crnich 2003). Gabriel *et al.* (2005) highlight the potential reduction in sharps injuries that may be achieved by the use of a sutureless device. Crnich and Maki (2002b) support the development of novel technologies such as sutureless devices in an attempt to reduce the incidence of CRBSI.

The Infusion Nurses Society no longer recommend sutures for catheter stabilization and instead recommend manufactured stabilization devices, sterile tape and surgical strips. If tapes of surgical strips are used they recommend that they are only placed over the catheter adaptor and not directly on the catheter–skin junction (INS 2006).

Catheter position

Fatal complications resulting from misplacement of CVCs have been reported for more than three decades (Brandt *et al.* 1970; Adar & Mozes 1971; Sheep & Guiney 1982; Maschke & Rogove 1984; McGee *et al.* 1993; Collier *et al.* 1998). There are also multiple reports of non-fatal complications such as dysrhythmia, hydrothorax, hydromediastinum, tamponade and tissue injury from extravasation.

The position of the CVC is usually confirmed by X-ray, although many experienced operators express confidence in catheter position based on the ease of insertion and free aspiration of blood from all lumens. Despite this confidence it is advisable to obtain X-ray confirmation of catheter tip position before use as the catheter may be malpositioned in an arm vein or a head vein, or it may have been advanced too far and be located within the chambers of the heart. Gladwin *et al.* (1999) undertook a prospective cohort study of 107 patients requiring elective internal jugular CVC insertion. Following catheter insertion the operator was required to complete a complex questionnaire designed to detect complications and to predict the need for a chest X-ray. All patients received a chest X-ray to compare operator perceptions with catheter location. The incidence of catheter tip malposition was 14% and operator intuition was not adequate to predict catheter location, even for experienced operators (Gladwin *et al.* 1999).

It is generally accepted that the catheters should be located in the distal third of the SVC 2 cm superior to the right atrium in adults and children who weigh more than 20 kg, and 1 cm superior to the right atrium in children weighing less than 20 kg (Albrecht *et al.* 2004). Catheter tip position is a complex and controversial subject and Vesely (2003) concludes that the scientific literature has so far failed to provide sufficient evidence to indisputably support or condemn the placement of a catheter tip into the right atrium. Identifying the catheter tip location from external landmarks is not easy, and visualization of the exact position of the catheter tip on an anterior–posterior chest X-ray can also be difficult. A number of authors have suggested using the carina as a marker for CVC tip location when interpreting the chest X-ray (Albrecht *et al.* 2004; Stonelake & Bodenham 2006). Vesely (2003) believes the right tracheobronchial angle to be the best radiographic landmark to delineate the borders of the SVC and the SVC/atrial junction. Weisenberg *et al.* (2005) proposed the use of external topographic landmarks to determine the correct length of catheter to be inserted. In their study the catheters were inserted to a length equal to a line obtained by uniting two transversal lines, one passing at the thyroid notch level and the other between the superior and middle thirds of the manubrium bone. In this study, 100 patients were randomized to receive a CVC inserted either to the full 15-cm depth of the catheter or to a depth determined by external topographic landmarks. The results demonstrated that 2% of the study group required an alteration in catheter position compared to 78% in the traditional placement group. In a randomized controlled trial Chu *et al.* (2004) compared intravenous electrocardiography with traditional landmark techniques for Port-A Catheter placement. By priming the Port-A Catheter with 0.8 mEq/ml of sodium bicarbonate and attaching a sterile electrode to a non-coring needle placed in the septum of the port they were able to monitor the size of the 'p' wave of the standard electrocardiogram (ECG) to determine the proximity of the catheter tip to the sinoatrial node. The placement was then evaluated using a transoesophageal echo probe. Correct catheter placement occurred in 100% of the intravenous ECG group while approximately 50% of the landmark group had successfully positioned catheters.

The use of topographical landmarks is solely to determine the catheter length; a check X-ray is still required to ensure that the catheter has not been misplaced into a head or arm vessel.

A number of authors report a change in catheter position as a consequence of patient movement (Kasten *et al.* 1985; Seneff 1987a; Soni 1989; Vesely 2003) which would suggest that catheter tip position should be checked if the healthcare worker has any doubt about patency of the CVC. Vesely (2003) notes that the majority of catheters will exhibit a range of movement extending 2–3 cm and that a catheter placed in the inferior segment of the SVC will more than likely move in and out of the right atrium. Catheter tip location should be determined radiographically and documented in the patient's notes before use (RCN 2005).

Catheter removal

This is an important aspect of the management of CVCs, and perhaps receives the least attention. The risks associated with catheter removal are not new, and the most significant is perhaps air embolism.

Air embolism has been reported to occur up to 72 hours after the removal of a CVC (Hanley *et al.* 1984; Phifer *et al.* 1991). The development of a fibrin tract between the skin entry site and the vessel is thought to be the cause of air embolism post central venous catheter removal (Roberts *et al.* 2003). The longer the catheter is *in situ* the more established the tract is likely to be (Mennim *et al.* 1992).

A survey demonstrated that nurses were more aware of the risks of embolism following catheter removal than were doctors. Nurses were better informed about the preventative strategies which could be employed during and after CVC removal (Mennim *et al.* 1992).

To prevent air embolism, it is recommended that patients who can tolerate lying flat are asked to do so during the catheter removal procedure. Failing this, they may be asked to breathe in and hold their breath for the few seconds required to remove the catheter. Following removal of the CVC and achievement of haemostasis, an occlusive transparent dressing (not moisture permeable) should be applied and left in place for 72 hours.

It is important to inspect the integrity of the catheter after removal. There are reports in the literature of catheter separation from the hub and catheter rupture following high-pressure injectates or excessive negative pressure during catheter aspiration (Scott 1988). Separation of a catheter fragment leads to catheter embolism and may result in the catheter lodging in the central circulation or the right side of the heart (Liu *et al.* 2004). Scott (1988) reported a mortality incidence of 30% if the catheter fragment is not retrieved. Domino *et al.* (2004) reported the litigation and claims relating to CVCs and pulmonary artery catheters between 1970 and 2000 recorded in the American Society of Anesthesiologists closed claims database. There were 110 claims for injuries related to CVCs, 20 of which were for wire or catheter embolus. Liu *et al.* (2004) reported a total of 20 patients with central embolization of Port-A Catheter fragments over a 5-year period and concluded that improper procedure handling by inexperienced surgeons was the most frequent cause of embolization.

The nurse should be aware of the potential for catheter embolus. If the catheter is not intact on removal, a medical officer should be informed. It is usual practice to perform a chest X-ray to locate the radio-opaque fragment. Retrieval of the fragment is performed percutaneously using loop snare catheters or baskets (Liu *et al.* 2004). The risk of catheter embolus is increased if a stylet (needle) has been reintroduced into a catheter during the insertion procedure. If the fragment is a result of a catheter defect it should be reported locally within the organization as well as to the manufacturer and to national bodies responsible for medical devices. In the UK this is the Medicine and Healthcare products Regulatory Agency (MHRA) and the National Patient Safety Agency (NPSA) (RCN 2005).

Microbiological assessment

Following removal of a CVC it may be necessary to send the catheter tip to microbiology for bacterial culture and sensitivity assessment. If this is clinically indicated, the tip of the catheter should be cut off, using sterile scissors, placed in a sterile container, labelled and sent to microbiology. This is usually a routine procedure for high-risk patients, who are generally defined as:

- those who are actively immunosuppressed
- those who are immunocompromised by their disease process (e.g. ITU patients of all ages)
- those with pyrexia of unknown origin
- those in whom catheter-associated infection is suspected
- those in whom septicaemia would be potentially life-threatening.

Microbiological assessment is traditionally carried out in one of two ways. The first method is to roll the catheter tip several times across a bacterial culture plate, incubate the plate and then analyse the number of bacterial colonies. This technique was established by Maki. The second method is to flush the catheter tip with culture broth and to culture the fluid (Cleri *et al.* 1980). These techniques facilitate assessment of extraluminal and intraluminal bacterial colonization, the two most important routes for catheter-related septicaemia (Elliott 1993).

However, as Elliott (1993) stated, the drawback of this method is that diagnosis is made after the catheter has been removed, and therefore some catheter removal may prove to be unnecessary. Markus and Buday (1989) proposed a brush culture technique to facilitate catheter culture *in situ*. This technique is not routinely used in the UK and may prove inappropriate if the catheter to be sampled contains inotropes or other vasoactive agents. The acridine orange leucocyte cytospin (AOLC) test has been developed to provide microbiological guidance whilst the catheter remains *in situ* and is reported by Rushforth *et al.* (1993) to provide a microbiological diagnosis of catheter-related bloodstream infection within 1 hour and to be highly sensitive when compared to traditional blood cultures. However, Hodge and Puntis (2002) suggest that due to the labour-intensive nature of the test it is unlikely to be widely embraced by laboratories.

In acute care, when faced with a septic, critically ill patient, it is often considered to be more prudent to presume the CVC to be the cause of the sepsis and to remove it, rather than leave the potential source of infection *in situ* for 3 days while awaiting the results of the catheter culture. As Maki and Crnich (2003) point out, failure to remove an infected CVC puts the patient at risk of developing septic thrombosis of a central vein or even endocarditis.

Complications of Central Venous Catheterization

Some complications have already been alluded to in association with particular access routes. This section will discuss the most common hazards of central venous

Section 2

catheterization, the mechanisms by which they occur, and any remedial or preventative action that can be taken to avoid or minimize their impact upon the patient.

Air embolism

This complication is almost exclusively limited to central rather than peripheral access. The veins of the thorax are under the influence of the changing pressures within the thoracic cavity. The pressure changes are due mainly to respiration, but pressure change is also seen in relation to gravity, i.e. lying down vs. sitting up.

Atmospheric air pressure at sea level is 760 mmHg. At the end of expiration, the intrathoracic pressure is in equilibrium with atmospheric pressure. As inspiration occurs and the chest expands, the intrathoracic pressure falls, causing a pressure gradient between the atmosphere and the lungs. Air rushes into the lungs until the pressure inside the chest is again in equilibrium with the atmosphere. When an individual begins to exhale, the chest wall compresses the lungs, causing the intrathoracic pressure to rise. Intrathoracic pressure is now greater than atmospheric pressure and this causes air to leave the lungs until the intrathoracic pressure is again in equilibrium with atmospheric pressure. These changes in pressure are only mild; however, the movement of gas along a pressure gradient is very efficient.

The central veins experience these pressure changes, with their internal pressure alternating subtly between being just above or just below atmospheric pressure. If a cannula is inserted into a central vein and left open to the atmosphere, each time the pressure in the vein falls below atmospheric pressure, air will be sucked into the circulation (i.e. during the inspiratory phase of the respiratory cycle). Air can be entrained into the circulation in this way at a rate of 100 mL/s (Phifer *et al.* 1991; Wysoki *et al.* 2001).

Prevention

To reduce the risk of air embolism during the CVC insertion procedure the patient is required to lie flat and is positioned head down (Trendelenburg's position). This causes the neck veins to fill, making them easier to palpate, but also making them less likely to experience negative pressure and entrain air. It is usual practice during catheter insertion for the operator to occlude the end of the catheter whenever the syringe or guidewire is removed. Poterack and Aggarwal (1991) describe a venous air embolism during a guidewire exchange of a CVC. The air embolism is reported to have occurred after the old catheter had been removed and before placement of the new catheter when only the guidewire was in the vessel.

Vigilance is essential to prevent air embolism during the use of a CVC. Most catheters include in-line clamps to allow them to be safely disconnected during administration set changes or any other procedure involving disconnection. All staff who handle CVCs must ensure that bungs are replaced correctly, that only luer-lock fittings are employed (Morton *et al.* 2005; RCN 2005) and that the luer-locks are screwed together tightly. When taking over the care of a patient, it is important to check the safety of the connections on a CVC (RCN 2005).

All burettes have in-built air inlets to allow the fluid to flow out. When using burettes on CVCs, it is essential that the product selected contains an air occlusion device to prevent air being entrained down the tubing and into the patient.

If an infusion is being delivered from a bottle (e.g. human albumin, antibiotics or clotting agents), an air inlet is usually inserted into the bottle so that the fluid can flow out. If a bottle is used on a CVC, it is essential that the patient and the infusion are constantly observed so that the infusion can be switched off when complete, thus preventing air embolism through the empty bottle. If the bottle is being delivered via a volumetric pump it is essential that the pump contains an air-in-line detector.

In both these situations, air embolism is much more likely in a patient whose blood volume is reduced, for example as a result of dehydration or haemorrhage (Vesely 2001). A patient whose circulation is empty may experience negative pressure in the central veins throughout the entire respiratory cycle. The more laboured a patient's breathing, the greater the range of pressure change within the chest and the greater the risk of air embolism.

The risk of air entrainment from a bottle or burette is of even greater significance if the infusion is being administered into a pumped extracorporeal circuit, such as in haemofiltration or haemodialysis. The pumped circuit has the capability to entrain air in proportion to the pump speed. Most (but not all) of these systems have methods of air detection, but despite these features entrained air can jeopardize the patient's treatment, create delays and increase nursing workload.

The risk of air embolism is often underestimated by healthcare staff. The longer a catheter remains *in situ*, the more likely it is that a tract will be established around the catheter into the vessel (Mennim *et al.* 1992). There are reported cases of patients experiencing air embolism through entrainment of air around catheters and transvenous pacing wires whilst the device is still *in situ* (Johnson *et al.* 1991).

The removal of a CVC is also a time of high risk because, for a brief period, the vein is again open to the atmosphere. To reduce this risk patients should be asked to lie flat for the removal of a central venous catheter (Mennim *et al.* 1992; RCN 2005). Some patients may not be able to tolerate lying flat and alternative strategies are required in order to prevent air embolism. Wysoki *et al.* (2001) compared three physiological manoeuvres for the prevention of air embolism: breath-holding, humming and valsalva. Pressure measurements were obtained at normal respirations and then during each of the three manoeuvres. Their survey revealed that 40% of patients had a negative venous pressure at rest, 25% had negative venous pressures during breath-holding, 20% had negative pressures whilst humming and 2.5% had negative pressures during a valsalva manoeuvre. The results were statistically significant and they concluded that the valsalva was the manoeuvre most likely to prevent air embolism.

The risk of air embolism is influenced by the clinical condition of the patient as well as the type and location of the VAD. For example, the literature reports that CVC removal in patients who have undergone lung transplantation carries an increased risk of air embolism (McCarthy *et al.* 1995). Wysoki *et al.* (2001) report that a 14-gauge cannula can entrain air at a rate of 100 mL/s, and suggest that a wide-bore catheter such as a dialysis catheter can entrain air at a rate of 300 mL in 0.5 s. They point out that a deep inspiration would increase the air entrainment rate significantly. Introducer sheaths used for the insertion of intravascular devices such as pulmonary artery catheters and pacing wires are also wide bore and carry a recognized risk of air embolism (Darovic 2002).

A practical nursing problem arises when multiple CVCs are placed in the same vessel and a decision is taken to remove only one CVC. It is difficult to achieve an airtight seal over the puncture site when another catheter remains *in situ*. It may be more prudent to delay removal until both catheters can be removed simultaneously and an airtight dressing can be successfully applied.

Many staff are unaware of the continued risk of embolism after the cannula has been removed and haemostasis achieved. The literature demonstrates that air embolism is possible up to 72 hours after catheter removal (Hanley *et al.* 1984; Phifer *et al.* 1991) and that the likelihood of embolism is proportional to the length of time during which the catheter was *in situ*. This would appear to be due to persistency of the skin tract down to the vein (Hanley *et al.* 1984; Phifer *et al.* 1991). It is therefore recommended that an occlusive dressing is applied to the site for 72 hours following removal of a CVC (RCN 2005).

Section 2

Management

An air embolism is a medical emergency and is associated with significant mortality. Nurses who care for patients with CVCs should be aware of this hazard, how to recognize it and the best course of action to deal with the problem.

Patients who experience air embolism may present with a range of symptoms, including:

* shortness of breath
* chest pain
* visual disturbance.
  Physical examination may reveal the following signs:
* altered consciousness
* tachycardia/bradycardia
* tachypnoea
* dysrhythmias
* a low cardiac output state
* pulmonary hypertension
* pulmonary oedema
* cyanosis
* a 'mill-wheel' murmur (a loud, churning, machinery-like murmur heard over the precordium) (Muth & Shank 2000a)
* seizures.

Any cause of the embolus should be found and rectified, for example by turning off any open three-way taps, replacing missing bungs, closing in-line clamps, applying pressure to any central puncture sites. The patient should receive 100% oxygen via a face mask which will improve their oxygenation and also help to reduce the size of the air embolus (Muth & Shank 2000a). The positioning of the patient in a left lateral Trendelenburg's position was recommended by Durant *et al.* (1947) and subsequent advice has been based upon this original research. More recent papers suggest that there is no additional benefit from this position (Mehlhorn *et al.* 1994; Geissler *et al.* 1997). Muth and Shank (2000b) point out that positioning the patient in a supine position affords the physician better opportunity to provide supportive interventions such as intubation, ventilation, resuscitation and vascular access. That the patient should be laid down is not disputed.

The object of Trendelenburg positioning is to facilitate entrapment of the air embolus in the apex of the ventricles. If the air is successfully trapped in the ventricles, it is unlikely to be pumped into the aorta and consequently through the carotid arteries and up to the brain where it may induce ischaemia, blindness or stroke. If the air is successfully trapped in this manner, it can be aspirated from the ventricles under image intensity.

In the event that the air does circulate to the brain, there are case reports of successful treatment with hyperbaric oxygen therapy, which causes the gas bubble to reduce in size and to be forced into solution in the blood (Halliday *et al.* 1994). Few centres, however, have the ability to deliver hyperbaric oxygen therapy.

Throughout this time, the patient will need calm reassurance and prompt decisive action from the practitioner. An emergency call should be put out to obtain assistance as quickly as possible. Emergency equipment should be available.

Pneumothorax

A pneumothorax occurs when air enters the pleural space between the visceral and parietal pleurae, producing partial or complete lung collapse (Morton *et al.* 2005). Pneumothorax can occur following central vein cannulation, and the mechanism is not dissimilar to that described in air embolism.

During the central venous catheterization process, the operator must locate the vessel which is under the surface of the skin. If, whilst probing with their needle, the operator punctures the pleural membrane it is possible for environmental air to be entrained down the needle and into the pleural space. This is most commonly seen following subclavian vein cannulation, but can also be seen following a low approach to the internal jugular vein (Seneff 1987b). In a study by Eisen *et al.* (2006) the subclavian route was associated with a pneumothorax rate of 1%.

Pleural pressure is the pressure of the fluid in the pleural space; pleural pressure is negative throughout the breathing cycle (Guyton & Hall 2006). Because the pleural pressure is negative air can be sucked into the pleural space which causes the two pleural membranes to separate and the normal mechanics of breathing to be impaired. If the air can enter the pleural space (via the needle puncture) but cannot escape again this is termed a tension pneumothorax (Morton *et al.* 2005).

Small pneumothoraces rarely cause complications unless the patient is already compromised by respiratory disease. A small pneumothorax in an asymptomatic patient will usually be left to resolve spontaneously (Laronga *et al.* 2000). If the pneumothorax is large or the patient compromised, the condition will be treated by the insertion of a pleural underwater seal drain. It is possible to entrain large quantities of air into the pleural space. This causes lung compression and can, in extreme circumstances, lead to a state of pulseless electrical activity (PET) or electromechanical dissociation of the heart. This is a medical emergency which will require resuscitation. In this situation, the PET results from the large pneumothorax causing a mediastinal shift, kinking of the SVC and/or IVC and acutely obstructing the venous return to the heart (Morton *et al.* 2005). The lack of venous return causes reduced preload, reduced contractility, reduced stroke volume and subsequently reduced CO.

The patient will usually complain of dyspnoea, will often become agitated or restless and may experience a sense of foreboding. They will usually require oxygen via a face mask, psychological support and positioning to optimize their respiratory function. Help should be summoned and the nurse will need to assist with the insertion of a chest drain, which is connected to an underwater drainage system. It is common practice to check the position of the drain on X-ray.

Hydrothorax

Hydrothorax may occur if the central venous catheterization process results in a catheter being placed in the pleural space. If the cannulation process is traumatic, it is possible for the operator to puncture the pleura and to think that they have located the vessel when really the cannula is in the pleural space. Due to local tissue trauma, the operator may even experience relatively free flow of blood when the cannula is aspirated.

If the placement of the catheter is not checked by X-ray prior to its use, a practitioner may inadvertently infuse intravenous fluids into the pleural space, thus causing a hydrothorax.

There are also reports of hydrothorax formation following erosion of the SVC as a result of poorly positioned external jugular catheters (Ghani & Berry 1983). More recently, Hohlrieder *et al.* (2004) reported hydrothorax as a consequence of SVC perforation during the CVC insertion procedure. Hohlrieder *et al.* (2004) postulated that the J wire was the cause of the SVC perforation despite the initial aspiration of blood via the syringe. They concluded that aspiration of an insufficient blood volume led to the erroneous conclusion that the catheter was correctly placed (Hohlrieder *et al.* 2004).

The presentation and treatment are the same as for pneumothorax. The speed of presentation may depend on the speed of infusion of intravenous fluids. The misplaced catheter should be removed.

Section 2

Haemorrhage

Most CVCs are large-bore devices. If a patient has a high central venous pressure (CVP), they will be at risk of bleeding from the catheter should it become dislodged or if a connection is inadvertently left open to the air. This is, in effect, the opposite situation to an air embolism. Air embolism will be a risk for patients with low CVP who experience subatmospheric pressure in their vessels during respiration.

Haemorrhage will be a risk for patients whose CVP is higher than atmospheric pressure. This may occur in a range of patients, including those:

- with chronic obstructive airways disease
- with acute pulmonary embolism
- with liver failure
- with right heart failure or congestive heart failure
- with vasoconstriction
- who are overhydrated or overtransfused (Guyton & Hall 2006).

Because of the diameter of the catheter and its placement in a large, high-flow vessel, it is possible for substantial haemorrhage to occur via a CVC. Nurses must be aware of this complication: all connections must be luer-locked (RCN 2005) and the security of the catheter must be checked regularly.

Monitoring

Haemodynamic monitoring

Bedside haemodynamic monitoring allows continuous surveillance of the cardiovascular system and provides the physiological data to guide therapy (Daily & Schroeder 1995).

In order to undertake haemodynamic monitoring, the vascular system must be cannulated and the pressure within the circulation interpreted. All electronic equipment for measuring haemodynamic information has three fundamental components:

- a transducer to detect physiological activity
- an amplifier to increase the size of the signal
- a recording device to display the information, either on a screen or as a paper recording.

Using high-pressure manometer tubing, it is possible to transmit pressure with minimal distortion. In connecting the manometer tubing to a central or arterial catheter, the effect is to artificially increase the length of the vessel so that it can be attached to the monitoring equipment.

By connecting the manometer tubing to a transducer, it is possible to convert mechanical energy (pressure) into electrical energy (the waveform) (Daily & Schroeder 1995).

The electrical signal produced by the transducer is transmitted through a cable to the monitor. The monitor contains an amplifier which modifies the signal by increasing the voltage and filtering the signal. The improved quality signal is then displayed as a waveform on the monitor.

Transduced, electronic information has the advantage of a rapid response time. There is no time lag between a physiological event and the information received on the monitor. Waveforms can be analysed and this may supply the practitioner with additional information. Mean values can also be calculated.

In order to perform haemodynamic monitoring, three conventions are observed.

1. Haemodynamic recordings are expressed in millimetres of mercury (mmHg) (except for CVP recordings which can be expressed in mmHg or cm H_2O).

2. Most haemodynamic recordings are referenced to the heart, in particular to the atria, to eliminate the effects of hydrostatic pressure.
3. All haemodynamic pressure monitoring devices are zeroed to ambient atmospheric pressure so that the actual pressure measured reflects pressure above atmospheric pressure (McGhee & Bridges 2002).

To improve the accuracy of pressure recordings, the weight of air or 'atmospheric pressure' must be eliminated from the recording. Atmospheric pressure will vary with altitude and environmental factors such as humidity and temperature. Elimination of the influence of environmental pressure is achieved by opening the transducer to air and adjusting the display system to read zero (Daily & Schroeder 1995).

Thus atmospheric pressure is described as zero, rather than 760 mmHg, which is the true value at sea level. If the true value was used in medical practice, then any pressure recordings, such as blood pressure, would have to be added to atmospheric pressure. A normal blood pressure would, in truth, be 880/840 mmHg. The normal range for blood pressure would also vary depending upon the altitude at which a person lived. In an attempt to reduce the complexity of reality, medicine adjusts its equipment so that atmospheric pressure is read as zero, and records all pressure values in relation to this.

In order for a transducer to be accurate, the user must ensure that the transducer recognizes atmospheric 'zero'. To test this, the transducer tap is turned off to the patient and opened to air and if the monitor fails to record zero, the zero button is pressed to reset the monitor.

Purely calibrating a machine to a single value is less accurate than calibrating it to a range of values. Most reusable transducers are recalibrated when they are serviced; the modern transducer is disposable and is precalibrated by the manufacturer. Practitioners who work with reusable transducers should check that they are regularly calibrated to at least two electronically known values, such as 50 and 100 mmHg or 100 and 200 mmHg. Calibration is a quality control measure.

Transducers are very sensitive and easily damaged, and the calibration to zero should be checked regularly throughout the day to ensure accuracy of the equipment.

For accuracy of results, transducers are usually positioned at a standard level in relation to the patient's position. This is traditionally level with the patient's right atrium. Anatomically this is either the intersection of the midaxillary line with the fourth intercostal space or the sternal notch. The latter point is more consistent for recordings as it is a geographical reference point which is easy to find. It is, however, only in line with the right atrium when a patient is sitting up. The intersection of the midaxillary line with the fourth intercostal space is a more universal reference point and is called the phlebostatic axis (Morton *et al.* 2005). The phlebostatic axis most accurately reflects the level of the atrium in both upright and supine patients (Kee *et al.* 1993). The practitioner should make a note of whichever site is selected so that readings are consistent; some authors advocate marking the reference point on the patient for consistency (Morton *et al.* 2005). The equipment should be levelled with the patient's right atrium every time the patient is repositioned and after patient transfers. The zero and the level should be checked before clinical decisions in relation to CVP, for example before giving volume replacement. Transducers that are positioned higher than the level of the right atrium gives falsely low readings while a transducer that is too low gives falsely high readings (Morton *et al.* 2005).

Accuracy can only be assumed if the equipment is well maintained and the patient is well positioned. Connections should be tightly luer-locked to ensure that there is no 'leakage' of pressure into the lower-pressured environment. The pressure signal from the patient is transmitted through fluid-filled manometer tubing. This fluid is usually 0.9% saline or heparinized saline, delivered via a pressurized flush device. The flush device is maintained at a constant pressure of 300 mmHg in adults, which produces a continuous flush of approximately 3 mL/h through the system (Daily & Schroeder 1995). The pressurized system prevents backflow of blood from entering the catheter and prevents the catheter from clotting (Morton *et al.* 2005). Modern disposable transducer systems include an in-line rapid flush device that can be manually activated (Morton *et al.* 2005). Lower pressures and smaller volumes are usually used in paediatrics. It is not uncommon in paediatrics to use volume-controlled pumps and syringes to administer a continuous flush to monitoring devices; this prevents volume overload from uncontrolled in-line flush devices (Daily & Schroeder 1995).

Heparinized saline has traditionally been used to maintain the patency of the system which would otherwise be at risk of clotting. The use of heparin is not without risk and there have been several papers investigating the need for it in a pressurized system (Taylor *et al.* 1989; Peterson & Kirchhoff 1991; Tuncali *et al.* 2005). Some studies have small sample sizes (Hook *et al.* 1987; Leighton 1994), but their data suggest that heparin is not required to maintain the patency of transduced catheters. Hook *et al.* (1987) concluded that it was probably the consistent pressurized flush that maintained the patency rather than the presence of heparin. Chow and Brock-Utne (2005) concluded that the incidence and implications of heparin-induced thrombocytopenia (HIT) outweighed any benefit that might be derived from the use of heparin in maintaining the patency of VADs, particularly in paediatrics and concluded that the pressurized transducer system would be adequate.

The responsiveness of the transduced system depends on its resonant frequency (Daily & Schroeder 1995), i.e. the speed with which the system oscillates. To ensure the greatest accuracy, the practitioner should consider the following issues.

Tubing length Where possible this should not exceed a metre, as increased tubing length reduces the system's responsiveness. The length of the pressure tubing should be kept to a minimum (Morton *et al.* 2005).

Tubing material It is essential to use dedicated manometer tubing which is non-compliant. Soft intravenous tubing is distensible and can reduce the quality of the transmitted pressure wave, resulting in a recording of reduced pressure (Morton *et al.* 2005).

Diameter of the catheter The smaller the diameter of the catheter, the more resistance it presents to flow through it. It is best to use the largest catheter possible to obtain accurate results. However, this must be tempered by the risks of large-bore cannulation and the device selected should be the best option for the patient. If, for example, a practitioner uses a multilumen catheter to record CVP, it is important that the largest lumen is selected. This creates the least resistance and produces the most accurate recording (Daily & Schroeder 1995).

Prevention of air bubbles The presence of air bubbles in the fluid-filled tubing will cause a reduction in the accuracy of the recordings. Air, like most gases, is compressible. If air bubbles are present in the system they will be compressed by the pressure wave that is being transmitted through the fluid-filled tubing. This will cause the pressure signal to weaken because some of the pressure has been absorbed by the gas bubbles.

A physical property of a liquid is that it is unable to be compressed. It is therefore a good medium to transmit a pressure signal, provided there are no gas bubbles in the liquid to distort the accuracy. Care must be taken when priming the system to eradicate all air bubbles. If a transducer set has been primed and then left to stand before use, many microbubbles will have come out of solution and will be attached to the walls of the tubing. It is essential to eliminate all these and to flush the system prior to use. Careful priming of all parts of the fluid-filled system, including taps, injection caps and the transducer is essential (McGhee & Bridges 2002).

Prevention of clots Small clots in the intravascular catheter can also cause a distortion in the transmission of the pressure wave. Regular flushing of the system and the use of a continuous flush device can contribute to reducing this risk (Daily & Schroeder 1995).

Distortions of the pressure wave caused by bubbles, clots, distensible tubing, over-long tubing, etc. is called damping. The features of a damped trace are loss of waveform dynamics, lower peak pressures and higher trough pressures (referred to as a narrow pulse pressure), and rounding of the waveforms with a loss of definition, e.g. loss of the dicrotic notch on an arterial wave.

A square-wave test (Figure 10.4) helps the nurse at the bedside to determine whether the haemodynamic monitoring is optimized. If the rapid flush device is activated for 1–2 seconds the arterial pressure wave will be replaced by a square-wave. In an optimized system the square-wave will have a vertical upstroke and a horizontal segment where the pressure is maintained for the duration that the flush device is activated, and then when the flush device is released there should be a vertical down stroke, the lowest point of which is lower than the patient's diastolic pressure; this is followed by a couple of sharp small oscillations of pressure (Morton *et al.* 2005). In an overdamped system the upstroke is not a true vertical, the downstroke does not fall below the level of the patient's diastolic pressure and there are no oscillations before the next arterial pressure wave (Morton *et al.* 2005). Leaks, clots and air bubbles are all possible causes of an over-damped system. If the system is underdamped it will demonstrate multiple, sharp and more extreme oscillations at the end of the square-wave (Morton *et al.* 2005).

Staff should be familiar with normal haemodynamic waveforms in order to interpret the abnormal or to detect change in the quality of the information.

Measurement of right atrial or central venous pressure

The central venous pressure is the pressure in the great veins supplying the venous return to the heart. As these vessels are in continuity with the right atrium, CVP is usually the same as right atrial pressure (RAP).

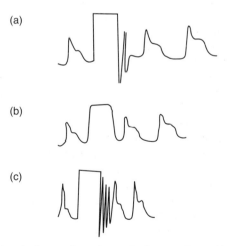

(a)

(b)

(c)

Figure 10.4 Square wave test for haemodynamic monitoring to support. (a) Optimally damped system. Activation of the rapid flush device produces a rapid upstroke, a horizontal line as the flush is maintained at the preset pressure of the flush bag (300 mmHg in adults), followed by a vertical downstroke with a minor oscillation before returing to the baseline. (b) Overdamped system. Activation of the rapid flush device produces an upstroke that is not truly vertical, followed by the horizontal wave which does not produce a 90° angle, and a downstroke that is not a true vertical. There are no oscillations after the flush. (c) Underdamped system. Activation of the rapid flush device produces a square wave followed by several oscillations above and below the baseline before the resumption of the normal pressure wave which appears excessively peaked with a sharp anacrotic shoulder.

Section 2

The CVP or RAP usually reflects the filling pressure of the heart, in particular the right atrium. This usually gives an indication of the quality of filling of the right ventricle; hence practitioners sometimes refer to the patient's 'filling pressure'. In health, the CVP is also assumed to be an indication of the filling of the left ventricle. There are certain circumstances when the behaviour of one ventricle may not have any bearing on the function of the other, such as in right or left heart failure. CVP is often used to assess the circulating volume. If the CVP is low, the circulating volume may be low. It is not possible, however, to assume this correlation as other factors must be considered, such as the patient's vascular tone. A profoundly peripherally dilated patient may have a normal circulating volume despite recording a low CVP. Peripheral dilation is seen in pyrexia, sepsis and anaphylaxis, and in patients in whom vasodilators are being used (Morton *et al.* 2005). The opposite is also true: if a patient is dehydrated, the sympathetic nervous system will increase the vascular tone to maintain the intravascular pressure; thus a hypovolaemic patient may record a normal CVP. A CVP recording on its own, without context, is meaningless and must be used in conjunction with other clinical information (Morton *et al.* 2005).

The CVP is not therefore a true measurement of intravascular volume, but rather a measure of the pressure in the central veins, and can only contribute to the assessment of intravascular volume (Soni 1989).

If a CVC is connected to a pressure transducer, it should be possible to record the CVP. A typical CVP waveform is illustrated in Figure 10.5. Alterations in CVP traces are seen in disease. For example, if a patient experiences atrial fibrillation (AF), their CVP trace will not usually demonstrate 'a' waves. Patients who have been overfilled or who have tricuspid valve regurgitation (TVR) will have very dominant 'v' waves, typical of TVR.

The CVP can also be measured using a water manometer. A water manometer measures the CVP in cmH$_2$O whilst haemodynamic monitoring records the CVP in mmHg so the information is not directly comparable. The normal value of a CVP obtained using a water manometer is 5–8 cmH$_2$O, whilst the normal value of a transduced CVP is 0–5 mmHg if taken from the sternal notch and 5–10 mmHg if taken from the intersection of the midaxillary line with the fourth intercostal space. To convert cmH$_2$O to mmHg the value in cmH$_2$O is divided by 1.36; to convert mmHg to cmH$_2$O the value in mmHg is multiplied by 1.36 (Morton *et al.* 2005). Isolated CVP readings are of little clinical value and more importance is placed on the trends that are recorded (Morton *et al.* 2005).

Left atrial pressure

Left atrial waveforms are usually similar to right atrial waveforms, but with less definition because of the distensibility of the pulmonary venous system. True left atrial

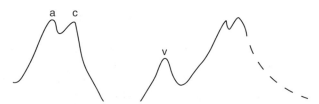

Figure 10.5 A typical central venous pressure waveform. (a) The increase in venous pressure seen during atrial systole. Because the atria have contracted, the venous return cannot enter the atria and accumulates in the great veins, causing an increase in pressure. (c) The transient increase in pressure caused by the bulging of the tricuspid valve during the isovolumetric contraction of the ventricles. (v) The change in pressure seen as the atria fill while the tricuspid valve is closed.

recordings are only obtained by the insertion of a direct left atrial catheter. This is usually restricted to post-cardiac surgical situations because the fine cannula must be placed through the chest wall and into the left atrium. This method of monitoring is not without risk. Gentle traction is placed on the catheter when it is ready to be removed. The catheter is usually removed relatively easily, but there is a risk that a patent hole will remain in the left atrium. This can result in tamponade and the patient must be monitored and observed during and after left atrial catheter removal. It is usual practice to remove the left atrial catheter before removing the cardiac drains so that any bleeding can be detected (Leitman *et al*. 1992). However, the catheter may be left in for several days if it is assisting with haemodynamic management and in this circumstance the drains may be removed before the left atrial catheter.

It is more common to pass a pulmonary artery flotation catheter in order to obtain information about the left side of the heart. This is a transvenous system without the inherent risks of bleeding from an atrial puncture site.

Arterial pressure recording

Continuous monitoring of intra-arterial blood pressure can be performed by placing a catheter in an artery and connecting it to a pressure monitoring system. As well as providing real-time blood pressure measurements an arterial catheter also provides vascular access for obtaining blood samples (Morton *et al*. 2005). Arterial blood pressure monitoring is indicated for patients receiving vasoactive infusions such as inotropes and vasodilators and for patients with unstable blood pressure (Morton *et al*. 2005). Real-time haemodynamic information allows nurses to titrate vasoactive agents within given clinical parameters.

Contraction of the left ventricle produces a pulse wave of blood that is transmitted through the arterial system. These pulses can be palpated at certain anatomical points; for example, the pulse can be felt in the brachial artery in the cubital fossa and in the radial artery in the distal forearm (Drake *et al*. 2005). It is this pulse wave that is sensed by the arterial catheter connected to the haemodynamic monitoring.

Arteries have forward flow and, as a result, waveforms are usually characterized by systolic waves followed by diastolic waves. Systole of the left ventricle produces a high-velocity ejection of blood through the aortic valve and into the aorta. The outflow of blood from the left ventricle produces the upstroke of the normal arterial waveform; this is also known as the anacrotic limb of the arterial pressure wave (McGhee & Bridges 2002). The aorta slows the pulse wave slightly by the distensibility of the aortic wall and by the curve of the aortic arch. The displacement of blood in the aorta produces the rounded top to the arterial pressure wave, also known as the ancrotic shoulder (McGhee & Bridges 2002). The downstroke of the arterial pressure wave is called the dicrotic limb and is characterised by a dicrotic notch which is a small change in pressure generated by the closing of the aortic valve at the end of systole (Morton *et al*. 2005). The shape and length of the diastolic run-off that follows the dicrotic notch changes with arterial compliance and heart rate (McGhee & Bridges 2002). Figure 10.6 illustrates an arterial waveform in health.

When systemic vascular tone is normal, the arterioles generate resistance to blood flow, and pressure within the arteries is sustained for relatively long periods of time. This creates a large area under the curve of the wave, and the top of the wave, although clearly defined, is not excessively peaked; there is a clear anacrotic shoulder to the wave.

In patients whose vascular tone is abnormally dilated, perhaps due to sepsis, the vasculature has less tone and is relatively unresistant, and pressure is allowed to dissipate very rapidly. This produces a much narrower pressure wave with less area under its curve, indicating that perfusion pressure has not been sustained for any length of time. This produces an overall reduction in mean pressure. The dicrotic notch is still seen, but

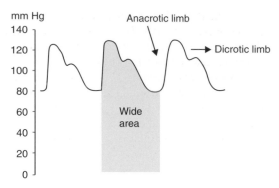

Figure 10.6   A normal arterial waveform.

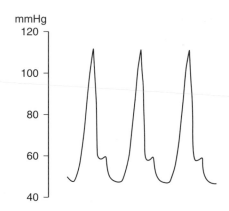

Figure 10.7   Arterial waveform in sepsis or conditions that lower systemic vascular resistance. Note the narrow, sharply peaked waveform and the lower dicrotic notch. Note the reduced area under the curve and the consequent reduction in perfusion.

appears to be in a different position (Figure 10.7). Its timing will not have changed (it is still produced by the closure of the aortic valve at the end of systole), but the amount of pressure left in the aorta when the dicrotic notch occurs is much reduced. This means that by the time the aortic valve closes, systolic pressure has already disappeared. The arterial pressure trace also appears much more peaked.

The arterial wave form produced on the monitor is not just the result of the forward pulse of blood along the artery, it is also influenced by a phenomenon known as 'wave reflection'. Wave reflection is caused by the impedence of the arteries and the branching of the arterial vessels; the impedence causes backward or retrograde reflection of the pressure wave (O'Rourke & Yaginuma 1984). McGhee and Bridges (2002) compare this phenomenon with the waves on a beach: the forward or antegrade waves and the reflected waves collide. The combination of the two types of wave serves to increase the systolic blood pressure the further down the arterial system it is measured; the blood pressure recorded in the radial artery or the dorsalis pedis artery may in fact be higher than the pressure recorded in the aorta (McGhee & Bridges 2002).

Some cardiac conditions cause abnormal arterial pressure waves. For example, in aortic regurgitation the aortic valve is dysfunctional and the blood that is pumped into the aorta is able to flow back into the ventricle. This produces an exceptionally low diastolic pressure, which may be nearly zero, and an absence of a dicrotic notch (Guyton & Hall 2006).

In ill health, where vascular tone is altered, arterial waves can appear less consistent and may even appear to be out of sequence. Shock waves of blood can appear to rebound up an artery, giving the appearance of either a double wave or a wave which is back to front, i.e. diastole before systole.

Arterial waveforms which are transduced from positional arterial catheters or from partially occluded arterial catheters can appear damped (Figure 10.8). This is the term used to describe loss of definition of the waveform. It can also be seen when the manometer tubing contains bubbles.

It is also possible to have a transduced arterial pressure wave which is underdamped. The waveform appears to have an exaggerated peak, and often the systolic wave appears to have two peaks. This is commonly described as 'overshooting' (Figure 10.9). To reduce the likelihood of overshooting, inaccuracies related to the tubing length and material, the diameter of the cannula, air bubbles and clots should be eliminated (*See* page 298). Commercial damping devices are available if the problem cannot be resolved.

Risk factors

Arterial catheters present significant risks to patients and should only be used when the benefits of patient management outweigh the disadvantages of catheter placement.

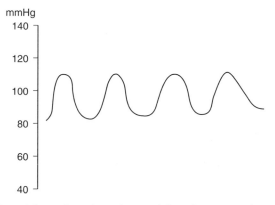

Figure 10.8 Damped arterial waveform. Note the raised diastolic pressure, the narrowed pulse pressure and the loss of definition to the wave.

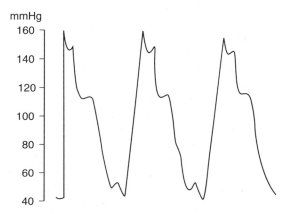

Figure 10.9 Arterial waveform with 'overshoot', the result of underdampening. Note the abnormally high peak pressure, the double peak at the top of the wave and the additional diastolic activity.

One of the most significant contraindications to arterial cannulation is coagulopathy. However, an arterial catheter placed at first attempt by an experienced practitioner may offer lower risk than numerous puncture sites to monitor gases or chemistry.

Insertion site and procedure

The most popular insertion site is the radial artery (Morton *et al.* 2005). This is one of two arteries which supply the hand, the other being the ulnar artery. By cannulating the radial artery, there is still another artery to guarantee adequate blood supply to the distal limb (Figure 10.10).

It is good practice to ensure that limb perfusion can be achieved using the other artery. This is called an Allen's test. Both the ulnar and radial arteries are occluded. The patient then clenches and unclenches their fist until the hand has blanched. Pressure on the ulnar artery is released and the hand is observed to ensure that colour returns to the entire hand, despite the radial artery still being occluded (Morton *et al.* 2005). If the hand remains blanched for longer than 15 seconds the ulnar circulation is considered to be inadequate and the radial artery should not be cannulated (Morton *et al.* 2005).

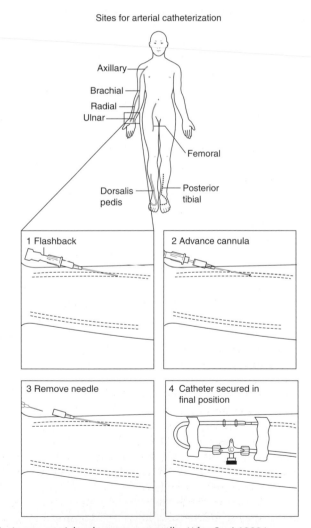

Figure 10.10   Placing an arterial catheter over a needle. (After Soni 1989.)

In clinical practice, in intensive care a modified Allen's test is often used as many patients are unconscious and therefore unable to comply with the test. In the modified Allen's test the artery which is intended to be used is occluded using digital pressure. The hand is observed to determine whether collateral supply is adequate to maintain perfusion to the limb. If it is not it would be prudent to select another site (Soni 1989). Despite collateral circulation to the hand there are reports in the literature of ischaemic injury resulting from the short-term use of radial artery catheters (Lee *et al.* 2001).

The brachial artery is rarely a first choice because it is the only artery supplying the arm at that point; it divides lower down to form the radial and ulnar arteries. Long-term usage of the brachial artery is not recommended (Daily & Schroeder 1995). The dorsalis pedis and posterior tibial arteries can also be used and both benefit from collateral circulation.

There are two methods of placement for a radial artery catheter: over a guidewire (Seldinger's technique), and the catheter-over-needle technique—similar or identical to the technique used for peripheral venous cannulation (Gerber *et al.* 1996). There is a significant cost difference between the two techniques and there are usually differences in the catheter tip design. Standard peripheral venous cannulae have an end hole design, whilst arterial catheters usually have side holes as well as an end hole. Gerber *et al.* (1996) sought to establish whether the success rate and time required to place the catheter via the Seldinger technique justified the cost. Whilst they found an increased success rate in some subsets, for example the patient with poorly palpable pulses, the overall success rate was no better and they concluded that the cost of guidewire catheters did not justify their routine use. They did, however, recommend the use of the guidewire catheter for difficult radial artery catheterizations. They did not study the impact of the catheter design. Side holes are contraindicated in umbilical artery catheterization in the newborn as they are associated with aortic thrombosis (Barrington 1999).

A number of techniques are used to secure arterial catheters. For short-term use, for example perioperatively, the catheter may be secured with steristrips at the entry site and covered with a transparent dressing. The extension set attached to the catheter is usually formed into a loop to prevent direct traction on the catheter. For more long-term use, for example in an ITU, the catheter may be sutured in an attempt to reduce the hazard of exsanguination should the catheter become dislodged. This is a particularly important issue in the agitated or confused patient. Whatever method is chosen, the securement device must be sterile. Maki and Crnich (2003) remind us that, contrary to popular belief, arterial catheters have a similar incidence of catheter-related bloodstream infection to non-tunnelled CVCs.

A transparent, moisture-permeable dressing is usually selected to secure the catheter and promote observation of the site. Care must be taken to ensure that luer-lock fittings are used and that they are tightly connected. Whilst the arterial catheter is *in situ*, the practitioner must carefully observe the patient, the catheter site and the distal limb. The catheter site should be observed in the same way as a venous cannula, looking for signs of erythema; oedema, leakage, bleeding, discharge or tracking along the arterial route.

The distal limb must be inspected and compared with the other non-cannulated limb; the nurse should assess the limb for colour, warmth, sensation, movement and capillary filling (Morton *et al.* 2005). Deterioration in any of these features is indicative of impaired perfusion to the distal limb. The signs must be reported immediately and it is good practice to electively replace the device.

In the event that a femoral artery site has been used, where there is no collateral supply, any signs of limb ischaemia could have devastating complications. Removal of the catheter is essential and it may be necessary to perform a Fogarty embolectomy to restore circulation to the limb (Daily & Schroeder 1995).

The femoral artery is a common site for paediatric arterial monitoring and is the only site for the placement of intra-aortic balloon pumps. In patients whose femoral arteries have been catheterized, particularly when the catheter is a large-bore device, it is important to monitor pedal pulses in addition to the range of arterial observations previously listed (Morton *et al.* 2005). It may be necessary to use a portable Doppler to confirm pulses in a patient whose pulses are difficult to palpate. Patients with intra-aortic balloon pumps *in situ* will require heparinization (Morton *et al.* 2005). Some units choose to monitor foot temperatures as an early indication of deterioration in peripheral arterial flow.

Complications
Complications of arterial catheterization include limb ischaemia, haematoma and aneurysm formation. The latter may require surgical repair. A significant complication is disconnection, which can have devastating results if not detected early. All connections must be luer-locked (Morton *et al.* 2005), and it is considered good practice to be able to observe the arterial catheter at all times (Garretson 2005), The arm should not, therefore, be left under the bedclothes where haemorrhage could go undetected. Femoral arterial catheters have a risk of occult haemorrhage as bleeding may track into the groin and can go unnoticed, and so the femoral catheter site should be checked regularly (Garretson 2005).

Management
It is considered good practice to clearly label an arterial catheter to prevent accidental drug administration. Other than the pressurised flush solution, no fluids or drugs should be injected into an arterial catheter. The exception to this rule might be the instillation of a thrombolytic agent to restore perfusion to a thrombosed artery. Eradication of all air from the continuous flush system of an arterial catheter is essential. Even small air bubbles in an arterial system can cause local air embolism and subsequent tissue ischaemia.

Removal
As with all intravascular devices, arterial catheters should be removed when they are no longer clinically useful. Care must be taken when removing an arterial catheter; non-sterile gloves should be worn and it would be good risk management to wear goggles to prevent blood splashes to the eye (RCN 2005). The flush device should be switched off, arterial alarms on the monitor disabled, any sutures removed and, using sterile gauze, pressure should be applied to the site while the catheter is gently pulled out. Firm pressure should be applied to the puncture site for at least 3 minutes, or longer if there is a known coagulopathy. After 3 minutes, the edge of the gauze should be tentatively lifted to observe whether the site has stopped bleeding. If it has not, firm pressure must be applied for a further 3 minutes. This process should be repeated until the bleeding is arrested.

A sterile pressure dressing should be applied and left in place for about an hour. The site should be inspected regularly for bleeding or haematoma formation. The distal limb perfusion should also be assessed in case the pressure dressing is too tight. If an arterial catheter has been removed in preparation for discharge of the patient to a ward, it would be prudent to tell the ward nurse where the arterial puncture was, and when any dressings should be removed.

Intra-aortic balloon pump removal is usually a medical task and carries a significant risk of blood contamination. Apron, gloves and eye protection should be worn (RCN 2005). Pressure is applied in a similar manner to the removal of an angioplasty catheter (although intra-aortic balloon pump catheters are of a significantly larger gauge), usually for about 20 minutes. Again, the site is cautiously inspected and further pressure applied if indicated. A pressure dressing is applied and usually left *in situ* for 24 hours. Pedal pulses should be checked to ensure that the pressure dressing does not cause reduced perfusion to the distal limb.

Special pressure-controlled devices are available for controlled removal of large-bore femoral catheters (e.g. the 'FemoStop'). These reduce the risk of both blood contamination and underperfusion of the limb from inappropriate pressure application. Due to the transparent nature of the device, observation of the site is possible even during the application of continuous pressure. However, haemostasis may be achieved more rapidly by the use of traditional manual compression (Walker *et al.* 2001).

Pulmonary artery pressure monitoring

Pulmonary artery (PA) flotation catheters can be used to measure pulmonary artery pressure. PA catheters were developed in the first half of the 20th century and Bradley (a British physician) was the first to describe the clinical use of the PA catheter in the management of sick adult patients in 1964. Branthwaite and Bradley (1968) then reported the use of the PA catheter to measure CO and later Swan *et al.* (1970) reported the use of balloon-tipped, flow-directed PA catheters.

By attaching the catheter to a pressure transducer it is possible to measure the pressure changes in the pulmonary circulation. An inflatable balloon is incorporated into the design of the catheter tip. The balloon is inflated with air which makes the tip of the catheter light-weight and buoyant. The tip of the catheter floats within the intracardiac blood flow and is carried forward through the right side of the heart with the direction of the blood flow. The operator advances the catheter with the balloon inflated and the tip of the catheter is carried into progressively smaller pulmonary arteries until finally it becomes wedged in a small pulmonary artery. The balloon obstructs the artery, preventing blood flow past the catheter. The transducer is then able to record the pressure in the pulmonary vascular bed, which is in direct continuity with the left atrium. Whatever pressure is present in the left atrium is transmitted back through the pulmonary vascular bed and interpreted by the wedged pulmonary artery catheter. This technique permits monitoring of left heart pressure without catheterization of the left side of the heart. The pulmonary artery wedge pressure (PAWP), also known as the pulmonary capillary wedge pressure (PCWP), provides a reflection of the pressure in the left side of the heart. Once the wedge pressure has been recorded it is important to deflate the balloon and to re-establish blood flow to the segment of the pulmonary arterial system that the balloon had obstructed. It is therefore important for the nurse to be able to recognize a wedged and an unwedged waveform.

Image intensity is often used to assist with the placement of this type of catheter. Some centres, however, rely solely on pressure changes to identify the placement of the catheter tip. The pressure changes recorded by the monitoring equipment will reflect the pressure changes in the heart as the catheter passes through the various chambers (Figure 10.11). The pressure waveforms corresponding to these chambers are shown in Figure 10.12.

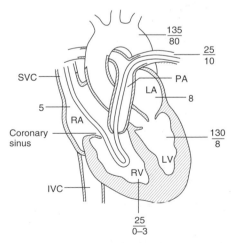

Figure 10.11 Normal pressure values in the heart. IVC, inferior vena cava; LA, left atrium; LV, left ventricle; PA, pulmonary artery; RA, right atrium; RV, right ventricle; SVC, superior vena cava. (After Soni 1989.)

Section 2

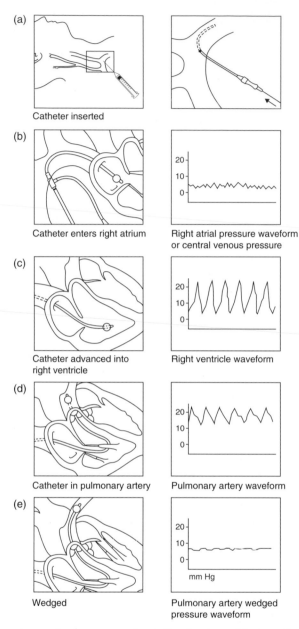

Figure 10.12 Pressure waveforms corresponding to the chambers of the heart through which the PA catheter is passing. (After Soni 1989.)

There are several designs of pulmonary artery catheter.

- *Simple*, incorporating a balloon and a distal lumen through which pulmonary pressure will be measured.
- *Intermediate*, incorporating a balloon, a distal lumen for PA pressure measurements and a proximal lumen through which the CVP may be measured.
- *Complex*, incorporating a balloon, distal and proximal lumens, plus a thermistor and electronic connections for cardiac output studies. This catheter can be used to measure CO, cardiac index, systemic vascular resistance and pulmonary vascular

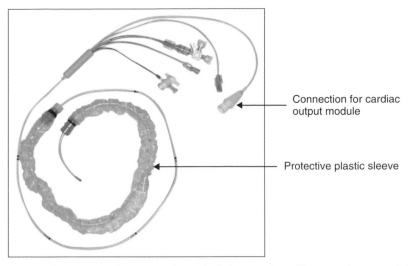

Figure 10.13   Cardiac output catheter. Note the multiple lumens; the red lumen is the port to inflate the balloon on the tip of the catheter. Note the plastic sleeve that protects the catheter, allowing it to be manipulated within the vein. The sleeve locks on to the top of the introducer and the cardiac output catheter is fed through the introducer to the correct position within the pulmonary artery.

resistance, as well as the traditional pulmonary artery pressure, PCWP and CVP. The most complex catheters have up to seven lumens (*see* Figure 10.13).

It is also possible to purchase CO catheters which can pace the myocardium, catheters which monitor mixed venous oxygenation as sampled from the pulmonary artery, and catheters with additional lumens for fluid administration. Cardiac output catheters have also been developed with ion electrodes at their tips for *in situ* measurement of pH.

The distal or PA lumen is always connected to a transducer and continuous flush device. This lumen transmits continuous real-time pulmonary artery pressure results and the PA systolic, diastolic and mean are displayed on the monitor (Morton *et al.* 2005). The proximal or right atrial lumen opens into the right atrium and provides continuous right atrial pressure or CVP measurements; this lumen can be used for drug or fluid infusions. The right atrial lumen is also used for the injectate to measure CO (Morton *et al.* 2005).

The balloon inflation port is usually supplied with its own volume-limited syringe to inflate the balloon on the distal end of the catheter. The balloon capacity of most PA catheters is 1.5 mL (Morton *et al.* 2005). If too much air is injected into the balloon the balloon will rupture, and the catheter will no longer be flow directed and can no longer measure wedge pressures.

If the PA catheter is also a CO catheter then the tip of the catheter will contain a thermistor. The thermistor is temperature sensitive and measures the temperature of the blood in the pulmonary artery. A cold or room-temperature solution is injected via the right atrial lumen of the catheter and the thermistor continuously detects the temperature of the blood flowing past it. The thermistor is connected electronically to a CO module in the bedside monitor or to a CO computer. The computer is programmed with the temperature of the solution that will be injected via the right atrial port. The computer continuously records the change in temperature of the blood and generates a temperature curve; the CO is calculated from the curve based on thermodilution (Morton *et al.* 2005).

Because the PA catheter passes through the heart and into the pulmonary artery it is subject to the rhythmical contractions of the heart and the position of the catheter can change. If the catheter moves too far forward it may become wedged even when the balloon is not inflated, making it necessary to pull the catheter back. The catheter will then have to be re-advanced until the correct wedge position is obtained. Because of the mobility of the catheter it is necessary to confirm the position of the catheter before measuring the PA or wedge pressure. To facilitate the manipulations of the catheter without compromising sterility the catheter is encased in a sterile plastic sleeve that locks onto the introducer sheath of the catheter. The plastic sleeve has been shown to reduce the incidence of catheter-related bloodstream infection associated with the PA catheter (Mermel 2000). *See* Figure 10.13.

Pulmonary artery and CO monitoring carry an intrinsic risk of morbidity (Valtier *et al.* 1998). If the information obtained will not improve the management of the patient then the procedure should not be carried out. When the catheter is no longer clinically useful, it should be removed. When using the PA catheter it is important to recognize the unwedged and wedged pressure waveforms. When inflating the balloon to measure a wedge pressure, a section of the pulmonary bed will be deprived of blood flow. Were the catheter to remain wedged for prolonged periods of time, ischaemia would occur. The practitioner at the bedside must be able to recognize the waveform in order to act in the best interest of the patient either by seeking assistance or by repositioning the catheter if trained to do so. The majority of units now prefer to use the less invasive oesophageal Doppler to monitor cardiac output, although most ITUs have at least two methods of CO measurement at their disposal (Esdaile & Raobaikady 2005).

Removal of the PA catheter is similar to removal of other central venous catheters. It must be remembered, however, that this catheter is much longer and less easy to handle. The practitioner should wear gloves and may require a surface on which to place the catheter when it is removed, such as a disposable absorbent pad. Before removing the catheter, the practitioner must check that the balloon at the end of the catheter has been deflated. Significant valvular damage could occur if the catheter were removed with the balloon inflated. There are reports of the PA catheter becoming entangled within the chordae tendonae of the tricuspid valve (Arnaout *et al.* 2001). On occasions, this has led to chordae rupture. As the catheter is removed it will pass through the pulmonary and tricuspid valves. This can often cause electrical irritability, with atrial and ventricular ectopics being seen on the ECG. In this event it is prudent to continue to remove the catheter rather than to stop pulling and run the risk of leaving the catheter tip positioned within the ventricle or against a valve which may cause further dysrhythmias. The patient's ECG should be observed during catheter removal. In the event that significant resistance is felt the procedure should be stopped and medical assistance sought. Emergency drugs and equipment must be available during catheter insertion and removal (Morton *et al.* 2005).

Due to the design of the catheter, it will have been inserted through an introducer sheath. The hole in the vessel will be large and pressure will need to be applied for several minutes. As with other CVCs, an occlusive dressing should be placed on the site and left *in situ* for 72 hours.

Temporary endocardial pacing

Patients in acute, life-threatening heart block or profound, persistent bradycardia will require a temporary, transvenous pacing wire. Some tachycardias may also be managed with overdrive pacing (Gammage 2000), although this is less common.

To pace the heart successfully, a current must be passed through it, and therefore an electrical circuit must be formed (Soni 1989). This is achieved by having two electrodes with heart muscle in between. The electrodes may be built into the same pacing wire, in which case it is termed bipolar, or one electrode may be in the wire whilst the other is placed on or in the skin. This type of wire is classified as unipolar. Modern temporary wires are usually bipolar.

These wires are inserted through an introducer sheath in a central vein, usually under X-ray guidance. In the case of heart blocks, the wire is positioned past the point of block, in the ventricles. In the case of bradycardia, an atrial wire may be used.

It can be difficult to secure the pacing wire against the myocardial wall; an atrial wire in particular may be difficult to position. As a result, the majority of temporary pacing wires are ventricular because the wire can be positioned up against the apex of the ventricle. The wire is connected to a pacing box; the battery should have been tested in advance. All pacing boxes are battery-controlled—the patient is never connected to 240 volts!

It is common to see a coil of pacing wire at the skin entry site. It is hoped that if undue traction is placed on the wire, the coil will tighten, rather than the wire become dislodged. Pacing wires are usually sutured in place at the skin entry site.

Temporary pacing wires are more rigid than i.v. catheters and fairly thin, commonly 5 or 6 Fr, it is not unusual for them to penetrate or perforate the right ventricular wall and the patient may present with pericarditic pain or a pericardial rub (Gammage 2000). This is usually resolved by withdrawing the wire back into the ventricle and repositioning it. However, on rare occasions tamponade may occur which requires urgent intervention (Gammage 2000). As with other central venous devices there are case reports of device fracture with the fractured portion of the transvenous pacing wire lodging in the heart and being retrieved radiologically (Deutsch *et al.* 1991). Pacing wires are removed in the same way as PA catheters with similar attention to dysrhythmias.

Vascular Access for Acute Renal Failure

The human kidney has several functions, the main one of which is excretory. The kidney is responsible for the excretion of water-soluble wastes, excess electrolytes, drugs, hormones and water (Berne *et al.* 2004). In the event that the kidneys should fail, the excretory role of the kidney can be mimicked by the artificial filtration of blood through a semipermeable membrane. This is most commonly achieved through a hollow fibre filter. The filtration that occurs is determined by the pore size of the membrane, the surface area of the membrane and the volume of blood passing through the filter.

Small dissolved electrolytes pass across the membrane easily, and as a result clearance of these substances is determined by blood flow and the surface area of the filter.

In haemodialysis, blood and a physiological solution (dialysate) flow in opposite directions through the filter, separated by a semipermeable membrane. Solutes transfer across the membrane down their concentration gradients. This process is termed diffusion. The transfer of small molecules less than 200 daltons (Da) is efficient and is determined by the rate of flow of the blood or the dialysate, whichever is slower. Transfer of molecules becomes progressively less as molecular size increases.

In haemofiltration, blood alone flows past one side of the membrane. The hydrostatic pressure gradient across the membrane results in ultrafiltration of water and an accompanying solute loss through convection (solute drag). This system permits the passage of molecules up to 10–20 000 Da almost as freely as water, in a process very similar to glomerular filtration.

The filtrate is discarded and a physiological substitution fluid replaces lost plasma volume. Fluid balance is manipulated by controlling the amount of substitution fluid. Whichever technique is utilized, vascular access will be necessary to deliver blood to the filter and subsequently return the filtered blood to the body.

If the patient is in an intensive care unit, haemofiltration will usually be the treatment of choice. Haemofiltration can be carried out as a slow continuous therapy, avoiding large fluid losses which might make an already sick patient more cardiovascularly unstable. Haemofiltration machines are very portable and require no special facilities. They are designed for continuous or intermittent use. Chemistry and fluid balance can be independently manipulated with the modern machines that are currently available. Modern haemofiltration is venovenous, which carries a lower mortality than arteriovenous haemofiltration.

Haemodialysis, in comparison, requires an environment with soft water plumbing, which is not always available outside a renal unit. Dialysis is designed as an intermittent treatment and is only suitable in patients who are cardiovascularly stable and fit enough to be transferred to the renal unit.

Catheters

Schwab and Beathard (1999) suggest that evolution of clinical practice has led to the development of two distinct classes of dialysis catheter access: temporary acute catheters and chronic tunnelled cuffed catheters. Temporary catheters are characteristically composed of rigid materials such as polyurethane or polyvinyl. These materials are fairly rigid at room temperature which allows for easy insertion over a guidewire without the incorporation of a sheath into the design (Schwab & Beathard 1999). Catheter rigidity decreases at body temperature within the bloodstream. Some newer catheters have used silicone which is much more flexible and consequently the catheters require a trochar or a peel-away sheath to facilitate insertion (Schwab & Beathard 1999). Peel-away sheath designs have been associated with venous air embolism during the insertion procedure (Vesely 2001; Wysoki 2001).

There are several designs of dialysis catheter in clinical use. Dialysis catheters may have stepped or staggered lumens, split lumens, parallel lumens or circumferential lumens; some require the use of twin catheters; many of the designs incorporate side holes. Twardowski and Moore (2001) believe that side holes are not beneficial because the manufacturing process produces a roughened surface that encourages clot formation (*See* Figure 10.14).

These catheters are traditionally 8 FG and are inserted using a Seldinger technique. As large vessels are required to tolerate such large catheters, access is usually restricted to the internal jugular, subclavian and femoral veins. Given the known association of venacaval thrombosis, the jugular vein often remains the first-line choice. Special catheters have been designed for the jugular site. They are the same diameter as for the SVC or femoral vein, but their extension ends have been curved back towards the tip of the catheter. This change in direction of the extensions allows the connections to be positioned away from the hair and the side of the face and is more comfortable for patients (Oliver 2001) (Figure 10.15).

In acute ITU or ward settings, these catheters are used as long as the patient's renal failure is deemed to be reversible. As with all CVCs, the catheter will be replaced regularly and, where appropriate, the access site will be rotated. Patients who are ambulatory will prefer not to have femoral vein catheters, both for comfort and for ease of dressing.

Dialysis catheters are usually dedicated to filtration or dialysis only, rather than being accessed for convenience. If a patient needs additional vascular access this should be

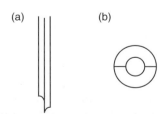

Figure 10.14   Catheter designs (a) Side profile of catheter. (b) Catheter in cross section.

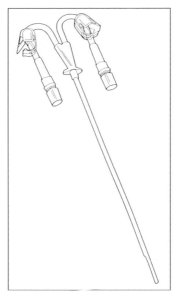

Figure 10.15 Haemofiltration catheter modified for the internal jugular site.

established rather than using the higher-risk dialysis catheter. Dialysis catheters are of no use if they are not fully patent as the dialysis team will be unable to establish adequate flow rates to perform the treatment. Most renal units maintain patency of their catheters with heparin to ensure that they are available for the next access. A dialysis catheter with a poorly controlled i.v. infusion will undoubtedly clot off, rendering the access useless. This means not only that renal treatment will be delayed, but also that the patient will have to go through unnecessary recannulation in order to continue their treatment. Given the diameter of this type of catheter, it is wise not to remove the catheter if the patient is actively heparinized as haemostasis can be difficult to achieve. Clotting agents may need to be given to patients with coagulopathies prior to removing this type of catheter.

Management
For removal, as with all CVCs, the patient should be correctly positioned, pressure should be applied until haemostasis is achieved and an occlusive dressing should be applied and left in place for 72 hours. In view of the wide-bore nature of this VAD it would be prudent to check clotting before removal of the catheter. If the cannula has been in for 5 days or more, or if catheter-related infection is suspected, the tip of the catheter should be sent for microbiological culture and sensitivity assessment. Catheters used for renal management are associated with an increased risk of septicaemia (Pearson 1995).

Arteriovenous fistulae

Once acute renal failure appears irreversible it will be necessary to consider alternative access for continued renal treatment. The gold standard for chronic dialysis patients is the establishment of a successful arteriovenous (AV) fistula. An AV fistula is an anastamosis between an artery and a vein, which is a surgical procedure. Connecting an artery to a vein creates extreme turbulence within the fistula, which causes the vessel to dilate. An AV fistula takes time to mature, sometimes more than a year, and it is necessary to use temporary vascular access in the interim. This usually takes the form of a tunnelled dialysis catheter with an implanted cuff (Schwab & Beathard 1999).

Conclusion

As the range of usage for acute vascular access continues to widen, the complexity of the devices continues to increase. This expansion of i.v. therapy is crossing more boundaries and has a progressively wider implication for the scope of nursing practice than ever before. Once seen as a last resort or reserved only for the critically ill, the central venous catheter has become commonplace in a variety of care settings. A minority of nurses have expanded their practice to include the placement of CVCs and Hamilton (2004) believes that this has led to reductions in cost and medical time and, more importantly, improvement in the patient experience. The nurse involved in the care of these patients is increasingly challenged to be familiar with the growing range of devices available. In addition, the management of these devices can vary between centres. By the development of a coordinated, national approach to i.v. therapy, based on sound principles rather than anecdotal rituals, nurses will develop the knowledge base from which to expand their individual scope of practice in order to respond to this increasingly challenging discipline.

References

Abi-Nader JA (1993) Peripherally inserted central venous catheters in critical care patients. *Heart and Lung* 22(5): 428–434.

Adar R, Mozes M (1971) Fatal complications of central venous catheter. *British Medical Journal* 3: 746.

Albrecht K, Nave H, Breitmeier D, Panning B, Tröger HB (2004) Applied anatomy of the superior vena cava—the carina as a landmark to guide central venous catheter placement. *British Journal of Anaesthesia* 92(1): 75–77.

Arnaout S, Diab K, Al-Kutoubi A, Jamaleddine G (2001) Rupture of the chordae of the tricuspid valve after knotting of the pulmonary artery catheter. *Chest* 120: 1742–1744.

Aubaniac R (1952) L'injection intraveneuse sousclaviculare advantage et technique. *Presse Medicale* 60: 1456.

Banton J, Banning V (2002) Impact on catheter-related bloodstream infections with the use of the Biopatch® dressing. *Journal of Vascular Access Devices* Fall: 1–6.

Baranowski L (1993) Central venous access devices: current technologies, uses, and management strategies. *Journal of Intravenous Nursing* 16(3): 167–194.

Bard www.accessabilitybybard.co.uk [accessed 21 June 2006]

Barrington KJ (1999) Umbilical artery catheters in the newborn: effects of catheter design (end vs side hole). *Cochrane Database of Systematic Reviews* 1 (CD000508).

Barton BR, Hermann G, Weil R III (1983) Cardiothoracic emergencies associated with subclavian haemodialysis catheters. *Journal of the American Medical Association* 250: 2600–2662.

Bartorelli AL, Trabattoni D, Agrifoglio M, Galli S, Grancini L, Spirito R (2001) Endovascular repair of iatrogenic subclavian artery perforations using the Hemobahn stent-graft. *Journal of Endovascular Therapy* 8: 417–421.

Berne RM, Levy NL, Koeppen BM, Stanton BA (2004) *Physiology*, 5th edn. Mosby, St Louis, Missouri.

Borow M, Crowley JG (1985) Evaluation of central venous catheter thrombogenicity. *Acta Anaesthesiologica Scandinavica* 198 (Suppl): 59–64.

Bosman M, Kavanagh RJ (2006) Two-dimensional ultrasound guidance in central venous catheter placement; a postal survey of the practice and opinions of consultant paediatric anaesthetists in the United Kingdom. *Paediatric Anaesthesia* 16(5): 530–537.

Brady HR, Fitzcharles B, Goldberg H *et al.* (1989) Diagnosis and management of subclavian vein thrombosis occurring with subclavian cannulation for haemodialysis. *Blood Purification* 7: 210–217.

Bradley RD (1964) Diagnostic right heart catheterisation with miniature catheters in severely ill patients. *Lancet* 2: 941–2.

Brandt RL, Foley WJ, Fink GH *et al.* (1970) Mechanisms of perforation of the heart with production of hydropericardium by a venous catheter and its prevention. *American Journal of Surgery* 119: 311–316.

Branthwaite MA, Bradley RD (1968) Measurement of cardiac output by thermodilution in man. *Journal of Applied Physiology* 24: 434–438.

Cardella JF, Fox PS, Lawler JB (1993) Interventional radiologic placement of peripherally inserted central catheters. *Journal of Vascular and Interventional Radiology* 4(5): 653–660.

ChloraPrep (2007) Information leaflet (www document) www.medi-flex.com/chloraprep_com/260700_label.pdf [accessed 7 January 2007]

Chow JL, Brock-Utne JG (2005) Minimizing the effect of heparin-induced thrombocytopenia: to heparinize or not to heparinize vascular access. *Pediatric Anesthesia* 15: 1037–1040.

Chu K, Hsu J, Wang S *et al.* (2004) Accurate central venous port-A catheter placement: intravenous electrocardiography and surface landmark techniques compared by using transesophageal echocardiography. *Anaesthesia and Analgesia* 98: 910–4.

Cicalini S, Palmieri F, Petrosillo N (2004) Clinical review: New technologies for the prevention of intravascular catheter-related infections. *Critical Care* 8: 157–162.

Cimochowski GE, Worley E, Rutherford WE, Sartain J, Blondin J, Harter H (1990) Superiority of the internal jugular over the subclavian access for temporary dialysis. *Nephron* 54: 154–161.

Cleri DJ, Corrado ML, Seligman SJ (1980) Quantitative culture of intravenous catheters and other intravenous inserts. *Journal of Infectious Diseases* 141: 781–786.

Collier PE, Blocker SH, Graff DM, Doyle P (1998) Cardiac tamponade from central venous catheters. *American Journal of Surgery* 176: 212–4.

Collin J, Collin C, Constable FL, Johnstone ID (1975) Infusion thrombophlebitis and infection with various cannulas. *Lancet* 2: 150–153.

Collins JL, Lutz RJ (1991) In vitro study of simultaneous infusion of incompatible drugs in multilumen catheters. *Heart and Lung* 20(3): 271–277.

Conly JM, Grieves K, Peters B (1989) A prospective randomised study comparing transparent and dry gauze dressings for central venous catheters. *Journal of Infectious Diseases* 158: 310–319.

Costerton JW, Stewart PS, Greenberg EP (1999) Bacterial biofilms: a common cause of persistent infections. *Science* 284 (5418): 1318–1322.

Craven DE, Lichtenberg DA, Kunches LM *et al.* (1985) A randomized study comparing a transparent polyurethane dressing to a dry gauze dressing for peripheral intravenous catheter sites. *Infection Control* 6: 361–366.

Crawford AG, Fuhr JP, Rao B (2004) Cost–benefit analysis of chlorhexidine gluconate dressing in the prevention of catheter-related bloodstream infections. *Infection Control and Hospital Epidemiology* 25(8): 668–674.

Crnich CJ, Maki DG (2002a) The promise of novel technology for the prevention of intravascular device-related bloodstream infection. 1. Pathogenesis and short-term devices. *Clinical Infectious Diseases* 34: 1232–1242.

Crnich CJ, Maki DG (2002b) The promise of novel technology for the prevention of intravascular device-related bloodstream infection. 1. Pathogenesis and short-term devices. *Clinical Infectious Diseases* 34: 1362–1368.

Dahlberg PJ, Agger WA, Singer JR *et al.* (1995) Subclavian haemodialysis catheter infections: a prospective randomized trial of an attachable silver impregnated cuff for prevention of catheter-related infections. *Infection Control and Hospital Epidemiology* 16: 506–511.

Daily EK, Schroeder JS (1995) *Techniques in Bedside Haemodynamic Monitoring*, 5th edn. Mosby, St Louis.

Darouiche RO, Raad I, Heard SO *et al.* (1999) A comparison of two antimicrobial-impregnated central venous catheters. *New England Journal of Medicine* 340: 1–8.

Darovic GO (2002) Ask the experts: percutaneous sheath introducer systems used for venous access. *Critical Care Nurse* 22: 1.

De Cicco M, Matovic M, Balestreri L *et al.* (1997) Central venous thrombosis: an early and frequent complication in cancer patients bearing long-term silastic catheter. A prospective study. *Thrombosis Research* 15; 86(2): 101–113.

Dennis AR, Leeson-Payne CG, Langham BT, Aitkenhead AR (1995) Local anaesthesia for cannulation; has practice changed? *Anaesthesia* 50: 400–402.

Dezfulian C, Lavelle J, Nallamothu BK, Kaufman SR, Saint S (2003) Rates of infection for single-lumen versus multilumen central venous catheters: A meta-analysis. *Critical Care Medicine* 31(9): 2385–2390.

Deutsch L, Dang H, Brandon JC, Ott R, Allen B, Futerman C (1991) Percutaneous removal of transvenous pacing lead perforating the heart, pericardium and pleura. *American Journal of Roentgenology* 156: 471–473.

Doğan E, Erkoç R, Sayarlıoğlu H, Etlik O, Uzun K (2005) A rare complication of internal jugular vein cannulation: Horner's syndrome. *European Journal of General Medicine* 2(4): 167–168.

Domino KB, Bowdle TA, Posner KL, Spitellie PH, Lee LA, Cheney FW (2004) Injuries and liability related to central vascular catheters: a closed claims analysis. *Anesthesiology* 100(6): 1411–1418.

Drake RL, Vogl W, Mitchell AWM (2005) *Gray's Anatomy for Students*. Elsevier Inc., Philadelphia.

Durant TM, Long J, Oppenheimer MJ (1947) Pulmonary (venous) air embolism. *American Heart Journal* 33: 269–281.

Eisen LA, Narasimhan M, Berger JS, Mayo PH, Rosen MJ, Schneider RF (2006) Mechanical complications of central venous catheters. *Journal of Intensive Care Medicine* 21(1): 40–46.

Elliott TSJ (1988) Intravascular device infections. *Journal of Medical Microbiology* 27: 161–167.

Elliott TSJ (1993) Line-associated bacteraemias. *Communicable Diseases Report* 3(7): R91–R96.

Elliott TSJ, Faroqui MH, Armstrong RF, Hanson GC (1994) Guidelines for good practice in central venous catheterization. *Journal of Hospital Infection* 28: 163–176.

Esdaile B, Raobaikady R (2005) Survey of cardiac output monitoring in intensive care units in England and Wales from *25th International Symposium on Intensive Care and Emergency Medicine*, Brussels, Belgium, 21–25 March 2005. *Critical Care* 9 (Suppl 1): P68.

Fabri PJ, Mirtallo JM, Ruberg RL *et al.* (1982) Incidence and prevention of thrombosis of the subclavian vein during total parenteral nutrition. *Surgery, Gynecology & Obstetrics* 155(2): 238–240.

Farber TM (1993) *ARROWgard Blue Antiseptic Surface: Toxicology Review*. A-76 20M. Arrow International, Inc., USA.

Fuller TJ, Mahoney JJ, Juncos LI *et al.* (1976) Arteriovenous fistula after femoral vein catheterization. *Journal of the American Medical Association* 236: 2943–2944.

Gabriel J (2000) Patients' impressions of PICCs. *Journal of Vascular Access Devices* 5(4): 26–29.

Gabriel J, Bravery K, Dougherty L, Kayley J, Malster M, Scales K (2005) Vascular access: indications and implications for patient care. *Nursing Standard* 19(26): 45–54.

Gammage MD (2000) Electrophysiology: temporary cardiac pacing. *Heart* 83: 715–720.

Garretson S (2005) Haemodynamic monitoring: arterial catheters. *Nursing Standard* 19(31): 55–64.

Gaukroger PB, Roberts JG, Manners TA (1988) Infusion thrombophlebitis: a prospective comparison of 645 Vialon and Teflon cannulae in anaesthetic and postoperative use. *Anaesthesia and Intensive Care* 16(3): 265–271.

Geissler HJ, Allen SJ, Mehlhorn U, Davis KL, Morris WP, Butler BD (1997) Effect of body repositioning after venous air embolism: an echocardiographic study. *Anesthesiology* 86: 710–717.

Gerber DR, Zeifman CWE, Khouli HI, Dib H, Pratter MR (1996) Comparison of wire-guided and nonwire-guided radial artery catheters. *Chest* 109(3): 761–764.

Ghani GA, Berry AJ (1983) Right hydrothorax after left external jugular vein catheterization. *Anesthesiology* 58: 93–94.

Gianino MS, Brunt LM, Eisenberg PG (1992) The impact of a nutritional support team on the cost and management of multilumen central venous catheters. *Journal of Intravenous Nursing* 15(6): 327–332.

Gil RT, Kruse JA, Thill-Baharozian MC, Carlson RW (1989) Triple vs single-lumen central venous catheters. A prospective study in a critically ill population. *Archives of Internal Medicine* 149: 1139–1143.

Gladwin MT, Slonim A, Landucci DL, Gutierrez DC, Cunnion RE (1999) Cannulation of the internal jugular vein: Is postprocedural chest radiography always necessary? *Critical Care Medicine* 27(9): 1819–1823.

Gopal K, Fitzsimmons L, Lawrance JAL (2006) Nurse-led central venous catheter service: Christie experience. *British Journal of Radiology* 79: 762–765.

Groeger JS, Lucas AB, Coit D *et al.* (1993) A prospective, randomized evaluation of the effect of silver impregnated subcutaneous cuffs for preventing tunneled chronic venous access catheter infections in cancer patients. *Annals of Surgery* 218: 206–210.

Gutierrez JA, Bagatell R, Samson MP, Theodorou AA, Berg RA (2003) Femoral central venous catheter-associated deep venous thrombosis in children with diabetic ketoacidosis. *Critical Care Medicine* 31(1): 80–83.

Guyton AC, Hall JE (2006) *Textbook of Medical Physiology*. 11th edn. Elsevier Saunders Company, Philadelphia.

Hadaway LR (2001) Anatomy and physiology related to intravenous therapy. In: Hankins J, Lonsway RA, Hedrick C, Perdue MB, eds. *Infusion Therapy in Clinical Practice*, 2nd edn, pp. 65–97. WB Saunders, Philadelphia.

Halliday P, Anderson DN, Davidson AI, Page JG (1994) Management of cerebral air embolism secondary to a disconnected central venous catheter. *British Journal of Surgery* 81: 71.

Hamilton HC (2004) Advantages of a nurse-led central venous vascular access service. *The Journal of Vascular Access* 5: 109–112.

Hanley PC, Click RL, Tancredi RG (1984) Delayed air embolism after removal of venous catheters. *Annals of Internal Medicine* 101: 401–402.

Hansen EK, Christensen KM (1983) Fatal thrombosis after subclavian catheter. *Anaesthesia* 38: 765–766.

Hibbard J (2005) Analyses comparing the antimicrobial activity and safety of current antiseptic agents: a review. *Journal of Infusion Nursing* 28(3): 194–207.

Hill RL, Fisher AP, Ware RJ, Wilson S, Casewell MW (1990) Mupirocin for the reduction of colonization of internal jugular cannulae a randomized controlled trial. *Journal of Hospital Infection* 15: 311–321.

Hoar PF, Wilson RM, Mangano DT *et al.* (1981) Heparin bonding reduces thrombogenicity for pulmonary artery catheters. *New England Journal of Medicine* 305: 993–995.

Hodge D, Puntis JWL (2002) Diagnosis, prevention, and management of catheter related bloodstream infection during long-term parenteral nutrition. *Archives of Disease in Childhood Fetal and Neonatal Edition* 87: F21–F24.

Hoffman KK, Western SA, Kaiser DL, Wenzel RP, Groschel DHM (1988) Bacterial colonization and phlebitis-associated risk with transparent polyurethane film for peripheral intravenous site dressings. *American Journal of Infection Control* 16: 101–106.

Hohlrieder M, Schubert HM, Biebl M, Kolbitsch C, Moser PL, Lorenz IH (2004) Successful aspiration of blood does not exclude malposition of a large-bore central venous catheter. *Canadian Journal of Anesthesia* 51: 89–90.

Hook ML, Reuling J, Leuttgen ML, Norris SO, Elsesser CC, Leonard MK (1987) Comparison of the patency of arterial lines maintained with heparinized and nonheparinized infusions. *Heart and Lung* 16: 693–699.

Horowitz HW, Dworkin BM, Savino JA, Byrne DW, Pecora NA (1990) Central catheter related infections: comparison of pulmonary artery catheters and triple lumen catheters for the delivery of hyperalimentation in a critical care setting. *Journal of Parenteral and Enteral Nutrition* 14: 588–592.

Hughes RE, Magovern GJ (1959) The relationship between right atrial pressure and blood volume. *Archives of Surgery* 79: 238–243.

Infusion Nurses Society (INS) (2006) Infusion nursing standards of practice. *Journal of Infusion Nursing* 29: 1S (Suppl).

Johnson CW, Miller DL, Ognibene FP (1991) Acute pulmonary embolism associated with guidewire change of a central venous catheter. *Intensive Care Medicine* 17(2): 115–117.

Jones A (2004) Dressings for the management of catheter sites. *Journal of the Association for Vascular Access* 9(1): 26–33.

Kamal GD, Pfaller MA, Rempe LE, Jebson PJ (1991) Reduced intravascular catheter infection by antibiotic bonding. A prospective, randomized, controlled trial. *Journal of the American Medical Association* 265: 2364–2368.

Kasten GW, Owens E, Kennedy D (1985) Ventricular tachycardia resulting from central venous catheter tip migration due to arm position changes: report of two cases. *Anesthesiology* 62: 185–187.

Kee L, Simonson J, Stotts N, Skov P, Schiller N (1993) Echocardiographic determination of valid zero reference levels in supine and lateral positions. *American Journal of Critical Care* 2: 72–78.

Kovacevich DS, Faubion WC, Braunschweig CL *et al.* (1988) Prevalence of catheter sepsis in parenteral nutrition patients with triple vs. single lumen. *Journal of Parenteral and Enteral Nutrition* 12 (Suppl): 23S.

Kristinsson KG (1989) Adherence of staphylococci to intravascular catheters. *Journal of Medical Microbiology* 28: 249–257.

Laronga C, Meric F, Truong MT, Mayfield C, Mansfield P (2000) A treatment algorithm for pneumothoraces complicating central venous catheter insertion. *American Journal of Surgery* 180(6): 523–526.

Lee MK, Lee IO, Kong MH, Han SK, Lim SH (2001) Surgical treatment of digital ischemia occurred after radial artery catheterisation. *Journal of Korean Medical Science* 16(3): 375–377.

Leighton H (1994) Maintaining the patency of transduced arterial and venous lines using 0.9% sodium chloride. *Intensive and Critical Care Nursing* 10: 23–25.

Leitman BS, Naidich DP, McGuiness G, McCauley DI (1992) The left atrial catheter: its uses and complications. *Radiology* 185(2): 611–612.

Levin A, Mason AJ, Jindal KK, Fong IW, Goldstein MB (1991) Prevention of haemodialysis subclavian vein catheter infections by topical povidone iodine. *Kidney International* 40: 934–938.

Liu J, Tseng H, Chen C, Chern M, Chang C (2004) Percutaneous retrieval of 20 centrally dislodged Port-A catheter fragments. *Journal of Clinical Imaging* 28(2004): 223–229.

Lopez-Lopez G, Pascual A, Perea EJ (1991) Effect of plastic catheter material on bacterial adherence and viability. *Journal of Medical Microbiology* 34(6): 349–353.

Loughran SC, Borzatta M (1995) Peripherally inserted central catheters: a report of 2506 catheter days. *Journal of Parenteral and Enteral Nutrition* 19(2): 133–136.

Lowenthal MR, Dobson PM, Starkey RE, Dagg SA, Peterson A, Boyle MJ (2002) *Anaesthesia and Intensive Care* 30(1): 21–24.

MacGregor DA, Smitherman KO, Deal DD, Scuderi PE (1998) Testing the competency of the hemostasis valve in introducer catheters (Laboratory report). *Anesthesiology* 88(5): 1404–1406.

Maki DG, Band JD (1981) A comparative study of polyantibiotic and iodophor ointment in the prevention of vascular catheter-related infection. *American Journal of Medicine* 70: 739–744.

Maki DG, Crnich CJ (2002) The promise of novel technology for the prevention of intravascular device-related bloodstream infection. II Long-term devices. *Clinical Infectious Diseases* 34: 1362–1368.

Maki DG, Crnich CJ (2003) Line sepsis in the ICU: prevention, diagnosis, and management. *Seminars in Respiratory and Critical Care Medicine* 24(1): 22–36.

Maki DG, Ringer M (1987) Evaluation of dressing regimens for prevention of infection with peripheral intravenous catheters. *Journal of the American Medical Association* 258: 2396–2403.

Maki DG, Weise CE, Sarafin HW (1977) A semi quantitative culture method for identifying intravenous catheter-related infection. *New England Journal of Medicine* 296: 1305–1309.

Maki DG, Ringer M, Alvarado CJ (1991) Prospective randomized trial of povidone-iodine, alcohol, and chlorhexidine for prevention of infection associated with central venous and arterial catheters. *Lancet* 338: 339–343.

Markus S, Buday S (1989) Culturing indwelling central venous catheters *in situ*. *Infections in Surgery* May: 157–162.

Maschke SP, Rogove HJ (1984) Cardiac tamponade associated with a multilumen central venous catheter. *Critical Care Medicine* 12: 611–613.

Maurer AH, Au FC, Malmud LS *et al.* (1984) Radionuclide venography in subclavian vein thrombosis complicating parenteral nutrition. *Clinical Nuclear Medicine* 9: 397–399.

McCarthy PM, Wang N, Birchfield F, Mehta AC (1995) Air embolism in single-lung transplant patients after central venous catheter removal. *Chest* 107: 1178–1179.

McGhee BH, Bridges MEJ (2002) Monitoring arterial blood pressure: what you may not know. *Critical Care Nurse* 22(2): 60–79.

McGee WT, Ackerman BL, Rouben LR, Prasad VM, Bandi V, Mallory DL (1993) Accurate placement of central venous catheters: a prospective, randomized, multicenter trial. *Critical Care Medicine* 21(8): 1118–1123.

Medical Defence Union (1996) *Informed Consent*. Medical Defence Union, London.

Mehlhorn U, Burke EJ, Butler BD *et al.* (1994) Body position does not affect the hemodynamic response to venous air embolism in dogs. *Anesthesia & Analgesia* 79: 734–739.

Mennim P, Coyle CF, Taylor JD (1992) Venous air embolism associated with removal of central venous catheter. *British Medical Journal* 305: 171–172.

Mercer-Jones MA, Wenstone R, Hershman MJ (1995) Fatal subclavian artery haemorrhage. A complication of subclavian vein catheterization. *Anaesthesia* 50(7): 639–640.

Section 2

Mermel LA (2000) Prevention of intravascular catheter-related infections. *Annals of Internal Medicine* 132: 391–402.

Mermel LA, McCormick RD, Springman SR, Maki DG (1991) The pathogenesis and epidemiology of catheter-related infection with pulmonary artery Swan–Ganz catheters: a prospective study utilizing molecular subtyping. *American Journal of Medicine* 91(Suppl 3B): 197S–205S.

Mermel LA, Stolz SM, Maki DG (1993) Surface antimicrobial activity of heparin-bonded and antiseptic-impregnated vascular catheters. *Journal of Infectious Diseases* 167: 920–924.

Mermel LA, Farr BM, Sherertz RJ *et al.* (2001) Guidelines for the management of intravascular catheter-related infections. *Clinical Infectious Diseases* 32: 1249–1272.

Merrer J, De Jonghe B, Golliot F *et al.* (2001) Complications of femoral and subclavian venous catheterization in critically ill patients: A randomized controlled trial. *Journal of the American Medical Association* 286(6): 700–707.

Morton PG, Fontaine DK, Hudak CM, Gallo BM (2005) *Critical Care Nursing: A Holistic Approach*, 8th edn. Lippincott Williams & Wilkins, Philadelphia.

Moss HA, Tenns SE, Faroqui M H *et al.* (2000) A central venous catheter coated with benzalkonium chloride for the prevention of catheter-related microbial colonization. *European Journal of Anaesthesiology* 17: 680–687.

Muhm M (2002) Editorial—ultrasound-guided central venous access. *British Medical Journal* 325: 1373–1374.

Murga R, Miller JM, Donlan RM (2001) Biofilm formation by Gram-negative bacteria on central venous catheter connectors: Effect of conditioning films in a laboratory model. *Journal of Clinical Microbiology* 39(6): 2294–2297.

Muth CM, Shank ES (2000a) Gas embolism. *New England Journal of Medicine* 342(7): 476–482.

Muth CM, Shank ES (2000b) Correction to Muth and Shank, *New England Journal of Medicine* 342(7): 476–482. 17 February 2000. Correspondence. Gas embolism. *New England Journal of Medicine* 342(26): 2000.

Nahum E, Levy I, Katz J *et al.* (2002) Efficacy of subcutaneous tunneling for prevention of bacterial colonization of femoral central venous catheters in critically ill children. *Pediatric Infectious Disease Journal* 21(11): 1000–1004.

National Institute for Health and Clinical Excellence (NICE) (2002) The clinical effectiveness and cost effectiveness of ultrasound locating devices for the placement of central venous lines. *Technology Appraisal Guidance No. 49*. National Institute for Health and Clinical Excellence, London.

National Kidney Foundation DOQI (1997) *Clinical Practice Guidelines for Vascular Access*. National Kidney Foundation, USA.

Oda T, Hamasaki J, Kanda N, Mikami K (1997) Anaphylactic shock induced by an antiseptic-coated central venous catheter. *Anesthesiology* 87: 1242–1244.

Oliver MJ (2001) Acute dialysis catheters. *Seminars in Dialysis* 14(6): 432–435.

O'Grady NP, Alexander M, Dellinger EP *et al.* (2002) Guidelines for the prevention of intravascular catheter-related infections. *Clinical Infectious Diseases* 35: 1281–1307.

O'Rourke MF, Yaginuma M (1984) Wave reflections and the arterial pulse. *Archives of Internal Medicine* 144: 366–371.

Padberg FT, Ruggiero J, Blackburn GL, Bistrian BR (1981) Central venous catheterization for parenteral nutrition. *Annals of Surgery* 193(3): 264–270.

Pearson ML (1995) Guideline for prevention of intravascular-device-related infections. *Infection Control and Hospital Epidemiology* 17(7): 438–473.

Pellowe CM, Pratt RJ, Loveday HP, Harper P, Robinson N, Jones SRLJ (2004) The *epic* project. Updating the evidence-base for national evidence-based guidelines for preventing healthcare-associated infections in NHS hospitals in England: a report with recommendations. *British Journal of Infection Control* 5(6): 10–16.

Peterson FY, Kirchhoff KT (1991) Analysis of the research about heparinized versus nonheparinized intravascular lines. *Heart and Lung* 20(6): 631–640.

Phifer TJ, Bridges M, Conrad SA (1991) The residual central venous catheter track—an occult source of lethal air embolism: a case report. *Journal of Trauma* 31: 1558–1560.

Poterack KA, Aggarwal A (1991) Central venous air embolism without a catheter. *Canadian Journal of Anesthesia* 38: 338–340.

Powell C, Fabri PJ, Kudsk KA (1988) Risk of infection accompanying the use of single-lumen vs double-lumen subclavian catheters: a prospective randomized study. *Journal of Parenteral and Enteral Nutrition* 12: 127–129.

Pratt RJ, Pellowe CM, Wilson JA *et al.* (2007) epic 2 – National evidence-based guidelines for preventing healthcare-associated infections in NHS hospitals in England. *Journal of Hospital Infection* 65(1): Suppl 1.

Raad II, Hohn DC, Gilbreath BJ *et al.* (1994) Prevention of central venous catheter-related infections by using maximum sterile barrier precautions during insertion. *Infection Control and Hospital Epidemiology* 15: 231–238.

Raad I, Darouiche R, Dupuis J *et al.* (1997) Central venous catheters coated with minocycline and rifampin for the prevention of catheter-related colonization and bloodstream infections: a randomized, double-blind trial. *Annals of Internal Medicine* 127: 267–274.

Reynolds MG, Tebbs SE, Elliott SJ (1997) Do dressings with increased permeability reduce the incidence of central venous catheter related sepsis? *Intensive and Critical Care Nursing* 13: 26–29 .

Ricard P, Martin R, Marcoux JA (1985) Protection of indwelling vascular catheters: incidence of bacterial contamination and catheter-related sepsis. *Critical Care Medicine* 13: 541–543.

Roberts S, Johnson M, Davies S (2003) Near-fatal air embolism: fibrin sheath as the portal of air entry. *Southern Medical Journal* 96(10): 1036–1038.

Ross AH, Griffith CDM, Anderson JR, Grieves DC (1982) Thromboembolic complications with silicone elastomer subclavian catheters. *Journal of Parenteral and Enteral Nutrition* 6(1): 61–63.

Royal College of Nursing IV Therapy Forum (2005) *Standards for Infusion Therapy*. Royal College of Nursing, London.

Ruesch S, Walder B, Tramer M (2002) Complications of central venous catheters: internal jugular versus subclavian access—a systematic review. *Critical Care Medicine* 30(2): 454–460.

Rushforth JA, Hoy CM, Kite P, Puntis JW (1993) Rapid diagnosis of central venous catheter sepsis. *Lancet* 342: 402–3.

Ryder M (2001) The role of biofilm in vascular catheter-related infections. *New Developments in Vascular Disease* 2: 15–25.

Scales K (2005) Vascular access: a guide to peripheral venous cannulation. *Nursing Standard* 19(49): 48–52.

Schwab SJ, Beathard G (1999) The hemodialysis catheter conundrum: hate living with them but can't live without them. *Kidney International* 56: 1–17.

Scott WL (1988) Complications associated with central venous catheters: a survey. *Chest* 94(6): 1221–1224.

Seldinger SI (1953) Catheter replacement of the needle in percutaneous arteriography: a new technique. *Acta Radiologica* 39: 368–375.

Seneff MG (1987a) Central venous catheterization: a comprehensive review, Part 1. *Journal of Intensive Care Medicine a* 2: 163–175.

Seneff MG (1987b) Central venous catheterization: a comprehensive review, Part II. *Journal of Intensive Care Medicine b* 2: 218–232.

Shapira M, Stern WZ (1967) Hazard of subclavian vein cannulation for central venous pressure monitoring. *Journal of the American Medical Association* 201: 327–329.

Sheep RE, Guiney WB Jr (1982) Fatal cardiac tamponade. *Journal of the American Medical Association* 248: 1632–1635.

Soni N (1989) *Anaesthesia and Intensive Care: Practical Procedures*, 1st edn. Heinemann, Avon, UK.

Spiers AF, Taylor KH, Joanes DN, Girdler NM (2001) A randomised, double-blind, placebo-controlled, comparative study of topical skin analgesics and the anxiety and discomfort associated with venous cannulation. *British Dental Journal* 190(8): 444–449.

Stephens R, Mythen M, Kallis P, Davies DW, Egner W, Rickards A (2001) Two episodes of life-threatening anaphylaxis in the same patient to a chlorhexidine-sulphadiazine-coated central venous catheter. *British Journal of Anaesthesia* 87: 306–308.

Stickle BR, McFarlane H (1997) Prediction of a small internal jugular vein by external jugular vein diameter. *Anaesthesia* 52(3): 220–222(3).

Stonelake PA, Bodenham AR (2006) The carina as a radiological landmark for central venous catheter tip position. *British Journal of Anaesthesia* 96(3): 335–340.

Sung JP, Bikangaga AW, Abbott JA (1981) Massive hemorrhage to scrotum from laceration of inferior epigastric artery following percutaneous femoral vein catheterization: case report. *Military Medicine* 146: 362–363.

Swan HJC, Ganz W, Forrester J *et al.* (1970) Catheterization of the heart in man with use of a flow-directed balloon-tipped catheter. *New England Journal of Medicine* 283: 447–451.

Taylor N, Hutchison E, Milliken W, Larson E (1989) Comparison of normal versus heparinized saline for flushing infusion devices. *Journal of Nursing Quality Assurance* 3(4): 49–55.

Timsit JF, Bruneel F, Cheval C, Mamzer MF, Garrouste-Org, Wolff M *et al.* (1999) Use of tunneled femoral catheters to prevent catheter-related infection. A randomized, controlled trial. *Annals of Internal Medicine* 130(9): 729–35.

Trerotola SO, Kuhn-Fulton J, Johnson MS, Shah H, Ambrosius WT, Kneebone PH (2000) Tunneled infusion catheters: increased incidence of symptomatic venous thrombosis after subclavian versus internal jugular venous access. *Radiology* 217: 89–93.

Tuncali BE, Kuvaki B, Tuncali B, Capar E (2005) A comparison of the efficacy of heparinized and nonheparinized solutions for maintenance of perioperative radial arterial catheter patency and subsequent occlusion. *Anesthesia & Analgesia* 100: 1117–1121.

Twardowski ZJ, Moore HL (2001) Side holes at the tip of chronic hemodialysis catheters are harmful. *Journal of Vascular Access* 2: 8–16.

Valtier B, Cholley BP, Belot J, de la Coussaye JE, Mateo J, Payen DM *(1998) Noninvasive monitoring of cardiac output in critically ill patients using transesophageal Doppler.* American Journal of Respiratory and Critical Care Medicine 158(1): 77–83.

Vanherweghem JL, Cabolet P, Dhaene M *et al.* (1986) Complications related to subclavian catheters for haemodialysis. *International Journal of Artificial Organs* 5: 297–309.

Vesely TM (2001) Air embolism during insertion of central venous catheters. *Journal of Vascular and Interventional Radiology* 12: 1291–1295.

Vesely TM (2003) Central venous catheter tip position: a continuing controversy. *Journal of Vascular Interventional Radiology* 14: 527–534.

Walker SB, Cleary S, Higgins M (2001) Comparison of the FemoStop device and manual pressure in reducing groin puncture site complications following coronary angioplasty and coronary stent placement. *International Journal of Nursing Practice* 7(6): 366–375.

Weiner P, Sznajder I, Plavnick L *et al.* (1984) Unusual complications of subclavian vein catheterization. *Critical Care Medicine* 12: 538–539.

Section 2

Weisenberg M, Szmuk P, Sessler DI, Evron S, Ezri T (2005) *External Topographic Landmarks for Correct Positioning of Central Venous Catheters Inserted through the Right Jugular Vein*. American Society of Anaesthesiology, Annual Meeting Abstracts. 14–18 October, Chicago.

Wilcox MH, Kite P, Mills K, Sugden S (2001) *in situ* measurement of linezolid and vancomycin concentrations in intravascular catheter-associated biofilm. *Journal of Antimicrobial Chemotherapy* 47: 171–175.

Woodburne RT, Burkel WE (1994) *Essentials of Human Anatomy*, 9th edn. Oxford University Press, New York.

Worly JM, Fortenberry JD, Hansen I, Chambliss CR, Stockwell J (2004) Deep venous thrombosis in children with diabetic ketoacidosis and femoral central venous catheters. *Pediatrics* 13(1): 57–60.

Wysoki MG, Covey A, Pollak J, Rosenblatt M, Aruny J, Denbow N (2001) Evaluation of various manoeuvres for prevention of air embolism during central venous catheter placement. *Journal of Vascular Interventional Radiology* 12: 764–766.

CHAPTER 11

Long-term Central Venous Access

Janice Gabriel

Introduction

As more patients become recipients of a vascular access device (VAD), especially for intermediate- to long-term parenteral therapies, it is important to ensure that the device selected not only meets their clinical needs, but is also acceptable to them and can become a part of their life (Chernecky *et al.* 2002; Petersen 2002).

This chapter will look at the types of central venous access device (CVAD) available for meeting the individual patient's intermediate- to long-term needs, i.e. skin-tunnelled catheters, implantable ports and peripherally inserted central catheters (PICCs). The indications for each device, placement techniques and management, together with the overall advantages and disadvantages, will be discussed, not only in relation to meeting the patient's clinical needs, but also in relation to how they can affect an individual's lifestyle.

Overview of Central Venous Access Devices

Recent years have seen an expansion in the numbers of patients receiving parenteral therapies. Medical research is resulting in an ever-expanding range of treatments, many of which are required to be administered intravenously (i.v.) (RCN 2005).

At the beginning of the 21st century the majority of patients admitted to hospital will receive a VAD at some point during their stay (Petersen 2002; Masoorli 2005). However, intravenous therapy is not confined solely to the hospital environment. Increasing numbers of patients who are not acutely ill, such as those who have chronic conditions such as cystic fibrosis requiring intermittent parenteral antibiotics, or those who have cancer and require the continuous infusion of, or intermittent treatment with, cytotoxic chemotherapy, are successfully being managed away from the hospital environment, providing they have a suitable VAD and fulfil the criteria for community/home-based treatment (Kayley 2003).

While a peripheral i.v. device can still meet the clinical requirements of many patients requiring venous access for a few days, there has been an increasing patient population requiring longer-term parenteral therapy and/or the administration of vesicant fluids/ drugs (Barbone & Rockledge 1995; Petersen 2002; Masoorli 2005). This has led to the development of a range of CVADs. Each type of CVAD has its advantages and potential limitations, depending on the requirements of the individual patient.

Defining Central Venous Access

Goodwin and Carlson (1993) defined a CVAD as a catheter which has its tip located in the superior vena cava (SVC). Other shorter catheters inserted by similar techniques, but whose tips do not extend as far as the SVC should not be described as CVADs, for example peripherally inserted catheters (PICs) (Dougherty 2006). A PIC does not extend beyond the axillary vein and should be described as a midline catheter (Goodwin & Carlson 1993). 'Long lines' extend beyond the axillary vein but not as far as the SVC. Dougherty (2006) stresses the importance of using the correct terminology, and advocates that generic terms should be used to avoid confusion and minimize the risk of inappropriate infusions/medicines being administered via VADs which are not centrally placed. Some practitioners prefer to place CVADs into the right atrium using fluoroscopy or ultrasound guidance. Gormon and Buzby (1995) suggested this position for long-term catheter placement, especially if the practitioner has easy access to the use of fluoroscopy and/or ultrasound guidance. Ultrasound guidance is now recommended by the National Institute for Health and Clinical Excellence (NICE) for the placement of all CVADs (NICE 2002; Dougherty 2006). The position of all CVADs should be confirmed directly after placement by chest X-ray (Hadaway 1989; RCN 2005).

Indications for a Central Venous Access Device

CVADs can be used for the administration of blood products, parenteral antibiotics and antiviral agents, cytotoxic drugs and parenteral nutrition. As many of these agents are vesicant or highly irritant to a patient's veins, their administration directly into the SVC ensures their rapid dilution by the large volume of blood flowing through this vessel (Richardson & Bruso 1993; Lowel & Bothe 1995; Masoorli 2005; RCN 2005).

Patients with poor peripheral venous access, requiring parenteral therapy for a short period of time or in an emergency situation may automatically become recipients of a CVAD because they have no accessible vein for a peripheral cannula. Apart from these patients, Shapiro (1995) identified five other groups of patients who could potentially benefit from the use of a CVAD as those requiring:

- continuous infusions of cytotoxic drugs
- prolonged/intermittent parenteral therapies
- prolonged blood product support
- administration of vesicant drugs
- parenteral therapies in paediatrics.

Vein Selection

Before discussing the specific devices available, it is important to identify which veins are commonly used for placement of a central venous access catheter (Gormon & Buzby 1995; Dougherty 2006):

- bilateral cephalic veins
- external jugular veins
- internal jugular veins
- axillary vein
- subclavian vein
- saphenous veins

- inferior epigastric vein
- gonadal veins
- lumbar veins
- intrathoracic veins
- femoral veins
- innominate (brachiocephalic) veins.

The basilic and median cubital veins can also be used (RCN 2005) (Figure 11.1).

Selection of a particular vein is dependent upon the individual patient's anatomy and medical condition and the reason for wishing to establish venous access. CVADs can be placed either percutaneously, i.e. by 'puncturing' the patient's skin to obtain access to a blood vessel, or surgically, i.e. by surgical cutdown through the patient's skin to identify the desired blood vessel for introduction of the CVAD (Dougherty 2006).

Bilateral cephalic veins/external and internal jugular veins

The cephalic and jugular veins can be accessed peripherally or by surgical cutdown. The tip of the CVAD is then threaded into the SVC or right atrium, via the subclavian or innominate (brachiocephalic) veins. Gormon and Buzby (1995) suggested that these are the preferred routes for establishing central venous access by a percutaneous or surgical cutdown approach, as the incidence of pneumothorax is minimal and the risk of subsequent bleeding from arterial injury is greatly reduced.

Mallory (2006) advocates the internal jugular vein as the preferred vein of choice for CVAD placement as it takes a shorter and more direct route to the subclavian vein. However, the disadvantages associated with using this vein include the potential for damage to the carotid artery and a challenge for dressing securement and comfort (Dougherty 2006; Hadaway 2006; Mallory 2006; Weinstein 2007).

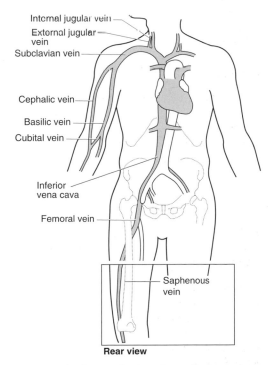

Figure 11.1   Venous access points for the introduction of central venous catheters.

Section 2

Axillary veins

The axillary vein is a continuation of the basilic vein. As it ascends the arm it increases in diameter and receives the cephalic vein as it passes beneath the clavicle (Figure 11.1). This vein can be used for CVAD insertion, and the more widespread use of ultrasound-assisted insertions has facilitated infraclavicular axillary vein cannulation (Dougherty 2006; Mallory 2006).

Subclavian veins

The subclavian vein is a continuation of the axillary vein. It extends from the outer edge of the first rib to the inner end of the clavicle, where it joins with the internal jugular vein (Figure 11.1).

The apex of the lung is very close to this vein and can therefore pose an increased risk for pneumothorax when the subclavian vein is punctured during cannulation. There is also the potential for a condition arising known as 'pinch-off' syndrome. This syndrome can occur if the CVAD is compressed between the clavicle and first rib (Galloway & Bodenham 2004).

Saphenous veins

The saphenous veins can be used successfully as a means of establishing central venous access using a cutdown procedure. It is essential that the skin surrounding the surgical cutdown is healthy and free from infection, as this will reduce the risk of infection for the patient. First, a surgical cutdown procedure is used to identify the saphenous vein. The catheter is then advanced under fluoroscopic guidance to the SVC/right atrium. Once in position, the catheter is secured to the patient's skin to prevent it from becoming dislodged (Gormon & Buzby 1995). While this technique will ensure central venous access for the patient, it is associated with a high risk of infection and is disliked by patients for long-term use due to its position (Gormon & Buzby 1995).

Inferior epigastric vein

The use of the inferior epigastric vein requires an involved surgical cutdown procedure through the patient's abdominal wall into the peritoneum. Once in the peritoneum, the inferior epigastric vein is identified. The CVAD is then tunnelled under the skin to the umbilicus. An incision is made into the inferior epigastric vein; the catheter is passed through it and advanced, under fluoroscopic guidance, to the right atrium. The CVAD is then secured to the blood vessel and the incision closed (Gormon & Buzby 1995). Although this procedure for central venous access is involved, it can be relied upon for long-term access. However, its position is associated with a high risk of infection and patient dissatisfaction for long-term use (Gormon & Buzby 1995).

Gonadal and lumbar veins

The technique for placing a CVAD via the gonadal vein requires the patient to be lying supine on the operating table. The patient's flank is then elevated by use of a sandbag or beanbag. An incision is made through the abdominal wall into the retroperitoneum and the gonadal vein identified. As with the inferior epigastric approach, the CVAD is tunnelled under the patient's skin and the catheter is advanced through the gonadal vein, under fluoroscopic guidance, until the right atrium is reached (Gormon & Buzby 1995).

Gormon and Buzby (1995) suggested the lumbar veins be used as an alternative if the gonadal vein is unsuitable. However, if the patient has experienced a central venous thrombosis, the lumbar veins are often enlarged, making them readily identifiable for easier access.

Intrathoracic veins

Gormon and Buzby (1995) discussed how the intrathoracic veins can be used when other options for placing CVADs have been eliminated. Two techniques can be used: a thoracotomy and a transthoracic approach. With the advancements in ultrasound techniques to facilitate CVAD placements these veins are seldom used today (Dougherty 2006)

Thoracotomy

The thoracotomy approach involves entering the patient's chest through the fourth intercostal space. The surgeon then decides which blood vessel to cannulate, depending upon the patient's anatomy. Once the CVAD has been placed, the device is then secured, a chest drain is inserted and the chest closed. There is a high degree of morbidity associated with this procedure due to the possible complications arising from the insertion procedure and it is rarely used today (Gormon & Buzby 1995).

Transthoracic approach

The transthoracic approach is considered to be the easiest and safest approach for placing a CVAD into an intrathoracic blood vessel. This technique involves a surgical incision into the parietal pleura to expose an upper intercostal vein. The CVAD is then tunnelled under the skin on the patient's chest wall, and the catheter advanced through the intercostal vein into the right atrium under fluoroscopic guidance. The incision is closed once the CVAD has been secured and a chest drain is left *in situ* during the postoperative period (Gormon & Buzby 1995). Again, this technique is seldom used today.

Femoral veins

The femoral vein approach can be performed relatively quickly, under local anaesthetic, by a percutaneous or surgical cutdown technique. However, it is associated with an increased incidence of iliofemoral thrombosis (Gormon & Buzby 1995). The procedure involves tunnelling the CVAD under the patient's skin from the umbilicus to the femoral vein. The CVAD is then introduced into the vein and advanced to the IVC or SVC/right atrium under fluoroscopic guidance.

Although this approach can be used for long-term use, it is associated with an increased risk of infection and disliked by many of its recipients due to the position of the catheter. Technology has also improved so it is seldom necessary to consider these veins today for patients requiring long-term central venous access (Mallory 2006).

Types of Central Venous Access Device

CVADs can be constructed from either polyurethane or silicone rubber. They are available in a variety of gauge sizes and can be single, dual or triple lumen, depending upon the device selected. The multilumen devices can have their exit points staggered at the proximal end of the CVAD to ensure that there is no mixing of the drugs/fluids as they exit the catheter and enter the venous circulation (Figure 11.2). Where the exit points are not staggered, concurrent administration of drugs/infusates should be avoided to prevent the potential for mixing as they exit the catheter into the venous circulation (Dougherty 2006).

Gauge sizes

The size of the CVAD will be described by the various manufacturers in terms of length and gauge size. The length will be expressed in either millimetres or centimeters,

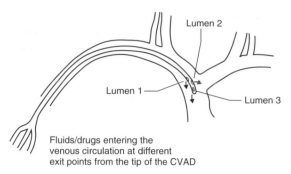

Figure 11.2   Multilumen vascular access devices. Staggering of lumens ensures that fluids/drugs do not mix as they exit the catheter and enter the venous circulation.

Table 11.1   External diameter sizes of central venous access devices.

Gauge (G)	French (Fr)
23 G	2.0 Fr
20 G	3.0 Fr
18 G	4.0 Fr
16 G	5.0 Fr

e.g. 36 mm or 60.0 cm. The gauge size will refer to the external diameter of the device and not the internal diameter. The external diameter can be expressed in either 'French' (Fr) or 'gauge' (G) size, e.g. 4.0 Fr or 18 G (Table 11.1). With multilumen devices it is the overall diameter of the device which is stated, e.g. 5 Fr (16 G) (Gabriel *et al.* 2005).

For the individual internal lumen size of a CVAD one would need to consult the specific product information supplied by manufacturers.

The flow rate through the CVAD will depend upon the internal diameter of the particular device. Individual manufacturers will be able to provide specific information on their products about the gravity flow rates and rates achieved by the use of a pump.

Catheter design and construction material

CVADs are commonly constructed from either polyurethane or silicone rubber (Gabriel *et al.* 2005; Dougherty 2006).

Polyurethane
CVADs constructed from polyurethane are more rigid than those constructed from silicone rubber. Consequently, in the longer term, they are more likely to break, due to an inability to recover from kinking and bending (Strumpfer 1991; Wickham *et al.* 1992; Sansivero 1997). This material does not soften when it comes into contact with body fluids (e.g. blood), and can cause irritation to the wall of the blood vessel, resulting in phlebitis and a higher incidence of thrombosis (Wickham *et al.* 1992; Sansivero 1997; Gabriel *et al.* 2005) Higher flow rates can be achieved through polyurethane CVADs than through those constructed from silicone rubber, as polyurethane is a more robust material and the walls are thinner, which in turn results in a lumen with a larger internal diameter (Gabriel *et al.* 2005).

Silicone rubber

Silicone rubber is a very flexible material which has the ability to recover from kinking and bending. The softness of this material means that any resulting phlebitis is less severe than that which can occur with polyurethane CVADs (Wickham *et al.* 1992). The incidence of thrombosis is also reduced in recipients of CVADs constructed from silicone rubber (Sansivero 1997). However, a disadvantage is that silicone rubber can be easily damaged by sharp instruments, such as toothed forceps used for clamping (Gabriel *et al.* 2005).

'Open-ended' and valved CVADs

Tunnelled catheters, implantable ports and PICCs can be either 'open-ended' or valved. An 'open-ended' CVAD can allow blood to reflux into the lumen(s) of the device (Mayo & Pearson 1995; Dougherty 2006). When the injection cap is removed, the catheter should be clamped to prevent air entering the patient's venous circulation (Gabriel *et al.* 2005; RCN 2005). There have been further modifications to the tips of CVADs; for example, Dr Groshong, an American clinician, developed a three-position slit valve as an integral part of the catheter's tip. In the absence of a negative or positive pressure, this valve remains closed, preventing air from entering the lumen(s) of the CVAD or blood refluxing. The design of this valve dispensed with the necessity of having to use a clamp to prevent air entry or the reflux of blood (Delmore *et al.* 1989; RCN 2005). A range of CVADs, including PICCs, are now available with non-return valves incorporated into either the distal or proximal tip of the catheter (Dougherty 2006) (Figure 11.3).

Skin-tunnelled catheters

In the 1970s, J. Broviac, an American clinician, developed a long-term skin-tunnelled catheter for patients requiring prolonged parenteral nutrition (PN) (Broviac *et al.* 1973). These catheters were tunnelled under the patient's skin, along the chest wall, and accessed the central venous system via the external jugular or cephalic veins. These devices had a

Section 2

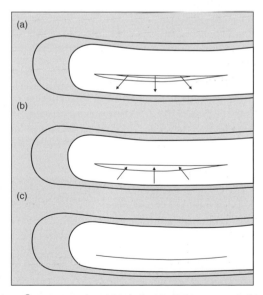

Figure 11.3   The Groshong® two-way valve. (a) Infusion (positive pressure); (b) aspiration (negative pressure); (c) closed (neutral pressure). (Reprinted by permission of Bard UK. Groshong® is a registered trademark of C. R. Bard or an affiliate.)

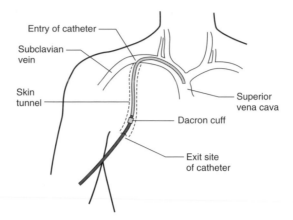

Figure 11.4 Placement of skin-tunnelled catheter.

dacron cuff attached to the portion of catheter that was tunnelled under the skin (Figure 11.4). The aim of the dacron cuff was twofold: firstly, it facilitated the growth of the surrounding tissue in and around the cuff, and therefore stabilized the catheter without the need for long-term additional securement; and secondly, the ingrowth of tissue coupled with the skin tunnelling technique created additional barriers, thus minimizing the potential for infection (Harris *et al.* 1987; Gabriel *et al.* 2005).

In the late 1970s, an American haematologist, Dr Hickman, realized the potential of a skin-tunnelled catheter for patients undergoing bone marrow transplantation. By modifying 'Broviac's' catheter, i.e., by increasing the internal diameter and creating a thicker wall, he increased the durability of the device (Harris *et al.* 1987; Mallory 2006).

All skin-tunnelled catheters are available today with one, two or three lumens, with or without non-return valves (Gabriel *et al.* 2005).

Implantable injection ports

An implantable injection port is a tunnelled CVAD attached to an injection port (a reservoir covered by a silastic membrane) which is totally implanted under the patient's skin. The injection port is secured to underlying muscle to prevent it from moving and the catheter tunnelled via a subcutaneous tunnel until the desired venous entry point is reached (Gabriel 2005; RCN 2005; Mallory 2006) (Figure 11.5). The first implantable injection port was introduced into clinical practice in 1982 (Gullo 1982; Boothe *et al.* 1984; Mallory 2006). Today, these devices are available either with the catheter already attached to the injection port or unassembled, in which case the individual placing the device must securely attach the catheter to the port (Gullo 1982). The unassembled system allows the catheter to be inserted before attaching the injection port. However, this technique can occasionally result in the catheter becoming detached from the injection port (Gullo 1982). These catheters are either open-ended or have a non-return valve.

Implantable injection ports are accessed by palpating the device through the patient's skin and using a 'Huber' needle to puncture the port's silastic membrane (Figure 11.5). It is vital that the individual accessing the injection port ensures that the needle has passed through the silastic membrane and into the port's reservoir. If the tip of the needle is not in the reservoir, extravasation of fluids/drugs could occur (Gabriel *et al.* 2005; Lokich *et al.* 1985; Masoorli 2005; Hadaway 2006).

The design of the 'Huber' needle minimizes the risk of 'coring' to the silastic membrane and therefore reduces the incidence of leakage (Gullo 1982; Gabriel *et al.* 2005; RCN 2005). However, the life of the port is limited by the overall number of punctures

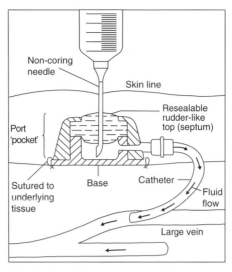

Figure 11.5   Cross-section of an implantable port accessed with a non-coring needle.

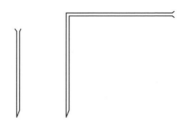

Figure 11.6   Huber needles.

to the silastic membrane. In time, even with the use of a 'Huber' needle, leakage becomes a possibility. 'Huber' needles are available in a variety of gauge sizes and lengths. They can be straight or right-angled. The choice of which to select is dependent upon what is to be administered and the duration of administration. A 'Huber' needle greater than 24 G should be used for the administration of blood products, as the internal diameter of the needle is large enough not to cause potential damage to the platelets as they are infused (Acquillo *et al.* 2006). If the patient is to receive an infusion as opposed to a bolus injection, an angled 'Huber' needle will probably be more comfortable and easier to secure when an i.v. administration set is attached to it (Figure 11.6).

All ports should be flushed thoroughly with sodium chloride 0.9% after each use to ensure that no drugs/infusates are retained in the reservoir. This will prevent any drug remaining in the reservoir from being 'flushed' into the venous circulation when the device is next used (Ben-Arush & Berant 1996; Gabriel *et al.* 2005; RCN 2005; Dougherty 2006).

Peripherally inserted central catheters

Peripherally inserted central catheters (PICCs), a group of single-, dual- and triple-lumen CVADs, were developed in the late 1970s in the USA (Gabriel 1996b; Nakazawa 2006). Venous access is achieved by cannulating a peripheral vein in the arm, i.e. the cephalic, basilic or median cubital vein. The catheter is then advanced through the cannula, or introducer, until it reaches the SVC/right atrium (Figure 11.7).

Section 2

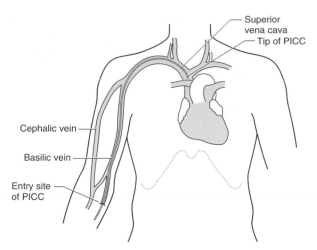

Figure 11.7   Entry site and position of peripherally inserted central catheter (PICC).

PICCs are available in a variety of gauges, but as the diameter of the arm veins is narrower than those of the larger veins in the chest, PICCs with a gauge size greater than 5 Fr cannot be accommodated by these smaller vessels. If too large a device is placed it will lead to mechanical phlebitis. Therefore triple-lumen PICCs should be placed in either the upper cephalic or basilic vein using a Seldinger technique (Nakazawa 2006).

PICCs were originally designed for intermediate-length parenteral therapies, but with good initial patient assessment and management they have been demonstrated to meet the clinical needs of patients for in excess of 6 months (Gabriel 2006). As venous access is achieved via cannulation or Seldinger technique, they have the advantage of minimal blood loss and can be placed in patients with low platelet counts (Gabriel 1996a). (The advantages and disadvantages of each device are summarized in Table 11.2 overleaf.)

Placement of CVADs

Patient assessment

Before a CVAD is placed for intermediate to long-term use it is important that the patient's clinical condition and lifestyle are assessed. This will help to ensure that the patient will 'accept' the device and complications are minimized (Gabriel 2000; Chernecky 2002). Firstly, the clinical needs of the patient should be assessed to determine which CVAD(s) will meet their needs. Secondly, if the patient is expected to spend time away from the hospital environment, or indeed become actively involved in the care and management of their own CVAD, the selected device should be acceptable to them and they should be able to manage it (*See* Quality of life on page 347) (Gabriel 2000; Chernecky 2002; Dougherty 2006). The patient should receive written and verbal information about the device selected. This information should include the following:

- rationale for the device
- advantages
- disadvantages/potential complications
- insertion procedure
- aftercare required
- 24-hour support information.

Table 11.2   Advantages and disadvantages of central venous access devices (CVADs).

Type	Features	Advantages	Disadvantages
Skin-tunnelled catheters	*Lumens available:* one, two or three, either open-ended or valved *Insertion technique:* surgical cut-down or percutaneous approach *Anaesthetic required:* either local or general *Dressings:* only required while incision and skin tunnel are healing *Limitations on patient's lifestyle:* some, e.g. no swimming and bathing unless waterproof dressing is worn *Removal technique:* surgical cut-down or gentle but firm traction *Long-term scarring:* some, i.e. from skin tunnel and insertion site	Available with one, two or three lumens. Ideal for patients who are needle-phobic Can be used long term	Increased infection risk compared with ports and PICCs Some limitations on patient's lifestyle
Implantable injection ports	*Lumens available:* one or two, either open-ended or valved (open-ended only available with multilayered septum) *Insertion technique:* surgical cut-down *Anaesthetic required:* either local or general *Dressings:* only required while skin incision is healing and to secure needle/cannula when *in situ* *Limitations on patient's lifestyle:* none *Removal technique:* minor surgical procedure *Long-term scarring:* from incision for placement/removal of reservoir	Suitable for long-term use for individuals requiring intermittent venous access	Not ideal for patients who are needle-phobic Only available with two lumens, unless more than one device is placed, e.g. a single + a dual Huber needles required for all types except the port with multilayered septum
PICCs	*Lumens available:* one or two, either open-ended or valved *Insertion technique:* cannulation of a peripheral vein *Anaesthetic required:* not always, but topical anaesthetic cream is usually applied *Dressings:* required to be changed weekly while PICC is *in situ* *Limitations on patient's lifestyle:* some, e.g. no swimming and soaking in bath *Removal technique:* gentle traction *Long-term scarring:* no	Quick and easy to place with minimal discomfort to the patient Can be used long term Lower rate of infection and associated insertion complications than other CVADs	Only available with two lumens, unless more than one device is placed, e.g. a single + a dual Dressing required the whole time the PICC remains *in situ* Some limitations on lifestyle

PICC, peripherally inserted central catheter.

Before the patient consents to the procedure the nurse must ensure that the patient has had sufficient opportunities to ask any questions about and to seek clarification on any aspect of the procedure, and what living with a CVAD may entail (Gabriel 2000).

Before placement of the CVAD the patient's blood count should be checked to ensure that the platelet count is adequate for the procedure (Gabriel *et al.* 2005). If appropriate, a clotting screen should also be undertaken. Where necessary, a thrombocytic patient can have the CVAD placed whilst receiving a platelet infusion. Patients with an elevated INR can have their anticoagulant therapy adjusted accordingly (Richardson & Bruso 1993; Hamilton 2000; Dougherty 2006).

For all insertions in the patient's upper body, except in the case of a PICC, they should be placed in the Trendelenburg position. This will ensure that the venous access point is below the level of the heart and therefore minimizes the risk of an air embolus. As PICCs are placed in an arm vein, the Trendelenburg position can be dispensed with, providing the person placing the device ensures that the patient's arm remains below the level of the heart (Richardson & Bruso 1993; Dougherty 2006).

CVADs can be placed under either local or general anaesthesia in order to minimize the discomfort of the procedure for the patient. The exception to this are PICCs, which can be successfully placed using a topical anaesthetic ointment or without any anaesthetic at all (Gabriel 2006). This is because the procedure involves accessing an arm vein with a conventional wide-gauge cannula, or an introducer of a similar size (RCN 2005).

The use of ultrasound guidance is recommended for placement of all CVADs where placements are undertaken without the assistance of imaging (i.e. usually outside of the imaging department or theatre) (NICE 2002). The use of ultrasound will not only help to locate veins that are difficult to palpate, but will also allow the practitioner to readily assess the patency and condition of the vessel (Mallory 2006; Marshalleck 2006).

Skin-tunnelled catheters

Skin-tunnelled catheters can be placed either by a cutdown technique or by a 'percutaneous' approach (Gormon & Buzby 1995). The cutdown procedure involves tunnelling a few centimeters of the catheter under the patient's skin using a trocar. A cutdown is then made into the vein, and the 'tunnelled' catheter threaded through the vessel until the tip of the CVAD reaches the SVC/right atrium (Figure 11.4). The percutaneous technique involves using a cannula to directly access the vein; no cutdown is used. Similar to the cutdown approach, a trocar is used to tunnel the catheter under the skin so that its exit site is away from where it enters the vein (Marshalleck 2006) (Figure 11.4).

Implantable injection ports

The implantable injection port is placed by making an incision into the patient's skin and creating a subcutaneous pocket. The device is then anchored with sutures to the underlying muscle, and the catheter tunnelled under the skin until it reaches the desired venous access point. The skin overlying the port is then surgically closed. The commonest area for siting these devices is on the patient's chest wall (Gullo 1982; Boothe *et al.* 1984). However, they can be placed more peripherally, e.g. on an arm. These devices are available with one or two ports. Each port is attached to a single-lumen catheter. If a patient requires more than two lumens to meet their clinical needs, there is no reason why two devices cannot be placed, e.g. a single and a dual lumen (Sansivero 1997).

Peripherally inserted central catheters

As with all CVADs, clinical assessment of the patient is important to minimize problems associated with the insertion procedure (Gabriel *et al.* 2005). As PICCs are placed by cannulation of the basilic, cephalic or median cubital vein, it is important that the clinical assessment of the patient takes into account any underlying condition which could result in pressure on the venous anatomy of the arm, axilla or supraclavicular fossa, such as a previously fractured clavicle, presence of a cardiac pacemaker, previous surgery or radiotherapy to that part of the body, or a history of axillary vein thrombosis. If the assessment of the patient does reveal any of these, for example left axillary node dissection, then the other arm should be considered; in this example, the right arm (Richardson & Bruso 1993).

The basilic vein is the ideal vein as, anatomically, it is the largest of the three vessels and provides the straightest route leading to the SVC (Hadaway 1989; Sansivero 1997). In the majority of patients, even if this vein cannot be readily visualized, there is usually no problem in palpating it. For patients who do not have a readily accessible antecubital fossa vein, fluoroscopy and/or ultrasound can be used to identify the vessel and therefore allow cannulation to take place using a micropuncture (Seldinger)

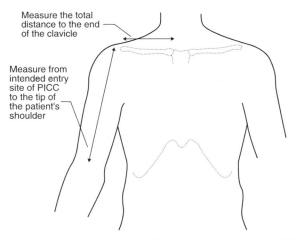

Figure 11.8 Preinsertion measurement of peripherally inserted central catheter (PICC).

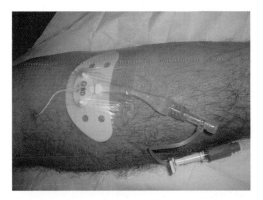

Figure 11.9 Peripherally inserted central catheter *in situ*.

technique (Sansivero 1997; NICE 2002; RCN 2005). The micropuncture or Seldinger technique was first developed in the 1950s by Dr. Seldinger. It involves accessing the vein with a fine hollow bore needle/cannula; threading a wire through the needle/cannula into the vein; removing the needle without dislodging the wire, and then threading the catheter over the wire before removing the wire (Mallory 2006).

Once the vein has been selected for placement of the PICC, the distance from the intended insertion site to the proximal end of the clavicle should be measured (Figure 11.8). Up to 3 cm should be added to the length of the catheter for placements in the left arm to ensure the device reaches the SVC. This additional length takes into account the position of the SVC (Gabriel 1996a).

When cannulation has been achieved, the PICC should be threaded through the cannula/introducer until the required length has been inserted (some PICCs are available with 'depth' markings printed onto the device to ensure the correct length is placed, whilst others are provided with a sterile tape measure). By asking the patient to place their chin on their shoulder on the placement side, the passage of the PICC into the subclavian vein is enhanced as this position gently distorts the venous anatomy and reduces the potential for the PICC to be passed into the jugular vein as opposed to the subclavian (Marshalleck 2006). The cannula/introducer is then withdrawn and the PICC secured with a self-adhesive anchoring device and/or steristrips (Figure 11.9). As with all CVADs,

> **BOX 11.1**
>
> **Steps involved in placing a PICC using a cannulation technique**
>
> Explain the procedure to the patient.
> - Assess the patient's clinical needs and lifestyle.
>   — Will a PICC meet the patient's clinical needs?
>   — Has the patient had any axillary/supraclavicular fossa (SCF) surgery/radiotherapy?
>   — Does the patient have a history of axillary vein thrombosis?
>   — Does the patient have a cardiac pacemaker?
>   — Is there a history of a fractured clavicle?
>   — Will the patient's condition prevent him from coping with a PICC?
>   — Does the patient have inaccessible antecubital fossa veins?
>   — Is the patient's blood count satisfactory for a PICC placement?
>   — Is the patient on anticoagulants? If yes, what is the clotting screen?
>
> If the answer to any of the above is 'yes', further assessment will be necessary to ensure that a PICC is the most appropriate CVAD. For example, can the opposite arm be used if the patient has had axillary/SCF surgery/radiotherapy (see text)?
> Gain the patient's consent for the procedure.
> - Select a vein and apply local anaesthetic cream as prescribed before commencing the procedure.
> - Measure the distance from the intended site of insertion to the proximal end of the clavicle, adding up to 3 cm for insertion on the left-hand side (see text).
> - Prepare your equipment for the procedure.
> - Lie the patient flat on a bed and extend the selected arm for the PICC placement at right angles to the patient's body (a couch may be too narrow to support the patient's arm comfortably during the procedure).
> - Wearing sterile gloves and gown, clean the skin around the intended entry site with an appropriate antiseptic.
> - Cannulate the selected vein with the cannula or introducer supplied with the PICC to gain venous access and release tourniquet.
> - Remove the stylet from the cannula/introducer and begin to thread the PICC.
> - Ask the patient to place his chin onto his shoulder on placement side.
> - Continue to thread the PICC through the cannula/introducer until the required length has been placed (check with the markings on the PICC or using a sterile tape measure).
> - Remove the cannula/introducer.
> - Flush with sodium chloride 0.9% for valved PICCs, or heparinized saline for open-ended PICCs.
> - Attach the injection hub.
> - Stabilize with a sterile self-adhesive anchoring device and/or steristrips.
> - Apply the dressing.
> - Confirm the position of the PICC by chest X-ray if not placed under fluoroscopic guidance.

a chest X-ray will be required to confirm the position of the PICC if it was not placed under fluoroscopic guidance (RCN 2005) (*See* Box 11.1).

Insertion complications

The possible complications other than infection that could be encountered during the insertion procedure and in the first 7 days are summarized in Table 11.3.

Air embolus

Air embolus is a potentially preventable complication of CVAD placement and removal. It is a result of air entering the venous circulation and travelling to the pulmonary vein. The risk of this complication can be minimized by placing the patient in the Trendelenburg position if the CVAD accesses the circulation in the patient's upper body, or, in the case of PICC placements, by ensuring that the patient's arm is kept below the level of the heart (Richardson & Bruso 1993; Dougherty 2006).

Table 11.3 Complications (other than infection) of catheter insertion.

	Valved skin-tunnelled	Open-ended skin-tunnelled catheter	Open-ended injection port	Valved injection port (chest placement)	Open-ended PICC and injection port (peripheral placement)	Valved PICC
Air embolus	Not once device is *in situ*	✓	✓	Not once device is *in situ*	✓	X
Pneumothorax	✓	✓	✓	✓	X	X
Catheter malposition	✓	✓	✓	✓	✓	✓
Pinch-off syndrome	✓	✓	✓	✓	X	X
Thrombosis	✓	✓	✓	✓	✓	✓
Chemical phlebitis	Very rare	Very rare	Very rare	Very rare	Very rare	Very rare
Mechanical phlebitis	Very rare	Very rare	Very rare	Very rare	✓	✓
Atrial fibrillation	✓	✓	✓	✓	✓	✓

PICC, peripherally inserted central catheter.

Clinical features of an air embolus can include:

- chest pain
- dyspnoea
- tachycardia
- hypotension.

Pneumothorax

Pneumothorax occurs if air enters the space between the pleural lining and the lung. Hadaway (2006) reported this potential complication in patients who have their CVAD placed directly into the subclavian vein.

Clinical features of a pneumothorax can include:

- pain on inspiration and expiration
- dyspnoea.

Haemothorax

Haemothorax can be a result of puncturing the subclavian vein or artery during the insertion procedure. Blood then leaks into the pleural cavity (Richardson & Bruso 1993; Dougherty 2006; Hadaway 2006).

Clinical features of a haemothorax can include:

- dyspnoea
- tachycardia.

Arterial puncture

Arterial puncture will result if an artery is cannulated or punctured during the insertion procedure. This complication is readily identifiable by the pulsation/spurting of bright-red blood, i.e. arterial blood, into the syringe or through the cannula/introducer. If the subclavian artery has been punctured, a chest X-ray should be performed to assess whether a mediastinal haematoma has occurred (Richardson & Bruso 1993; Dougherty 2006).

Nerve injury

The ulnar and median nerves can be damaged during PICC placement if they accidentally come into contact with the cannula/introducer. Similarly, damage to the radial cords of the brachial plexus can also result from subclavian placements of other types of CVAD (Richardson & Bruso 1993; Dougherty 2006; Cassutt 2006; Hadaway 2006).

Clinical features of nerve injury may include:

- tingling
- loss of movement down part or all of the affected arm.

Catheter malposition

A chest X-ray should be performed after the placement of any CVAD to verify its position, if it was not placed under fluoroscopic guidance (RCN 2005). A CVAD may become malpositioned not only as a result of the insertion procedure, but also through spontaneous migration or following a repair procedure (Gabriel 2006; Hadaway 2006).

Clinical features A malpositioned CVAD may present the patient with no symptoms, but if clinical features are present, they may include:

- continuous backflow of blood into the catheter
- coughing
- ear/neck pain on the side of insertion
- palpitations/arrhythmias
- inability to aspirate blood (or difficulty in doing so).

Atrial fibrillation

Atrial fibrillation can result if the catheter extends beyond the SVC and into the heart (Hadaway 2006).

Thrombosis

Wickham *et al.* (1992) reported that the formation of thrombosis following CVAD placement is probably multifactorial. They discussed how the catheterization of the vein causes damage to the wall of the blood vessel. This initial trauma leads to the release of thromboplastic substances which cause platelets to collect at the site of the injury. These initial thrombi can then go on to develop into larger areas, or break away causing occlusion elsewhere in the venous system (Droullard 2000; Dougherty 2006; Hadaway 2006).

Clinical features can include:
- swelling of the neck, chest or arm/leg (depending on insertion site)
- skin discoloration
- skin temperature changes
- infusion difficulties
- inability to aspirate blood (or difficulty doing so).

Pinch-off syndrome

Hadaway (2006) described pinch-off syndrome (POS) as a condition which can arise when the CVAD is compressed between the clavicle and the first rib. This phenomenon was first discussed by Hinke *et al.* (1990).

Clinical indications of POS can include:

- inability to infuse fluids
- difficulty in aspirating blood.

If these signs are ignored, the catheter can go on to rupture and migrate through the blood vessels and into the heart (Hadaway 2006).

Routine Management

Skin cleansing before catheter placement

Elliott (1993) was one of the earliest to emphasize the importance of appropriate and effective skin cleaning before the placement of any vascular access device. He stated that contamination of the intravenous catheter by bacteria on the patient's skin could result in infection of the CVAD. The resulting infection might be confined to the insertion site, with the patient complaining of localized pain, and could be associated with erythema, oedema and even a purulent discharge. A systemic infection resulting from an infected CVAD may be more difficult to diagnose. The patient might present with a low-grade pyrexia and have only a slightly elevated white cell count (Elliott 1993).

Maki *et al.* (1991) carried out a randomized trial of skin cleansing agents for the prevention of catheter-associated infections. They concluded that aqueous chlorhexidine 2% used for cutaneous disinfection before insertion of an i.v. device and for post-insertion site care substantially reduced the incidence of device-related infection, compared with povidone-iodine 10% and alcohol 70%. Recently published/updated national and international guidelines now advocate the use of chlorhexidine-based solutions for cutaneous disinfection (RCN 2005; INS 2006; Pratt *et al.* 2007).

Accessing the injection hub

Linares *et al.* (1985), and more recently Maki (2005), suggested that the commonest cause of catheter-related septicaemia was catheter hub colonization by microorganisms. It is therefore vital to ensure that injection hubs of CVADs are adequately cleaned before they are accessed or removed. This can be achieved by cleaning with chlorhexidine 0.5% in industrial methylated spirits (IMS) or a presaturated alcohol wipe. The hub should be cleaned for a minimum of 30 seconds and allowed to dry before being accessed/removed (Gabriel *et al.* 2005; RCN 2005). A strict aseptic technique should be used when accessing the CVAD.

Dressings

Skin-tunnelled catheters

With skin-tunnelled catheters, the rationale for applying dressings permanently over the insertion site has been questioned. The reason for this is that after 14–21 days the skin tunnel has formed in the majority of patients and tissue has begun to grow into the dacron cuff, thereby creating a barrier against infection (Masoorli 1993; Dougherty 2006). Many patients opt for no dressing but if a dressing is used, such as a transparent dressing, it should be changed every 7 days if intact and exhibiting no visible accumulation of exudate (RCN 2005; Dougherty 2006).

Implantable ports

Once the wound overlying the skin incision has healed, there is obviously no need for further dressings, unless the patient requires a continuous infusion. In this latter case, a dressing will be required to stabilize the infusion device while it remains *in situ*. In the study by Young *et al.* (1988), a sterile, transparent semipermeable dressing was shown to be more effective in minimizing the risk of infection than conventional gauze dressings. If a patient requires continuous access to the injection port, the needle/cannula can be secured by a sterile, transparent semipermeable dressing with a piece of sterile gauze placed, if required, under the needle/cannula. This will prevent movement of the needle/cannula and minimize the possibility of a pressure sore developing on the patient's skin unless there is any exudate (Dougherty 2006).

PICCs

As there is usually some slight oozing of blood immediately after the placement of a PICC, a small piece of sterile gauze can be placed over the insertion site. This can then be covered with a sterile, transparent semipermeable dressing. The following day the whole dressing should be removed and the patient's skin cleaned with chlorhexidine in IMS (RCN 2005). The PICC should then be secured with a sterile, self-adhesive anchoring device and/or steristrips (according to the manufacturers' directions), and a sterile, transparent semipermeable dressing applied. If the patient does not require access to the PICC continuously (e.g. for intermittent cytotoxic drug therapy), the injection cap can be wrapped in sterile gauze, to prevent it causing a pressure sore on the forearm, and a second dressing can be applied, to overlap with the first. This will create a waterproof barrier to allow the patient to shower. Unlike skin-tunnelled catheters and implantable injection ports, PICCs require being continually dressed while they are *in situ*. Following the first dressing change 24 hours after insertion, a weekly dressing change interval is recommended (RCN 2005; Dougherty 2006).

Maintaining patency

Goodwin and Carlson (1993) drew attention to the importance of the flushing technique in preventing occlusion of all CVADs. They recommended a rapid push–pause or pulsated flushing technique. This creates turbulence within the lumen(s) of the catheter, thereby decreasing the risk of fibrin and platelets becoming adhered to the internal wall(s) of the CVAD and minimizing the risk of occlusion. If the CVAD has more than one lumen, each one should be flushed separately, i.e. treated as if it were a separate device (Masoorli 1993; Gabriel *et al.* 2005; RCN 2005; Dougherty 2006).

There has been great debate over the flushing frequencies and flushing solutions for all CVADs (Masoorli 1993). The general consensus is that CVADs with a valve should be flushed with sodium chloride 0.9%. Despite the results of a study by Barbone and Rockledge (1995) suggesting that sodium chloride 0.9% is as effective as heparinized saline in maintaining the patency of 'open-ended' CVADs, there is no uniformly agreed protocol. Whether to use sodium chloride 0.9% or varying strengths of heparinized saline, and at what intervals, appears to be very much dictated by individual departments and hospitals (Dunn 1987; Geritz 1992; Kelly 1992; Masoorli 1993; RCN 2005 Pratt *et al.* 2007). If the CVAD is open-ended and has a lumen smaller than a 21 G, it will require more frequent flushing than a wider-gauge device to ensure that it remains patent (Masoorli 1993). (Individual catheter manufacturers will provide guidance relating to their specific product range.)

There is a consensus of opinion that injection ports should be flushed monthly with heparinized saline. However, the strength of the heparinized saline used still varies among individual departments and hospitals.

Results of various studies have suggested rates of CVAD-related thrombosis of between 3% and 37% for patients with solid tumours and haematological malignancies. In an attempt to reduce the risk of a thrombosis developing, therapeutic and low doses of warfarin have been used as prophylaxis (Bern *et al.* 1986, 1990; Boraks *et al.* 1998; Heaton *et al.* 2002). More recent studies have shown the incidence of thrombosis in this group of patients is less common than previously perceived, and that 1 mg/day of warfarin does not appear to reduce the incidence of thrombosis in these recipients of CVADs (Couban *et al.* 2005).

Blood sampling

Blood samples should not be taken through the lumen of a CVAD which has recently been used for the administration of drugs or fluids, as this could result in inaccurate biochemistry results or drug-level analysis. If this is the only route available for obtaining such blood samples, infusions should be stopped for a minimum of 20 minutes and flushed with 0.9% sodium chloride before aspirating, and twice the prime volume of the CVAD should then be discarded before aspirating the blood sample for testing (RCN 2005).

Blood samples can be obtained from CVADs, providing the lumen of the device is greater than 24 G. Withdrawing blood through a CVAD with a lumen smaller than 21 G had previously been thought to damage the blood cells and result in altered laboratory results (Scott 1995). However, a study undertaken by Acquillo *et al.* (2006), using 24-G needles, has suggested this not to be the case.

To obtain a blood sample, it is important to ensure that all the materials are prepared in advance and are within easy reach. A delay in flushing the CVAD directly after obtaining a blood sample can lead to occlusion. It is also important to ensure that a strict aseptic technique is maintained at all times to minimize the risk of infection to the patient (RCN 2005). If there is residual blood visible following blood sampling via an injection cap/needle-free cap, the cap should immediately be replaced to minimize the potential for infection. Individual hospital policies and procedures may vary, but the general principles of obtaining a blood sample from a CVAD are presented in Box 11.2.

Aspiration of blood from a PICC is a much slower procedure than from other types of CVAD, due to the length of the catheter and the size of the lumen. Providing the individual is aware of this, and flushes the PICC as soon as the blood sample is obtained, there is no reason why PICCs cannot be used successfully for this purpose (Scott 1995). A syringe smaller than 10 mL and vacuum blood collection systems should not be used on PICCs without consulting individual manufacturers, as there is the potential for the pressure that they create to lead to rupture of the catheter (Conn 1993; Richardson & Bruso 1993; Sansivero 1997; RCN 2005; Dougherty 2006).

Conn (1993) highlighted that the smaller the syringe size, the higher the pressure generated. She demonstrated that the average person injecting a 1-mL syringe can exert a pressure in excess of 300 pounds/square inch (psi), which can result in catheter rupture.

BOX 11.2

Blood sampling

- Following a strict aseptic technique, remove the injection hub and aspirate twice the prime volume of the lumen of the CVAD and discard. This will ensure that the stagnant contents of the CVAD lumen do not contaminate the blood sample and possibly lead to an inaccurate laboratory analysis.
- Aspirate the required amount of blood and decant into the relevant collection tube(s)/bottle(s). Do not use vacuum collection bottles directly onto the CVAD or syringes smaller than 10 mL without consulting the advisory literature for the individual catheter's manufacturer, as there is a potential for the pressure to be too high and rupture of the device could result (Conn 1993, Richardson & Bruso 1993, Gabriel *et al.* 2005).
- Using a rapid push–pause method, flush the CVAD with 10–20 mL of 0.9% sodium chloride to minimize the risk of occlusion (Goodwin & Carlson 1993, Masoorli 1993, RCN 2005; Dougherty 2006). Open-ended CVADs should then be flushed with heparinized saline (according to individual department/hospital policies and manufacture guidance), finishing with positive pressure.

Management of Complications

Occlusion

Occlusion of a CVAD may be either intraluminal or extraluminal (Wickham *et al.* 1992). Both intraluminal and extraluminal occlusions prevent blood from being aspirated back from the CVAD. However, with an extraluminal occlusion, it is sometimes possible to continue with the infusion of drugs/fluids without realizing that there is a problem (Gabriel *et al.* 2005; Mayo & Pearson 1995; Dougherty 2006; Hadaway 2006).

Intraluminal occlusion

Intraluminal occlusions are more commonly a consequence of clotted blood. A CVAD can become occluded by a blood clot in a relatively short period of time, especially if it has a small lumen (e.g. smaller than 21 G). Total occlusion can also develop over several days as a result of a clot of blood gradually increasing in size, resulting in progressively slower infusion of fluids/drugs (Wickham *et al.* 1992; Dougherty 2006). Precipitation of incompatible drugs and of parenteral nutrition can result in sudden occlusion of the CVAD.

Extraluminal occlusion

Extraluminal occlusion should be considered when it is possible to infuse drugs/fluids into a CVAD, but impossible or difficult to aspirate blood. This condition has been described by Mayo and Pearson (1995) as 'persistent withdrawal occlusion' (PWO). PWO can result from malposition of the CVAD, an anatomical obstruction, or fibrin sheath formation (Tschirhart & Rao 1988; Gabriel *et al.* 2005; Dougherty 2006).

A chest X-ray to confirm the correct positioning of the CVAD at the time of placement will minimize the risk of PWO as a result of malpositioning. However, subsequent migration of the tip of the CVAD into a smaller vessel or perforation of the SVC/endocardium can occasionally occur (Wickham *et al.* 1992; Gabriel *et al.* 2005; Dougherty 2006). Malposition of a CVAD can also result if the device is shortened during a repair procedure.

An anatomical obstruction (e.g. a fractured clavicle), presence of a cardiac pacemaker, enlarged/removed axillary nodes or previous radiotherapy to the axilla/supraclavicular fossa can all result in pressure on the venous system and possibly lead to PWO, especially if a CVAD was placed through a vessel underlying one of these conditions (Tschirhart & Rao 1988; Gabriel *et al.* 2005; Dougherty 2006).

Fibrin sheath formation is the commonest cause of PWO and has been reported in the majority of CVADs left *in situ* for more than 7 days (Wickham *et al.* 1992; Mayo & Pearson 1995). Fibrin sheath formation occurs as a result of fibrin and platelets being deposited along the external wall of the CVAD. When this sheath reaches the tip of the CVAD, it can act as a 'one-way' valve, allowing drugs/fluids to be infused, but preventing the withdrawal of blood (Mayo & Pearson 1995). Sometimes this fibrin sheath can totally envelope the CVAD, i.e. from tip to entry site, resulting in extravasation of drugs/fluids (Wickham *et al.* 1992; Gabriel *et al.* 2005; RCN 2005; Dougherty 2006).

If precipitation has been excluded as a possible cause of the occlusion, the pathway in Figure 11.10 could be used to assess whether the CVAD is malpositioned, or, if occluded, to restore it to patency.

A cathetergram can be useful, depending upon an individual hospital's policies and procedures, to confirm or exclude the presence of a fibrin sheath if PWO is experienced. If fibrin sheath formation is suspected, it can be treated initially in the same manner as if the CVAD was occluded by blood, i.e. instillation of 5000 i.u./mL of urokinase or 2 mg of tissue plasminogen activator (TPA), and left for between 10 and 60 minutes before being aspirated back (Gabriel *et al.* 2005). A syringe smaller than 10 mL should never be used for this purpose, as the potential pressure is too high and could lead to rupture of the CVAD (Conn 1993; RCN 2005; Dougherty 2006). If difficulty is encountered with injecting the urokinase, a three-way tap can be attached to the end of the CVAD. Two syringes, one empty and one containing the urokinase, are then attached to the tap (Figure 11.11). A gentle rocking action between the two syringes will then ensure that the urokinase is instilled into the lumen of the CVAD.

If the bolus injection of urokinase is unsuccessful in restoring the patency of the CVAD, Haire and Leiberman (1991) suggest that a urokinase infusion of 40 000 i.u./h over 6 hours can be used. Out of 19 CVADs in which Haire and Leiberman used a urokinase infusion, 15 responded and patency was restored. Of the four devices that remained occluded, two were malpositioned and the patency was restored in the remaining two after they responded to a further 6-hourly infusion of urokinase. In the USA, TPA has also been used successfully in place of urokinase to restore the patency of CVADs (Droullard 2000).

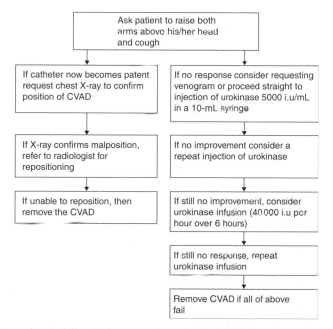

Figure 11.10   Procedure to follow in the event of extraluminal occlusion.

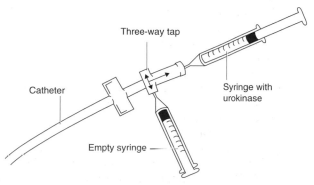

Figure 11.11   Three-way tap and two syringes used to overcome difficulty with injection of urokinase in the event of a fibrin sheath formation.

Section 2

Thrombosis

Patients with certain types of malignancies, i.e. mucin-secreting adenocarcinomas, pro-myelocytic leukaemia and myeloproliferative disorders, are more at risk of thrombosis as a result of CVAD placement than other groups (Brothers *et al.* 1988; Wickham *et al.* 1992; Couban *et al.* 2005). Camp-Sorrell (1992) highlighted a study which recorded a 40% risk of thrombosis in patients with adenocarcinoma of the lung that had a CVAD, compared with 17% in patients with small-cell lung cancer or squamous cell carcinoma. However, from a review of previous studies looking at the incidence of CVAD-related thrombosis in this patient population, Couban *et al.* (2005) identified that the incidence is probably lower than previously believed and recommended a further trial involving larger numbers of patients.

The process of developing a thrombosis related to CVADs is believed to be linked to a series of events (Wickham *et al.* 1992; Ryder 1995; Dougherty 2006). The process of introducing the catheter into the vein causes trauma, which results in thromboplastic substances and platelets collecting at the site of venepuncture. Obviously, the larger the size of the puncture or cutdown, the greater the injury to the vein. This trauma to the vein may result in the development of small thrombi which can adhere to the wall of the damaged vein, or possibly migrate, increasing in size and leading to occlusion of a larger vessel (Camp-Sorrell 1992; Wickham *et al.* 1992; Hadaway 2006).

The size and rigidity of the CVAD can also cause further trauma to the vein. Large, rigid catheters are associated with a higher risk of thrombosis than finer, more supple devices (Camp-Sorrell 1992; Wickham *et al.* 1992; Ryder 1995; Gabriel *et al.* 2005).

The rapid administration of vesicant/highly irritant drugs or infusates can lead to chemical phlebitis, which may result in the development of thrombosis (Ryder 1995; Wickham *et al.* 1992; RCN 2005).

The clinical features of thrombosis formation are variable and may not become apparent until there is total occlusion of the blood vessel. Early symptoms may include erythema of the skin overlying the CVAD, oedema, discomfort, pyrexia and pain radiating down the arm on the side the device has been placed. Later symptoms tend to be more indicative of the underlying problem, with facial swelling, neck vein distension and arm swelling. Diagnosis is usually confirmed by cathetergram or ultrasound examination (Wickham *et al.* 1992; Dougherty 2006).

It is possible to treat a patient's thrombosis without removing the CVAD, but this depends upon the severity of the symptoms and the patient's general condition (Wickham *et al.* 1992; Sansivero 1997; Dougherty 2006). Management of the thrombosis is more effective if treatment is initiated early. Treatment can include the surgical removal of the clot, but more commonly urokinase, heparin or TPA is administered as a continuous infusion through the CVAD. A review of the literature has identified that although these agents have been used with varying degrees of success, there are no uniform doses or lengths of infusion (Brothers *et al.* 1988; Wickham *et al.* 1992; Gabriel *et al.* 2005; Dougherty 2006). Brothers *et al.* (1988) highlighted that, once the patient's thrombosis has resolved, parenteral therapy can be resumed through the original CVAD.

Phlebitis

Richardson and Bruso (1993) identified three types of phlebitis: chemical, mechanical and infective.

Chemical phlebitis

As the tip of a CVAD terminates in a large blood vessel, i.e. the SVC, it would be rare to see this type of phlebitis in recipients of skin-tunnelled catheters, implantable ports or PICCs. This is because the drugs or fluids infused are quickly diluted by the volume of blood flowing through the SVC, so they have little opportunity to irritate the lining of the vein's wall.

Mechanical phlebitis

Mechanical phlebitis is more likely to occur within the first 7 days following insertion of the CVAD. It commonly results from too large a device being placed into an individual with small blood vessels. As the blood is restricted from flowing around the catheter, phlebitis results. This type of phlebitis is more obvious in recipients of PICCs and peripheral implantable ports, where too large a device has been placed in a small cephalic, basilic or median cubital vein. It can usually be resolved within 48 hours by the application of heat to the upper arm for 20 minutes three times a day (Richardson & Bruso 1993).

Goodwin and Carlson (1993) investigated the incidence of mechanical phlebitis in male and female recipients of PICCs and concluded that women were almost twice as likely to be affected as men. They reasoned that this was because women had smaller blood vessels, resulting in a decreased blood flow around the catheter.

Infective phlebitis

If phlebitis presents more than 7 days after insertion of a CVAD, or if a suspected case of mechanical phlebitis is not resolved by the application of heat, infection could be the cause (Richardson & Bruso 1993). A swab should be taken from the insertion site and sent to microbiology for culture and sensitivity. If considered appropriate, blood should also be aspirated from the lumen(s) of the CVAD and sent for culture and sensitivity.

Management of infection

CVAD-related infection is probably very much underestimated in its associated morbidity and mortality (Elliott 1993; Maki 2005). Press *et al.* (1984) investigated the incidence of infections in 922 patients with skin-tunnelled catheters and identified that 14.4% had a catheter-related infection from which four died (i.e. four out of 922 patients).

Maki (1993, 2005) suggested that the incidence of infection from catheters inserted via the antecubital fossa was far lower than that from catheters inserted via the chest and trunk areas. The reason he identified was the lower number of skin commensal organisms present on the arm (10 colony-forming units [CFUs] per site) compared with the chest (10 000 CFUs) per site). The skin temperature is also lower on the arm, thus presenting a less hospitable environment for bacteria to multiply.

If there is redness and/or discharge around the insertion site, a swab should be taken and sent to microbiology for culture and sensitivity. The site should then be cleaned with an appropriate skin-cleansing agent, e.g. chlorhexidine in IMS, and dressed daily (Maki *et al.* 1991; Maki 2005). When the results of the swab culture are known, an antibiotic may be prescribed, depending upon the infection and the individual clinician's preference.

The development of unexplained pyrexia in a patient with a CVAD is not an indication for removing the device (Goodwin & Carlson 1993; Ray 1999; Baron 2006). To confirm, or indeed eliminate, the CVAD as the cause of the infection, blood cultures should be taken from both the CVAD and a peripheral vein. The microbiology results of both cultures should then be compared. The decision to remove an infected CVAD very much depends upon what the infection is, how ill the patient is, and the individual hospital's policies and procedures (Maki 2005). If the CVAD is removed as a proven or suspected focus of infection, its tip should be sent for microbiological culture and sensitivity.

Brothers *et al.* (1988) reported that, in a study of 300 patients with implantable injection ports, 26 experienced an infection resulting in tissue necrosis in the skin overlying the port. Of these 26 patients, 23 were successfully treated with either parenteral or enteral antibiotics. The three patients whose infection did not respond to antibiotic therapy had their devices removed.

Damaged catheters

Rupture of a CVAD can be minimized by ensuring that high-pressure methods of drug/fluid administration are avoided, i.e. needles smaller than 21 G and syringes smaller than 10 mL (Conn 1993; RCN 2005; Dougherty 2006). Vacuumed blood collection bottles and infusion pumps should not be used without consulting the manufacturer's literature for each individual CVAD (Conn 1993; RCN 2005).

Pinch-off syndrome (POS) can occur as a result of a CVAD placed via the subclavian vein becoming compressed between the clavicle and the first rib. This can lead to fracture and migration of the catheter's tip. POS can be prevented by ensuring that the CVAD is placed correctly and performing a post-insertion X-ray to confirm the position of the device (Gabriel *et al.* 2005; Cassutt 2006; Hadaway 2006)

More commonly, damage or complete rupture of skin-tunnelled catheters or PICCs occurs in the portion of catheter exiting from the patient (Gabriel 1996a; Sansivero 1997; Dougherty 2006).

With open-ended CVADs, care should be used when clamping the catheter to minimize the risk of damage. 'Non-toothed' clamps, or the clamp supplied by the manufacturer, should be used on the catheter when removing the injection hub. Valved CVADs do not necessitate the use of clamps when removing the injection hub, because the absence of either a negative or positive pressure will prevent the opening of the non-return valve (RCN 2005). However, if the catheter is not securely anchored to the patient's skin when connected to an infusion, the device can twist. The increasing stress from the twisting can result in damage and possibly a complete rupture of the CVAD. The location of the damage will determine whether it is possible to repair the catheter (Dougherty 2006).

Generally speaking, single-lumen CVADs are the easier to repair. The complexity of construction of multilumen CVADs makes repair more difficult. (Individual manufacturers will be able to provide specific information relating to their products.) If damage to the CVAD has occurred in the portion of the catheter that is actually *in situ*, it may not be possible to repair it without shortening the device or replacing it (*See* Box 11.3).

The manufacturers of valved devices do supply repair kits. The procedure involves removing the damaged part of the device, which necessitates shortening the exposed length of catheter containing the damage, and replacing the injection hub. If it is suspected that

---

BOX 11.3

Procedure for replacing a PICC (Sansivero 1997)

- Explain the procedure to the patient.
- Following a strict aseptic technique, clean the catheter and surrounding skin with an appropriate antiseptic.
- Using a pair of sterile scissors, cut off the length of PICC attached to the injection hub of the catheter.
- Pass the sterile guidewire through the remaining PICC.
- Gently pull on the PICC to facilitate its removal over the wire.
- *Either* place a new PICC over the wire and advance both along the vein until the desired length has been advanced and remove wire *or* make a small incision and insert an introducer, remove the wire and advance the catheter through it, removing introducer once catheter inserted to desired length.
- Secure and dress the PICC as if it were a primary insertion.
- Request a chest X-ray to confirm the position of the PICC.
- Document the procedure in the patient's notes.

the tip of the catheter could have moved during the repair procedure, a chest X-ray should be performed before use of the device is resumed.

Many of the manufacturers of the open-ended CVADs also supply repair kits with comprehensive instructions. Some of these kits involve the use of sterile glue to mend the CVAD, so the catheter cannot be used until the glue has thoroughly dried.

With PICCs, it may be possible to attempt to replace the catheter by adopting the procedure outlined in Box 11.3.

Removal of CVADs

Before removal of a CVAD other than a PICC, the patient should have a full blood count and, if appropriate, a clotting screen performed, to ensure there is no increased potential for haemorrhage. As for the insertion procedure, CVADs can be removed under a local or general anaesthetic to minimize the discomfort of the procedure for the patient. The exceptions to this are PICCs, which can easily be removed without anaesthesia (Gabriel 1996b).

PICCs

PICCs can easily be removed by applying gentle traction to the device once the steristrips and/or self-adhesive anchoring device have been removed. If difficulty is encountered, the application of heat to the patient's upper arm will increase the blood flow and the diameter of the vein, and therefore aid the removal of the PICC (Gabriel 1996a; Sansivero 1997). An alternative to this approach is to apply gentle traction to the PICC and use a piece of adhesive tape to secure it to the patient's forearm. This should be left for approximately 30 minutes before a further attempt is made to remove the catheter (Sansivero 1997; RCN 2005).

Skin-tunnelled catheters

Whether these devices have been placed by a surgical cutdown technique or by a percutaneous approach, the removal procedure is the same (Gabriel 1996b; RCN 2005). It is common practice to use a local anaesthetic to infiltrate the area around the dacron cuff, usually 5 cm along the skin tunnel (Figure 11.4). The skin can then be incised and the dacron cuff identified. Once the cuff has been located, the surrounding tissue is dissected until the cuff is 'free'. Gentle traction is then applied to the catheter to remove it. An alternative approach involves applying gentle but firm traction to the catheter. In some instances this will prove sufficient to 'free' the dacron cuff and therefore release the catheter without dissecting the cuff. There is, however, a risk of applying too much traction and snapping the catheter, which may then result in its migration (Sansivero 1997). A transparent pressure dressing should be applied to the skin overlying the site where the catheter entered the vein (RCN 2005). Sutures or steristrips are commonly used to close the skin after the catheter has been removed, and a dressing applied (Drewett 2000; Gabriel *et al.* 2005).

Implantable injection ports

Either a general anaesthetic or local anaesthetic is used for the removal of injection ports. The procedure involves locating the injection port and making an incision into the overlying skin. Once the device is identified, the sutures securing it to the underlying tissue are removed. Gentle traction is then applied to remove the port and catheter. The skin is usually closed with sutures and a dressing applied (Gabriel 1993).

Section 2

The Nurse's Role in Placing CVADs

The introduction of PICCs into clinical practice in the USA has resulted in all States now allowing nurses to place these catheters, provided that i.v. therapy is an integral part of their practice and they have the necessary skills (Gabriel 1996b). PICCs were not introduced into the UK until 1994 and it is a procedure which has been nurse driven (Gabriel 1996b; Dougherty 2006).

The Nursing and Midwifery Council (NMC) has produced a number of documents providing professional guidance to nurses including *The Code of Professional Conduct* (NMC 2004). This document emphasizes that it is the individual nurse who is professionally accountable for her clinical practice. Any nurse must be prepared to be accountable for her own care of a patient to that patient, her employer and the NMC. With more nurses now taking on specialist and 'extended' roles, it is inevitable that they will encounter new developments which could be of potential benefit to individual patients (Gabriel 1996b). The NMC has clearly indicated that there is no objection to nurses specializing and broadening their individual area of practice, providing the nurse concerned possesses the necessary knowledge and skills, is acting in the interest of the patient and is accountable for her own actions (NMC 2004).

In the USA, as long ago as 1983, Mansell reported that the introduction of a nurse-led PICC insertion programme into his hospital resulted in increased numbers of patients becoming recipients of a CVAD. On the surface this may appear to have been a negative aspect of the programme, but the nurses' assessment and education of the individual patients not only ensured that they received the appropriate i.v. catheter for their clinical needs and lifestyle at the outset of treatment, but also decreased the incidence of problems associated with the management of the CVADs, such as catheter malposition, infection, etc. The need for constantly resiting peripheral cannulae was greatly reduced, as was the incidence of chemical phlebitis associated with the inappropriate use of peripheral cannulae for some parenteral therapies.

In the UK, Hamilton and Gabriel (2005) have shown that suitably skilled nurses assuming responsibility for the placement of skin-tunnelled catheters and PICCs has improved the overall CVAD service to patients. The nurses delivering these services not only achieve a lower rate of insertion complications than their medical colleagues (catheter malposition, infection, etc.), but also provide a quick response time for the placement of CVADs. The nurses also undertake an assessment of the patient's needs before placing the CVAD, and provide the necessary education and training for both patients and staff (Hamilton & Gabriel 2005).

There are also financial savings in nurses assuming responsibility for the placement of CVADs (Mansell 1983; Hamilton *et al.* 1995; Hamilton & Gabriel 2005). A nurse's time may be less expensive than that of a senior medical colleague. A quick response time and adequate assessment of the patient ensure that they receive the most appropriate CVAD at the earliest opportunity, with minimal complications (Hamilton *et al.* 1995) (Hamilton & Gabriel 2005). Boland *et al.* (2003) examined the clinical and cost-effectiveness of blind compared with image-guided insertion by nurses in 470 adult cancer patients. There was no statistically significant difference in mean cost. The only statistically significant difference in clinical outcomes was the frequency of catheter tip misplacement, being higher in the blind arm where 14% had misplaced tips compared with 1% under image guidance. It was also evident that nurses previously inexperienced in the procedure could be trained within a 3-month period to insert tunnelled catheters successfully.

Where i.v. therapy is an integral part of a nurse's practice, she has the opportunity to augment her knowledge and skills to assume responsibility for placing a patient's CVAD. Not only is this financially attractive to health service managers, but it also provides continuity of care for individual patients. Patients have the opportunity to discuss the implications of life with a CVAD with a nurse who knows them. The nurse can then use her knowledge of the patient (e.g. their underlying medical condition, proposed treatment and lifestyle) to suggest the most suitable CVAD (Gabriel 1996b, 2000).

Quality of Life

Safe, simple and reliable venous access has to be beneficial for any patient requiring intermediate- to long-term parenteral therapy. In recent years, developments in technology have increased the range of CVADs able to meet the clinical needs of individual patients. It is also the case that the range of treatments is increasing, so that in future more and more patients will require a vascular access device (Petersen 2002; RCN 2005). Whichever catheter is selected, it will become a part of that patient's life for the foreseeable future and the patient should be involved in the device selection process (Loughran & Borzatta 1994; Gabriel 2000; Chernecky *et al.* 2002).

CVADs are now becoming necessary devices for the treatment and management of patients with chronic disease (RCN 2005). Patients who are recipients of such devices will be expected to 'live' with their CVAD, and in many instances will assume responsibility for its care and management. In this situation, it is important not only to match the clinical needs of the individual to the CVADs available, but also to consider the impact such a device could have on the patient's lifestyle (Gabriel 2000). If the patient will not psychologically accept the CVAD that has been placed, they will be less likely to accept it as part of their life. As mentioned above, this potential problem can be overcome by involving the patient in the decision-making process and by ensuring that he is provided with knowledge and training to manage the CVAD selected (Gabriel 2000).

The placement of a CVAD for intermediate- to long-term parenteral therapy is rarely an emergency procedure. Assessment of the individual patient's clinical needs, and assessment and understanding of their lifestyle will often yield more than one suitable CVAD. If there is such a choice, the final decision should rest with the patient. If they are aware of the care and maintenance required for any proposed CVADs, and any lifestyle restrictions that could be imposed, they will be able to decide which device they prefer. This will help to ensure that they can safely 'live' with their device, with the minimum of disruption to their lifestyle (Gabriel 2000; Chernecky *et al.* 2002).

As long ago as 1966, Henderson believed that health education was an essential part of a nurse's role if she was to become a health promoter (Henderson 1966). With the delivery methods of healthcare changing, especially in relation to parenteral therapies, the role of the nurse is becoming more complex (DH 1989). With more nurses assuming greater responsibility for establishing venous access, they must ensure that they are able to advise their patients appropriately, so that all patients receive a CVAD that is acceptable to them and undertake any necessary care safely (Gabriel 1996b, 2000; NICE 2003).

Fallowfield (1990) identified that disruption to an individual's life can cause depression and anxiety, which may result in a decline in overall quality of life. What an individual perceives as a 'disruption' is obviously open to debate (Thompson *et al.* 1989). For example, does an implantable injection port which is noticeable when wearing certain clothes constitute a disruption? Or a PICC preventing the individual from swimming; or a skin-tunnelled catheter acting as a visual reminder to the patient and his partner that there is an underlying medical condition?

Thompson *et al.* (1989) undertook a survey of 24 recipients of skin-tunnelled catheters and implantable injection ports. Part of the questionnaire dealt with the effects of the CVAD on clothing, personal hygiene, body image, relationships, employment and leisure activities. Many of the recipients of skin-tunnelled catheters considered the device and its integral clamp to be bulky. This caused problems with clothing, especially for the female recipients who stated that the device caught on their bras. Nine of the 24 patients would have preferred a lower insertion site. None of the patients was prevented from driving because of their CVAD, although it was found that right-sided placements were more comfortable. Only five out of the 24 patients in the study perceived their CVAD as having an adverse effect on body image, a proportion similar to that found by Daniels (1996). Both studies highlighted that recipients of CVADs viewed them as part of their treatment process. Thompson *et al.* (1989) cautioned against healthcare professionals becoming complacent about CVADs. Nurses must be aware of the developments in this area which could potentially benefit patients, especially as more become recipients of CVADs (Gabriel 2000).

Education and information are key to assessing any patient who will be a potential recipient of a CVAD. The two go hand in hand. When the patient has had their clinical needs assessed, often several CVADs will meet their clinical requirements. This is where a nurse can play a key role in helping the patient through their treatment. If a patient has already experienced a change to their physical appearance the last thing they may want is an additional visual reminder of their ongoing treatment while they are away from the hospital environment, so an injection port may be the solution for them? Another patient may feel that they would do anything to avoid needles, so may prefer a skin-tunnelled catheter or PICC? For example, a cystic fibrosis patient requiring intermittent courses of parenteral antibiotics may prefer to opt for a PICC each time he has a chest infection. This would ensure that there were no visual reminders of his underlying medical condition during periods of good health, and no necessity to maintain the patency of a CVAD when it was not in continual use. Another patient with cystic fibrosis may prefer an implantable injection port, to provide 'peace of mind' by knowing that he had ready venous access when required. A third patient may opt for a skin-tunnelled catheter, because he has a dislike of needles and is not prepared to undergo a PICC insertion each time parenteral antibiotics are required.

The assessment does not stop here. The patient requires additional information regarding the care and management of a particular device and any possible limitation(s) it may impose on their lifestyle. If they have young children or pets at home, a PICC may be a little more challenging to care for and have an increased risk of becoming accidentally damaged, unless it is protected carefully. With the support of local anaesthetic creams and the low maintenance required for a port, the initial concerns of an individual with needle phobia may be overcome and they may ultimately find such a device more beneficial to them. Another patient may prefer a PICC because it will leave no long-term scarring.

Education and information must be appropriate for the individual and include the following.

- Why the need for a CVAD.
- Length of time required.
- Alternatives (if any).
- Types of CVAD available.
- Advantages and disadvantages of each.
- Insertion procedure.
- Potential risks of insertion.
- Maintenance required.
- Limitations on lifestyle.
- Ongoing support available.
- Removal procedure.
- Opportunities for questions.
- Opportunity to speak to other patients.

Where appropriate, the patient's carer, with the patient's consent, should also be involved in the assessment. They may be required to help with the maintenance of the CVAD selected, or indeed help to administer any medications/infusions. Time invested in the assessment process will enable the patient to be informed about the CVAD they are to receive and what it will mean to have that CVAD as part of their life, whether it is for a few weeks or for many years.

Conclusion

In recent years, the range of reliable CVADs has been expanding and it is anticipated that the number of patients using such devices will continue to grow. Nurses are becoming increasingly familiar with these devices in relation to both their management and their placement. Through education of healthcare professionals, we can work towards ensuring that each recipient of a CVAD receives the most appropriate device for him as an individual. Education and assessment must be an ongoing commitment. Nurses play a crucial role in the management of today's patient by contributing to the longevity of a CVAD though careful patient assessment, and ongoing care of the patient and their CVAD.

References

Acquillo G, Reiner J, Valenty K (2006) *Blood Transfusion Flow Rate Study*. Poster presentation, 20th Annual Association of Vascular Access (AVA) Conference, Indianapolis, USA.

Barbone M, Rockledge PA (1995) *VAD Patency*. Paper presented at 9th National Association of Vascular Access Networks (NAVAN) Conference, Salt Lake City. NAVAN Program no. 9506.

Baron E (2006) *Laboratory Diagnosis of Catheter-Related Bloodstream Infections*. Oral presentation, 20th Annual Association of Vascular Access (AVA) Conference, Indianapolis, USA.

Ben Arush M, Berant M (1996) Retention of drugs in venous access port chamber: a note of caution. *British Medical Journal* 312: 496–497.

Bern MM, Bothe A, Bristrain B (1986) Prophylaxis against central venous thrombosis with low-dose warfarin. *Surgery* 99: 216–221.

Bern M, Lokich J, Sabina R *et al.* (1990) Very low doses of warfarin can prevent thrombosis in central venous catheters. *Annals of Internal Medicine* 112: 423–428.

Boland A, Haycox A, Bagust A, Fitzsimmons L (2003) A randomised controlled trial to evaluate the clinical and cost effectiveness of Hickman line insertions in adult cancer patients by nurses. *Health Technology Assessment* 7(36).

Boothe A, Piccione W, Ambrosino J, Benotti PN, Lokich JJ (1984) Implantable central venous access system. *The American Journal of Surgery* 147: 565–569.

Boraks P, Seale J, Price J *et al.* (1998) Prevention of central venous catheter associated thrombosis using minidose warfarin in patients with haematological malignancies. *British Journal of Haematology* 101: 483–486.

Brothers TE, Von Moll LK, Arbor A *et al.* (1988) Experience with subcutaneous infusion ports in three hundred patients. *Surgery, Gynaecology & Obstetrics* 6(4): 295–301.

Broviac J, Cole JJ, Scribner BH (1973) A silicone rubber atrial catheter for prolonged parenteral alimentation. *Surgery, Gynaecology & Obstetrics* 136(4): 602–606.

Camp-Sorrell D (1992) Implantable ports: everything you always wanted to know. *Journal of Intravenous Nursing* 15(5): 262–272.

Cassutt C (2006) *Needle And Nerves: A Legal Connection*. Oral presentation, 20th National Association of Vascular Access (AVA) Conference, Indianapolis, USA.

Chernecky C, Macklin D, Nugent K, Waller JL (2002) The need for shared decision making in the selection of vascular access devices: an assessment of patients and clinicians. *Journal of Vascular Access Devices* 7(3): 34–39.

Conn C (1993) The importance of syringe size when using implanted vascular access devices. *Journal Vascular Access Network* 3(1): 11–18.

Couban S, Goodyear M, Burnell M *et al.* (2005) Randomized placebo-controlled study of low-dose warfarin for prevention of central venous catheter-associated thrombosis in patients with cancer. *Journal of Clinical Oncology* 23(18): 4063–4069.

Daniels LE (1996) Exploring the physical and psychosocial implications of central venous devices in cancer patients—interviews with patients. *Journal of Cancer Care* 5: 45–48.

Delmore J, Horbett DV, Jack BL (1989) Experience with the Groshong long-term venous catheter. *Gynaecologic Oncology* 2(34): 216–218.

Department of Health (DH) (1989) *Working For Patients*. HMSO, London.

Dougherty L (2006) *Central Venous Access Devices: Care and Management*. Blackwell Publishing, Oxford.

Drewett S (2000) Central venous catheter removal: procedures and rationale. *British Journal of Nursing* 9(22): 2304–2315.

Droullard A (2000) An activase primer. *Journal of Vascular Access Devices* 5(2): 21–26.

Dunn DL (1987) The case for the saline flush. *American Journal of Nursing* 6: 798–799.

Elliott TS J (1993) Line-associated bacteraemias. *Communicable Diseases Report* 3(7): R91–R96.

Fallowfield L (1990) *The Quality of Life—The Missing Measurement in Health Care*. Souvenir Press (E & A) Ltd, London.

Gabriel J (1993) *Long Term Vascular Access Devices—Education for Patients to Choose and Care For Their Own Venous Catheters*. National Florence Nightingale Memorial Committee Scholarship, RCN Library, London.

Gabriel J (1996a) Care and management of peripherally inserted catheters. *British Journal of Nursing* 5(10): 594–599.

Gabriel J (1996b) Peripherally inserted central catheters: expanding UK nurses' practice. *Surgical Nurse* 5(2): 71–74.

Gabriel J (2000) Patients' impressions of PICCs. *Journal of Vascular Access Devices* 5(4): 26–29.

Gabriel J (2006) Vascular access. In: Grundy M, ed. *Nursing in Hematological Oncology*, 2nd edn, pp. 295-320. Baillière Tindall Elsevier, Edinburgh.

Gabriel J, Bravery K, Dougherty L *et al.* (2005) Vascular access: indications and implications for patient care. *Nursing Standard* 19(6): 45–54.

Galloway S, Bodenham A (2004) Long-term central venous access. *British Journal of Anaesthesia* 92: 722–734.

Geritz MA (1992) Saline versus heparin in intermittent infuser patency maintenance. *Western Journal of Nursing Research* 14(2): 131–141.

Goodwin M, Carlson (1993) The peripherally inserted catheter: a retrospective look at 3 years of insertions. *Journal of Intravenous Nursing* 12(2): 92–103.

Gormon C, Buzby G (1995) Difficult access problems. *Surgical Oncology Clinics of North America* 4(3): 453–473.

Gullo SM (1982) Implanted ports. Technologic advances and nursing care issues: *Nursing Clinics of North America* 28(4): 850–871.

Hadaway LC (1989) An overview of vascular access devices inserted via the antecubital area. *Journal of Intravenous Nursing* 13(5): 297–306.

Hadaway L (2006) *Infiltration and Extravasation from Vascular Access Devices*. Oral presentation, 20th Annual Association of Vascular Access (AVA) Conference, Indianapolis, USA.

Haire W, Lieberman R (1991) Thrombosed central venous catheters: restoring function with six hour urokinase infusion after failure of bolus urokinase. *Journal of Parenteral and Enteral Nutrition* 16: 129–132.

Hamilton H (2000) Selecting the correct intravenous device: nursing assessment. *British Journal of Nursing* 9(15): 968–978.

Hamilton H, Gabriel J (2005) *When, why and how we insert Long Term Central Lines for Chemotherapy in the Oncologic Patient*. GAVeCeLT Meeting. Rome, November.

Hamilton H, O'Byrne M, Nicholai L (1995) Central lines inserted by clinical nurse specialists. *Nursing Times* 91(17): 38–39.

Harris LC, Rushton CH, Hale SJ (1987) Implantable infusion devices in the paediatric patient: a viable alternative. *Journal of Paediatric Nursing* 2(2): 174–179.

Heaton DC, Han DY, Inder A (2002) Minidose (1 mg) warfarin as prophylaxis for central vein catheter thrombosis. *Internal Medicine Journal* 32: 84–88.

Henderson V (1966) *The Nature Of Nursing—A Definition and its Implication for Practice, Research and Education*. MacMillan, New York.

Hinke DH, Zandt-Stastny MD, Goodman LR, Quebbeman EJ, Kyzywda EA, Andris DA (1990) Pinch-off syndrome: a complication of implantable subclavian venous access devices. *Radiology* 177: 353–356.

Infusion Nurses Society (INS)((2006) *Infusion Nursing Standards of Practice*. JIN, 29 (1S) Lippincott Williams and Wilkins, Philadelphia.

Kayley J (2003) An overview of community intravenous therapy in the United Kingdom. *Journal of Vascular Access Devices* 8(2): 22–26.

Kelly C (1992) A change in flushing protocols of central venous catheters. *Oncology Nursing Forum* 19(4): 599.

Linares J, Sitges-Serra A, Garau J (1985) Pathogenesis of catheter sepsis: a prospective study with quantitative and semi-quantitative cultures of catheter hub and segments. *Journal of Clinical Microbiology* 21(3): 357–360.

Lokich J, Bothe A, Benotti P, Moore C (1985) Complications and management of implanted venous access catheters. *Journal of Clinical Oncology* 3(5): 710–717.

Loughran SC, Borzatta M (1994) Peripherally inserted central catheters: a report of 2506 catheter days. *Journal of Parenteral and Enteral Nutrition* 19(2): 133–136.

Lowel JA, Bothe A Jr (1995) Central venous catheter related thrombosis. *Surgical Oncology Clinics of North America* 4(3): 479–491.

Maki DG (1993) *Complications Associated with Intravenous Therapy*. Paper presented at the 7th NAVAN Conference, Washington, DC.

Maki DG (2005) *The Promise of Novel Technology*. First Leading Edge Symposium. La Jolla, California.

Maki DG, Ringer M, Alvarado CJ (1991) Prospective randomised trial of povidone-iodine, alcohol, and chlorhexidine for prevention of infection with central venous and arterial catheters. *Lancet* 338: 339–343.

Mallory B (2006) *Assessing Venous Access Needs in the Pediatric Patient.* Oral presentation, 20th Annual Association of Vascular Access (AVA) Conference, Indianapolis, USA.

Mansell C (1983) Peripherally inserted central venous catheterization by IV nurses—establishing a procedure. *National Intravenous Therapy Association* 6: 355–356.

Marshalleck F (2006) *Venous Access in Interventional Radiology.* Oral presentation, 20th Annual Association of Vascular Access (AVA) Conference, Indianapolis, USA.

Masoorli S (1993) *Cost containment program for IV nursing.* Paper presented at 7th NAVAN Conference, Washington, DC.

Masoorli S (2005) *Infusion Therapy Standards: Clinical and Legal Implications.* Paper presented at RCN IV Forum conference. Brighton. 4th and 5th November.

Mayo D, Pearson D (1995) Chemotherapy extravasation: a consequence of fibrin sheath formation around venous access devices. *Oncology Nursing Forum* 22(4): 675–680.

Nakazawa N (2006) Difficult peripherally inserted central catheter (PICC) insertions. *Journal of the Association for Vascular Access* 11(3): 124–128.

National Institute for Health and Clinical Excellence (NICE) (2002) *Ultrasound Imaging for Central Venous Catheter Placement.* National Institute for Health and Clinical Excellence, London.

National Institute for Health and Clinical Excellence (2003) *Infection Control: Prevention of Healthcare Associated Infection in Primary and Community Care.* Clinical guideline 2. National Institute for Health and Clinical Excellence, London.

Nursing and Midwifery Council (NMC) (2004) *The Code of Professional Conduct.* Nursing and Midwifery Council, London.

Petersen B (2002) *Stepping Into the Future: Who Will Care for Healthcare?* Presentation at NAVAN Conference, San Diego California, September.

Pratt RJ, Pellowe CM, Wilson JA *et al.* (2007) ePIC 2 National evidence-based guidelines for preventing healthcare associated infection in NHS hospitals in England. *Journal of Hospital Infection* 655 (Suppl): S1–S64.

Press OW, Ramsey PG, Larson EB, Fefer A, Hickman RO (1984) Hickman catheter infections in patients with malignancies. *Medicine* 63: 189–200.

Ray CE (1999) Infection control: principles and practices in the care and management of central venous access devices. *Journal of Intravenous Nursing* 22(65): S18–S25.

Richardson D, Bruso P (1993) Vascular access devices—management of common complications. *Journal of Intravenous Nursing* 16(1): 44–49.

Royal College of Nursing (RCN) (2005) *Standards for Infusion Therapy.* Royal College of Nursing, London.

Ryder MA (1995) Peripheral access options. *Surgical Oncology Clinics of North America* 4(3): 395–427.

Sansivero GE (1997) *Update on Advanced PICC Placement.* Paper given at Bard PICC Workshop, London.

Scott WL (1995) Central venous catheters: an overview of food and drug administration activities. *Surgical Oncology Clinics of North America* 4(3): 377–390.

Shapiro CL (1995) Central venous access catheters. *Surgical Oncology Clinics of North America* 4(3): 443–451.

Strumpler A (1991) Lower incidence of peripheral catheter complications by the use of elastomeric hydrogel catheters in home intravenous therapy patients. *Journal of Intravenous Nursing* 14(4): 261–267.

Thompson AM, Kidd E, McKenzie M, Parker AS, Nixon SJ (1989) Long term central venous access: the patient's view. *Intensive Therapy and Clinical Monitoring* May: 142–144.

Tschirhart J, Rao M (1988) Mechanism and management of persistent withdrawal occlusion. *The American Surgeon* 54: 326–328.

Weinstein SM (2007) *Plumer's Principles and Practice of Infusion Therapy*, 8th edition. Lippincott Williams & Wilkins, Philadelphia.

Wickham R, Purl S, Welker D (1992) Long-term central venous catheters: issues for care. *Seminars in Oncology Nursing* 2(8): 133–147.

Young GP, Alexeyeff M, Russell DR (1988) Catheter sepsis during parenteral nutrition: the safety of long-term Opsite dressings. *Journal of Parenteral and Enteral Nutrition* 12(4): 365–370.

Section 2

CHAPTER 12

Intravenous Therapy in the Community

Jill Kayley

Introduction

Intravenous therapy is routine practice in hospital in the UK, and the requirement for intravenous (i.v.) therapy is frequently a reason for admission to hospital. However, the constant demand for hospital beds has led to pressure on acute hospitals to find ways to reduce the number of admissions and the length of hospital stays (Hardy *et al.* 2001). It is a natural and necessary development therefore for some i.v. therapies to take place outside the hospital inpatient setting (Kayley 2004). Current government initiatives promote the provision of healthcare in the community rather than in acute hospitals (Lane 2000; Department of Health (DH) 2006): '90% of patient journeys begin and end in primary care and it is where most contacts with the NHS take place' (*Liberating the Talents*, DH 2002).

Whilst reducing the number of acute admissions and reducing the length of hospital stays is part of current government policy, the NHS plan (DH 2000) and *Our Health, Our Care, Our Say: a New Direction for Community Services* (DH 2006) also set out a vision of a patient-centred NHS. The government's aim is to ensure that patients and communities are involved in service changes and are provided with greater choice (DH 2002; Billingham 2003; DH 2006). Patients now have a greater influence on the choice and location of treatment, and in many circumstances prefer the comfort and familiarity of their own home environment (Kayley 2004).

Community i.v. therapy in the UK is now an area of healthcare provision that is expanding to cover not only a wider range but more complex treatments too. However, acceptance of community i.v. therapy in the UK has been slow because of the way healthcare is funded, the lack of incentives to change current practice, and the existence of other priorities (Nathwani and Davey 1996). For example, it is not uncommon for ambulant patients to remain in hospital purely to receive i.v. antibiotics, because oral therapy is contraindicated, or there is no suitable oral alternative (Nathwani and Morrison 2001).

However, recent developments in technology, and drugs with pharmacokinetic profiling, such as some antimicrobials that allow once- or twice-daily dosing, have enabled community i.v. therapy to be a realistic and viable option. The administration of i.v. therapy either on an outpatient basis or in the home reduces the cost of inpatient care (Nathwani and Morrison 2001), frees acute hospital beds, enables patients to return to work, school or family life (Kayley 2000), and reduces the risk of acquiring nosocomial infections (Nathwani 2001).

Carrying out this form of treatment safely and effectively within the community requires comprehensive organization, multidisciplinary working and refinement of technical skills to ensure that all the coordination required takes place smoothly and efficiently.

Table 12.1   Established intravenous therapies.

Condition	Treatment	Started
Haemophilia A and B	Factors VIII and IX	1971
Intestinal failure	Total parenteral nutrition	Late 1970s
Primary antibody deficiency	Immunoglobulin	Mid 1980s
Cystic fibrosis	Antibiotics	Mid 1980s

Definition of Intravenous Therapy in the Community

It is important to define what is understood by the phrase 'i.v. therapy in the community'. In the context of this chapter i.v. therapy in the community is classified as any intravenous treatment administered at home, or in GP surgeries, community hospitals, outpatient clinics, day units and nursing or residential homes.

'Community nurse' is the generic term used to identify healthcare professionals in the community who are involved in the administration of i.v. therapy and/or support of the patient and carer. 'Patient' is used consistently throughout this text for convenience to mean any of the following : client, user, consumer, person or individual. 'Carer' means any individual who is involved in the administration of the i.v. therapy and support of the patient in a non-professional capacity and could be a family member, friend or neighbour.

Background

Community i.v. therapy itself is not a new concept. It has been a well-established practice for some years for a very small number of chronic conditions that require long-term i.v. therapy such as parenteral nutrition (PN), factors VIII and IX for haemophilia, immunoglobulin therapy and i.v. antibiotics for cystic fibrosis (Kayley 2003) (Table 12.1). These practices have evolved because it is impractical both socially and economically for them to be carried out in hospital or on an outpatient basis (Kayley *et al.* 1996).

More Recent Intravenous Therapies

Over the past 5 years there has been a general increase in the range and complexity of i.v. treatments administered in the community (Table 12.2). However, the main growth areas have been i.v. antimicrobial therapy for acute and chronic infections (Kayley 2000; Deagle 2001; Nathwani 2001; Nathwani and Morrison 2001; Cooper *et al.* 2003; Seaton *et al.* 2005) and ambulatory chemotherapy (Daniels 1996; Dougherty *et al.* 1998; Aston 2000). Despite recent growth and development of these services, the availability, standard, uniformity and organization of community i.v. therapy services still varies considerably throughout the UK.

Organizational Issues

In the USA the first adult outpatient and home parenteral antibiotic therapy (OHPAT) service was described in 1978 (Poretz 1998). OHPAT services in the USA now have a well-developed infrastructure for delivering a high-quality service to a large number of patients (Tice *et al.* 2004). The experience in the USA in relation to community

Table 12.2   More recent intravenous therapies.

Condition	Treatment
Acute or chronic infection	Antibiotics
Cytomegalovirus	Antivirals
Serious fungal infection	Antifungals
Haematological disorders	Blood products/platelets
Cancer	Chemotherapy
Nausea/vomiting	Antiemetic
Acute/chronic pain	Analgesia
Thalassaemia Sickle cell disease	Desferal
Gaucher's disease	Ceredase
Dehydration	Intravenous fluid
Hyperemesis	Intravenous fluid
Hypercalcaemia/bone pain	Bisphosphonates
Rheumatoid arthritis, Crohn's, ankylosing spondylitis, psoriatic arthritis and psoriasis	Monoclonal antibodies, for e.g. Infliximab

i.v. therapy has shown that patients having a wide range of i.v. therapies can be managed in the community safely and effectively (Cox and Westbrook 2005).

There is little doubt that most patients would prefer to be at home rather than in hospital. Patients are now wanting and expecting to go home to have their i.v. treatment, especially when they are aware of patients in other areas having similar treatments in the community.

Community i.v. therapy is a viable and manageable concept but the success of i.v. therapy services depends on having a motivated, multidisciplinary team and good communication between the hospital and community. The UK and US OHPAT practice guidelines recommend that a lead nurse with experience in i.v. therapy is an essential part of the multidisciplinary team (Tice 1997; Nathwani and Conlon 1998; Tice *et al.* 2004). This role has been described using a variety of terms such as infusion nurse specialist (Tice 1997; Tice *et al.* 2004), community specialist nurse (Kayley *et al.* 1996), community liaison nurse (Nathwani and Conlon 1998), nurse practitioner (Nathwani *et al.* 1999), and lead nurse (Cooper *et al.* 2003). It is certainly evident from well-established OHPAT services in the UK that the lead nurse role is key to the day-to-day running and overall management of the service.

Whilst it is not possible to list every aspect of the lead nurse's role, many are responsible for:

- patient selection, screening and assessment
- home assessment
- selection, placement and care of the vascular access device
- documentation of all plans and decisions made
- education and training for patients/carers and community nurses
- organization of drugs, equipment and ancillary items
- communication and liaison with the multidisciplinary team, patient/carer, GP, community nurse and primary healthcare team
- administering i.v. therapy
- discharge planning
- monitoring and follow-up

- problem-solving
- audit.

(Kayley 2004)

The planning, organization and ongoing support for community i.v. therapy should be acknowledged as an important process, with the quality of care provided being as high as, or higher than, in hospital (Nathwani and Conlon 1998). If problems occur due to poor organization and communication this can cause untold anxiety, confusion, isolation and anger for patients/carers and their families on top of coping with an illness, its treatment and a new skill (Dobson 2001). It also means that the day-to-day management and logistics of i.v. therapy are made so much harder for community nurses and other members of the primary care team (PCT). This is unacceptable practice and can be avoided with careful planning, thorough assessment and good communication.

Vascular Access Devices

The administration of any i.v. therapy treatment, regardless of the setting, requires a vascular access device (VAD). Patients may have courses of treatment for the short term (days), medium term (weeks) or long term (months or years), and the choice of VAD must meet the patient's clinical needs and be acceptable to them (Gabriel 2000; Kayley 2000; Dougherty 2006).

There are many factors that need to be taken into consideration before placing a VAD for i.v. therapy in the community. An accurate and detailed patient assessment is essential to ensure that patients requiring i.v. therapy have a suitable, reliable, safe and simple VAD, especially if they are to become actively involved in the care and management (Hamilton and Fermo 1998; Dougherty 2006). It is equally important that patients are involved and have a choice in the decision-making process (Gabriel 2000; Sarpal *et al.* 2004; Dougherty 2006). They need to be aware of the different types of VADs that are suitable, and understand any restrictions the VAD may have on normal daily activities such as bathing, swimming and other sporting activities, thus enabling them to make an informed choice (Gabriel 2000; Dougherty 2006).

Community nurses can play an important role in providing support, advice and information for patients with a VAD in relation to:

- activities of daily living, especially bathing and showering
- sporting activities
- sexual activity
- exemption from wearing a seat belt in a car
- altered body image
- preventing external catheters getting caught in clothing.

(Daniels 1995; Gabriel 2000; Dougherty 2006)

The type of VAD and location of vein used to administer the i.v. therapy is dependent on:

- the pH and osmolarity of the drug
- the nature and duration of the treatment
- the patient's lifestyle
- who is administering the treatment
- how the therapy is administered in the community.

For a detailed description of and information about each VAD, *See* Chapter 11.

Peripheral cannulae are appropriate for patients in the community with good vein status who will receive a short course of i.v. therapy (less than 2 weeks) with an agent that has low potential for causing phlebitis or tissue damage if infiltrated (Tice *et al.* 2004). In many

PCTs peripheral i.v. therapy is not part of the core community nursing service provided. If a patient is discharged home with a peripheral cannula it can be problematic to find someone in the community to take on responsibility for resiting the cannula (Kayley and Finlay 2003). Whilst peripheral cannulae may be suitable for some specific situations, there is a growing acceptance that peripherally inserted central catheters (PICCs) or midline catheters are more appropriate for community i.v. therapy (Hamilton 2000; Tice *et al.* 2004).

Nurses working in the community will be asked to accept patients for community i.v. therapy, and therefore need to be aware of the different types of VADs and the possible advantages and disadvantages of each (Table 12.3). It is also important to know of any particular aspects related to the care and management of the VAD, as well as

Table 12.3 Advantages and disadvantages of alternative vascular access devices (Kayley and Finlay 2003; Dougherty 2006).*

Vascular access device	Advantages	Disadvantages
Steel winged infusion device	Can be inserted and then removed after IV therapy	Very limited use for community IV therapy
Peripheral cannula	Less invasive to place than midline and PICC	Requires someone in the community to resite or patient has to travel back to hospital Not user friendly for patients who want to self-administer Limited dwell time – 48–96 h Pain and discomfort for patient
Midline catheter	Easy to remove No discomfort with use Easy to conceal under clothing No scar once removed Suitable for needle-phobic patients	Can be dislodged/pulled out Not recommended if patient wishes to go swimming Need to avoid heavy lifting and excessive use of arm Difficult for self-administration without extension set More liable to occlude than wider lumen catheters Dressing required for the whole time the catheter remains *in situ*
Valved midline	As above Only requires flushing with sodium chloride 0.9% to maintain patency (Perucca 2001; Weinstein 2007)	As above for midline catheters
Open-ended PICC	As above for midline catheters	As above for midline catheters
Valved PICC	As above for midline catheters. Only requires flushing with sodium chloride 0.9% to maintain patency (Perucca 2001; Weinstein 2007)	As above for midline catheters
Tunnelled uncuffed central catheter	Easy to remove No discomfort with use Easily accessible Can be used for blood sampling	Can be dislodged/pulled out Vulnerable to activities that may catch or pull catheter Exit site suture must remain *in situ* Altered body image Discomfort with car seat belts Requires very secure waterproof protection for swimming
Open-ended tunnelled cuffed central catheter	Dacron cuff anchors catheter in place No discomfort with use Easily accessible Can be used for blood sampling	Altered body image Can get caught in clothing and bedding Vulnerable to activities that may catch or pull catheter External clamps (if required) are bulky May require minor surgical procedure to remove Discomfort with car seat belts Requires very secure waterproof protection for swimming

(Continued)

Table 12.3   (*Continued*)

Vascular access device	Advantages	Disadvantages
Valved tunnelled catheter	As above Only requires flushing with sodium chloride 0.9% to maintain patency (Weinstein 2007; Perucca 2001)	As above
Implantable port	Concealed under skin—only small, raised area visible No restrictions on physical activities Suitable for bathing, showering and swimming No dressing required	Requires a surgical procedure to remove Each use requires a needle puncture (unless non-coring needle with extension tubing left *in situ*. Needle can be left *in situ* for 7 days) More difficult to access, particularly when patient is accessing own port Skin can become sore with frequent accessing Not suitable for needle-phobic patients

* Vascular access devices vary between different manufacturers. The table is a general guide only, and not an exhaustive or inclusive list.
PICC, Peripherally inserted central catheter.

Table 12.4   Vascular access device problems/complications, possible causes and suggested action.

Problem/complication	Possible cause	Suggested action for community nurses
Inability to administer medication, flush catheter and/or aspirate blood	Position of clamp Venous thrombosis Drug precipitate Catheter tip position Pinch-off syndrome Intraluminal clotting	Check clamp, if this does not resolve problem refer patient back to hospital unit for review/assessment
Inability to aspirate blood but ability to administer medication, flush catheter	Fibrin sheath	Take blood sample peripherally Contact referring unit and ask for review/assessment of patient's catheter at their next hospital appointment
Difficulty administering medication, flushing catheter and/or aspirating blood	Position of clamp Venous thrombosis Catheter tip position Pinch-off syndrome	Check clamp, if this does not resolve problem refer patient back to hospital unit for review/assessment
Redness and/or exudate at exit site	Exit site infection	Check whether patient is pyrexial. Clean exit with chlorhexidine with alcohol 70% solution and apply new dressing. Ask GP to visit and contact referring unit for advice. Take a swab
Redness at exit site of skin tunnelled cuffed catheter spreading along and around subcutaneous tunnel area, with/without exudate at exit site	Exit site and tunnel infection	Check whether patient is pyrexial. Clean exit with chlorhexidine with alcohol 70% solution and apply new dressing. Take a swab. Refer patient back to hospital unit for review/assessment
Patient unwell and/or has any of the following signs and symptoms: pyrexia, rigors, tachycardia, hypotension, sore throat, aching, headache, nausea, diarrhoea	Catheter infection Bacteraemia Septicaemia	Refer patient back to hospital unit **immediately** for review/assessment. If patient very unwell, based on vital signs and/or signs and symptoms, dial 999 and ask for an ambulance

Section 2

(*Continued*)

Table 12.4 (*Continued*)

Problem/complication	Possible cause	Suggested action for community nurses
Signs of redness, warmth, swelling, pain, induration and a hard, palpable venous cord in the upper arm above PICC, occurring within first 7 days following PICC insertion	Mechanical phlebitis	Ask GP to visit and contact referring unit for advice Monitor daily Apply heat to affected area 4 times per day Elevate affected arm and advise only gentle movement. Use of prescribed non-steroidal anti-inflammatory drugs
Purulent discharge from exit site and above signs and symptoms but occurring more than 7 days after insertion of PICC. Patient may be unwell and pyrexial	Infective phlebitis	Check whether patient is pyrexial. Refer patient back to hospital unit immediately for review/assessment
Fluid leaking from the catheter or exit site on administration of flush/drugs/infusion	Damaged, split or ruptured catheter	The damage/split part of the catheter may be external and therefore visible or the catheter may be damaged/split internally. Clamp catheter (if possible) above damaged portion using non-toothed forceps or by manually pinching the catheter. Refer the patient back to hospital immediately for review and catheter repair
Fluid or blood leaking from injection cap	Damage to injection cap possibly caused by use of a needle into a needle-free injection cap	Do not use. Remove injection cap (as per guideline) and replace with a new sterile injection cap
Length of external portion of PICC is longer than original measurement	PICC may not have been secured properly. PICC may have been pulled or caught in clothing	Redress PICC as per guideline. Contact referring unit for advice explaining by how much (cm) the PICC has come out. Do not use CVAD until advice has been sought
PICC has come out completely	PICC may not have been secured properly. PICC may have been pulled or caught in clothing	If PICC has just come out apply pressure to exit site. Clean exit site with chlorhexidine with alcohol 70% solution and apply a sterile dressing (as per guideline). Contact referring unit to inform them that PICC has come out
Dacron cuff visible at exit site of skin-tunnelled cuffed catheter	Catheter may not have been secured properly. Exit site sutures may have been removed too soon or catheter may have been pulled or caught in clothing	Check original measurement. Redress catheter as per guidelines ensuring it is well secured and supported. Contact referring unit for advice explaining by how much catheter has come out (if appropriate). Patient may need to return to hospital for repeat chest X-ray and resuturing at exit site
Skin tunnelled cuffed catheter has come out completely	Catheter may not have been secured properly. Exit site sutures may have been removed too soon or catheter may have been pulled or caught in clothing	If catheter has just come out apply pressure to exit site and incision site for 5 minutes. Clean exit with chlorhexidine with alcohol 70% solution and apply a sterile occlusive dressing to exit site (as per guideline). Contact referring unit to inform them that skin tunnelled catheter has come out. Patient may need to be reviewed in hospital
Blood visible in the external portion of PICC	Blood has back tracked down PICC—cause may not be known/obvious	Flush PICC (as per guideline) using push–pause technique, ending with positive pressure. Ensure all blood is cleared from PICC

PICC, peripherally inserted central catheter.

understanding any possible complications that could develop, and how those complications might be recognized and dealt with appropriately in the community (Table 12.4).

When a referral is made there are a number of questions that need to be answered by the referring unit related to the VAD before accepting the patient for community i.v. therapy.

- What type of VAD does the patient have?
- Is the VAD suitable for the prescribed i.v. therapy?
- When was the VAD placed/inserted?
- If centrally placed, where is the tip positioned?
- What is the external measurement of the VAD (not peripheral cannulae)?
- What are the common complications associated with this type of VAD?
- What are the signs and symptoms of these complications?
- Are there any policies (local or hospital) for the management of the VAD?
- Who should be contacted if any problems occur and what are their contact details?
- Does the patient/family/carer understand about the treatment and the VAD, how to recognize and deal with any complications, and whom to contact throughout the day or night?
- Is there a planned date for removal of the VAD?
- Who will remove the VAD and where?

(Kayley and Finlay 2003)

Methods of Administration and Equipment

The method of administration of any i.v. therapy falls into three categories.

A continuous infusion   is the infusion of a volume of drug or fluid continuously at a constant rate, over a prescribed period of time ranging from 24 hours to days. A pump or prefilled device is required to ensure the safe and correct administration rate (Lister and Sarpal 2004). The volume of actual drug or fluid can be anything from a small volume to a large volume depending on the treatment. Examples of continuous infusions administered in the community are total parenteral nutrition, chemotherapy, analgesia and rehydration fluid.

An intermittent infusion   is the administration of a small volume of drug or fluid (i.e. 50–250 mL) over a period of between 20 minutes to 2 hours which is then stopped until the next dose is due (Lister and Sarpal 2004). The frequency of administration could be daily or more often. Examples using this method of administration are antimicrobials, antivirals, antifungals, chemotherapy, immunoglobin, factor VIII/IX, blood and blood products.

A direct intermittent injection   (also known as a bolus or i.v. push) is the injection of a smaller volume of drug/fluid from a syringe directly into a VAD. Most direct intermittent injections are administered over a period of 3–10 minutes (Lister and Sarpal 2004). Example of this method of administration are antimicrobials, chemotherapy, analgesics, antiemetics and catheter flushes.

The method and rate of administration of any i.v. drug is dictated by the manufacturers' recommendations (Lister and Sarpal 2004; NMC 2004a). Any i.v. therapy administered in the community requires equipment—the amount, complexity and cost depends on the drug or treatment and how it has to be administered (Table 12.5).

The equipment and supplies required for a direct intermittent injection are considerably easier to obtain and organize than those required for a continuous or intermittent infusion. This should therefore be an important consideration when planning to discharge a patient into the community for i.v. therapy—the aim should be to find the safest and most straightforward method of administration that complies with the manufacturers' recommendations, regardless of who is administering it in the community.

Section 2

Table 12.5 Equipment required for the three methods of administration.

Continuous infusion	Intermittent infusion	Direct intermittent injection
Pump to regulate infusion	Prefilled device OR	Syringes and needles (for reconstitution)
Designated administration set	Small ambulatory pump with designated administration set OR	Needle-free device
Drip stand if volumetric pump used	Infusion bags, drip stand and administration sets	Small sharps bin
Infusion bags	Large sharps bin	
Needle-free device		
Large sharps bin		

The provision and availability of more 'high-tech' equipment (e.g. pumps) for community i.v. therapy can be a difficult and not easily resolved issue. For some i.v. therapies administered in the community, for example PN and chemotherapy, a pump is a prerequisite for safe and accurate administration, and one is therefore provided as part of the whole package.

Pumps

PCTs do not generally have resources to purchase pumps for i.v. therapy, especially when the demand for them is low and infrequent. Acute hospitals have pumps for use on the wards but they do not generally have surplus available to loan to the community. Pumps can be hired from commercial companies, and some of the pump manufacturers offer more flexible options apart from outright purchase.

If a pump is required for the safe and accurate administration of the i.v. therapy then the provision of training related to these pumps for all those involved, especially the operators, must feature as a very high priority (MDA 2003). All operators of pumps must be well trained and fully understand all aspects and workings of the pump (Quinn 2000; MDA 2003; NPSA 2003).

If patients or carers are going to be responsible for operating the pump they should be well trained before the patient is discharged into the community (MDA 2003). If community nurses are involved in the administration they should have the opportunity to undertake training before the patient is discharged, or training should be provided in the community by a designated person (MDA 2003). Any training must be supported by written information and the product user manual should always be available (MDA 2003; RCN 2005).

Any pump, whether battery or electrically operated, must be maintained and serviced by a medical engineering department at defined intervals (MDA 2003). PCTs will need to make arrangements to ensure all equipment is maintained and serviced on a regular basis. Such arrangements are often made through acute hospitals which all have a medical engineering department.

Ambulatory Infusion Devices

Ambulatory infusion devices were developed to allow patients more freedom and enable them to continue with normal activities of daily living (Sarpal *et al.* 2004).

They are ideal for community i.v. therapy and can be used for a range of therapies, such as administration of antimicrobials, analgesia, PN and chemotherapy (Schleis and Tice 1996; Tice 1997).

They can loosely be divided into two categories: mechanical, for example elastomeric devices/mechanical single dose infusors, and battery-operated infusion devices (Sarpal *et al.* 2004).

Elastomeric devices

Elastomeric infusion devices consist of an inflatable 'balloon' reservoir which is surrounded by a protective outer shell of hard or soft plastic. There is a port to enable the balloon reservoir to be filled with medication, and attached tubing for infusion. The flow rate is controlled either by the length and bore of the tubing or by a flow-restricting device situated near the end of the tubing (Sarpal *et al.* 2004). When the clamp is released on the infusion tubing the positive pressure created by the filled balloon reservoir forces the medication through the tubing. Before infusion the device should be removed from the fridge and allowed to warm to room temperature. Each elastomeric infusion device is for single use only and can be used for a range of i.v. medication (e.g. antimicrobials, chemotherapy and analgesia).

Mechanical single-dose infusors

These consist of a two-part cylindrical housing which is spring loaded and reusable. The round infusion pouch with attached tubing is prefilled with medication and placed in the lower half of the housing, and the other half of the housing which contains the spring is then screwed on (Perucca 2001). Once the clamp on the tubing is released the infusion will commence and flow rate is controlled by the proprietary flow-regulating tubing.

Battery-operated infusion devices

These small ambulatory pumps can offer a wide range of infusion systems, such as intermittent, continuous, patient-controlled analgesia and PN (Sarpal *et al.* 2004). They all require designated administration sets/cassettes/tubing and are usually powered by either mains current, batteries or a battery pack. The flow rates can range from 0.05 to 500 mL/h, but this varies depending on the make of pump.

For detailed descriptions of and information about the range of different pumps, *See* Chapter 8.

Patient Assessment and Discharge Planning

Community nurses are accountable for their own practice, and once they accept a patient for i.v. therapy in the community they are accepting accountability for the treatment and care they provide to that patient.

The NMC *Code of Professional Conduct: Standards for Conduct, Performance and Ethics* states:

> 1.3 You are personally accountable for your practice. This means that you are answerable for your actions and omissions, regardless of advice or directions from another professional.
> 1.4 You have a duty of care to your patients and clients, who are entitled to receive safe and competent care.

> (NMC 2004b)

It is important that an early and thorough assessment of any patient being considered for i.v. therapy in the community is carried out, whether the plan for community i.v. is to facilitate early discharge or prevent hospital admission.

Section 2

The assessment will help to ascertain at an early stage whether the treatment is manageable and appropriate for the community. The assessment should involve a multidisciplinary team comprising the physician, community specialist nurse, hospital nurse, pharmacist, social worker (if needed), general practitioner, patient and carer (Tice *et al.* 2004). The UK and US OHPAT practice guidelines recommend that a lead nurse with experience in i.v. therapy is an essential part of the multidisciplinary team (Tice 1997; Nathwani and Conlon 1998; Tice *et al.* 2004).

Each patient should be considered on an individual basis in relation to established assessment criteria, which may be drawn up at local level. This assessment should be balanced against the treatment options available in order to form a judgement of suitability (Nathwani and Conlon 1998; Dobson 2001; Tice *et al.* 2004).

The assessment should cover all the following aspects.

Patient and carer

1. Is the patient able to comply with the treatment regimen? Consider the following.
   - Age
   - Physical disability
   - Pain
   - Disease
   - Side-effects of medication
   - Poor vision
   - Poor manual dexterity
   - Exhaustion.
2. Does the patient and their carer/family understand the implications of the treatment, the VAD, how to recognize and deal with any complications and whom to contact throughout the day or night?
3. Does the patient want to have i.v. therapy treatment in the community?
4. Is the patient medically and psychologically fit for discharge?
5. Is the patient's home situation suitable; do they have a telephone and running water and is there anyone else in the house?
6. Are there any wider family issues and responsibilities?

Intravenous therapy treatment

1. Does the treatment need to be given i.v. rather than by another route?
2. Are there any implications in relation to allergies/anaphylaxis?
3. Who will administer the i.v. therapy, what training will they require, where will that training be done, and by whom?
4. Is the treatment regimen appropriate and manageable for the community?
5. What equipment supplies are required and where will they come from?
6. Will any blood monitoring be required, what and how often, and who will assimilate the results?

Availability of community support

1. What ongoing support is available, from whom, and what are the follow-up arrangements?
2. Is the GP happy to accept the patient home for this treatment?
3. What level of support and involvement are the community nurses and GPs able to provide?
4. As part of the overall assessment, specific questions need to be asked about the vascular access device (*See* section on VADs on Page 355), and the i.v. therapy treatment (*see* section on prescribing on Page 354).

5. There are circumstances where community i.v. therapy may not be suitable for patients, and some examples are listed below:
   - patient is confused/has dementia
   - patient is elderly or frail and lives alone
   - patient may abuse venous access, for example intravenous drug user
   - patient's home situation is unsuitable, for example no telephone, no running water, no electricity, isolated, dirty
   - patient has no insight into/comprehension of the treatment
   - patient is not suitable to administer the therapy and no-one else is able to
   - patient cannot give informed written or verbal consent.

(Dobson 2001)

Discharge planning begins with the initial assessment of the patient and is an ongoing process until the point of discharge from hospital. It should ideally be coordinated by one person as this encourages continuity, avoids duplication, minimizes the likelihood of problems occurring and ensures all the necessary aspects are considered and dealt with as appropriate (Tice 1997; Nathwani and Conlon 1998; Tice *et al.* 2004). It should involve the following.

- Communication and liaison with:
  - patient/carer
  - members of the multidisciplinary team
  - GP, community nurse and PCT.
- Documentation of all plans and decisions made.
- Organization of drugs, equipment and ancillary items.
- A treatment plan—duration of treatment, review date and/or completion date.
- Follow-up arrangements.
- Planning a realistic discharge date that is satisfactory to all those involved.

Good communication and careful discharge planning are an integral part of the whole process and essential for a smooth, trouble-free transition from hospital to the community (Kayley 2000).

Who Delivers?

The decision as to who will administer the i.v. therapy in the community should involve the patient/carer. Their role must not be underestimated and they should play a part in planning for community i.v. therapy and follow-up (Tice *et al.* 2004). There are a range of people or combination of people who could be involved in the administration, subject to the following considerations (*See* Table 12.6).

- Availability of resources, for example i.v. trained community nurses
- Patient/carer choice
- Dexterity of patient/care
- Concordance and understanding
- Length of i.v. therapy treatment—frequency/duration
- Ease of administration
- Type of vascular access device
- Wider picture of home situation, condition of patient.

(Kayley 2004)

Patient/carer administration

If it is appropriate for the patient/carer to administer the i.v. therapy then they require training (NMC 2004a; RCN 2005). In most circumstances it is preferable that this is

Section 2

Table 12.6 Who delivers?

	Advantages	Disadvantages
Patient carer	Patient autonomy/control Available 24 hours/day Technique good Methodical and thorough	Training is time consuming therefore possible delayed discharge from hospital More difficult to monitor patient/carer technique
Community nurse	Works in the community Able to monitor patient Works 7 days a week Flexible hours (am and pm) in some areas	Requires training and support Several nurses may be involved in the administration
Rapid response intermediate care team	Flexible hours May be able to prevent hospital admission or facilitate early discharge Intensive input Able to monitor patient	Requires training and support Several nurses may be involved in the administration Period of input may be time limited
Private home i.v. company	Flexible service Experienced nurses Able to monitor patient 24 hour back up support	Cost Patient could have care from several different agencies
Practice nurse	Limited number of nurses involved (1 or 2) Able to monitor patient Enables patient	Requires training and support 5/6 day service during daytime
Outpatient nurse	Medical back-up available Able to monitor patient	Patient has to travel 5-day service 9 am–5 pm
Specialist community i.v. nurse	Experienced nurses Able to monitor patient	Not feasible for long distances, large numbers of patients and frequent dosing
General practitioner	May be prepared to cannulate (if needed) Would increase knowledge about community i.v. therapy	Requires training and support for all GPs in the practice Limited knowledge about vascular access devices and community i.v. therapies Not enough time or resources

carried out in hospital before discharge so that the patient/carer is fully trained and competent when finally discharged into the community. It is not realistic or acceptable to start the training in hospital and then to expect a community nurse, who may not have been involved, to continue the training and supervision.

Training a lay person is time consuming, requires patience and consistency and should be provided by a limited number of trainers (Cox and Westbrook 2005).

Guidelines for training patients/carers

- Limit the number of trainers to two or three.
- Draw up written guidelines (step by step) of how to administer the therapy and be very specific, starting with a list of equipment and supplies required.
- The trainers should go through the guidelines thoroughly together so they are all teaching the same method.
- Give the patient/carer a copy of the guidelines to read before starting the training.
- Find a suitable environment which is comfortable, with room for all persons involved.
- Set aside plenty of time.

- Ensure there are no distractions and that a calm/quiet environment is available with no interruptions.
- Start with basics—handling equipment, connecting needles to syringes, drawing up sodium chloride for flushing.
- Demonstrate each stage, then let them try.
- Keep explanations simple and short. Emphasize what to do rather than what not to do.
- Encourage the patient/carer to write their own additional instructions on the guidelines.
- Give feedback and allow plenty of time for questions.
- Do not suggest alternative procedures or short cuts. Stick rigidly to the guidelines until a routine is established.
- Cover side-effects and complications, what to do, and whom to contact.
- Move slowly from dependence to independence and appreciate it may take a number of teaching sessions.
- Observe the patient/carer doing the whole procedure from start to finish, without intervention, before discharge.
- Ensure the patient/carer feels confident about the administration.
- Document all training undertaken.
- Try and arrange for someone competent to be with them the first time they do it in the community.

(Cox and Westbrook 2005; RCN 2005)

Note:

- Trainers need to feel confident about their own skills/knowledge about the therapy/treatment.
- The trainers must be able to present the information in an orderly and understandable manner.
- Trainers must be able to work on the same level as the patient/carer.
- The patient/carer must be able to learn.
- It is important to recognize that not all patients/carer want to take on the administration of their i.v. therapy, not all are suitable and not all are teachable.

(Cox and Westbrook 2005; RCN 2005)

It is impossible to safeguard against every eventuality, and once patients are discharged into the community they do not necessarily have anyone monitoring their technique. The majority of patients who self-administer i.v. therapy are highly motivated, understand the importance of the treatment and have a sense of self-control and autonomy (Tice *et al.* 2004). At the same time, it is important to provide good, regular communication and ongoing support to monitor how they are coping in the community.

The role of community nurses

Community nurses are ideally placed to provide i.v. therapy as well as support to patients and carers in the community. However, in order to provide this care and support they do need access to a community-based theoretical i.v. training programme, supervised practice and ongoing support. The RCN *Standards for Infusion Therapy* (RCN 2005) provide clear guidance on the aspects that should be covered in theoretical and practical training. All staff have a professional obligation to maintain their knowledge and skills (NMC 2004b) and 'it is also the responsibility of the organization to support and provide staff with training and education' (RCN 2005).

Whilst i.v. therapy is now more routine practice in many areas of the UK, some community nurses may only encounter it on an infrequent basis and this makes it difficult for them to maintain their practical skills and have the confidence to use them. Community

Section 2

nurses may also come across a range of different i.v. therapies and vascular access devices and therefore require the specific knowledge and practical skills to enable them to cope with each situation (Turner and Pateman 2000). Therefore it must be recognized that community nurses need to keep updating their practical skills and theoretical knowledge. This may be achieved by visiting the hospital unit when a patient is referred, although time and distance constraints may make this difficult. A number of areas of the UK now have specialist community i.v. nurses and part of their role is to provide practical training and ongoing support for nurses within the community setting (Kayley *et al.* 1996; Nathwani *et al.* 1999; Deagle 2001; Cooper *et al.* 2003; Kayley 2004).

Rapid response/intermediate care teams

Rapid response and intermediate care teams have been developed to prevent the need for hospital admission, or to enable early discharge from hospital. Most areas in the UK are providing some form of rapid response/intermediate care service (Shepperd and Iliffe 1998; Shepperd *et al.* 1998). The care they provide often covers a 24-hour period but their overall input may be time-limited (e.g. 2 weeks). Most of these services accept patients who require i.v. therapy for example for antimicrobials (Shepperd *et al.* 1998), and less commonly for blood transfusions (Phillips 2000).

Commercial home-care companies

There are a number of commercial home-care companies in the independent sector who can provide a range of services for patients requiring i.v. therapy in the community, and many of these services are listed below.

- Assessment and discharge planning.
- Specialist nurses to administer i.v. therapy, and monitor and support the patient.
- Cannulation and venepuncture.
- PICC insertion.
- Intravenous infusion clinics for specific therapies.
- 24-hour access for specialist advice.
- Liaison with hospital.
- Training and support for community nurses and other members of the PCT.
- Liaison with GPs.
- Reconstitution or preparation of i.v. therapy in device/form/pump of choice.
- Delivery of drugs plus all ancillary equipment to patients on a regular basis.
- Collection of sharps bins and clinical waste.

The number of commercial home-care companies has increased over the last 5 years and some of the well-established companies have expanded significantly. Whilst a considerable proportion of their work is for patients with private healthcare insurance, many now have contracts with the NHS to provide a range of therapies, which are not all intravenous. The cost of using a commercial home-care company can be a significant constraint to use by the NHS. However, this factor has to be balanced with the constant pressures on NHS hospitals such as the need for acute hospital beds. In some areas of the UK there is no existing system within the community to support patients having i.v. therapy, so using commercial home-care companies may currently be the only way of enabling these patients to be supported in the community.

Practice nurses

Practice nurses are health-centre/surgery based, and therefore patients have to come to them for treatment. This encourages ambulant patients to be more independent rather than having to wait in at home for a nursing visit. The service that practice nurses provide is generally daytime Monday to Friday with some early evening cover.

Practice nurses generally are not i.v. trained, but if they were trained they could offer a service to patients who required i.v. therapies that are administered over a relatively short period of time such as antimicrobials as direct intermittent injections.

Outpatient

Intravenous therapy administered on an outpatient basis is rapidly becoming an option for treating patients and freeing up acute hospital beds, especially where there is no existing infrastructure in the community to support i.v. therapy (Deagle 2001). This method of delivery is most commonly used for patients requiring short-term i.v. antimicrobial therapy, and follows the principles of the US office/infusion centre model of outpatient delivery (Tice *et al.* 2004).

Community i.v. specialist nurses

Specialist nurses may be available to administer i.v. therapy to patients under their care but as specialist nurses are few in number this is not sustainable or feasible:

- for long-term treatment
- for frequent dosing
- if large numbers of patients are involved
- if there are long distances to travel.

GPs

The majority of GPs support the principle of community i.v. therapy but are concerned about being asked to provide medical responsibility for i.v. treatments with which they are unfamiliar, and which have been prescribed by the hospital (Kayley *et al.* 1996; Parker *et al.* 1998). The ever-increasing workload of GPs means that their involvement in the administration of i.v. therapy is only realistic for infrequent, short-term, preagreed therapy that could be shared with other professionals.

Prescribing and Funding of Intravenous Therapies

Before 1995, some GPs prescribed i.v. therapy for their patients, and some i.v. therapies were organized and funded by secondary or tertiary care (the hospitals, or NHS trusts). In April 1995, a UK Department of Health executive letter *EL (95)5: Purchasing High Tech Healthcare for Patients at Home* was implemented (DH 1995). This document shifted the funding of high-tech packages of care from the GP prescribing system to the purchasers (health authorities, HAs). Patients whose i.v. treatments at home included 'the delivery of drugs together with other products and equipment needed to administer them' were classified as packages of care (DH 1995). The NHS Executive identified the amount that was currently being spent on these high-tech packages of care through GP prescribing, and those funds were shifted to the purchasers.

The document listed the main groups of patients who were receiving high-tech i.v. packages of care at home, some of which were being prescribed by GPs.

- Cystic fibrosis patients receiving intravenous antibiotics.
- Cancer patients receiving i.v. chemotherapy agents.
- HIV patients receiving i.v. anti-infectives.
- Patients receiving parenteral nutrition.

However, the HAs only contracted for those patients for whom GPs were previously prescribing, which were generally patients with cystic fibrosis receiving i.v. antibiotics, and patients with Crohn's disease or short bowel syndrome requiring parenteral nutrition. Hospitals therefore continued to pay out of their own budgets for patients they were already treating with home i.v. therapy. The funding of drugs, equipment and supplies for community i.v. therapy initiatives that have developed since 1995 (e.g. i.v. antimicrobials), tends to have come from hospital budgets and this lack of additional and identified funding is often a major stumbling block in the development of community i.v. therapy services.

The interpretation of the *EL (95)5* varies from area to area in the UK, so despite the fact that the *EL (95)5* has been implemented for 12 years there is still a lack of coordination and clarity with respect to purchasing, funding and provision of community i.v. therapy (Loader *et al.* 2000). Although responsibility for purchasing healthcare passed to PCTs in 2002, there has so far been no noticeable change in the funding mechanisms for community i.v. therapy (Kayley 2003).

At the national level, the DH sets guidelines and targets for prescribing, which filter down to the local level via strategic health authorities (SHAs), PCTs and practices (Royal College of General Practitioners (RCGP) 2006). Each PCT has an area prescribing committee (APC), which has representatives from primary care (GPs and prescribing advisors) and secondary care (chief pharmacists, consultants and medical information pharmacists) (National Prescribing Centre (NPC) 2000; RCGP 2006). The purpose of the APC is to manage local prescribing issues, and in many areas a 'traffic light system' operates which is determined by the APC (NPC 2000; Burrill 2003). Medication is classified according to traffic light colours, although different APCs may put the same drug in different categories and this can lead to cross-county problems (Burrill 2003).

- Green—anyone can prescribe.
- Amber—suitable only for prescribing by GPs/primary care clinicians following a shared-care protocol involving a consultant and approved by the APC.
- Red—only suitable for consultants/specialists to prescribe due to specialist nature.
- Brown—not suitable for prescribing because of limited evidence base.

(Burrill 2003; NPC 2000)

The NMC *Guidelines for the Administration of Medicines* (NMC 2004a) provides clear guidelines in relation to the prescription of medication. Therefore, if community nurses are involved in the administration of the i.v. therapy, the treatment should be clearly written on a community drug chart stating the drug name, dose, route, frequency, timing of administration and review or completion date of the treatment (Scales 1996; Hyde 2002). The patient's name must be clear and the drug chart should be signed and dated by the prescribing doctor. This can then be countersigned by the GP once the patient is home.

It is important to obtain as much relevant information as possible about the i.v. therapy treatment before accepting a patient and this information should be clearly documented.

- What is the name of the drug/treatment?
- What is the drug/treatment for?
- What are the side-effects?
- How should it be administered?
- At what rate should it be administered?
- Is the dose prescribed the correct dose for that patient (weight, height etc.)?
- Does the patient have a history of any allergies or anaphylaxis?
- Does the patient have any relevant past medical history?
- Has the patient had any problems/side-effects with the treatment so far?

- How many doses of drug treatment has the patient had?
- Is any blood monitoring required and how often, and who will assimilate/communicate the results?
- Is there a finish or review date for the drug/treatment?

In Glasgow, patient group directions (PGDs) have been developed and used for the management of patients requiring i.v. antibiotic therapy for specific conditions (Seaton *et al.* 2005). This has meant that community i.v. nurse specialists can manage the clinical episode themselves without recourse to hospital admission or the need for any routine medical review, and without compromising clinical care (Seaton *et al.* 2005).

Allergic/Anaphylactic Reactions

All drugs possess the potential to cause hypersensitivity reactions. Although these are not common they do occur and therefore their prevention and treatment should be an important consideration for i.v. therapy in the community (Dobson *et al.* 2004).

Hypersensitivity reactions can range from a skin rash and itching to a severe anaphylactic reaction which can occur with any dose (Henderson 1998; Jordan and Tait 1999). The intensity and severity of the response is thought to be related to administration and the rate of absorption of the drug (Henderson 1998; Jordan and Tait 1999). Anaphylaxis is a rare complication with an estimated incidence of 1 in 1000 to 10000 treatment courses of beta-lactam antibiotics (McEntee 2004). Dobson *et al.* (2004) reported no life-threatening reactions in 1000 courses of community i.v. antimicrobial therapy. In this study all patients had at least the first dose of therapy under direct supervision (Dobson *et al.* 2004).

Adrenaline is regarded as the most important drug for any severe anaphylactic reaction and is generally the only drug available for community nurses (Resuscitation Council 2002). It is very important to teach patients or carers who are administering i.v. therapy in the community about the possible signs and symptoms of an allergic/anaphylactic reaction and this should be incorporated into the teaching programme (Dobson 2001; Cox and Westbrook 2005). For some specific i.v. therapies (e.g. i.v. immunoglobulin) patients are taught about how to treat an anaphylactic reaction as part of their training programme. They are issued with a prefilled syringe of adrenaline (EpiPen) and taught to give it in the event of a reaction and then to seek medical help (Chapel and Brennan 1988).

The issue about whether first or second doses of i.v. drugs, in particular i.v. antimicrobials, should be given in the community setting has more recently been the source of considerable discussion amongst both acute hospital and community-based healthcare professionals. Guidelines from the USA and Australia support the administration of first doses being administered in a supervised setting with the availability of personnel trained in resuscitation and appropriate equipment (Dobson 2001; Dobson *et al.* 2004; Tice *et al.* 2004).

In the UK there is no legislation that requires the first dose of an antimicrobial to be given in hospital (McEntee 2004). An assessment of a random selection of summaries of product characteristics (SPCs) for i.v. antimicrobials found no mention of a requirement to initiate treatment in hospital, except for linezolid (McEntee 2004). It is unlikely that any i.v. antimicrobial would be prescribed to a patient with a documented known allergy to it, or an agent in the same family (McEntee 2004). This would mean that it is more likely that the antibiotic is being used for the first time in a patient and therefore the risk following the first dose would be low (McEntee 2004). In this situation, the risk of anaphylaxis would be greater following administration of the second dose so it would seem advisable, in view of this, that treatment is initiated and continued for a few doses in hospital where resuscitation facilities are available (McEntee 2004).

The issue of possible allergic reactions or anaphylaxis highlights the importance of asking relevant questions as part of the assessment process and documenting all this information even if there is nothing of note to report. Local i.v. policies should clearly address the position about the administration of first, second and third doses of medication in the community. It is also relevant to get into perspective that a severe anaphylactic reaction is very rare. However, it is still essential to concentrate on educating patients and carers about early signs and symptoms of an allergic reaction, and the importance of seeking advice immediately. Once the patient is discharged into the community they should be monitored closely and assessed on a regular basis. They need to be encouraged to report anything, however insignificant they may feel it is. The practitioner should always listen to the patient and if in doubt seek advice.

Drug Storage and Transportation

Intravenous drugs for administration in the community can come in a range of preparations, from dry powder in vials to ready prepared syringes, cassettes, bags and prefilled devices. Any drug preparation should be labelled by either the pharmacy department, compounding unit or drug manufacturer, and this label should state:

- patient's name
- name and dose of the drug
- the expiry date of the drug
- how it should be stored
- at what temperature it should be stored
- any reconstitution directions
- any administration directions.

If drugs do not require refrigeration then the label will state the temperature they should be stored at, and this is usually below 25°C. Drugs should be stored in a coolish, dust-free environment, away from direct heat and sunlight and out of reach of children (Dobson 2001).

The majority of drugs that require refrigeration are those that have been reconstituted and prepared in an aseptic services department or compounding unit. The recommended storage temperature in the fridge is usually between 2 and 5°C. For many of these drugs a fridge is provided as part of the package of care, especially when the patient has considerable stock which would be unreasonable or impractical to store in a domestic fridge. The drug fridges supplied are regularly maintained and checked by the provider and usually contain a fridge thermometer so that the correct temperature can be maintained, and some have a door locking system.

Some prepared i.v. drugs require storage in a frozen form, generally at –2°C, and the pharmaceutical companies who prepare/reconstitute the drug usually provide a temperature-controlled freezer with the drugs.

If drugs are to be stored in a domestic fridge it is important to consider the following before the patient is discharged.

- Is there room in their fridge for the drugs?
- Is the fridge working properly?
- Do they have a fridge thermometer? If not, suggest they buy one.
- Do children have access to the fridge?
- Do they have a hard container with a lid they could store the drug/s in ?
- Do they have a tray they could store the drug/s on?

(Dobson 2001)

Drugs that are stored in a refrigerator may need to be removed from the fridge before administration for a period of time varying from 30 minutes to 4 hours. If the drug is going to be removed from the fridge for longer than the recommended ' warming up' period then the length of time of the drug stability should be checked with a pharmacist. It is also useful to know this information in case there is a power cut.

Before discharge the following considerations should be discussed with, explained to, and understood by the patient/carer.

- How and where the drug should be stored.
- At what temperature the drug should be stored.
- Is it out of reach of children and animals?
- Where to dispose of the drug/device/equipment once used.
- What to do in the event of a spillage of drug.
- Whom to contact if there are any problems or queries.

(Dobson 2001)

If commercial home-care companies are used, they will usually provide all the ancillary equipment required as well as the drug and take responsibility for ensuring that the patient has sufficient stock at all times. If drugs and ancillary equipment are provided by the hospital, the patient needs to know when more supplies will be needed and where to obtain these.

Commercial home-care or pharmaceutical companies which prepare or reconstitute drugs for transport usually deliver them directly to the patient's home in an appropriate container—often in a cool box. They always check that someone is at the property and able to receive the drugs, and to transfer them to the fridge as soon as possible.

If patients are transporting their own drugs home from hospital, in whatever form, they should be advised to bring a cool box or rigid container for transportation and they must not leave the drugs in a hot car or in direct sunlight (Dobson 2001). Patient-ready cytotoxic drugs must be transported in a sealed, labelled, rigid container and handled in accordance with local policy (Cooper and Depledge 2004).

Some drugs, not cytotoxic drugs (Health and Safety Executive (HSE) 2003), may require reconstituting in the home setting. This should be done in a clean, well ventilated room with sufficient space to organize and prepare the drug. Care must be taken not to spill or splash any drug on surfaces that may be damaged, for example varnished or polished wood. Using a melamine or plastic tray is advisable as this can easily be wiped and cleaned before and after each use. The drugs can be prepared on a sterile field on the tray and safely carried to the patient for administration.

Disposal of Waste

Anyone involved in the administration of community i.v. therapy should be aware of the correct disposal procedure for the equipment and drugs they are using. Patients, carers and healthcare professionals must have access to sharps bins (conforming to UN3291 and BS 7320 standards) (NICE 2003) and clinical waste bags, and know how and where these are to be disposed of safely once full (DH 2005). Any unused drugs or solutions should ideally be returned to a pharmacy department so they can be disposed of appropriately.

Local policies must identify systems for the collection and disposal of cytotoxic drug waste and sharps in the community (Daniels 1996; HSE 2003; Cooper and Depledge 2004). Community personnel must be aware of and informed about these policies and the relevant documentation required. All drug containers, unused drugs and equipment (including gloves and aprons) should be disposed of in a 100% leak-proof container that is clearly marked as containing cytotoxic waste (Ferguson and Wright 2002; HSE 2003). There are a number of possible disposal methods.

- The leak-proof container is returned to the dispensing hospital by the patient/carer at the next visit, but the process of transportation needs careful consideration.
- The leak-proof container is collected by a designated courier service.
- The leak-proof container is collected from designated collection points and disposed of by local clinical waste services.

(Cooper and Depledge 2004)

In the case of incomplete administration, all of the i.v. system should be disposed of (Cooper and Depledge 2004). Any unused prepared syringes should be placed into the leak-proof container and returned to the compounding centre with the contents clearly and precisely labelled, and an explanation of why it has been returned (Cooper and Depledge 2004).

Conclusion

Community i.v. therapy services in the UK are being developed in many areas, building on the experience of existing and established programmes elsewhere (Kayley 2000). Patients now often expect to have the choice to return home and continue their i.v. treatment, enabling them to go back to work or school, and to their families. Together with the pressure for acute hospital beds and advances in technology and treatments, this means that there is likely to be a continuing and increasing demand for community i.v. therapy services. Community i.v. therapy is a viable and manageable concept but the success of i.v. therapy services depends on having a motivated, multidisciplinary team and good communication between the hospital and community. There needs to be an established procedure for outcome monitoring, feedback and audit in order to ensure a high level of service and patient care.

There is still a lot of work that needs to be done nationally within both the acute and the community setting to ensure that this type of treatment is organized and managed safely and effectively. Funding is often the critical issue for such services, and at some stage in the further development of i.v. therapy in the community issues around the source, allocation and distribution of funding need to be addressed.

References

Aston V (2000) Community management of peripherally inserted central catheters. *British Journal of Community Nursing* 5(7): 318, 320–325.

Burrill P (2003) Area prescribing committees—what is their role in the new NHS? *The Pharmaceutical Journal* 270(7241): 409.

Billingham K (2003) The reality of liberating the talents. *Primary Health Care* 13(1): 21–22.

Chapel HM, Brennan V (1988) Immunoglobulin replacement therapy for self infusion at home. *Clinical and Experimental Immunology* 73: 160–162.

Cooper C, Depledge J (2004) Cytotoxic chemotherapy: what do community nurses need to know? *British Journal of Community Nursing* 9(1): 26–32.

Cooper C, Coward M, Lessing MPA (2003) An outpatient/home parenteral antibiotic service. *Primary Health Care* 13(8): 20–22.

Cox JA, Westbrook LJO (2005) Home infusion therapy. essential characteristics of a successful education process: a grounded theory study. *Journal of Infusion Nursing* 28(2): 99–107.

Daniels L (1995) The physical and psychological implications of central venous access in cancer patients—a review of the literature. *Journal of Cancer Care* 4: 141–145.

Daniels LE (1996) Innovations in cancer care in the community; home therapy. *British Journal of Community Health Nursing* 1(3): 163–168.

Deagle J (2001) Administering antibiotic therapy at home. *Nursing Times* 97(38): 62–63.

Department of Health (DH) (1995) Executive Letter EL(95)5. Purchasing high-Tech Health Care for Patients at Home. HMSO, London.

Department of Health (2000) *The NHS Plan: A Plan for Investment, A Plan for Reform*. TSO, London.

Department of Health (2002) *Liberating the Talents*. Department of Health, London.

Department of Health (2005) *Safe Management of Healthcare Waste: A Public Consultation*. Department of Health, London.

Department of Health (2006) Our Health, Our Care, Our Say: a New Direction for Community Services. TSO, London.

Dobson PM (2001) A model for home infusion therapy initiation and maintenance. *Journal of Infusion Nursing* 24(6): 385–394.

Dobson PM, Boyle M, Loewenthal M (2004) Home intravenous antibiotic therapy and allergic drug reactions. *Journal of Infusion Nursing* 27(6): 425–430.

Dougherty L (2006) *Central Venous Access Devices. Care and Management. Essential Clinical Skills for Nursing*. Blackwell Publishing, Oxford.

Dougherty L, Viner C, Young J (1998). Establishing ambulatory chemotherapy at home. *Professional Nurse* 13(6): 356–358.

Ferguson L, Wright P (2002) Health and safety aspects of cytotoxic services. In: Allwood M, Stanley A, Wright P, eds. *The Cytotoxics Handbook*, 4th edn, pp. 35–63. Radcliffe Medical Press, Oxford.

Gabriel J (2000) What patients think of a PICC. *Journal of Vascular Access Devices* 5(4): 26–29.

Hamilton HC (2000) Selecting the correct IV device: nursing assessment. *British Journal of Nursing* 9(15): 968–978.

Hamilton HC, Fermo K (1998) Assessment of patients requiring IV therapy via a central venous route. *British Journal of Nursing* 7(8): 451–460.

Hardy C, Whitwell D, Sarsfield B, Maimaris C (2001) Admission avoidance and early discharge of acute hospital admissions: an accident and emergency based scheme. *Emergency Medical Journal* 18: 435–441.

Health and Safety Executive (HSE) (2003) *Safe handling of cytotoxic drugs*. HSE information sheet MISC615. HSE Books, Suffolk.

Henderson N (1998) Anaphylaxis. *Nursing Standard* 12(47): 49–55.

Hyde L (2002) Legal and professional aspects of intravenous therapy. *Nursing Standard* 16(26): 39–42.

Jordan S, Tait M (1999) Antibiotic therapy. *Nursing Standard* 13(45):49–54.

Kayley J (2000) Home IV antibiotic therapy. *Primary Health Care* 10(6): 25–30.

Kayley J (2003) An overview of community intravenous therapy in the United Kingdom. *Journal of Vascular Access Devices* 8(2): 22–26.

Kayley J (2004) A Qualitative Study to Explore Patients' Understanding and Experience of Short-Term IV Antibiotic Therapy Outside the Hospital Inpatient Setting. Unpublished MSc dissertation, Oxford Brookes University, Oxford.

Kayley J, Finlay T (2003) Vascular access devices used for patients in the community. *Community Practitioner* 76(6): 228–231.

Kayley J, Berendt AR, Snelling MJM *et al.* (1996) Safe intravenous antibiotic therapy at home: Experience of a UK based programme. *Journal of Antimicrobial Chemotherapy* 37(5): 1023–1029.

Lane L (2000) Client centred practice: is it compatible with early discharge hospital-at-home policies? *British Journal of Occupational Therapy* 63(7): 310–315.

Lister S, Sarpal N (2004) Drug administration: general principles. In: Dougherty L, Lister S, eds. *Royal Marsden Manual of Clinical Nursing Procedures*, 6th edn, pp. 184–227 . Blackwell Publishing, Oxford.

Loader J, Sewell G, Gammie S (2000). Survey of home infusion care in England. *American Journal of Health-System Pharmacy* 57: 763–766.

McEntee J (2004) *Enquiry Number 156022004. First Dose of Antibiotics*. Hope Hospital Medicines Information Centre, Salford, Manchester.

Medical Devices Agency (MDA) (2003) *Infusion System Device Bulletin*. Medical Devices Agency, London.

Nathwani D (2001) The management of skin and soft tissue infections: outpatient parenteral antibiotic therapy in the United Kingdom. *Chemotherapy* 47 (suppl 1): 17–23.

Nathwani D, Conlon C (1998). Outpatient and home parenteral antibiotic therapy (OHPAT) in the UK: a consensus statement by a working party. *Clinical Microbiology and Infection* 4: 537–551.

Nathwani D, Davey P (1996) Intravenous antimicrobial therapy in the community: underused, inadequately resourced, or irrelevant to health care in Britain? *British Medical Journal* 313: 1541–1543.

Nathwani D, Morrison J (2001) Parenteral therapy in the outpatient or home setting: evidence, evaluation and future prospects. *Journal of Infection* 42: 173–175.

Nathwani D, Morrison J, Seaton RA, France AJ, Davey P, Gray K (1999) Out-patient and home parenteral antibiotic therapy (OHPAT): Evaluation of the impact of one year's experience in Tayside. *Health Bulletin* 57(5): 332–337.

National Institute for Health and Clinical Excellence (NICE) (2003) *Infection Control: Prevention of Healthcare-Associated Infection in Primary and Community Care*. Clinical Guideline 2. National Institute for Health and Clinical Excellence, London.

National Patient Safety Agency (NPSA) (2003) *Risk Analysis of Infusion Devices*. National Patient Safety Agency, London.

National Prescribing Centre (NPC) (2000) *Area Prescribing Committees—Maintaining Effectiveness in the Modern NHS. A Guide to Good Practice*. National Prescribing Centre, Liverpool.

Nursing and Midwifery Council (NMC) (2004a) *Guidelines for the Administration of Medicines*. Nursing and Midwifery Council, London.

Section 2

Nursing and Midwifery Council (NMC) (2004b) *The NMC Code of Professional Conduct: Standards for Conduct, Performance and Ethics*. Nursing and Midwifery Council, London.

Parker SE, Nathwani D, O'Reilly D, Parkinson S, Davey PG (1998) Evaluation of the impact of non-inpatient IV antibiotic treatment for acute infections on the hospital, primary care services and the patient. *Journal of Antimicrobial Chemotherapy* 42: 373–380.

Perucca R (2001) Obtaining vascular access. In: Hankin J *et al.*, eds. *Infusion Therapy in Clinical Practice*, 2nd edn, pp. 375–388. WB Saunders, Philadelphia.

Phillips L (2000) Devising a nurse-led home blood transfusion service. NT/3M 1999 National Nursing Awards. *Nursing Times* 96(4): 40–41.

Poretz D (1998) Evolution of outpatient parenteral antibiotic therapy. *Infectious Disease Clinics of North America* 12(4): 827–834.

Quinn C (2000) Infusion devices: risks, functions and management. *Nursing Standard* 14(26): 35–41

Resuscitation Council (UK) (2002) The Emergency Medical Treatment of Anaphylactic Reactions for First Medical Responders and for Community Nurses. Resuscitation Council, London.

Royal College of General Practitioners (RCGP) (2006) *Prescribing in Primary Care. RCGP Information Sheet*. Royal College of General Practioners, London.

Royal College of Nursing (RCN) (2005) *Standards for Infusion Therapy*, 2nd edn. Royal College of Nursing and Becton Dickinson, London.

Sarpal N, Dougherty L, Laverty D (2004) Drug administration: delivery (infusion devices). In: Dougherty L, Lister S, eds. *Royal Marsden Manual of Clinical Nursing Procedures*, 6th edn, pp. 259-274 . Blackwell Publishing, Oxford.

Scales K (1996) Legal and professional aspects of intravenous therapy. *Nursing Standard* 11(3): 41–48

Schleis TG, Tice AD (1996) Selecting infusion devices for use in ambulatory care. *American Journal of Health-System Pharmacy* 53: 868–877.

Seaton AR, Bell E, Gourlay Y, Semple L (2005) Management of cellulitis in the community: evaluation of a protocol incorporating a patient group direction for intravenous antibiotic therapy. *Journal of Antimicrobial Chemotherapy* 55: 764–767.

Shepperd S, Iliffe S (1998) The effectiveness of hospital at home compared with in-patient hospital care: a systematic review. *Journal of Public Health* 20(3): 344–350.

Shepperd S, Harwood D, Jenkinson C, Gray A, Vessey M, Morgan P (1998) Randomised controlled trial comparing hospital at home care with inpatient hospital care. I: 3-month follow up of health outcomes. *British Medical Journal* 316: 1786–1791.

Tice AD (1997) *Handbook of Outpatient Parenteral Therapy for Infectious Diseases*. Scientific American, New York.

Tice A *et al.* (2004) Practice guidelines for outpatient parenteral antimicrobial therapy. *Journal of Infusion Nursing* 27(5): 338–359.

Turner C, Pateman B (2000) A study of district nurses' experiences of continuous ambulatory chemotherapy. *British Journal of Community Nursing* 5(8): 396–400.

Weinstein SM (2007) *Plumer's Principles and Practice of Intravenous Therapy*, 9th edn. Lippincott, Philadelphia.

Section 3
Specialities

CHAPTER 13

Blood Transfusion Therapy

Liz Bishop

The right blood to the right patient at the right time for the right reasons.

(RCN 2004)

Introduction

Approximately 3.4 million blood components are transfused every year in the UK (RCN 2004) and transfusion is an essential component of clinical care. The safety of blood transfusion has improved significantly over the past 20 years, primarily due to improvements in donor-blood screening and stringent quality-control measures. In spite of these improvements risks remain with blood transfusion (Williamson *et al.* 1999). Errors at the point of administration of blood are the most frequently documented mistakes leading to the transfusion of the wrong blood. However, preceding errors in blood sampling, laboratory procedures, storage, handling and withdrawal of blood components are also contributory factors in many transfusion incidents (Serious Hazards of Transfusion (SHOT) 2004). Because of the risks associated with transfusion, procedures are continually changing in order to improve safety. In addition, there is a drive to conserve blood, not only to reduce costs but also to minimize the risk to patients. One of the most important ways of avoiding risks of transfusion is to prescribe blood products only when they are really needed, for example if there is life-threatening haemorrhage or to prevent symptoms of anaemia, and to keep the number of units transfused to a minimum (McClelland 2007).

Alternatives to allogeneic transfusion are being developed and some of these are described in this chapter. However, until there are safe and effective alternatives to blood component therapy, it is important to understand the risks and benefits associated with transfusion and the processes to improve safety. The nurse plays a vital role through all the stages of blood transfusion therapy including the initial venesection, the identification of clinical need, blood product administration, monitoring, assessment and documentation. It is therefore essential that the nurse understands and adheres to her local blood transfusion product policies.

History of Blood Transfusion

Historically, there has always been a fascination with blood, but in spite of this, blood transfusion is quite a recent phenomenon. Two major developments occurred at the beginning of the 20th century that were to revolutionize blood transfusion. The first was the discovery in 1900 by Karl Landsteiner of the ABO blood group system. The second was the independent development by Alexis Carrel and George Crile of methods by which a donor's artery could be attached to a recipient's vein; the so-called 'direct method'. Both of these events stimulated research for improved methods, culminating in the discovery by Agote, Hustin and Lewisohn that citrate was a safe and effective anti-coagulant, which dealt with the problems of clotting and storage (Thomas 2005).

In the 19th century, blood transfusion was used for the treatment of disease, rather than resuscitation, and its use to combat shock only appeared in World War I. As World War II loomed the need for blood storage was even greater. An Army Blood Supply Depot (ABSD) was developed, and the first donor panel was set up. After the war, it was realized that the structure which had proved to be so successful for blood collection should be preserved and so in 1946 the National Blood Transfusion Service was founded. Improved storage techniques were developed over the years, as were systems to fraction-ate blood components. Methods of testing for prevention of transfusion-transmitted infections (TTIs) progressed, including techniques for testing for viral hepatitis and human immunodeficiency virus (HIV) in 1985; human T-cell leukaemia virus (HTLV) in 1989; hepatitis C (HCV) in 1990, and HIV p24 antigen in 1996. Using the advances made in genetic engineering, nucleic acid amplification testing for HIV and HCV was introduced in 1999 (Howell & Barbara 2005).

The annual cost of provision and transfusion of blood products is increasing. The actual number of blood donations only increased by 2% in 2000–2001 but the cost of transfusion increased by 256% to £898 million (Varney & Guest 2003). Varney and Guest (2003) calculated the cost of the modern blood product taking into account hospi-tal stay, management of complications and cost to society. They estimated the NHS cost for an adult transfusion was £635 for red blood cells, £378 for fresh frozen plasma and £347 for platelets. It is inevitable that this cost will continue to rise as collection, testing, processing and administration systems become more complex (Thomas 2005).

Blood Components

Table 13.1 summarizes the range and features of blood products.

Red Blood Cell Transfusions

Red blood cells require ABO and Rhesus cross-matching to determine compatibility of the product with the patient. The majority of people in the UK are blood group O or A (*See* Table 13.2).

Whole blood is rarely transfused and the modern red blood cell transfusion consists of concentrated red blood cells, also known as 'packed red blood cells', because a propor-tion of plasma has been removed. Furthermore, in the UK all the blood is filtered to remove the white blood cells and therefore all blood is 'leukocyte-depleted' as a precau-tion against variant Creutzfeldt–Jakob (vCJD) disease (BCSH 1998). Red cells are usu-ally indicated when the haemoglobin is less than 7 g/dL but not above 10 g/dL (BCSH 2001). When ordering or administering blood products local policy should be adhered to but the following may provide some guidance. Red blood cell transfusions are indi-cated for the following.

1. Acute blood loss, which is generally defined as greater than 30% of blood volume (approximately 1500 mL) (BCSH 2001). This is an emergency where the blood loss is acute and rapid. The concentration of haemoglobin should be considered along with other factors such as the rate of blood loss and the clinical status of the patient.

Table 13.1 Range and features of blood products (Summarised from McClelland 2005).

Type of trans fusion	ABO/Rh cross-matching	Administration	Shelf-life /storage
Red blood cell transfusions	Required	Administer through a blood administration set containing an integral filter. It must be changed at least 12 hourly. A new giving set should be used if another fluid is to be administered following the blood component	Red blood cell storage life is 35 days if kept at 2–6°C. Infusion must start within 30 minutes of removing from the fridge and infusion of the pack must take no more than 4 hours. The longest time from leaving controlled storage to completing infusion should be 5 hours
Platelets	Preferably ABO compatible with patient. Rhesus negative females under the age of 40 years should be given Rh D-negative platelets	Administer through a blood or platelet administration set. Use a fresh administration set with each unit of platelets	At 20–24°C on platelet agitator. Shelf-life is 5 days. The infusion should start as soon as the pack is received from the blood bank. Infuse over no more than 30 minutes.
Fresh frozen plasma	Should be ABO compatible to avoid risk of haemolysis caused by donor anti-A and anti-B	Administer through a blood administration set containing an integral filter. It must be changed at least 12 hourly. A new giving set should be used if another fluid is to be administered following the blood component	Storage life of 1 year if stored at −30°C. Once thawed, infusion should be complete within 4 hours. Start infusion as soon as the pack of thawed plasma is received from the blood bank. Anaphylactoid reaction may be more of a risk with rapid infusion
Cryoprecipitate	Should be ABO compatible to avoid risk of haemolysis cause by donor anti- A and anti-B	Administer through a blood administration set containing an integral filter. It must be changed at least 12-hourly. A new giving set should be used if another fluid is to be administered following the blood component	Storage life of 1 year if stored at −30°C. Once thawed, infusion should be complete within 4 hours. Start infusion as soon as the pack of thawed plasma is received from the blood bank. Anaphylactoid reaction may be more of a risk with rapid infusion

Table 13.2 ABO groups and serology.

	A	B	AB	O
Plasma antibodies	Anti-B	Anti-A	No anti-A or -B	anti-A and anti -B
Frequency in the UK (%)	42	8	3	47

2. Surgical patients, particularly if the preoperative haemoglobin (Hb) is less than 8 g/dL and the surgery is associated with the possibility of major blood loss. It may be indicated postoperatively if the Hb falls below 7 g/dL. If possible, preoperative anaemia should be investigated, as medical management may prevent the need for transfusion. For example, if a patient has iron-deficient anaemia a course of iron therapy before surgery may be adequate to maintain the haemoglobin.

3. People with anaemia in active myocardial infarction (Hb less than 10 g/dL) are among the few patients who benefit from an Hb above 8 g/dL (Hill *et al*. 2002). The effects of each unit should be evaluated as each unit is transfused (McClelland 2007).

Section 3

4. Consider transfusion in normovolaemic patients only if they have symptoms of anaemia such as shortness of breath (other causes being excluded), ST depression on ECG due to hypoxia in the cardiac muscle, angina, tachycardia for no other reason, syncope or postural hypotension. Transfusion above 10 g/dL is rarely indicated (Hill *et al.* 2002). The decision to transfuse a patient should be taken only once the benefits and risks have been carefully assessed. The patient should be assessed after each unit is transfused and blood withheld if symptoms have resolved. Single-unit transfusions should be considered (Garrioch 2003) to minimize the risk to the patient because each unit of blood has a separate risk.

Platelet Transfusions

The use of platelet transfusions continues to increase; there was a 2.3% increase in the demand for platelet concentrates by hospitals in England in 2001–2002 resulting in 215 050 adult doses in total (BCSH 2003a). As for blood transfusion, the decision to transfuse platelets must also be based on assessment of risk versus benefit and the cause of the thrombocytopenia should be established prior to transfusion. Risks associated with platelet transfusions include alloimmunization, transmission of infection, allergic reactions and transfusion-related lung injury (BCSH 2003a). Potential benefits include reducing morbidity and/or mortality resulting from major bleeding. One pool of platelets is sufficient to increase the normal adult platelet count by approximately 50×10^9/L, but this is highly variable and if there are any concerns a repeat full blood count is advised following platelet transfusion. The thresholds for prophylactic platelet transfusion vary and hospitals should have a local policy. It is not necessary to transfuse patients with thrombocytopenia secondary to marrow failure if the platelets are more than 10×10^9/L, providing they are in a stable condition (BCSH 2003a). If the patient is septic and/or bleeding the threshold should be maintained above $25–50 \times 10^9$/L (BCSH 2003a). For invasive procedures such as central venous catheterization platelets should be maintained above 50×10^9/L. For invasive procedures of critical sites (e.g. eyes, central nervous system), the platelets should be maintained above 100×10^9/L (BCSH 2003a).

If the thrombocytopenia is due to peripheral consumption of platelets but the patient is stable then the threshold of 10×10^9/L is acceptable. Peripheral consumption of platelets can occur either because they are being destroyed, for example in autoimmune conditions such as idiopathic thrombocytopenic purpura (ITP) where antiplatelet antibodies destroy the platelets at a rapid rate; or because they are being consumed by abnormal clotting processes such as occur in disseminated intravascular coagulation (DIC).

For patients who are unstable, critically ill, bleeding or receiving anticoagulation a target of $25–50 \times 10^9$/L is recommended, depending on the individual patient and clinician decision (BCSH 2003a). In those with uncontrolled bleeding in a critical site it may be necessary to try to maintain the platelet count above 100×10^9/L (BCSH 2003a).

Massive blood loss is likely to cause haemodilution and platelet consumption after transfusion of more than 1.5 times the patient's blood volume (Hippala 1998). Platelet transfusion may be indicated to maintain the platelets above $50–100 \times 10^9$/L but this would depend on local policy and/or the clinical decision. Platelet function is reversibly affected by cardiopulmonary bypass and this abnormality persists for approximately 3–6 hours. Platelets may be indicated postoperatively in the presence of bleeding in these patients (BCSH 2003a).

Platelet transfusions should be avoided in some rare clinical conditions such as thrombotic thrombocytopenic purpura (TTP) as they can exacerbate the disease state. TTP involves a microangiopathic process whereby the patient develops small clots. If platelets are transfused it may contribute to further clot formation, worsening the patient's clinical status (Harkness *et al.* 1981; Gordon *et al.* 1987; BCSH 2003b). In patients with heparin-induced thrombocytopenia (HIT), platelet transfusion can cause acute arterial thrombosis with a similar pathogenesis to that of TTP (Cimo *et al.* 1979) Platelets should only be transfused under the guidance of a haematologist in either of these clinical conditions (BCSH 2003b).

Platelet refractoriness

This is defined as a repeated failure to increment platelet counts following platelet infusion (BCSH 2003a). It is usually seen in patients who have received multiple platelet transfusions and occurs because of the presence of antibodies to human leukocyte antigens (HLAs) and development of platelet autoantibodies, a process known as alloimmunization (Novotny 1999). Other causes of shortened platelet survival should be excluded; for example, patients often do not increment well if they have a fever, splenomegaly or DIC. Furthermore, some drugs may inhibit platelet response, for example antibiotics and amphotericin (Doughty *et al.* 1994). If the patient has HLA antibodies, HLA-matched platelets may improve response to platelet infusion. These are costly and transfusion must be negotiated with a haematologist because it involves apheresis collection of platelets from an HLA-matched donor. The incidence of platelet refractoriness has declined as a result of leukocyte depletion of blood components, which exposes the patient to fewer HLAs and therefore less antibody formation (Brand 2001)

Fresh Frozen Plasma (FFP) and Cryoprecipitate

FFP is indicated for treatment of significant coagulopathy, for example if the patient has an activated partial thromboplastin time (APTT) of more than 1.5 or an International Normalized Ratio (INR) of more than 1.5 (with age-appropriate normal ranges), or they are at significant risk of bleeding because they have to undergo an invasive procedure. Correction is often unreliable and a coagulation screen should always be rechecked. FFP is a human blood component which is screened for transmissible agents but is not virally inactivated. The exception is FFP for patients up to the age of 16 years, which is methylene blue-treated to inactivate viruses, and sourced from the USA. FFP is indicated for the replacement of clotting factors when no virally inactivated or recombinant factor is available. FFP should be group compatible but it is not cellular. Therefore it does not need to be irradiated in those requiring irradiated blood (see section on irradiated blood products) and does not transmit cytomegalovirus (CMV) or human T-cell lymphotrophic virus (HTLV). The dose of FFP for adults is usually 12–15 mL/kg and therefore the normal adult will require 4 units (BCSH 2004).

It should be noted that FFP is not indicated as first-line therapy for warfarin reversal, because usually vitamin K and/or prothrombin complex is used (BCSH 2004). Other points to consider are as follows.

- The risk of volume overload due to the large protein content.
- Anaphylactic reactions, especially with rapid infusion rates.
- FFP contains normal levels of plasma immunoglobulins, including red blood cell antibodies that can damage red blood cells, which is why it should be group compatible (McClelland 2007).

Cryoprecipitate is used as a source of fibrinogen and is now supplied pooled (5 units = 1 pool). If the patient has ongoing bleeding the use of fibrinogen concentrate should be considered. Cryoprecipitate is used in the bleeding patient when fibrinogen is less than 1.0 g/dL. The adult dose is 2–3 pools, which raises the fibrinogen level by approximately 1 g/dL (BCSH 2004).

Special Requirements

Cytomegalovirus-negative blood components

All cellular blood components have the potential to transmit CMV and although all blood is now routinely leukocyte depleted by the National Blood Service (NBS), this is not sufficient to substitute for CMV-negative components. Local guidance for CMV-negative components should be adhered to but generally CMV-negative components are required in the following situations:

- all CMV-negative patients who are potential candidates for stem cell/bone marrow transplant or solid organ (heart/lung/liver) transplant
- all CMV-negative patients who are within 6 months of an autologous stem cell/bone marrow transplant
- all CMV-negative patients whose allogeneic donor was CMV negative
- all intrauterine transfusions
- all components for neonates and infants up to 1 year of age
- all transfusions for pregnant women
- all HIV-positive patients who are CMV negative.

Irradiated blood components

Irradiation of cellular blood components (red cells, platelets and granulocytes) is performed to prevent the occurrence of transfusion-associated graft versus host disease (TA-GVHD), which is a fatal complication of transfusion (BCSH 1996). TA-GVHD can occur either when there is a considerable overlap in the HLA type of donor and recipient or when the recipient is immunocompromised. The transfused lymphocytes recognize the host as foreign, and can engraft and start attacking the host. The patient then develops classic signs of GVHD such as a skin rash, diarrhoea and raised liver function tests due to liver failure, and bone marrow failure and death from infection follow, usually within 2–3 weeks of the transfusion. Gamma irradiation (25 Gy) to the cellular blood components can prevent the development of TA-GVHD by inactivating the donor leukocytes (BCSH 1996).

Local guidance should be adhered to but generally irradiated blood components should be ordered for the following patients and situations.

- Allogeneic bone marrow/peripheral blood stem cell transplant:
  - transplant donors: for 14 days before the harvest
  - transplant recipient: from initiation of conditioning until 6 months after transplant or immunosppression has stopped.
- Autologous bone marrow/peripheral blood stem cell transplant:
  - For 14 days before the harvest and until 3 months after transplant, although 6 months if conditioning included total body irradiation.
  - All patients with Hodgkin's disease.
  - Patients who have received purine analogue therapy (fludarabine, cladribine or deoxy-coforomycin).
  - All granulocyte or buffy coat preparations.
  - All HLA-matched blood components or components donated by family members.
  - All blood for intrauterine transfusion.
  - All subsequent transfusions for babies who received intrauterine transfusions.
  - All blood for transfusion exchange in neonates.
  - All patients with known congenital immunodeficiency with the exception of chronic mucocutaneous candidiasis.

Blood Transfusion Service: from Donor to Patient

It is useful for the practitioner to understand the process whereby the donated blood finally reaches a patient because it affects the availability and safety of the final product. Donated blood is a raw material from which a range of blood products are derived, including packed red blood cells, plasma products and platelet concentrates. Donors can give approximately 450 mL of whole blood up to three times per year (McClelland 2007). Platelets, plasma and red cell concentrates can be either prepared from whole blood or collected from apheresis procedures. Donor screening is essential to minimize risk to the recipient and in the UK every blood donation is checked for hepatitis B and C, HIV-1 and HIV-2, and syphilis. Blood components may be further tested for CMV for infusion into neonates or immunosuppressed recipients, and all blood components have the white blood cells removed as a precaution against vCJD. All blood components in the UK are filtered within 48 hours of collection from the donor to reduce the risk of vCJD transmission by leukocyte depletion (McClelland 2007). This negates the need for bedside filtration.

The Transfusion Process

Every hospital must have policies and procedures in place for every step in the transfusion process (BCSH 1999). It is now a legal requirement for blood unit traceability at each step of the transfusion process. While it is a medical responsibility to prescribe blood components, the completion of the request form, the responsibility for taking a blood sample for pretransfusion testing and the administration of the component can be delegated to a nurse or midwife with the appropriate training (BCSH 1999). The patient should be informed of the intention to transfuse and wherever possible be given the opportunity to ask questions and raise any concerns (RCN 2004). Local patient information leaflets may exist, but there are leaflets available from the Blood Transfusion Service and patients should be given the patient information leaflet *Receiving a Blood Transfusion*. Other leaflets are also available, including:

- *Receiving a Plasma Transfusion*
- *Information for Patients Needing Irradiated Blood (with alert card and sticker)*
- *Blood Group and Red Cell Antibodies in Pregnancy*
- *Children Receiving a Blood Transfusion: a Parent's Guide.*

Every patient who has the potential to undergo a transfusion should wear an identity band on which is recorded legibly the patient's correct minimum identification data (BCSH 1999). Once the decision has been made to transfuse a patient this should be recorded in the patient's notes and the fact that the reason has been explained to the patient or responsible person for the patient (RCN 2005; McClelland 2007).

Taking a blood sample

Before sampling blood, the practitioner should ask the patient to state their first name, surname and date of birth, and check that it is the correct patient. If the patient is unconscious or a child, it is necessary to ask another member of staff, relative or carer to verify the patient details. The given details should always be checked with the patient's identity wristband. After taking the blood sample, and before leaving the patient, the practitioner must label the compatibility sample tube clearly and accurately with the patient details and sign the tube and request form as the person drawing the sample, checking that the tube and form details correspond (RCN 2005). Prelabelling of the tube is not good practice and has been identified as a major cause of patient identification errors that can lead to fatal transfusion reactions (O'Donovan 2005). Ensure the reason for the transfusion is documented on the request form and any relevant previous transfusion history and special requirements, for example, irradiated components.

Collection

Every blood component collection should be checked against the patient's minimum identification data set, including first name, surname, address, date of birth and hospital identity number (BCSH 1999; RCN 2004). The patient's details on the blood collection form (or local documentation) should be checked for compatibility against the blood component being collected. Systems should be in place to record the date, time and person removing it from the storage.

Preadministration

The transfusion should begin as soon as possible after arrival in the clinical area (BCSH 1999; RCN 2004). Inspection of the blood component must be carried out to check for leaks, haemolysis, discoloration, clots and expiry date. If there are any problems the unit must not be transfused and returned to the transfusion laboratory. It is important at this stage to make a final check with the patient that they understand the reasons for the transfusion and provide additional explanation if necessary. All blood components must be prescribed, ensuring additional requirements such as irradiated products, CMV-negative components or additional drugs such as diuretics or desferrioxamine have also been prescribed.

Administration

The unit must also have a final identity check at the bedside by asking the patient to provide their full name and date of birth (RCN 2004). If the patient is a child, or unconscious, or unable to provide their details, then where possible, confirm details with a relative or another member of staff. The wristband must be in place and checked against the blood component details and finally the labels checked with the blood group and any special requirement details. This should be repeated for each component transfused (RCN 2005). It is not uncommon in a busy clinical environment to be interrupted during these final checking procedures and if this happens the process should be repeated as it has been shown that distraction can lead to errors (Pape 2003). Finally, hand-washing and aseptic procedures should be followed when connecting any blood component to the patient as with any intravenous therapy (RCN 2005).

Patient monitoring

The clinical staff responsible for monitoring patients undergoing transfusion must be trained in and knowledgeable of the signs and symptoms of acute transfusion reactions as well as the technical aspects of blood product administration. It is also recommended that transfusions should be undertaken in an area where staff can easily observe the patients (BCSH 1999; RCN 2005). Before administration of the blood product baseline observations should be undertaken, including temperature, pulse, blood pressure and respiration rate. Fifteen minutes after the start of each unit of blood, these observations should be repeated and again at the completion of each unit transfused. This may detect a reaction of delayed onset and act as a baseline for the next unit (BCSH 1999). These are the minimum requirements, and the frequency of observations will need to be increased if the patient shows signs of a transfusion reaction or if they require monitoring for other clinical reasons (BCSH 1999), for example unconscious, disorientated or anaesthetized patients who are unable to communicate symptoms. This also applies to children. It may also be necessary to increase the frequency of observations in patients who are known to have had previous reactions and those who have known cardiac and/ or renal impairment. The start and finish times should also be recorded and the volume infused recorded on the fluid balance chart (RCN 2004).

Technical aspects

If the transfusion of blood is not commenced within 30 minutes of removal of the blood from the fridge, it should be returned to storage to minimize risk of bacterial proliferation. Once commenced it should be transfused within 4 hours of puncture of the bag (McClelland 2007; RCN 2005). Platelets should not be stored in the fridge but should be stored on an agitator to avoid platelet clumping. Again, these must be infused as soon as possible after arrival in the clinical area and infused over no more than 30 minutes (McClelland 2007). No drugs should be added to the blood component, but it is acceptable to simultaneously infuse intravenous desferrioxamine via a Y-connector (RCN 2005).

Blood components must be transfused through a blood administration set with an integral mesh filter (170–200 μm size) and this should be changed every 12 hours for a continuing transfusion and changed on completion of the transfusion (McClelland 2007; RCN 2005). Platelets can be infused through either a fresh blood administration set or a platelet administration set (McClelland 2007). It is acceptable to administer blood via an infusion pump providing the appropriate administration set is used and in accordance with manufacturer's recommendations (RCN 2005).

Blood warmers are not recommended unless infusing large volumes, for example during an automated exchange blood transfusion and/or rapid rates (more than 50 mL/kg/h) and in the paediatric setting when infants are undergoing exchange transfusions (BCSH 1999; McClelland 2007). A rare clinical condition where it is crucial to warm the infusion fluid is when patients are undergoing either blood transfusion or plasma exchange and they suffer from cold agglutinin disease, whereby intravascular haemolysis occurs in the presence of cold temperatures. With the exception of this clinical indication, blood warming is not recommended and usually keeping the patient warm is satisfactory. Certainly no other method of warming blood other than a controlled and alarmed blood warmer should be used and even these should be used according to the manufacturer's recommendations (RCN 2004).

Adverse Effects of Transfusion

Like most therapies, the benefits of the blood component therapy must be balanced against the risks and, inevitably in the modern healthcare setting, the costs. Both the blood products themselves and also the management of transfusion-related adverse events are expensive, with the total cost of blood transfusion-related complications estimated to be £20.6 million in 2000–2001 (Varney & Guest 2003).

Any adverse events, near-misses or suspected adverse events should be reported. The Serious Hazards of Transfusion (SHOT) system was established in 1996 to improve reporting of such events and is a voluntary system; however, initially all reports should be communicated to the hospital transfusion department. The aims of the SHOT system are to educate users in transfusion hazards, improve standards, and aid in the production of guidelines to improve safety. Among the complications arising from blood transfusion are transfusion-transmitted infection (TTI) and immune complications and incorrect blood component transfused (IBCT) errors. In the UK, SHOT data from 2004 revealed four deaths directly attributable to transfusion, 439 reports of IBCT and 1076 near-misses (SHOT 2004). Typical SHOT IBCT errors are shown in Box 13.1.

Section 3

BOX 13.1

Typical SHOT incorrect blood component transfused errors (SHOT 2004)

- The blood sample was taken from the wrong patient
- Patient details were recorded incorrectly on the blood sample label or the blood request form
- The incorrect unit was collected from the blood refrigerator
- The formal identity check at the bedside was not done or performed incorrectly at the time of the administration of the blood component

---

Acute transfusion reactions

These are potentially life-threatening, and immediate response is recommended for any suspected occurrence (BCSH 1999). It may be difficult to establish the cause of an acute transfusion reaction but essentially the initial management is the same, including stopping the infusion, seeking immediate medical assistance, monitoring vital signs closely and initiating resuscitation procedures. The haematologist and transfusion laboratory staff should also be informed immediately as they can provide expert advice.

An acute haemolytic transfusion reaction is where incompatible transfused blood cells react with the host's own anti-A and/or anti-B antibodies, resulting in destruction of red cells in the circulation (McClelland 2007), a process known as intravascular haemolysis (Weir 2001). The most common cause is the transfusion of ABO-incompatible blood, and it may be fatal. The reaction is most severe when group A red cells are transfused into a group O recipient. Free haemoglobin released from the haemolysis of the red blood cells filters through the kidneys, leading to haemoglobinuria. This is associated with DIC, hypotension, fever, chills, agitation, pain at cannula site, oozing from wound sites, haemoglobinaemia, haemoglobinuria, loin/lumbar pain (often severe) and facial flushing. A sense of 'impending doom' may be associated with cytokine release (Weir 2001), and the patient may become agitated. Immediate action is required, preventing any further transfusion of incompatible red blood cells. The transfusion must be stopped and the bag and administration set returned to the hospital transfusion laboratory. Samples should be taken from the patient for repeat group and screen, full blood count (FBC), clotting, biochemistry and urinalysis. The urine output should be monitored, with oxygen and fluid support as necessary. Appropriate therapy for DIC is also required (McClelland 2007).

Infusion of a bacterially contaminated blood product

The patient will become unwell very quickly with acute onset of rigors, hypotension and collapse. If this is suspected the transfusion must be stopped and the bag and administration set returned to the hospital transfusion laboratory. Blood cultures should be taken from the patient, and repeat group and screen, FBC, clotting, biochemistry and urinalysis should be performed. The urine output should be monitored and broad-spectrum antibiotics should be begun, with oxygen and fluid support as necessary (McClelland 2007).

Fluid overload

This can occur if the fluids have been transfused too quickly, if large volumes have been transfused, or if the patient has a degree of heart failure prior to transfusion. The patient may become dyspnoeic or tachypnoeic, there may be a non-productive cough, basal crackles and tachycardia with hypotension. The infusion should be stopped, and the patient monitored closely, including their oxygen saturation and assessed by the medical team. Usually oxygen therapy would be initiated with furosemide 40–80 mg intravenously to remove the excess fluid, depending on an assessment of the clinical status.

Severe allergic reaction or anaphylaxis

This usually occurs soon after beginning the infusion. It is rare and life-threatening. Typical severe allergic responses are observed, such as bronchospasm, angioedema, periorbital oedema, vomiting, chest pain, abdominal pain and hypotension. It is more common if large volumes of plasma such as FFP are being infused (McClelland 2007). As for the other acute transfusion reactions, the infusion must be stopped immediately and all blood products and administration sets must be returned to the hospital transfusion laboratory. It is recommended that repeat group and screen samples are taken. Immediate assessment by the medical team is required and it may be that chlorpheniramine 10 mg intravenously is given. Salbutamol nebulizer may assist with relief of the bronchospasm, and in the case of severe hypotension adrenaline may be considered (McClelland 2007).

Transfusion-related acute lung injury (TRALI)

This occurs when antibodies in the donor plasma mount an immune response against the recipient's leukocytes. The donors in confirmed cases of TRALI tend to be parous women (Weir 2001; McClelland 2007). It is important that such cases are reported to the BTS so these donors can be removed from the panel (McClelland 2007).

Infiltration of the lower lung fields gives rise to chills, fever, non-productive cough and dyspnoea, resulting in a chest X-ray with a typical 'white-out' appearance. Treatment is that for any acute respiratory distress syndrome. Again, the transfusion must be stopped and any blood products returned to the hospital transfusion laboratory. Expert help should be sought, with close monitoring of the patient, including oxygen saturation and/or blood gases and the administration of oxygen therapy and resuscitation procedures. Mechanical ventilation may be necessary. The mortality of TRALI was 20% of all cases reported to SHOT (McClelland 2007).

Reactions due to red cell antibodies other than anti-A and anti-B

This is rare and occurs when red blood cells become coated in antibody and complement and are destroyed in the spleen and liver by macrophage; in other words extravascular haemolysis. These antibodies can form against the ABO, S, Kell, Duffy and Kidd antigen systems. Up to 400 mL a day can be removed from the circulating blood volume, resulting in a decreasing Hb and increasing bilirubinaemia, with fever and chills (McClelland 2007).

Delayed haemolytic reaction

Again this is rare but typically occurs in patients who have been multiply-exposed to transfusion and in parous women. They develop antibodies to red cells, which may go unnoticed for many years but when exposed again to the same antigen at a subsequent transfusion a massive antibody reaction is triggered. This can be months or even years after the initial exposure and often involves the Kidd (Jk) system (McClelland 2007). Following the transfusion the Hb begins to fall, with a subsequent rise in bilirubin as haemolysis occurs. The haemolysis is not as rapid as intravascular haemolysis but if suspected can be confirmed with a positive direct antiglobulin test (Weir 2001).

Post-transfusion purpura (PTP)

This is a rare but serious delayed reaction following either blood or platelet transfusion. It is caused by alloimmunization and development of platelet-specific antibodies and typically presents as a falling platelet count with or without bleeding 5–9 days post transfusion. Treatment is with intravenous immunoglobulin (McClelland 2007).

Febrile non-haemolytic transfusion reactions

These are not as common as they were before the use of leukodepleted products. They typically present as a rising fever during transfusion, or following transfusion, occasionally with rigors and chills. Slowing the transfusion and administering paracetamol can manage most of these minor reactions.

Allergic reactions

These tend to occur during the transfusion and the patient can start to experience urticaria and/or itching, as an allergic response to foreign plasma proteins and is consequently more common with platelet or FFP or other plasma infusions. These should be reported to the medical team but slowing the infusion and/or administering chlorpheniramine 10 mg intravenously may help (Weir 2001). If it occurs frequently prophylactic chlorpheniramine along with along with the use of washed products may help if the reactions are severe and persistent.

Iron overload

Each unit of blood transfused contains 250 mg of iron, which the body cannot excrete. The human body is very efficient at reusing iron stores and therefore if a patient has undergone many red blood cell transfusions iron stores gradually increase and can eventually cause liver and cardiac damage. Iron chelation therapy with desferrioxamine can be initiated to reduce the iron stores before damage occurs, but it involves many hours of intravenous or subcutaneous infusion (McClelland 2007).

Transfusion-Transmitted Infections (TTIs)

The risk for a blood transfusion recipient of getting a TTI is relatively low, largely because of stringent pretesting and use of a selected donor panel. Other countries have higher rates of TTIs because they use a paid donor pool and their range of tests may not be so wide (Howell & Barbara 2005).

Which infections are relevant to transfusions?

The significance of these infections varies geographically so that each country should assess its own priorities and ascertain the risks involved.

Hepatitis B

The test for Hepatitis B surface (HBsAg) antigen is very efficient; however there is still a small chance of transference via blood transfusions from a donor with extremely low level infection. The estimated risk of transmission of hepatitis B per unit of blood transfused is 1 in 50–170 000 (Regan *et al.* 2000). It may be that in the future this risk will become negligible if either testing improves or postnatal screening and vaccination for hepatitis B is initiated (Howell & Barbara 2005).

Hepatitis C

Tests to detect Hepatitis C were introduced in 1990 and like the other screening methods have continued to improve since then, such that the chances of a blood component transmitting hepatitis C are less than 1 in a million if direct hepatitis C RNA is tested for (Howell & Barbara 2005).

HIV 1 and 2

The current risk of a blood component transmitting HIV is less than 1 in 2 million (Regan *et al.* 2000). Since the emergence of HIV in the early 1980s the screening of donors has improved dramatically. In 1985 the first HIV test was introduced. Since then the techniques of donor interviewing have been greatly improved, the test for HIV p24 antigen was introduced in 1996, and subsequent improvements in nucleic acid amplification testing for HIV and HCV were introduced in 1999 (Thomas 2005).

HTLV

HTLV can cause persistent, permanent infection by targeting the T-cells and causing an immune paresis, and can predispose a patient to developing a rare form of T-cell lymphoma leukaemia (ATLL) (Hjelle 1996). It is transmitted by the cellular component and not plasma. Japan was one of the first countries to introduce screening for this virus because of a high incidence in that population. All blood donations in the UK have been tested for the antibody to HTLVI and II since leukocyte depletion has been shown to lower the risk of transference (McClelland 2007).

CMV

Approximately 50% of UK donors carry CMV, although only a small proportion of donations can actually result in transference (Pomeroy & Englund 1987). As mentioned previously, CMV is a risk to immunocompromised patients, such as transplant recipients and low-birth-weight babies. It is usual for these patient groups to receive blood which has been screened for CMV, but although not proven by prospective studies, leukodepletion of blood components is likely to prove as safe as screening (Howell & Barbara 2005). FFP and cryoprecipitate do not transmit CMV.

Bacteria

The estimated risk for bacterial contamination of red cell components is 1 in 500 000 and for platelets 1 in 12 000 (Dodd 1994). It is difficult to estimate however, because many cases may be unrecorded if fevers are attributed to causes other than the transfusion, and therefore accurate data are not available. The only bacterium for which specific screening is implemented is the causative agent of syphilis, *Treponema pallidum*. Haemovigilance schemes continue to report morbidity and mortality associated with other bacterial transmissions, and although the numbers are low they are considerably higher than acute viral reactions. Bacterial contamination can either be endogenous or exogenous. For example, syphilis is an example of an endogenous transmission and there have been a few reports of *Yersinia enterocolitica* from red cells, usually when they are near the end of their shelf-life (Howell & Barbara 2005).

The pattern of exogenous contamination is changing. There have been improvements in manufacturing and processing leading to fewer contaminations with organisms such as *Pseudomonas*. More common is the identification of skin contaminants arising from inadequate skin cleansing before venepuncture to obtain the blood donation. Skin contaminants such as staphylococci may proliferate in platelet concentrates stored at 20–22°C. This is a factor limiting the safe storage of platelet concentrates, which is one of the reasons why platelets are more likely to be associated with bacterial transference than red blood cell components (McClelland 2007). As a result the National Blood Service has investigated different procedures for arm cleansing and introduced the practice of diverting the first 20 mL of the donation so that the skin bacteria contaminating the venepuncture needle are flushed away into a pouch separate from the collection bag. (McClelland 2007)

Parasites

Several parasitic diseases are potentially transmissible via blood transfusion, for example malaria, toxoplasmosis and leishmaniasis. Prevention of transmission of parasitic diseases by transfusion is by donor exclusion of those who have travelled to a malaria-prevalent area. There have been only four cases of transfusion-associated malaria in the past 25 years, all due to *Plasmodium falciparum* (Thomas 2005). This is becoming an increasing problem in all areas because of increased global travel.

Prions

The emergence of vCJD has led to issues relating to prions and blood safety. Cases suspected of being caused by blood transfusion transference have been reported

(Llewellyn *et al.* 2004; Peden *et al.* 2004). This fact, coupled with concerns over the prevalence of subclinical disease in the UK population (Clarke & Ghani 2005), has led to the introduction of further precautionary measures. For example, following a reported case, from April 2004 the UK excluded blood transfusion recipients as blood donors.

The disease is unusual clinically in that it presents with neuropsychiatric symptoms, such as anxiety or depression, dysaesthesia and ataxia (Ludlum & Turner 2005). Patients then deteriorate further, developing progressive dementia, myoclonus and choreoathetosis with an average clinical course to death of 6 months to 2 years (Will & Ward 2004). The emergence of vCJD resulted in the UK decision to source plasma from the USA and this practice currently continues for patients under 16 years old (Clarke & Ghani 2005; National Blood Service 2005).

Other emerging risks

Emerging pathogens will always challenge the safety of blood transfusion. West Nile virus (WNV) which is transmitted via mosquitoes, severe acute respiratory syndrome (SARS), Human Herpes Virus 8 (HHV8) and TT virus have all been suggested as a threat to the safety of the future blood supply; however, there is no consensus (Thomas 2005). It seems likely that new emerging infections will pose a threat to transfusion safety. Any additional testing introduced to improve safety will inevitably increase costs, which will add further impetus to the drive to develop alternatives to blood transfusion.

Blood Conservation Strategies

Blood conservation strategies are continually being developed because of the risks and cost of blood transfusion together with the future threat of a diminished donor pool. For example, if a screening test for vCJD is developed, the donor base may be diminished by anything from 5 to 20% (Thomas 2005). Blood conservation techniques include better preoperative preparation of patients, anaesthetic techniques, lowering the transfusion threshold and bloodless surgery techniques, for example the use of tourniquets for knee surgery, autologous transfusion and the use of erythropoietin therapy (Dobson 2005; Taylor & Torella 2005). The impetus for the use of autologous blood resulted from developments in cardiac surgery as it was recognized that this would be a major consumer of allogenic blood resources, but it does have its limitations. Patients scheduled for elective surgery where blood transfusion is anticipated can be considered for this option but not if they are febrile or have active infection (Weir 2001) and obviously it is not an option for emergency surgery.

Recombinant human erythropoietin is commercially available and has been evaluated in clinical trials for the treatment of chronic anaemia. Erythropoietin, a glycoprotein hormone produced by the kidney in response to tissue hypoxia, increases bone marrow erythroid (red blood cell) activity. Although erythropoietin is well tolerated and has largely negated the need for blood transfusion use in patients with renal failure, it is expensive and is not effective in all patients, including some cancer patients (Ludwig & Fritz 1998).

Clearly, the future of blood transfusion hangs in the balance and is dependent on further scientific developments, for example, oxygen-carrying resuscitation fluids. However, blood component transfusion will continue to remain an integral part of nursing practice, and it is therefore vital that nurses remain updated on transfusion practice because it is an area of rapid development and increasing complexity.

Box 13.2 summarizes current blood conservation strategies that are being either implemented or investigated. It is likely that combinations of these will be used to minimize allogeneic blood transfusion rather than a single method being adopted universally.

> **BOX 13.2**
>
> **Blood conservation strategies**
>
> - Autologous transfusion
> - Acute normovolaemic haemodilution
> - Erythropoietin and/or iron supplementation
> - Intraoperative cell salvage
> - Postoperative cell salvage
> - Oxygen carriers
> - Surgical methods to reduce blood loss (meticulous dissection, limb exsanguinations, diathermy, laser)
> - Anaesthetic methods to reduce blood loss (hypotensive anaesthesia, normothermia, fluid replacement strategies)
> - Pharmacological strategies (Desmopressin)

The British Committee for Standards in Haematology (BCSH) has issued guidelines for autologous transfusion and red blood cell salvage to help guide practice (BCSH 1993, 1997). Many larger trusts are employing staff specifically to implement some of these strategies and it likely therefore that it will become a growing subspecialism.

Patients who Refuse Blood Products

At one time it may have been the opinion that the only people who refuse transfusions are Jehovah's Witnesses. This cannot be assumed, however, and it may be that the more the public are made aware of the risks (e.g.of vCJD transmission), the more people will refuse blood products. Jehovah's Witnesses are the obvious group of people who may refuse blood products but generally they will accept recombinant erythropoietin therapy, crystalloid and some colloid volume expanders, controlled hypotension and oral or parenteral iron (Stevenson 2005). Jehovah's Witnesses will generally not accept blood components but each Witness makes a personal 'conscience choice' and therefore each patient needs to be managed independently. Furthermore, as Jehovah's Witnesses believe that blood removed from the body must be destroyed, they may not accept autologous transfusion. Intraoperative haemodilution, cell salvage and reinfusion may be acceptable but again this should be a subjective, informed choice. In summary, where possible the issue should be discussed and an agreement reached between clinician and patient.

The Role of the Hospital Transfusion Team and the Blood Transfusion Practitioner

The concept of the Hospital Transfusion Team (HTT) was outlined in the Department of Health circular *Better Blood Transfusion* (NHS Executive 2002). The role of the HTT is to:

- develop and meet the objectives of the hospital transfusion committee
- promote and provide advice and support to clinical teams on the appropriate and safe use of blood
- analyse and respond to any critical incident reporting
- actively promote the implementation of good transfusion practice and
- support the training of all hospital staff involved in the process of blood transfusion.

These points highlight the main aims of the HTT, which are to raise awareness amongst staff and very often to change outdated attitudes to transfusion practice. The team should consist as a minimum of a consultant haematologist, the blood bank manager and the Blood Transfusion Practitioner (BTP). The BTP is a new role created at the suggestion of *Better Blood Transfusion* (NHS Executive 2002), and it has now been recommended that every trust should have a BTP, with either a nursing or biomedical background (SHOT 2004). Blood Transfusion Practitioners work closely with laboratory staff and lead transfusion consultants to support and develop safer transfusion practices and participate in staff education and training. They also facilitate the implementation of national and local policy, follow up on any reported errors and near-misses, participate in the implementation of new technologies that improve patient safety and are involved in blood conservation strategies (Gray & Melchers 2002).

Conclusion

Blood component transfusion in the developed world is safe but never completely without risk. The greatest risk is due to clerical or identification errors, with transfusion-transmitted infections only being a small part of the risk. Haemovigilance schemes such as the SHOT scheme in the UK directly assess the residual risk of complications associated with transfusion, and these systems are helpful in ensuring continued improved safety, but management of the risk of transmission of pathogens by blood and plasma products remains highly problematic (Wilson & Ricketts 2004). Blood donor selection and screening assays offer a better chance of control but most new risk reduction measures are likely to be expensive and create different risks, including threat to blood supply. In this context it is of increasing importance that health services work to ensure that prescription of blood products occurs only when absolutely required (Hart *et al.* 2004; McClelland & Contreras 2005). Nurses can be involved at almost every point of the transfusion chain, from initiating the transfusion to administering it. Therefore it is important they are fully knowledgeable of the risks and benefits of blood component therapy so they can be involved in this decision-making process as well as ensuring that patient safety is maximized.

References

Brand A (2001) Alloimmune platelet refractoriness: incidence declines, unsolved problems persist. *Transfusion* 41: 724–6.
British Committee for Standards in Haematology (BCSH) (1993) Guidelines for autologous transfusion. I. Pre-operative autologous donation. *Transfusion Medicine* 3: 307–16.
British Committee for Standards in Haematology (1996) Guidelines on gamma irradiation of blood components for the prevention of transfusion-associated graft versus host disease. *Transfusion Medicine* 6: 261–271.
British Committee for Standards in Haematology (1997) Guidelines for pre-operative autologous transfusion. II. Perioperative haemodilution and cell salvage. *British Journal of Anaesthesia* 78: 768–71.
British Committee for Standards in Haematology (1998) Guidelines on the clinical use of leucocyte depleted blood components. *Transfusion Medicine* 8: 59–71.
British Committee for Standards in Haematology (1999) Guidelines for the administration of blood and blood components and the management of transfused patients. *Transfusion Medicine* 9: 227–38.
British Committee for Standards in Haematology (2001) Guidelines for the clinical use of red cell transfusions. *British Journal of Haematology* 113: 24–31. www.bcshguidelines.com
British Committee for Standards in Haematology (2003a) Guidelines for the use of platelet transfusions. *British Journal of Haematology* 122: 10–23. www.bcshguidelines.com
British Committee for Standards in Haematology (2003b) Guidelines on the diagnosis and management of thrombotic microangiopathic haemolytic anaemia. *British Journal of Haematology* 120: 556–73. www.bcshguidelines.com
British Committee for Standards in Haematology (2004) Guidelines for the use of fresh frozen plasma, cryoprecipitate and cryosupernatant. *British Journal of Haematology* 126: 11–28. www.bcshguidelines.com

Cimo PL, Moake JL, Weinger RS, Ben-Menachen Y, Khalil KG (1979) Heparin induced thrombocytopenia: association with a platelet-aggregating factor and arterial thromboses. *American Journal of Hematology* 6: 125–33.

Clarke P, Ghani AC (2005) Projections of the future course of the primary variant CJD epidemic in the UK: incidence of sub-clinical infection and the possibility of wider genetic susceptibility. *Journal of the Royal Society Interface* 17: 1–13.

Dobson PMS (2005) Anaesthetic method to minimise blood loss. In: Thomas D, Thompson J, Ridler B, eds. *The Manual for Blood Conservation*, pp. 65–74. tfm Publishing Ltd, Shrewsbury.

Dodd RY (1994) Adverse consequences of blood transfusion: quantitative risk estimates. In: Nance ST, ed. *Blood Supply: Risk Perceptions and Prospects for the Future*, pp. 1–24. American Association of Blood Banks, Bethseda, MD.

Doughty HA, Murphy MF, Metcalfe P, Rohatiner AZS, Lister TA, Waters AH (1994) Relative importance of immune and non-immune causes of platelet refractoriness. *Vox Sanguinis* 66: 200–205.

Garrioch M (2003) Red cell transfusion guidelines. *Transfusion Medicine* 16(5): 12–19.

Gordon LI, Kwaan HC, Rossi EC (1987) Deleterious effects of platelet transfusions and recovery thrombocytosis in patients with thrombotic microangiopathy. *Seminars in Haematology* 24: 194–201.

Gray S, Melchers RA (2002) Transfusion nurses—the way forward. In: *Serious Hazards of Transfusion Annual Report 2000–2001*. Serious Hazards of Transfusion Steering Group, Manchester.

Harkness DR, Byrnes JJ, Lian ECY, Williams WD, Hensley GT (1981) Hazard of platelet transfusion in thrombotic thrombocytopenic purpura. *Journal of the American Medical Association* 246: 1931–1933.

Hart J, Leier B, Nahirniak S (2004) Informed consent for blood transfusion: should the possibility of prion risk be included? *Transfusion Medicine Reviews* 18: 177–183.

Hill SR, Carless PA, Henry DA et al. (2002) Transfusion thresholds and other strategies for guiding allogeneic red blood cell transfusion. *Cochrane Database of Systematic Reviews* 2: CD 002042.

Hippala S (1998) Replacement of massive blood loss. *Vox Sanguinis* 74: 199–407.

Hjelle B (1996) Transfusion-transmitted HTLV-I and HTLV-II. In: Rossi EC, Simon TL, Moss GL, Gould SA, eds. *Principles of Transfusion Medicine*, 2nd edn, pp. 163–185 Williams & Wilkins, Baltimore.

Howell D, Barbara J (2005) Transfusion transmitted infections. In: Thomas D, Thompson J, Ridler B, eds. *The Manual for Blood Conservation*, pp. 13–23. tfm Publishing Ltd, Shrewsbury.

Llewellyn CA, Hewitt PE, Knight SR et al. (2004) Possible transmission of variant Creutzfeldt–Jakob disease by blood transfusion. *Lancet* 363: 417–21.

Ludlum CA, Turner ML (2005) Managing the risk of transmission of variant Creutzfeldt–Jakob disease by blood products. *British Journal of Haematology* 132: 13–24.

Ludwig H, Fritz E (1998) Anemia of cancer patients: patient selection and patient stratification for epoetin treatment. *Seminars in Oncology* 25(3): 35–38.

McClelland B, Contreras M (2005) Appropriateness and safety of blood transfusion. *British Medical Journal* 330: 104–5.

McClelland DBL (2007) *Handbook of Transfusion Medicine*, 4th edn. TSO, London. www.transfusionguidelines.org.uk National Blood Service (2005). http://www.blood.co.uk/hospitals/ . Accessed 20th July 2007

NHS Executive (2002) *Better Blood Transfusion : Appropriate Use of Blood*. Health Circular 2002/009. Department of Health, London.

Novotny VMJ (1999) Prevention and management of platelet refractoriness. *Vox Sanguinis* 76: 1–13.

O'Donovan M (2005) Mismatching errors in the blood transfusion process. In: Thomas D, Thompson J, Ridler B, eds. *The Manual for Blood Conservation*, pp. 225–240. tfm Publishing Ltd, Shrewsbury.

Pape TM (2003) Applying airline safety practices to medication administration. *Medsurg nursing* 12(2): 77–93.

Peden AH, Head MW, Ritchie DL, Bell JE, Ironside JW (2004) Pre-clinical vCJD after blood transfusion in a PRNP codon 129 heterozygous patient. *Lancet* 364: 527–529.

Pomeroy C, Englund JA (1987) Cytomegalovirus: epidemiology and infection control. *American Journal of Infection Control* 15(3): 107–119.

Regan FAM, Hewitt P, Barbara JAJ, Contreras M (2000) Prospective investigation of transfusion in transmitted infection in recipients of over 20 000 units of blood. *British Medical Journal* 320: 403–406.

Royal College of Nursing (RCN) (2004) *Right Blood, Right Patient, Right Time*. Royal College of Nursing, London.

Royal College of Nursing (2005) *Standards for Infusion Therapy*. Royal College of Nursing, London.

Serious Hazards of Transfusion (SHOT) (2004) *SHOT Summary 2004*. SHOT, Manchester. www.shotuk.org

Stevenson PM (2005) Assisting patients who refuse transfusion. In: Thomas D, Thompson J, Ridler B, eds. *The Manual for Blood Conservation*, pp. 189–202. tfm Publishing Ltd, Shrewsbury.

Taylor JV, Torella F (2005) Surgical methods to minimise blood loss. In: Thomas D, Thompson J, Ridler B, eds. *The Manual for Blood Conservation*, pp. 65–74. tfm Publishing Ltd, Shrewsbury.

Thomas MJG (2005) Blood letting and blood giving. A history of blood transfusion. In: Thomas D, Thompson J, Ridler B, eds. *The Manual for Blood Conservation*, pp. 1–12. tfm Publishing Ltd, Shrewsbury.

Varney SJ, Guest JF (2003) The annual cost of blood transfusions in the UK. *Transfusion Medicine* 13: 205–218.

Weir J (2001) Blood component therapy. In: Hankin J, Lonsay RAW, Hedrick C, Perdue MB, eds. *Infusion Therapy in Clinical Practice—Clinical Principles and Practice*, pp. 165–187. WB Saunders, Philadelphia.

Section 3

Will RG, Ward HJ (2004) Clinical features of variant Creutzfeldt-Jakob disease. *Current Topics in Microbiology and Immunology* 284: 121–32.

Williamson LM, Lowe S, Love EM *et al*. (1999) Serious Hazards of Transfusion (SHOT) initiative: analysis of the first two annual reports. *British Medical Journal* 319: 16–19.

Wilson K, Ricketts MN (2004) The success of precaution? Managing the risk of transfusion transmission of variant Creutzfeldt–Jakob disease. *Transfusion* 44: 1475–1478.

CHAPTER 14
Parenteral Nutrition
Clare Shaw

Introduction

Parenteral nutrition (PN) is the provision of nutrition support through intravenous administration of nutrients such as amino acids, glucose, fat, electrolytes, vitamins, minerals and trace elements (Furst *et al.* 2001). The most common route of administration is via a central venous access device (CVAD). Parenteral nutrition may also be infused via a peripheral vein. The solutions used for peripheral infusion have a lower osmolarity than those used in central administration, to help avoid phlebitis and thrombosis (Palmer & MacFie 2001).

Composition of parenteral nutrition

Amino acids are the principal protein substrate in PN solutions. Initial work centred primarily on the categorization of amino acids into essential and non-essential, with the former being necessary as the body is unable to make them from other nitrogen sources. However, more recent work has shown that the requirements for particular amino acids may change during times of metabolic stress, when the demand for such nutrients increases, making them 'essential' in certain clinical situations (Furst *et al.* 2001). The addition of some amino acids, such as glutamine, may be limited by their instability during the manufacturing process and solubility in the PN solution.

Glucose is the main carbohydrate source in PN. Glucose is utilized by all cells and serves as a metabolic fuel for muscle and for organs such as liver, kidney, gut and brain. D-glucose (dextrose) is used in PN and it is this that contributes most of the osmolarity of the PN solution. It provides 3.75 kcal/g (Furst *et al.* 2001).

Lipid in PN is provided in the form of an emulsion. It has a low osmolarity and due to its high energy value has a low volume when compared with an isocaloric solution of glucose. It is required to ensure that essential fatty acids are obtained by the body and is a good energy source, providing 9 kcal/g (Furst *et al.* 2001). Usually the non-protein energy component of PN is made of a combination of lipid and glucose. Several new formulations of lipid emulsions are being examined and some are now available on the market. These include lipids based on olive oil, medium-chain triglycerides and structured lipids (Furst *et al.* 2001).

Electrolyte content of parenteral nutrition

Parenteral nutrition solutions should aim to meet the electrolyte and fluid requirements of the patient. The actual composition must be calculated to avoid instability of the PN solution which is dependent on the types of cations, the concentration and the pH of the solution. Poor compatibility of solutions will result in precipitation of insoluble compounds such as calcium phosphate.

Standard PN, where the admixtures contain fixed formulations of nutrients, can be obtained in a prefilled triple-chamber bag. This system stores the solutions separately and in a stable condition until needed, thus providing a shelf-life of up to 12 months. When the feed is required for use, the operator squeezes and rolls the bag on a work surface, breaking the seals between the compartments and allowing the fat emulsion and solutions to mix. Vitamin, mineral and trace elements must be added to the bags under sterile conditions. Specialist PN bags, for example with varying levels of electrolytes or macronutrients such as amino acids, glucose or lipid, may be made to specific requirements by PN manufacturers or compounding units. These need to be stored in a refrigerator and used within the manufacturer's recommended time (Koletzko *et al.* 2005). They are often more expensive and have a limited shelf-life when compared to standard PN bags.

Addition of drugs to parenteral nutrition

In the past there has been interest in adding drugs to PN but generally this is to be discouraged. When medicines are added to PN solutions this may affect the stability of the solution, the stability of the drug and the bioavailability of the drug (Furst *et al.* 2001). Parenteral nutrition companies may hold limited data on this subject so it is essential to check with individual manufacturers before any such additions are made to the solution.

Indications for Parenteral Nutrition

Parenteral nutrition is required when the intestine cannot be accessed or is not functioning sufficiently to absorb or digest an adequate amount of nutrients (National Collaborating Centre for Acute Care 2006). Whenever possible, the gastrointestinal tract is the preferred route for the administration of nutritional support but PN should be considered when the patient cannot be adequately fed by other means. Indications for PN are:

- malnourished (body mass index < 18.5 kg/m^2 and unintentional weight loss of more than 10% within the previous 3–6 months) or
- at risk of malnutrition (eaten very little for more than 5 days and/or unlikely to eat more than very little amounts for the next 5 days).

(National Collaborating Centre for Acute Care 2006)

The patient may be able to take some nutrition via the enteral route, for example via enteral tube feeding or by diet orally, and this may help in preserving the function of the gastrointestinal tract and the gut integrity.

There is evidence that 40% of hospital inpatients are malnourished, and that malnutrition may increase during their hospital stay if it is not addressed at an early stage (McWhirter & Pennington 1994; National Collaborating Centre for Acute Care 2006). Therefore, it is important to identify these patients early and plan interventions to improve their nutritional status. Careful screening and assessment of nutritional status on or before admission to hospital can identify problems that, if left unchecked, may increase morbidity. Commonly, simple actions such as introducing oral supplements like nutrient-dense foods and commercially available sip feeds to at-risk surgical patients preoperatively can help improve outcomes after surgery. Parenteral nutrition is therefore not an intervention that is introduced without careful assessment of patient needs and equally careful assessment of the risks involved (National Collaborating Centre for Acute Care 2006).

Table 14.1 Nutrition screening in adults using Malnutrition Universal Screening Tool (MUST).

Step 1	Determine body mass index from height and weight and obtain score (using MUST tables)
Step 2	Note percentage unplanned weight loss and score (using MUST tables)
Step 3	Establish acute disease effect and score (using MUST tables)
Step 4	Add scores from steps 1, 2 and 3 together to obtain overall risk of malnutrition
Step 5	Use management guidelines and/or local policy to develop care plan

Assessment

All patients admitted to hospital must undergo nutritional screening, with appropriate intervention for those patients who are identified as being malnourished. This would include development of a plan of nutritional care depending on the patient's nutritional problems, disease state and anticipated future treatment or care. The Malnutrition Universal Screening Tool (MUST) was developed for the purpose of nutritional screening in adults and is based on the criteria of body weight, BMI, weight change and clinical condition (BAPEN 2003). Recent recommendations on screening suggest that MUST or a similar tool that assesses body weight, weight loss and anticipated nutritional problems in the near future should form a basis for screening patients in both an inpatient and outpatient setting. It involves a five-stage process (*See* Table 14.1).

Details of the screening tool can be obtained from www.bapen.org.uk/the-must.htm. An explanatory booklet is available to help interpretation of the screening results and gives advice for when height and weight cannot be measured. Other screening tools may be appropriate in specific clinical settings but these still rely on weight and changes in body weight.

Once the presence or risk of malnutrition has been established then an appropriate care plan should be commenced to ensure that nutritional support is provided in a timely and clinically appropriate way with enteral nutrition being used whenever possible.

Determining Nutritional Requirements

Healthy adults have basic daily requirements of essential nutrients such as protein, fats, carbohydrate, water, electrolytes, minerals and vitamins. Parenteral nutrition requirements must be estimated by healthcare professionals who are appropriately skilled and trained and have knowledge of nutritional requirements and nutrition support. Planning of the PN regimen must take into account any food or fluids taken via the enteral route (National Collaborating Centre for Acute Care 2006).

Important considerations are:

- total requirements for energy, protein, fluid, electrolytes, mineral and micronutrients
- activity levels and any clinical condition that may affect energy requirements
- metabolic instability and risk of refeeding syndrome
- clinical condition and potential tolerance to feed
- likely duration of nutrition support and route of intravenous access.

(PENG 2004)

For people who are not severely ill or injured, nor at risk of refeeding syndrome, the suggested nutritional prescription for total intake should provide all of the following:

- 25–35 kcal/kg/day total energy (including that derived from protein)
- 0.8–1.5 g protein (0.13–0.24 g nitrogen)/kg/day
- 30–35 mL fluid/kg (with allowance for extra losses from drains and fistulae)

• adequate electrolytes, minerals, micronutrients. Dietary fibre should be considered if nutrition is given via the enteral route.

(National Collaborating Centre for Acute Care 2006)

Alternative methods can be used to assess the nutritional requirements of severely ill or metabolically stressed patients (Schofield 1985; PENG 2004). Some examples of equations to calculate basal metabolic rate are given in Table 14.2. The requirements can then be adjusted with the use of factors for stress, activity and diet-induced thermogenesis to estimate total energy requirements (PENG 2004). Additional energy may be added or subtracted if an increase in energy stores is required, although it is inadvisable to aim to change body weight in this way during acute illness or trauma. Requirements should be reviewed on a regular basis as the patient's clinical condition changes and monitoring can indicate whether requirements are being met adequately.

In the seriously ill or injured then nutritional support, particularly PN, should be started at no more than 50% of the estimated target energy and protein needs. Parenteral nutrition should be introduced progressively and monitored closely. No more than 50% of estimated requirements should be given for the first 24–48 hours (National Collaborating Centre for Acute Care 2006).

Refeeding problems may occur in patients who are malnourished and have had a poor dietary intake. Refeeding problems may be characterized by metabolic instability and patients should be identified before starting nutritional support (*See* Table 14.3).

The compounding of specific bags to meet individual patient requirements requires careful liaison with pharmacy staff. They can comment and advise on the suitability and stability of suggested regimens. The prescription should be written clearly and precisely to ensure that the PN is administered correctly.

Table 14.2   Estimation of energy requirements for adults: equations for estimating basal metabolic rate (Schofield 1985; PENG 2004).

Age	Females (kcal/day) W=weight	Males (kcal/day) W=weight
10–17 years	13.4 W + 692	17.7 W + 657
18–29 years	14.8 W + 487	15.1 W + 692
30–59 years	8.3 W + 846	11.5 W + 873
60–74 years	9.2 W + 687	11.9W + 700
75 years +	9.8 W + 624	8.3 W + 820

Table 14.3   Criteria for determining patients at risk of refeeding problems (National Collaborating Centre for Acute Care, 2006).

Patient has one or more of the following	Patient has two or more of the following
BMI <16 kg/m^2	BMI <18.5 kg/m^2
Unintentional weight loss >15%	Weight loss >10%
Very little nutritional intake for >10 days	Very little nutritional intake for > 5 days
Low levels of potassium, phosphate or magnesium prior to feeding	A history of alcohol abuse or drugs including insulin, chemotherapy, antacids or diuretics
BMI, body mass index.	

The Nutrition Support Team

The delivery of PN is a complex process and is best managed by a multidisciplinary nutrition support team. There is strong evidence from research conducted throughout the world that complications are minimized and satisfactory outcomes reached when such a team manages PN (BAPEN 1994a; Schneider 2006). The team will usually consist of a:

- clinician
- nutrition nurse specialist
- dietitian
- pharmacist
- biochemist.

In a well-functioning team, these disciplines interlink with each other to provide the support needed to administer PN safely. The dynamics of each team, however, vary considerably. Within some teams the clinician takes the lead, in others it may be the pharmacist or the dietitian. Members of the nutrition support team will make their assessment through a variety of means:

- the patient's clinical history and planned treatment
- dietary history
- physical examination
- BMI
- anthropometric measurements such as weight or bioelectrical impedance
- biochemical status
- immunological status
- muscle function
- whether to be given peripherally or centrally.

Peripheral PN

Feeding via a peripheral vein is now becoming regarded as a viable option to central venous feeding (National Collaborating Centre for Acute Care 2006), particularly for patients requiring short-term PN of less than 14 days or when insertion of a central venous catheter is inadvisable or impossible (Burnett 2000). The main problems have been related to volume (usually 2–2.5 L) and composition (osmolarity and pH) which has resulted in thrombophlebitis (Burnett 2000). It may be possible to alter the solution by giving fewer calories in total, and a significant proportion as fat can reduce the overall osmolarity and further reduce the risk of phlebitis (Colagiovanni 1997a). The use of filters should also be considered (Burnett 2000; Palmer & MacFie 2001). Pharmaceutical methods of reducing phlebitis include use of glyceryl trinitrate patches, hydrocortisone and heparin (Burnett 2000; Palmer & MacFie 2001). Factors related to the device used can be found in the section on venous access. However, peripheral PN avoids the risks associated with central venous catheterization, there is no X ray required, it reduces cost, simplifies nursing care and prevents delay of initiation of therapy (Burnett 2000; Palmer & MacFie 2001).

Venous Access (*See* Table 14.4)

Peripheral access

As peripheral parenteral nutrition (PPN) is mildly hypertonic it should be delivered into a large peripheral vein via a peripheral cannula; midlines are also used more now for PPN (Phillips 2005). If a peripheral cannula is used, the device should be placed in the largest

Table 14.4   Advantages and disadvantages of peripheral and central venous routes for parenteral nutrition.

Type	Advantages	Disadvantages
Central venous catheter	Reliable long-term access to central venous system Allows the infusion of high-osmolarity feeds	Insertion associated with complications Needs experienced practitioner to insert Risk of catheter-related sepsis Central veins may not be available in critically ill patients because they are already in use
Peripheral venous catheter	Few insertion-related risks Less traumatic for patient Can be inserted by suitably trained staff Less risk of infection No chest X-ray	Suitable peripheral veins may not be available Possibility of development of phlebitis Requires routine resiting and rotation of venous sites Not suitable for those with high nutritional requirements

Table 14.5   Indications for central venous access devices for parenteral nutrition (National Collaborating Centre for Acute Care 2006).

Patients identified as likely to require parenteral nutrition for a period of more than 2 weeks

Patients already have suitable central venous access with a lumen which can be used solely for feeding (e.g. postoperative from theatre)

Patients with no suitable veins for peripheral feeding

Patients requiring specialized parenteral nutrition feeds that cannot be given into smaller peripheral veins, for example hypertonic feeds

vein possible (Palmer & MacFie 2001), usually in the forearm (Hamilton 2000) away from a joint (Burnett 2000). The use of a smaller device (22 G) in a large vein (National Collaborating Centre for Acute Care 2006) will allow good blood flow around the catheter and rapid circulation of the irritant solution in order to reduce the development of phlebitis. It is recommended that sites should be rotated every 48–72 hours (Wilson 2001; National Collaborating Centre for Acute Care 2006). All peripheral devices should be inserted with strict attention to aseptic technique, inspected at least once a day and removed at the first signs of phlebitis (National Collaborating Centre for Acute Care 2006).

Central venous access

The device selected should be comfortable, not limit mobility and be accessible enough to allow maintenance procedures by patients (Wilson 2001).

Short-term access is usually obtained by using a non-tunnelled central venous catheter or peripherally inserted central catheter (PICC). PICCs are often associated with higher incidence of placement and mechanical complications than other CVADs (De Legge *et al.* 2005) but are being used successfully for longer-term access (National Collaborating Centre for Acute Care 2006). Skin-tunnelled catheters and ports are suitable when access is required for longer than 30 days (Wilson 2001; National Collaborating Centre for Acute Care 2006) and must be inserted in optimum sterile conditions using full aseptic conditions including sterile drapes, gown and gloves (National Collaborating Centre for Acute Care 2006). For indications for central venous access, *See* Table 14.5.

It is recommended that these devices have the minimum number of lumens. A single lumen is preferable, but if a multilumen device is used then one lumen should be dedicated solely to the infusion of PN to reduce the risk of contamination (Hamilton 2000; Banton 2006; National Collaborating Centre for Acute Care 2006; Pratt *et al.* 2007;

Weinstein 2007). If using a single-lumen device, routine blood sampling and additional infusions should be carried out independently using a separate cannula if necessary (Davidson 2005).

Preparing the Patient

The need for PN and how this is administered must be explained to the patient. The discussion should include why the therapy is necessary, and where and how the catheter is to be inserted. The potential length of time that PN is to be administered may also be discussed. Once the patient understands the need for the treatment and how it will be managed, a consent is obtained (Balsdon 2000).

The patient should be made aware of the existence of a patient support group (e.g. Patients on Intravenous and Nasogastric Nutrition Therapy (PINNT)) particularly if home parenteral nutrition is being considered; this can help to ease many of the fears patients hold, and allows them to talk through their anxieties with someone in a similar position (DH 2002).

The patient must also be adequately prepared for the catheter insertion procedure. It is crucial that the relevant blood samples are taken (such as full blood count and clotting profile) and checked, particularly if there is a history of anticoagulant treatment or abnormal clotting results (Hamilton 2000).

Administration of Parenteral Nutrition

Parenteral nutrition should be connected to the CVAD using an aseptic technique. The lumen used to administer PN should not be used for other medicines or fluids but should be dedicated for PN only. If additional medicines or blood products are required then these should be given via a separate lumen or via a peripheral device (Shaw *et al.* 2004). Administration sets should be changed every 24 hours and should be labelled with the date and time of use (Pratt *et al.* 2007).

Monitoring

Monitoring of the patient receiving PN is essential in order to avoid clinical and biochemical complications of the therapy.

It is advisable to establish a local procedure for routine blood monitoring in order to recognize and treat any metabolic complications, and the biochemistry department plays a crucial role in helping to detect these changes quickly. Blood should not be taken from the PN line but should be taken from another lumen or peripheral access device. Biochemical aspects of monitoring are listed in Table 14.6.

Ongoing care and monitoring

Ongoing assessment of the patient's response to treatment is part of the clinical team's responsibility. Specific interventions are discussed below, and an example of a monitoring regimen is presented in Box 14.1 (PENG 2004; National Collaborating Centre for Acute Care 2006). Aspects of monitoring and care of the patient should be recorded according to local policy on patient records.

Fluid balance and body weight

Parenteral nutrition should be monitored to assess the nutrients obtained, actual volume of feed delivered and fluid balance. Fluid balance is particularly important to ensure that the patient is not over- or underhydrated (PENG 2004).

Section 3

Table 14.6 Biochemical monitoring of parenteral nutrition (National Collaborating Centre for Acute Care 2006).

Parameter	Frequency	Rationale	Interpretation
Sodium, potassium, urea, creatinine	Baseline Daily until stable then 1 or 2 times a week	Assessment of renal function, fluid status and Na and K status	Interpret with knowledge of fluid balance and medication
Glucose	Baseline 1 or 2 times a day (or more if needed) until stable then weekly	Glucose intolerance is common	Good glycaemic control is necessary
Magnesium, phosphate	Baseline Daily if risk of refeeding syndrome Three times a week until stable then weekly	Depletion is common and under-recognised	Low concentrations indicate poor status
Liver function tests including International Normalized Ratio	Baseline Twice weekly until stable then weekly	Abnormalities common during parenteral nutrition	Complex, may be due to sepsis, other disease or nutritional intake
Calcium, albumin	Baseline then weekly	Hypocalcaemia or hypercalcaemia may occur	Correct measured serum calcium concentration for albumin Hypocalcaemia may be secondary to magnesium deficiency Low albumin reflects disease not protein status
C-reactive protein (CRP)	Baseline then 2 or 3 times a week until stable	Assists interpretation of protein, trace elements and vitamin results	To assess the presence of an acute-phase reaction. The trend of results is important
Full blood count and mean cell volume	Baseline 1 or 2 times a week until stable then weekly	Anaemia due to iron or folate deficiency is common	Effects of sepsis may be important
Iron, ferritin	Baseline then every 3–6 months	Iron deficiency common in long-term parenteral nutrition	Iron status difficult if there is an acute-phase reaction as indicated by a rise in CRP (Fe decreases and ferritin increases)
Folate, B_{12}	Baseline then every 2–4 weeks	Iron deficiency is common	Serum folate/B_{12} sufficient, with full blood count

Monitoring of trace elements such as selenium, zinc, copper and manganese should be carried out if patients are on long-term parenteral nutrition, for example for periods longer than 1 month.

BOX 14.1

Monitoring of patients receiving parenteral nutrition (National Collaborating Centre for Acute Care 2006)

- Record daily weight and fluid balance initially, reducing to twice weekly when stable
- Record actual intake of parenteral nutrition on a daily basis, then twice a week when stable
- Inspect catheter entry site daily for signs of infection or inflammation
- Assess general condition daily
- Record temperature and blood pressure daily initially, then as needed.

All losses from urine, stoma, fistulae, vomit/nasogastric aspirate and diarrhoea must be recorded. The electrolyte content of each is different, and knowing volumes can help in planning replacement. Controlled infusion of PN is vital and a volumetric infusion pump should always be used (Shaw 2004). For a full discussion of the importance of monitoring fluid balance, *see* Chapter 3.

Daily weight should be taken, reducing to twice weekly when stable. This is a crucial part of monitoring. Weight gains of more than 0.5–1.0 kg/day may indicate problems. Such dramatic weight changes can only be attributed to unwanted accumulation of fluid, as it is not physiologically possible to gain lean body mass in such short time periods. Weight gain of this type signals a need to reassess the patient's clinical condition, volume of PN and rate of infusion (National Collaborating Centre for Acute Care 2006).

Metabolic complications of parenteral nutrition

Parenteral nutrition must be managed to minimize the risk from adverse metabolic effects of administering nutrients directly into the bloodstream.

Refeeding syndrome

Rapid and serious derangement of blood biochemistry may occur in refeeding syndrome. These can lead to cardiac, respiratory, neuromuscular, renal, metabolic, haematological, hepatic and gastrointestinal problems (PENG 2004). The patient should be assessed for the risks of refeeding syndrome before starting PN (*See* Table 14.3) and should be monitored closely when PN commences (PENG 2004). During nutritional repletion, electrolytes may be removed from the plasma and transferred into the body's cells which results in a fall in plasma levels. Phosphate and potassium are particularly susceptible to this shift and levels may need to be corrected with additional infusions.

Blood glucose

Hypo- or hyperglycaemia may be a problem in the stressed and critically ill patient. Hypoglycaemia is less common but is potentially life-threatening and so must be recognized and treated quickly. Hyperglycaemia may occur in the metabolically stressed or diabetic patient. Insulin resistance may contribute to hyperglycaemia and in all cases it should be treated with insulin using a sliding scale. Rebound hypoglycaemia may occur if PN is stopped abruptly. A reduction in the infusion rate to half the rate prior to stopping and careful adjustment of the sliding scale insulin, if used, should be adopted (Sobotka & Camilo 2004).

Mouth care

Patients receiving PN are commonly unable to take food or fluids by the oral route. Oral hygiene is therefore an important part of nursing assessment and care. Regular brushing of teeth is encouraged, refreshing mouth-washes are offered regularly, and an artificial saliva spray may be used to retain moisture in the mouth.

Malnutrition causes sore mouth and gums with cracking of the angles of the lips (cheilosis), all of which are distressing for the patient. Such problems are exacerbated when oral hygiene is poor. Aggressive *Candida* infections can be a particular problem, often leading to angular cheilitis (Soady 2004). Halitosis is also common and may be unpleasant for the patient. Competent assessment and regular attention to oral hygiene can prevent many of these unpleasant and uncomfortable sequelae of treatment.

Pressure area care

Skin and subcutaneous tissue are at risk of breaking down and becoming damaged when the patient is undernourished, so regular assessment of skin integrity and correct positioning of the patient are essential (Pancorbo-Hidalgo *et al.* 2005).

Longer-term patient monitoring

It is vitally important that the nurse establishes a partnership in care with the patient from the outset to achieve the most satisfactory outcome. Daily progress should be documented and the care plan regularly referred to and evaluated. A carefully designed care plan, if adhered to by all members of the multidisciplinary team, can almost completely eliminate the administrative problems associated with PN.

Care of Catheter and Intravenous Infusion System

Nurses play a major role during the insertion and care of CVADs, and written guidelines and protocols should be established regarding the care and management of the catheter and intravenous system, in order to reduce complications such as infection and occlusion (Wilson 2001; National Collaborating Centre for Acute Care 2006). Handling of the catheter by a minimum of carefully selected and specifically designated staff such as a nutrition team minimizes the risk of infection, which is the most common complication associated with PN (Tait 2000; Palmer & MacFie 2001; Banton 2006). Most contamination occurs during manipulations of intravenous systems, changing bags and drug administration and additives (Colagiovanni 1997b).

Insertion and any intervention should always be performed using good aseptic technique (National Collaborating Centre for Acute Care 2006). Intravenous tubing should be changed every 24 hours (RCN 2005; National Collaborating Centre for Acute Care 2006; Weinstein 2007) and the solution infused or discarded within 24 hours (RCN 2005; INS 2006). All sets should be of luer-lock design (INS 2006). Chlorhexidine 2% is recommended for site care, and the dressing of choice is a transparent dressing changed every 7 days (CDC 2002). Injection port care is equally important and many hospitals now use closed luer-lock needleless connection devices (Ryder 2006; Weinstein 2007). These devices allow access to the catheter while maintaining a closed system, reducing the risk of air embolism, bleeding and infection (INS 2006).

Occlusion can occur due to blood but also to lipid deposits or precipitates usually as a result of inadequate flushing. Occlusion can occur suddenly, either during or immediately after an infusion. Clearing agents such as hydrochloric acid or ethanol can be used for unblocking lipid deposits, and urokinase for blood (Davidson 2005; Weinstein 2007).

Discontinuing Parenteral Nutrition

It is more common to wean the patient off gradually in order to allow the gut time to adapt to the reception of oral food again (National Collaborating Centre for Acute Care 2006). To do this, the nutrient infusion may be administered at a reduced volume or over a reduced time period, or both, whilst the patient starts taking food and fluids orally. While the patient is receiving only PN, the gut atrophies, the villi flatten, gastric motility decreases, enzymes become less active, and release of gastric, intestinal, biliary and pancreatic secretions slows down. When oral nutrition is restored, the patient may experience feelings of fullness, altered taste and possibly altered bowel function. The healthcare team may find encouraging patients to eat a considerable challenge, as the patient will need to be tempted with appetizing meals and snacks. It is advisable not to stop the PN completely until the patient is eating sufficient food; for example there may be a target that 50% of nutritional requirements must be taken orally or via an enteral feeding tube before the PN is stopped (National Collaborating Centre for Acute Care 2006). An accurate food record and fluid chart must be maintained so that nutritional intake can be assessed and monitored by the dietitian.

Home Parenteral Nutrition

Home parenteral nutrition may need to be considered in patients whose gastrointestinal function is insufficient to maintain nutritional status (DH 2002). This may occur temporarily or permanently. In the UK the commonest reason for patients to require home parenteral nutrition is the development of short bowel syndrome. The causes for this

> **BOX 14.2**
>
> **Psychological considerations for home parenteral nutrition (Stilwell 1992)**
>
> - Interrupted sleep patterns:
>   - nocturnal polyuria
>   - alarms from pumps
> - Depression/grief:
>   - not being able to eat
>   - altered body image from central venous catheters
>   - bowel surgery patients who have lost most of their bowel may no longer feel whole people
> - Impairment of sexual function:
>   - fear of dislodgement of catheter
> - Issues related to communication with family/friends; anger

are Crohn's disease, mesenteric vascular disease, volvulus and surgical complications. Other indications include intestinal fistulae, motility disorders and sequelae of radiation damage. Providing and caring for PN at home requires considerable psychological adjustment by both patients and their families too. Depression and grief have been expressed by patients who have had to adjust to permanent loss of normal sleeping patterns, and marital and sexual relationships may be strained due to altered body image and feelings (Howard 2006). Patients must be carefully assessed for their suitability before any decision on home therapy is taken (Box 14.2). Those who are suitable should be referred to specialist centres with the experience and back-up facilities to support highly technological healthcare at home. The therapy is not without risk, so it is recommended that certain basic criteria are checked before beginning home parenteral nutrition.

- Do the patient and carer understand the reasons for long-term PN, and have they accepted that it is necessary?
- Are the patient and carer willing to receive this care in the home?
- Have they the mental and physical ability to learn and apply basic principles and techniques of care?
- Is there an appropriate long-term venous access device in place?
- Has appropriate funding been agreed?
- Is there an on-call system for providing expert advice to the patient by telephone day and night?

Home parenteral nutrition is regarded as a specialized service. Its management is associated with potentially life-threatening complications such as sepsis, and therefore requires specialist care and management. All patients requiring home parenteral nutrition have their programme initiated by a hospital who maintain clinical responsibility for the contents of the nutrients as well as the monitoring and care of the patient. The provision may be via a local hospital or a specialist centre. The majority of patients are taught to self-care for their CVAD and nutrients, although some may require support from a family member, carer or local community nurses. This involves an extensive training programme that requires patients to have clearly defined learning goals relating to the management of PN. The requirements for the provision of home parenteral nutrition are set out in detail in the Department of Health's *Specialised Services National Definitions Set* (2nd edition) (DH 2002). Care packages must be arranged by the centre responsible for the patient. These may also be negotiated and purchased from home-care companies if necessary. The standards of care and support required for such patients is described in detail in the national definitions set (DH 2002).

Section 3

References

Balsdon H (2000) Preparing the patient for central venous catheter insertion. In: Hamilton H, ed. *Total Parenteral Nutrition: A Practical Guide for Nurses*, pp. 83–100. Harcourt Publishers Limited, London.

Banton J (2006) Techniques to prevent central venous catheter infections: products, research and recommendations. *Nutrition in Clinical Practice* 21: 56–61.

British Association for Parenteral and Enteral Nutrition (BAPEN) (1994a) *Organisation of Nutritional Support in Hospitals*. BAPEN, Maidenhead.

British Association for Parenteral and Enteral Nutrition (1994b) *Enteral and Parenteral Nutrition in the Community*. BAPEN, Maidenhead.

British Association for Parenteral and Enteral Nutrition (1995) *Home Parenteral Nutrition*. BAPEN, Maidenhead.

British Association for Parenteral and Enteral Nutrition (1996a) *Standards and Guidelines for Nutritional Support of Patients in Hospitals*. BAPEN, Maidenhead.

British Association for Parenteral and Enteral Nutrition (1996b) *Current Perspectives on Parenteral Nutrition in Adults*. BAPEN, Maidenhead.

British Association for Parenteral and Enteral Nutrition (2003) *Malnutrition Universal Screening Tool 'MUST' Report*. BAPEN, Maidenhead .

Burnett C (2000) Patient assessment. In: Hamilton H, ed. *Total Parenteral Nutrition: A Practical Guide for Nurses*, pp. 31–54. Harcourt Publishers Limited, London.

Centers for Disease Control and Prevention (2002) Guidelines for the prevention of intravascular catheter-related infections. *Morbidity and Mortality Weekly Report* 51(RR-10): 1–29. Available from: www.cdc.gov/mmwr/PDF/rr/rr5110.pdf

Colagiovanni L (1997a) Parenteral nutrition. *Nursing Standard* 12(9): 39–45.

Colagiovanni L (1997b) Parenteral nutrition and in line filtration. *Nursing Times* 93(34): 76–78.

Davidson A (2005) Management and effects of parenteral nutrition. *Nursing Times* 101(42): 28–31.

De Legge MH, Borak G, Moore N (2005) Central venous access in home parenteral nutrition population – You PICC. *Journal of Parenteral and Enteral Nutrition* 29(6): 425–428.

Department of Health (2002) *Specialised Services National Definition Set. 12 Home Parenteral Nutrition (HPN) (Adult)*. Department of Health, London.

Furst P, Kuhn KS, Stehle (2001) Parenteral nutrition substrates. In: Payne-James J, Grimble G, Silk D, eds. *Artificial Nutrition Support in Clinical Practice*, 2nd edn, pp. 401–434. Greenwich Medical Media Ltd, London.

Hamilton H (2000) Choosing the appropriate catheter for patients requiring parenteral nutrition. In: Hamilton H, ed. *Total Parenteral Nutrition: A Practical Guide for Nurses*, pp. 55–82. Harcourt Publishers Limited, London.

Howard L (2006) Home parenteral nutrition: survival, cost and quality of life. *Gastroenterology* 130 (2 Suppl 1): S52–9.

Infusion Nursing Society (INS) (2006) *Infusion Nursing Society Standards for Infusion Therapy*. Infusion Nursing Society, Philadelphia.

Koletzko B, Agostoni C, Ball P *et al.* (2005) ESPEN/ESPGHAN Guidelines on Pediatric Parenteral Nutrition. *Journal of Pediatric Gastroenterology and Nutrition* 41: S19–S87.

McWhirter JP, Pennington CR (1994) Incidence and recognition of malnutrition in hospital. *British Medical Journal* 308(6934): 945–948.

National Collaborating Centre for Acute Care (2006) *Nutrition Support in Adults: Oral Nutrition Support, Enteral Tube Feeding and Parenteral Nutrition*. National Collaborating Centre for Acute Care, London. Available from www.rcseng.ac.uk

Palmer D, MacFie J (2001) Venous access for parenteral nutrition. In: Payne-James J, Grimble G, Silk D, eds. *Artificial Nutrition Support in Clinical Practice*, 2nd edn, pp. 379–400. Greenwich Medical Media Ltd, London.

Pancorbo-Hidalgo PL, Garcia-Fernandez FP, Lopez-Medina IM, Alvarez-Nieto C (2005) Risk assessment scales for pressure ulcer prevention: a systematic review. *Journal of Advanced Nursing* 54(1): 94–110.

The Parenteral and Enteral Nutrition Group of The British Dietetic Association (PENG) (2004) *A Pocket Guide to Clinical Nutrition*. The Parenteral and Enteral Nutrition Group of The British Dietetic Association, Birmingham.

Phillips L (2005) *Manual of IV therapeutics*, 4th edn. F A Davis, Philadelphia.

Pratt RJ, Pellowe C, Wilson JA *et al.* (2007) epic 2: national evidence-based guidelines for preventing healthcare-associated infections in NHS hospitals in England. *Journal of Hospital Infection* 655 (Suppl): S1–S64.

Royal College of Nursing (RCN) (2005) *Standards for Infusion Therapy*. Royal College of Nursing, London.

Ryder M (2006) Evidence-based practice in the management of vascular access devices for home parenteral nutrition therapy. *Journal of Parenteral and Enteral Nutrition* 30(1): S82–S93.

Schneider PJ (2006) Nutrition support teams: an evidence-based practice. *Nutrition in Clinical Practice: official publication of the American Society for Parenteral and Enteral Nutrition* 21(1): 62–67.

Schofield WN (1985) Predicting basal metabolic rate. *Clinical Nutrition* 44: 1–19.

Shaw C (2004) Nutritional support. In: Dougherty L, Lister S, eds. *The Royal Marsden Hospital Manual of Clinical Nursing Procedures*, 6th edn, pp. 420–441. Blackwell Publishing, Oxford.

Soady (2004) Mouth care. In: Dougherty L, Lister S, eds. *The Royal Marsden Hospital Manual of Clinical Nursing Procedures*, 6th edn, pp. 570–579. Blackwell Publishing, Oxford.

Sobotka L, Camilo ME (2004) Metabolic complications of parenteral nutrition. In: Sobotka L, ed. *Basics in Clinical Nutrition*, 3rd edn, pp. 275–280. Galen, Czech Republic.

Stilwell B (1992) TPN at home. *Community Outlook* August 2: 18–19.

Tait J (2000) Nursing management. In: Hamilton H, ed. *Total Parenteral Nutrition: A Practical Guide for Nurses*, pp. 137–172. Harcourt Publishers Limited, London.

Weinstein S (2007) *Plumer's Principles and Practice of IV Therapy*, 8th edn. Lippincott, Philadelphia.

Wilson JM, Jordan NL (2001) Parenteral nutrition. In: Hankins J, Lonsway RA, Hedrick C, Perdue MB, eds. *Intravenous Therapy: Clinical Principles and Practices*, 2nd edn, pp. 209–247. WB Saunders, Philadelphia.

CHAPTER 15

Paediatric Intravenous Therapy in Practice

Karen Bravery

Introduction

The aim of this chapter is to provide an overview of the different types of venous access devices (VADs) used for the administration of intravenous (i.v.) therapies to children. The focus will be on obtaining venous access (site selection and device placement), maintenance of VADs and management of complications associated with VAD use. Other topics covered in this chapter include the safety aspects of the administration of i.v. therapies and methods to reduce pain and anxiety associated with i.v. therapy procedures in children.

Peripheral Venous Access

The age and developmental level of the child will often dictate which site is used for peripheral venous access, which is more difficult to achieve in children as the veins are smaller and often obscured by subcutaneous fat (Frey 2000, 2001). This is complicated by the fact that the child will resist attempts to establish venous access and will not understand the need for a cannula. The nurse inserting peripheral venous cannulae (PVCs) in children needs technical skill and competency in approaching children at different stages of development (Sundquist Beauman 2001). This section covers obtaining peripheral venous access, the management of peripheral venous access devices and potential problems.

Intravenous sites used in children

The ideal site for peripheral venous access in children is the one that interferes least with the child's developmental level. The characteristics of the therapy to be infused and the child's developmental level should be considered when choosing a site for a cannula. In younger children, additional sites are utilized, including the foot or scalp (Frey 2001). *See* Table 15.1 and Figure 15.1 for details of i.v. sites and devices used in children.

Scalp

One advantage of this particular site is that the scalp veins are superficial and easily visualized, especially in the newborn (Frey 2001). These veins are readily accessible until the age of 12–18 months when the hair follicles mature and the skin thickens. Use of this site

Table 15.1 Intravenous sites used in children (Frey 2001, 2006).

Site	Age	Veins used
Scalp	Infant, toddler	Superficial temporal, frontal, occipital, posterior auricular, supraorbital
Foot	Infant, toddler	Greater or lesser saphenous, median marginal, dorsal arch
Hand	Toddler to adolescent	Metacarpal, dorsal venous arch, tributaries of cephalic and basilic
Forearm	All ages	Cephalic, basilic, median antebrachial
Antecubital fossa	All ages	Median basilic, median cephalic, median cubital

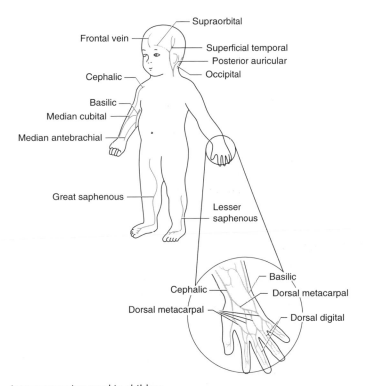

Figure 15.1 Intravenous sites used in children.

leaves the hands free. This is important for the child who sucks his fingers or thumb for comfort. However, there are several disadvantages associated with the use of scalp veins. The arteries of the scalp are located in close proximity to the veins and may be hidden within suture lines. This makes pulsation difficult to feel. Use of this site can be distressing to parents as the scalp is shaved. Without adequate explanation, parents may think that the infusion enters the brain (Frey 2001, 2007). Peripheral venous access devices placed in the scalp are difficult to secure and are associated with an increased risk of dislodgement and subsequent infiltration. If a scalp vein is used to infuse a solution or medication that is a vesicant, frequent site assessments should be made (Frey 2001). *See* section on prevention of infiltration and extravasation for further information.

Foot

This site can be used until the child is able to walk. However, a cannula placed in the foot of an active, mobile toddler may be difficult to maintain. Veins in the feet are sometimes used in older children (e.g. a child with spina bifida with little or no sensation in the foot), or in emergency/intensive care situations. Although the large veins of the foot are visible and accessible, the curve of the foot may make venous entry and catheter advancement problematic, especially at the ankle. The dorsum of the foot has little subcutaneous fat, making extravasation injury more likely. This site should be avoided unless absolutely necessary (Frey 2001). The foot can be used if other sites are not available (e.g. in burns or trauma) (Frey 2007).

Hand and arm

These are the most commonly used sites for peripheral venous access in children. The non-dominant arm should be used where possible, and the thumb-sucking hand of an infant avoided (Frey 2000). The antecubital veins can be difficult to access in chubby babies and toddlers, whereas the veins located on the hand are often easier to cannulate (Frey 2001). Antecubital veins are often the best sites to use for venepuncture. However care must be taken to avoid damaging the brachial artery (Willock *et al.* 2004). The veins of the forearm may be difficult to locate in children. If long-term venous access is anticipated, the antecubital veins may need to be reserved for phlebotomy or a peripherally inserted central catheter (Frey 2001).

Peripheral venous access devices

Winged infusion needles have largely been replaced by plastic, over-the-needle cannulae which can remain *in situ* for longer periods. Winged infusion needles are easily dislodged and are best reserved for blood sampling or for a one-time infusion of short duration (Frey 2001; INS 2006). It should be noted that as winged infusion needles are made of metal, they should not be used for vesicant infusions, because of the associated risk of damaging the vein during insertion and use (CDC 2002; Sauerland *et al.* 2006).

The most commonly used device for peripheral infusion therapy is the over-the-needle cannula. Some cannulae have wings to aid insertion and taping of the device. Current practice dictates that the smallest-gauge, shortest-length cannula capable of administering the prescribed therapy should be used (RCN 2005b; INS 2006). Blood and blood products can be infused via a 24- or 22-gauge cannula in children (Frey 2007). Catheters as small as 27 gauge have been used to administer blood, with no significant haemolysis (Hockenberry *et al.* 2006). Blood may need to be infused via a syringe pump or infusion pump that has been designed to deliver blood without increasing haemolysis (Frey 2007).

A midline catheter should be considered if therapy will last between 2 and 6 weeks. A midline catheter is commonly inserted via the basilic, cephalic or median cubital veins in the antecubital fossa in the arm. The catheter tip does not extend beyond the axilla in the upper arm (Frey 2001). In neonates and children additional insertion sites include veins of the head, neck and lower extremities (INS 2006). The midline catheter can be used for the administration of fluids and medications suitable for infusion via a peripheral vein. Therapies not suitable for administration via midline catheters are continuous vesicant infusions, parenteral nutrition, infusates with a pH of less than 5 or greater than 9, and infusates with an osmolality greater than 600 mOsm/L (INS 2006).

Research on the use of midline catheters in children is limited. Turner *et al.* (2002) illustrate how midline catheters can be used successfully for antibiotic administration in children with cystic fibrosis. In this UK study the midlines were inserted by paediatric i.v. therapy team nurses. Two studies describe the use of midline catheters in neonatal populations using solutions appropriate for infusion via peripheral veins. Both studies suggest that midline catheters are a safe alternative to peripheral venous cannulae. When compared

Table 15.2 Peripheral venous access devices used in children (Frey 2001, 2007; CDC 2002; Dawson 2002; INS 2006; Sauerland *et al.* 2006).

Device	Uses	Comments
Winged infusion set (butterfly needle, scalp vein needle) 27–19 gauge Steel	Infusions of short duration Blood sampling and single-bolus drug administration	Easily dislodged Increased risk of infiltration/ extravasation Should not be used for vesicant infusions
Cannula 26–14 gauge Teflon, Vialon, polyurethane	Neonates: 26 and 24 gauge Child: 24 and 22 gauge Intravenous fluid and drug administration	Can remain *in situ* longer than winged infusion device Less risk of infiltration/ extravasation
Midline catheter (long line, peripherally inserted catheter) 24, 22 gauge Length 3–6 inches Neonates 24, 28 gauge Length 8 cm	Used for i.v. therapies of 2–6 weeks duration Intravenous fluid and drug administration	Not suitable for continuous vesicant infusions, parenteral nutrition, infusate with pH < 5 or > 9 or infusate with an osmolality > 600 mOsm/L

with peripheral cannulae, midline catheters show lower infection rates, cost less, lead to reduced length of stay in hospital and reduce the pain and stress experienced by neonates by reducing the number of attempts at i.v. access (Mason Wyckoff 1999; Dawson 2002).

Refer to Table 15.2 for more information on peripheral venous access devices used in children.

Obtaining peripheral venous access in children

The principles of cannulation are detailed in Chapter 9. Specific considerations for achieving successful cannulation in children are discussed in the following section. Peripheral venous cannulation in children is usually considered to be an expanded role. It requires practical ability and dexterity underpinned by theoretical knowledge. The child's physical, developmental and psychological needs should be assessed before, during and after cannulation. The nurse should endeavour to utilize appropriate strategies to minimize pain and distress and take steps to ensure the safety of self, the child and others assisting with the procedure (RCN 2005a). Paediatric nurses are perhaps the best people to insert cannulae in children. Once trained, they achieve better success rates than doctors and possess greater knowledge of child development and distraction techniques (Frey 1998; Fitzsimons 2001). Strategies to minimize the pain and distress associated with peripheral venous cannulation are discussed in the section on methods to reduce pain and anxiety associated with i.v. therapy procedures on page 442.

Environment

The practitioner should ensure that a safe, comfortable, calm and child-focused environment is maintained throughout the procedure (RCN 2005a). The child's bed or room should be considered a 'safe' place and painful procedures performed elsewhere, such as in the treatment room (Frey 2007). Babies, especially premature infants, should be kept warm throughout the procedure as the infant's large surface area and thin layer of subcutaneous fat predispose to excessive heat loss. Cold stress can be life-threatening for premature infants (Duck 1997). This can be prevented by the use of incubators, cotton blankets, head coverings, an overhead heater (kept at a safe distance from the skin) and warm packs. Only the extremity where the cannula will be placed should be exposed (Frey 2007).

Section 3

Restraining and holding the child during cannulation

When inserting peripheral cannulae the principles of restraining, holding still and containing children should be applied (RCN 2005a). It may be necessary to hold a child during cannulation to maintain the child's safety and prevent injury (Willock *et al.* 2004). Restraint has been defined as the use of force with the intention of overpowering the child, without the consent of the child (RCN 2003), whereas holding still or immobilization uses limited force and is a method of helping children cope with a painful procedure, with the child's permission (RCN 2003). With good preparation, use of topical anaesthetics, sedation and distraction techniques available, undue force/restraint should not be necessary to cannulate a child and should be used as a last resort for essential, urgent venous access (*See* Section on methods to reduce pain and anxiety associated with i.v. therapy procedure on page 442).

The parents should be involved but should not restrain their child. The parents' role should be one of comfort and support throughout the procedure (Frey 2000). It should be agreed with the parents and child how holding still will be used. The parents' role should be explained before cannulation takes place and parents should have the option not to be present (RCN 2003). An infant or toddler can be held securely or wrapped in a blanket to aid immobilization and facilitate the procedure.

Cannulation is distressing for both the child and person performing the procedure, and the number of attempts should be limited (RCN 2005a). Multiple attempts at insertion in infants can lead to episodes of oxygen desaturation and apnoea (Pettit 2000). Older children may become progressively uncooperative as the number of unsuccessful attempts rises.

Consent

The informed consent of the parents and assent of the child should be sought before cannulation and holding still takes place. If the child is not legally competent, or does not posses capacity to give consent, this will need to be sought from someone who has parental responsibility for the child (DH 2001). Holding still without the consent or assent of a child may be necessary in urgent or emergency situations to perform a procedure in a safe and controlled way (RCN 2003).

Documentation

The procedure should be documented in the child's nursing and/or medical record along with the date of cannula insertion and removal (DH 2003a; RCN 2005b). All documentation should comply with the Nursing and Midwifery Council (NMC) guidelines for records and record-keeping (NMC 2005). Any agreement made with the parents and child about methods of holding still or restraint to be used and the event should also be documented (RCN 2003).

Techniques for successful paediatric cannula insertion

Scalp vein insertion

The scalp around the vein insertion site will need to be shaved or clipped before placing the cannula. Some parents may like to keep the infant's hair. The parents' informed consent should be sought before shaving an infant's head. In place of a tourniquet, a rubber band placed around an infant's head above the eyes and ears will aid distension of the scalp veins. Attach a piece of tape to the band to allow for easy removal. Alternatively, the vein may be occluded distally using a finger. The access device should always be inserted in the direction of venous flow, i.e. towards the heart (Frey 2007).

Skin decontamination before cannula insertion

An appropriate antiseptic should be used before cannula insertion. Adult guidelines advocate the use of chlorhexidine gluconate for insertion site preparation (RCN 2005b;

INS 2006). A combination of alcohol with either chlorhexidine or povidone iodine is the current preferred antiseptic (INS 2006). UK guidelines advocate the use of alcoholic chlorhexidine (Pratt *et al*, 2007).

There is very little research that considers the most effective antiseptic for skin preparation before cannula insertion in children. Caution should be exercised in the use of chlorhexidine in neonates (*See* below and Section on catheter site care, page 427). Alternatives to chlorhexidine for insertion site preparation include alcohol, povidone iodine and tincture of iodine (CDC 2002; INS 2006). However, it is suggested that chlorhexidine 0.5% in 70% alcohol is commonly used in paediatric practice in the UK (MacQueen 2005).

Skin preparation in neonates

The skin of a premature infant demonstrates increased potential for allowing the absorption of chemicals through the skin (Irving 2001a). If an occlusive dressing is used the rate of absorption may be increased (MacQueen 2005).

The use of alcohol for skin preparation in neonates and premature infants can cause burns and blisters, and so isopropyl alcohol is not recommended for access site care (Pettit 2000; INS 2006). Povidone iodine can be absorbed via the skin and lead to raised iodine levels (Linden *et al.* 1997; Pettit 2000).

The use of chlorhexidine gluconate has been associated with contact dermatitis in infants weighing less than 1000 g and it should be used with caution (Garland *et al.* 2001). The HIPAC/CDC guidelines state that there is no consensus on the use of chlorhexidine in children less than 2 months of age (CDC 2002).

Where used, povidone iodine or chlorhexidine gluconate solutions need to be completely removed from the skin after the procedure with sterile water or sodium chloride 0.9% to prevent absorption (Lund 1999; INS 2006).

Improving vein visibility

There are various methods that will aid visibility and distension of the child's veins. The extremities may be warmed by encouraging the child to play in warm water before the procedure, as warming causes the vein to dilate. Other methods to increase visibility include positioning the limb lower than the rest of the body and using a transilluminator placed beneath the limb (Frey 2001). Transillumination of the palm can facilitate the establishment of venous access in infants and can be achieved using an otoscope (Goren *et al.* 2001).

Ensuring the cannula is in the vein

Blood return in the flashback portion of the cannula may be poor in children. In addition, it may not be possible to feel the vein 'pop' on entering the vein. The cannula should be inserted gently, then slowly advanced. The needle should be advanced no more than 0.3 cm to ensure that the cannula is in the vein and avoid puncturing the vein wall.

Difficulty in advancing the catheter

The presence of valves or venous spasm may prevent advancement of the cannula into the vein. Venous spasm occurs frequently in small veins (Frey 2001). If flashback of blood ceases, wait for the child to calm down and venous spasm to decrease, then flush with sodium chloride 0.9% as the cannula is advanced (Frey 2007). Flushing will be facilitated by attaching a T-connector or low prime extension set to the cannula. If blood return is absent, often as a result of the small size of the vein and small gauge of cannula, the device can then be flushed with sodium chloride 0.9% to confirm correct placement. This method also reduces the risk of clotting of the device during the procedure (Frey 2007).

The child's understanding of peripheral venous cannulation

A study by Gordon *et al.* (2002) identifies how children may have difficulty in making sense of cannulation. Misunderstandings arise as children create their own version of events in the absence of alternative explanations. In this study children aged between 5 and 14 years had difficulty in understanding what tourniquets did and why armboards were used, and images of and beliefs about 'the needle'. Children believed that the tourniquet kept their arm still and controlled any pain. The cannula was a major area of misunderstanding; many children thought the needle remained in their arm and would be painful if moved. These misunderstandings emphasize the need for age-appropriate explanations to avoid distress and anxiety associated with cannulation.

Use and maintenance care of peripheral venous cannulae in children

Securing the cannula

Once the cannula has been placed, it is essential to secure it to prevent dislodgement. The device must also be protected from the child's attempts to manipulate or remove it. A young child or infant will be unable to comprehend the importance of not manipulating the device (Frey 2007).

Dressings

There is very little research that compares dressing types in paediatric populations, as research in this area has been focused on adults. Studies involving children with peripheral venous cannulae have concentrated on identification of the prevalence of risk factors and complications associated with this method of venous access and have not included device securement. Studies in adults have shown few differences between transparent and gauze dressings (Callaghan *et al.* 2002). In the absence of adequate research in paediatric populations it is suggested that adult 'best practice guidelines' are followed (Garland *et al.* 2002). Adult studies imply that either a sterile gauze or transparent semipermeable membrane (TSM) dressing can be used to protect and maintain security of cannulae. Gauze dressings should be changed routinely every 24–48 hours, TSM dressings changed when the cannula is replaced, and both changed immediately if the integrity of the dressing is compromised (CDC 2002; RCN 2005b; INS 2006). Peripheral cannulae should be secured with sterile tape (e.g. skin closure strips), and the sterile dressing can then be applied on top (MacQueen 2005).

Callaghan *et al.* (2002) compared adhesive tape with a combination transparent polyurethane film/soft cloth surgical tape dressing in children. There were few differences in the incidence of phlebitis or extravasation. However, the transparent dressing group demonstrated better site visibility and dressing adherence and less dressing reinforcement.

Transparent dressings offer several advantages over gauze and tape when used in children. They allow for site assessment without removal of the dressing, provide a waterproof barrier against contamination, reliably secure the cannula, and reduce the frequency of dressing changes required. A gauze dressing offers less protection from manipulation by the child. Children are naturally inquisitive and a gauze dressing may be easily removed, along with the cannula! An important consideration when choosing a dressing is whether paediatric sizes are available.

Neonates and dressings

Epidermal stripping occurs in premature infants when adhesive products are removed, if the bond between the product and the epidermis is greater than that between the epidermis and the dermis. The fibrils in preterm skin are fewer in number, and more widely spaced, allowing areas of epidermis to be easily removed (Irving 2001a). Application of an alcohol-free barrier film underneath transparent dressings has been shown to be beneficial in reducing the risk of epidermal stripping (Irving 2001b). Transparent dressings should be removed using the horizontal stretch method to prevent epidermal stripping (Irving 2001a).

Splints

A splint (armboard) is recommended if the cannula site is in or adjacent to an area of flexion (INS 2006). These are crucial to secure the extremity and insertion site in children (Hadaway 1999). The use of a splint will restrict the child's range of motion and help reduce the risk of dislodging the cannula (Frey 2007). Any splint used should not impede evaluation of the site and should be removed periodically for assessment of circulatory status (INS 2006).

The splint should be shaped and applied in a manner that will maintain joint configuration. Padding may be required under the foot to preserve the natural bend at the child's ankle and maintain normal joint position. This will help to prevent foot drop or contractures (Frey 2007).

If bandages are used to apply the splint, the child's fingers and toes should remain visible to allow checks of circulation as the bandages will reduce the visibility of the site. Cotton bandages with loose fibres should be avoided as they can be eaten by the child or become wrapped around fingers and toes causing restricted circulation and necrosis (MacQueen 2005). Stretch netting can be used as an alternative to a bandage; this will protect the site and allow it to be seen (Frey 2006). Some splints include a Velcro band that can be applied around the splint. The Velcro is easily removed and allows visualization of the site. Bandages make site assessment difficult and time consuming, and their use should be avoided where possible. *See* section on preventing infiltration and extravasation on page 419.

Maintaining patency of peripheral cannulae

Research in adult populations supports the use of sodium chloride 0.9% to maintain patency of peripheral cannulae (LeDuc 1997). Whether sodium chloride 0.9% or heparinized saline should be used to maintain patency of peripheral venous access devices in children is less clear. Four paediatric studies found sodium chloride 0.9% to be as effective as heparinized saline and found no difference in the duration of use and complication rates (Kleiber *et al.* 1993; McMullen *et al.* 1993; Hanrahan *et al.* 1994; Lombardi *et al.* 1998). Kleiber *et al.* (1993) maintained that the technique is as important as the flush solution and advocated the use of positive pressure whilst clamping the extension tubing or T-connector. In contrast, a study by Gyr *et al.* in 1995 found that there was more patency and less tenderness associated with the use of heparinized saline (Gyr *et al.* 1995). Pain and discomfort may be a feature of the use of heparinized saline (Kleiber *et al.* 1993; McMullen *et al.* 1993). In addition, sodium chloride 0.9% may be less effective in maintaining patency if 24-gauge cannulae are used (Danek & Noris 1992). More recently, LeDuc (1997) compared sodium chloride 0.9% with heparinized saline in children and found no significant difference in demographics or complications.

The effectiveness of heparin to prolong peripheral catheter life has been systematically reviewed in patients of all age groups. These reviews concluded that sodium chloride 0.9% was as effective as heparin in prolonging catheter life. Only one of these studies was in neonates (Shah *et al.* 2005). The effectiveness of heparin in the continuous infusion fluid or intermittent flush solution to prolong cannula use in neonates has not been determined despite a systematic review. More research is needed to determine the safety and effectiveness of heparin and the optimal dose in this age group (Shah *et al.* 2005). It is also unclear in this age group whether continuous infusion or intermittent flushes are better at maintaining cannula patency. However, the use of intermittent flushes was not found to be associated with decreased cannula life or other disadvantages, and its use is supported in neonates (Flint *et al.* 2005).

The use of heparin is not without risks, it can induce bleeding complications and immune-mediated heparin-induced thrombocytopenia (Klenner *et al.* 2003). The use of sodium chloride 0.9% in preference to heparin offers several advantages including the elimination of risks associated with heparin, reduced potential for infection and cost savings (LeDuc 1997). In the absence of definitive research the use of sodium chloride 0.9% to maintain patency in peripheral cannulae offers several advantages and reduction in risks. Preservative-free sodium chloride 0.9% is recommended in children (INS 2006).

The volume used to flush the cannula should be twice the volume capacity of the catheter and add-on device. The concentration of heparin, if used, should be the lowest possible that will maintain patency (RCN 2005b; INS 2006). More research is needed to confirm the optimal flush solution and volume in paediatrics.

Blood sampling and peripheral venous access

There are some studies that suggest that blood samples can be collected via PVCs *in situ*. The use of small syringes is recommended for specimen withdrawal to reduce the risk of haemolysis and releasing the tourniquet before withdrawing the blood specimen (Sliwa 1997; Seemann & Reinhardt 2000). It should be noted that neither of these studies was undertaken in children. However blood sampling from peripheralvenous cannulae is often employed in paediatrics in order to avoid additional venepuncture and trauma for the child. Blood samples are often collected immediately after insertion of the cannula through the device, before flushing.

In neonates several methods are used to obtain blood samples. These include the 'broken needle technique', via the cannula, Vacutte needle, butterfly needle (tubing cut short), syringe and needle, and heel lance. All of these methods entail risk to either the operator or the infant, cause pain and/or discomfort to the infant, or are associated with haemolysis/clot formation (Philip & Beckett 2000). The 'broken needle technique' has been specifically advised against by the Medicines and Healthcare products Regulatory Agency, as unsafe practice (MHRA 2001). Venepuncture has been advocated as the sampling method of choice in this age group (Shah & Ohlsson 2004). Safer devices have now been developed to aid venepuncture and blood sampling in neonates such as the Neo-safe®, Vygon, and blood sampling needle (Philip & Beckett 2000).

Complications of peripheral intravenous therapy in children

Phlebitis

Phlebitis can be described as inflammation of a vein often associated with infusion therapy (Taylor 2000). The cause of the inflammation can be chemical, mechanical or bacterial (Macklin 2003). Phlebitis rates in children have been reported as 1.1–13% (Garland *et al.* 1992; Shimandle *et al.* 1999; Foster *et al.* 2002).

Mechanical phlebitis

Mechanical phlebitis occurs when a catheter irritates or injures the vein wall. It is important to stabilize a cannula to minimize movement within the vein (Macklin 2003). Movement and activity or manipulation by the child may contribute to the development of phlebitis. To reduce the occurrence of mechanical phlebitis, the cannula should be secured adequately. The limb may be immobilized with a splint if the device is placed in an area of flexion (Frey 2007). However, when the cannula is stabilized it should not interfere with the flow rate or visualization of the site (*See* Section on securing the cannula) (Macklin 2003; Frey 2007).

A low prime extension set will allow manipulation of the device away from the insertion site and reduce movement of the cannula within the vein (Livesley 1996). This will reduce direct manipulation of the cannula during drug administration and flushing procedures. Either the extension tubing or the infusion tubing should be coiled and taped to the child's limb to reduce tension on the cannula site from inadvertent tugging and movement by the child (Frey 2007).

The smallest gauge necessary to achieve prescribed flow rate should be used, to minimize catheter–vein wall contact (Macklin 2003). In paediatric patients 22–24-gauge cannulae are commonly used (Frey 2006). As a 24-gauge cannula is capable of achieving flow rates of greater than 1400 mL/hour larger sizes are not strictly necessary. Even blood can be infused via a 22-gauge cannula without damaging red blood cells (Keller 1995).

Chemical phlebitis

Chemical phlebitis occurs when the infusate (drugs and solutions) damages the vein wall (Macklin 2003). Therapies not recommended for infusion via peripheral cannulae include parenteral nutrition containing more than 10% dextrose and/or 5% protein, solutions and/or medications with pH of less than 5 or greater than 9, and solutions and/or medications with osmolality greater than 500 mOsm/L (RCN 2005b).

Small veins may become inflamed when used for the infusion of irritating solutions. In this instance, the cannula occludes the lumen of the vein, obstructs the flow of blood and reduces the dilution of the infusate. The infusate then flows undiluted and irritates the wall of the vein (Weinstein 2006a). The smallest cannula placed in the largest vein available will allow a greater volume of blood to flow more quickly around the catheter tip and dilute the infusate (Macklin 2003).

Bacterial phlebitis

Bacterial phlebitis can have serious systemic consequences, although this rarely occurs with peripheral cannulae. Bacteria can be introduced via contamination of the infusate, tubing, cannula or insertion site (Macklin 2003).

Rotation of cannula sites

Phlebitis and catheter colonization have been associated with a greater risk for catheter-related infection, and routine replacement of PVCs has been suggested as a means of reducing the risk of infection and patient discomfort associated with phlebitis (CDC 2002). Contrary to adult studies, in children the risk for phlebitis and infection does not increase with the length of time a cannula remains in place (Garland *et al.* 1992; Shimandle *et al.* 1999; Oishi 2001). Current guidelines recommend that PVCs in children are left *in situ* until therapy is complete, unless complications develop (CDC 2002; INS 2006).

Infiltration and extravasation injury in children (peripheral devices)

Extravasation is the inadvertent administration of a vesicant medication or solution into the surrounding tissue instead of the intended vascular pathway. In contrast, infiltration involves inadvertent administration of a non-vesicant (RCN 2005b). Whilst infiltration is often viewed as the lesser injury, it can lead to nerve compression and compartment syndrome and compromise arterial circulation (Roth 2006). The consequences of extravasation can range from a burn to severe tissue damage that may require debridement or even amputation (Roth 2006). Both infiltration and extravasation injury in children can result in litigation claims (MacDonald 2001; Masoorli 2003; Quinn & Upton 2006; Roth 2006). Neonates in particular may be at greater risk of extravasation as they often require infusions of high concentrations of glucose and calcium for growth and maintenance of normal levels (Duck 1997).

Early detection and prompt treatment are essential to minimize the complications of extravasation and infiltration injury in children. Children may not be able to verbalize the pain and discomfort associated with infiltration/extravasation (Sauerland *et al.* 2006). Crying, whimpering or unusual movement of the extremity may indicate infiltration/extravasation (Roth 2006). The child or infant is therefore dependent on the nurse to detect and prevent infiltration/extravasation injuries. In addition, the child's activity and inability to comprehend the importance of not manipulating or tugging the infusion tubing increase the potential for cannula dislodgement and subsequent infiltration/extravasation.

It is essential that nurses are aware of the drugs or solutions that are capable of causing tissue damage and that policies are in place for the prevention and management of infiltration/extravasation injury in children.

Recognition of extravasation

The classic initial signs of extravasation include the following.

- A burning sensation.
- Tautness of the skin.
- Swelling of the tissues surrounding the infusion/cannula site.
- Discomfort or burning pain at the infusion/cannula site. Observe the child for facial expressions, crying and reluctance to use the affected limb which may indicate an extravasation.
- Coolness in the area where infusate has entered the tissue (Roth 2003).

It should be remembered that, apart from swelling, the visual signs of tissue damage may be delayed(Sauerland *et al*. 2006).

Management of extravasation

Early identification and prompt action can significantly reduce the complications associated with extravasation injury (Pettit & Hughes 1993). A combined approach to extravasation has been advocated, which includes early detection, cessation of further drug therapy, rapid administration of an appropriate antidote and surgical excision. Only experienced individuals should initiate peripheral venous access for vesicant therapy and be accountable for monitoring and assessment of the site (Kassner 2000). Many centres have produced extravasation protocols to help reduce the potential for serious injury (Roth 2003).

If extravasation is suspected, it is imperative that the infusion is stopped. This should be followed by an attempt to aspirate the extravasated fluid via the cannula (Banta 1992; Flemmer & Chan 1993; Pettit & Hughes 1993; Kassner 2000). The affected extremity may be elevated to facilitate fluid reabsorption (Zenk *et al*. 1981). More recent advice questions the effectiveness of this approach (Roth 2003).

The injection of hyaluronidase 15 units/mL either via the cannula or subcutaneously in a circular pattern around the affected area has been shown to reduce the severity of tissue damage (Few 1987; Banta 1992; Flemmer & Chan 1993). This should be carried out within 1 hour of injury to maximize the beneficial effect (Few 1987). Hyaluronidase is contraindicated if the cause of the extravasation injury is a vasopressor (e.g. dopamine, dobutamine) (Pettit & Hughes 1993). A number of wound contact materials (i.e. hydrocolloids, hydrogels and film dressings) have been found to be useful in the management of extravasation injuries in preterm infants (Irving 2001c).

Gault (1993, 2006) described a technique called 'saline flush-out'. First, the area of extravasation is infiltrated with hyaluronidase, which reduces the viscosity of the connective tissue, making it more permeable to the sodium chloride 0.9% that is flushed through the subcutaneous space. Following this, four small exit incisions are made around the periphery of the extravasation and a large volume of sodium chloride 0.9% (500 mL) is flushed through the subcutaneous space. This technique removes the damaged tissue and conserves the integrity of the overlying skin. In his study, 86% of patients treated with saline flush-out following extravasation injury healed without any subsequent skin loss (Gault 1993).

Documentation of an infiltration/extravasation event is vital for medicolegal purposes (Roth 2003). All information related to the event including photographs should be documented in the patient record and an incident form completed (Kassner 2000; RCN 2005b).

Prevention of extravasation and infiltration

- There should be hourly observation, and palpation of the insertion site for signs of extravasation/infiltration (MacDonald 2001; Masoorli 2003). More frequent observation of the site (i.e. every 30 minutes) is advised during vesicant infusions (Masoorli 2003).
- Consideration should be given to the appropriateness of administering vesicant solutions and drugs via peripheral venous access devices. It is recommended that these infusions are administered using central venous access devices (RCN 2005b; INS 2006).
- Use an electronic infusion pump that incorporates a variable pressure setting to monitor any rise in pressure. The occlusion alarm pressure should be set low to alarm quickly (Quinn 2000). Once the infusion has been started and pumping pressure established, the alarm limit can be lowered. The pump can be set at 30 mmHg higher than pumping pressure (Amoore & Adamson 2003). Limiting the occlusion pressure will not in itself prevent extravasation (Irving 2001c). It is imperative that the site is observed for signs of infiltration/extravasation (Amoore & Adamson 2003). The pressure reading should be monitored and recorded hourly (MacDonald 2001; McIntosh 2006).
- The use of steel needles should be avoided for the administration of medication/solutions that may cause tissue necrosis if extravasation occurs (CDC 2002).
- Ensure that the cannula is adequately secured and the limb immobilized with a splint if necessary. Any dressing, tape, splint or bandage used should facilitate visual inspection and palpation of the site and not obscure the insertion site. Any bandage or armboard should be completely removed when the site is checked and the circulation to the extremities assessed. This assessment should be documented to avoid litigation (MacDonald 2001; Masoorli 2003).
- Act promptly if the child exhibits signs of pain or discomfort, i.e. crying or holding the affected limb. Frequent observation of the site is paramount as children cannot be relied upon to communicate pain effectively (Sauerland *et al.* 2006).
- NB Not all patients experience discomfort with infiltration/extravasation (Hadaway 2002).
- Assess blood return before and at appropriate intervals during administration of vesicant agents (Sauerland *et al.* 2006).

Central Venous Access in Children

Central venous access devices (CVADs) have been used in the management and treatment of a number of conditions in children since Broviac *et al.* (1973) first described the use of a silicone central venous catheter (CVC) that could be used for long-term therapy almost 30 years ago. CVADs are commonly used to administer i.v. therapies to children with chronic diseases who may require lifelong treatment. CVADs may also be employed for children who require several weeks of i.v. access and/or therapy (*See* Table 15.3). Peripherally inserted central catheters (PICCs), tunnelled and non-tunnelled CVCs and implanted ports (IPs) are all used in children. CVADs have enabled some children to receive treatment at home and thus avoid repeated hospitalization (RCN 2001).

This section provides an overview of the use of CVADs and highlights the differences in maintenance care and management of complications specific to paediatrics.

Types of central venous access device used in children

Non-tunnelled central venous catheters

Percutaneously placed catheters are the most commonly used CVADs in critical care situations in children (Decker & Edwards 1988). Non-tunnelled percutaneously placed

Table 15.3 Uses of central venous access devices (CVADs) in children (Holden *et al.* 1996; Tweddle *et al.* 1997; Bravery & Wright 1998; Aitken & Tonelli 2000; McMahon *et al.* 2000; Hacking *et al.* 2003; Valentino *et al.* 2004; Ramage *et al.* 2005; Frey 2007; National Kidney Foundation 2006).

Condition	Intravenous therapies	Central venous access devices used
Cancer and leukaemia	Administration of chemotherapy, blood products, antibiotics, parenteral nutrition. Peripheral blood stem cell collection	Tunnelled catheter Implanted port PICC Apheresis/dialysis catheter (tunnelled or non tunnelled)
Haemophilia	Administration of prophylactic factor concentrate, blood products and immune tolerance therapy	Tunnelled catheter Implanted port
Cystic fibrosis	Administration of antibiotics	Implanted port Tunnelled catheter PICC
Gastrointestinal failure	Administration of parenteral nutrition	Tunnelled catheter Implanted port
Chronic renal failure	To facilitate maintenance haemodialysis	Cuffed haemodialysis catheter
Several weeks of antibiotics for infections (e.g. osteomyelitis, meningitis)	Administration of antibiotics	PICC
Several weeks of i.v. access for critical care patients (e.g. post trauma)	Administration of antibiotics and parenteral nutrition	Non-tunnelled central venous catheter

PICC, peripherally inserted central catheter.

CVCs are made of a stiff material e.g. polyurethane to aid insertion, and are often short. They can have between one and four lumens and range in size from 3 to 5 French. These catheters may be placed using the femoral, internal and external jugular and subclavian veins (in order of preference). Placement in children may require a local anaesthetic or sedative, and is usually undertaken by a doctor (Frey 2007).

Antimicrobial/antiseptic-impregnated catheters have been studied in adult critical care settings to determine their effectiveness in reducing catheter-related bloodstream infections (CRBSIs) (Pellowe 2004). It is recommended that these catheters are used (in adults) if the rate of CRBSI remains high despite the application of preventative measures. Currently, there is no such recommendation for the use of these catheters in children (CDC 2002).

Non-tunnelled CVCs are usually removed without sedation or general anaesthesia in children. This can be undertaken on the ward by a suitably trained nurse (Bravery & Wright 1998; RCN 2005b). Precautions should be taken to minimize the risks of air embolus (Drewett 2000; RCN 2005b).

Peripherally inserted central catheters (PICCs)

These small-gauge catheters were originally developed for use in neonates in the 1970s (Wiltgen-Trotter 1996). Since their introduction they have filled a niche between peripheral cannulae and long-term CVADs (Frey 2002). In the USA, PICCs have been used safely in both the hospital and home setting for short- and long-term i.v. therapies (Doellman 2003). A PICC is defined as a central venous catheter that is inserted into an extremity and advanced until the tip is positioned in the lower third of the superior vena cava (SVC) (RCN 2005b). Additional insertion sites in neonates and children include the veins of the head, neck and lower extremities (INS 2006). If the saphenous, popliteal or femoral veins are used the tip location will be the inferior vena cava (National Association of Vascular Access Networks 1998). In older children the median cubital, basilic and cephalic veins of the antecubital fossa are used. The PICC may be placed slightly above or below this site (Frey 2006). Veins used in neonatal PICC insertion include the basilic, cephalic, axillary, external jugular, temporal, posterior auricular, femoral, greater/lesser saphenous and popliteal veins (National Association of Neonatal Nurses 2001). Frey (2002) describes four methods of PICC insertion used in children and neonates. These are use of a winged steel needle, a winged breakaway needle, a peel-away i.v. catheter and a modified or unmodified Seldinger technique.

PICCs are available in both single- and dual-lumen configurations and the catheter tip may be open-ended or valved. PICC sizes in children vary (*See* Table 15.4).

Insertion is the same as in adults except that a child may be more anxious and lack the ability to cooperate (Frey 2007). PICC placement can cause psychological distress for both the child and parent. The stress of the procedure can be minimized if the child's and parent's coping abilities are enabled. Both should be appropriately prepared for the procedure. A combination of pharmacological and non-pharmacological techniques can be employed to minimize distress during PICC insertion. *See* Section on methods to reduce pain and anxiety associated with i.v. therapy procedures, page 442.

In the USA these catheters are placed by specially trained nurses in both adults (Egan-Sansivero 1995; Weinstein 2007) and children (Frey 2002; Doellmann 2003). In the UK PICC insertion began in the 1990s (Dougherty 2006). The placement of PICCs in adult patients has evolved to a nurse-led practice in the UK (Philpot & Griffiths 2003). In a study by Barber *et al.* (2002) it was concluded that trained nurses could successfully place the majority of PICCs. However, despite the increasing popularity of nurse placement of PICCs among adult nurses in the UK, this is yet to be mirrored in paediatrics. Kleidon (2004) describes the implementation of a nurse-led service for insertion of PICCs and tunnelled CVCs in an interventional radiology department, and appears to be the only nurse in the UK to place PICCs in children. There are reports of PICCs being used in children in the UK that are inserted by doctors for cystic fibrosis patients (Miall *et al.* 2001) and children with leukaemia (Hacking *et al.* 2003).

Ultrasound guidance is being used more widely for PICC placement in children's hospitals in the USA by nursing and medical staff (Crowley 2003; Frey 2007). In the UK two-dimensional ultrasound guidance is recommended for the placement of CVCs in both adults and children (NICE 2002). In the UK a clinical nurse specialist has successfully used ultrasound guidance to place PICCs and tunnelled CVCs in paediatric patients (Kleidon 2004).

Tunnelled cuffed central venous catheters

Tunnelled CVCs are often used for long-term venous access. They are the most commonly used CVAD in children (Wiener & Albanese 1998). Paediatric-sized tunnelled

Table 15.4 Peripherally inserted central catheter (PICC) sizes used in children (Frey 2006).

Single lumen	Dual lumen
28 gauge, neonatal 2 French (23 gauge) 3 French (20 gauge) 4 French (18 gauge)	3.5 French (18 gauge) to 5 French (16 gauge)

catheters are available in single- and dual-lumen varieties. Triple-lumen catheters are available but may be considered too large for some paediatric patients. Tunnelled catheters used in children may be open-ended or valved (Frey 2007). *See* page 327 for details of valved catheters.

In children, tunnelled catheters are usually placed in the operating theatre or interventional radiology suite under general anaesthesia, although local anaesthesia and sedation may be used in the older child (NICE 2005). These catheters are primarily placed by a surgeon or interventional radiologist (NICE 2005; Frey 2007). Insertion and removal of tunnelled catheters in children may be successfully undertaken by a trained clinical nurse specialist (Kleidon 2004; NICE 2005). Several procedures may be scheduled to coincide with CVC insertion to avoid unnecessary trauma for the child, such as biopsy, bone marrow aspiration and lumbar puncture (Frey 2007).

In a small number of children central venous access may be exhausted and the jugular, subclavian, SVC and femoral veins become occluded. This may occur in situations where the child requires numerous CVCs for continuous central venous access; for example a child with short bowel syndrome who requires lifelong total total parenteral nutrition (TPN) (Crowley 2003). Alternative sites can be employed such as the femoral vein to the inferior vena cava, the hepatic veins or a translumbar approach (Crowley 2003; Frey 2007). Some radiologists have developed techniques to recanalize chronically occluded neck and chest veins to allow CVC placement in these situations (Lorenz *et al.* 2001).

Implanted ports

Implanted ports were initially introduced in the 1980s for adult cancer patients and have been used successfully in children for the treatment of cancer and leukaemia, cystic fibrosis and haemophilia. They are ideal for children requiring intermittent venous access who can tolerate the needle access, and are most commonly used for the treatment and aftercare of children with leukaemia or cancer. The use of ports in children is not commonplace in the UK and is thought to be greater in the USA (Tweedle *et al.* 1997; Munro 1999). Tunnelled catheters have been the standard device used in the UK for children with cancer (Tweedle *et al.* 1997; Munro 1999). However, the largest study undertaken in childhood cancer patients in the USA recommends ports as the device of choice unless the child is to undergo bone marrow transplantation (Weiner *et al.* 1992).

A port consists of a catheter connected to a reservoir made of titanium or plastic. Above the reservoir is a dense, self-sealing silicone septum. To use the port a non-coring needle is pushed firmly through the skin and septum until the base of the port is felt by the operator (Bravery & Hannan 1997). Implanted ports are available in dual- and single-lumen configurations. The dual-lumen port has two reservoirs and septums, attached to a dual-lumen catheter. Each reservoir is accessed with a separate needle and is thus equivalent to a dual-lumen tunnelled catheter. There have been some reports of use of dual-lumen ports in older children (Lorenz *et al.* 2001).

Implanted port insertion requires vein access similar to that for tunnelled catheters (Crowley 2003). Ports can be placed by surgical cutdown (Ross *et al.* 1988; Munro *et al.* 1999) or using a percutaneous approach (Lorenz *et al.* 2001; Nosher *et al.* 2001). In children ports are usually placed under general anaesthesia, by a surgeon or interventional radiologist. However the use of conscious sedation has been reported (Lorenz *et al.* 2001). Ports are implanted in the chest, upper abdomen or forearm, with the catheter threaded into a central vein (Frey 2006). Arm placement avoids the risk of pneumothorax (Crowley 2003). A pocket is created to house the port reservoir and the catheter tunnelled to the site of vein insertion (Wiener & Albanese 1998). The device is secured with sutures to prevent it 'flipping' over (Crowley 2003).

Children below 1 year of age may not have enough subcutaneous fat to support an implanted port and the device may erode through the skin (Frey 2006). Both low-profile and adult-sized ports are used in children, but low-profile ports should be used in babies and small children, as the larger device may erode through the skin (De Backer *et al.* 1993; Frey 2007).

Selection of the appropriate central venous access device

Parents and children should be offered a choice of CVAD where appropriate (Hollis 1992). The NICE guideline (2005) for children with cancer recommends that the child and parents are involved in choosing the type and site for the CVAD and are provided with information necessary to inform that choice (NICE 2005). McInally (2005) notes that, in practice, it is often a medically driven decision as to which device is used. The nurse involved in preparing the child and family for insertion of a CVAD must be familiar with the wide range of devices available. In addition, she should be aware of the advantages and disadvantages associated with each type, in order to fully inform the child and family (Winslow *et al.* 1995; McInally 2005) (*See* Table 15.5 for an overview of advantages and disadvantages of CVADs used in children). Some centres may have a specialist nurse to assist families in the selection of the most appropriate device (Bagnall & Ruccione 1987; Frey 2007). In the UK, specialist nurses in the areas of paediatric oncology, i.v. therapy, haemophilia and cystic fibrosis may fulfil this role. The following factors should be addressed during the selection process.

- Disease.
- Type of therapy.
- Duration of therapy.
- Access to veins.
- Ability of child and family to care for the device at home.
- Child and family preference.
- Complications (Wiener & Albanese, 1998; McCloskey 2002; Frey 2007).

Disease

The choice of CVAD may be governed by expert opinion for patients with a specific diagnosis (Dougherty 2006). In children the type of CVAD used for different conditions is often determined by specialist tertiary care centres. There is a major difference between children requiring a CVAD for cancer treatment or antibiotic therapy for an infection (e.g. meningitis, osteomyelitis) who only need the device until completion of therapy, and children who require a CVAD for haemophilia, cystic fibrosis or gut disorders needing long-term parenteral nutrition who may require the CVAD for life. Whilst some degree of choice may be appropriate for a child with cancer, a child with a lifelong need for central venous access will require a long-term CVAD with the least risk of complications. *See* Table 15.3 for CVAD types used in specific diseases.

CVADs commonly used in paediatrics may differ according to the disease/condition of the child or change as the child grows and develops. For example, a child with haemophilia (as a baby) may have a tunnelled catheter or implanted port initially to administer coagulation factors. However, when either the parents or the child are able to cannulate and administer the coagulation factors themselves a CVAD is no longer required (Ewenstein *et al.* 2004; Liesner *et al.* 1995). For children with haemophilia peripheral venous access is the route of choice, to avoid the risk of infection associated with a CVAD. In contrast children with cystic fibrosis may start with peripheral venous access devices such as cannulae and midline catheters then switch to a CVAD (PICC or implanted port) once venous access becomes more frequent and the disease progresses (Hatchard & O'Leary 1999; Aitken & Tonelli 2000; Miall *et al.* 2001; Frey 2007). Home parenteral nutrition (HPN) for children with chronic intestinal failure requires central venous access as HPN solutions are hypertonic and irritant to peripheral veins (Hodge & Puntis 2002).

Table 15.5 Advantages and disadvantages of central venous access devices used in children (Reed & Phillips 1996; Wiener & Albanese 1998; Frey 1999; Schulmeister & Camp-Sorrell 2000; CDC 2002; McCloskey 2002; Doellman 2003; Ferguson & Costa 2004; Frey 2007).

Tunnelled catheter	Implanted port	Peripherally inserted central catheter
General anaesthetic usually required for insertion	General anaesthetic usually required for insertion	Inserted under sedation, general anaesthesia or neither. Topical anaesthetic used for insertion with/without sedation
Easily removed on completion of therapy. General anaesthetic required	Removal more complicated; larger scar. General anaesthetic required	Easily removed on completion of therapy without sedation/general anaesthesia
No needles required to access the device	Needles required to access device	No needles required to access the device
Can be repaired if damaged	Cannot be repaired if damaged	Can be repaired if damaged. More prone to damage as fragile
Frequent maintenance care	Minimal maintenance care	Frequent maintenance care
Family must learn some aspects of care e.g. prevention of damage/dislodgement, keeping catheter dry during bathing	Family need not learn care as device not accessed at home	Family must learn some aspects of care e.g. prevention of damage/dislodgement, keeping catheter dry during bathing
Clamps needed at all times	Clamps not required	Clamps needed at all times
Some activity restrictions e.g. swimming, contact sports	Few activity restrictions—child can swim and bathe freely; vigorous contact sports and direct pressure on the device should be avoided	Some activity restrictions e.g. swimming, contact sports
Outside the body	Under the skin	Outside the body
Visible reminder of the disease	Less impact on body image	Visible reminder of the disease
Risk of damage	Less risk of damage as under the skin	Risk of damage
Risk of dislodgement as it can be pulled out	Less risk of dislodgement; cannot be pulled out	Risk of dislodgement as it can be pulled out
Greatest risk of infection in comparison to implanted ports and PICCs	Lowest risk of infection	Less risk of infection than tunnelled catheter
Dressing required. Weekly dressing change if transparent dressing used	No dressing required unless device in use. If device accessed dressing replaced with routine needle change	Dressing required. Weekly dressing change if transparent dressing used
Weekly flush	Monthly flush	Weekly flush (valved catheter). More frequent flushing may be required for open-ended catheter
Low risk for extravasation—recommended for continuous vesicant infusions	Risk of extravasation secondary to needle dislodgement	
Recommended for long term, regular or continuous access	Recommended for long term, intermittent access	Recommended for short- or intermediate-term therapy, frequent or continuous access
	Lowest overall complication rates	
	Not suitable for obese child	

Tunnelled catheters are the most frequently used device in this population, with some limited use of ports (Holden *et al*. 1996).

Type of therapy

Therapies that require delivery via a CVAD rather than a peripheral VAD include continuous vesicant therapy, parenteral nutrition exceeding 10% dextrose and/or 5% protein, solutions and/or medications with a pH of less than 5 or greater than 9, and solutions and/or medications with osmolality greater than 600 mOsm/L (INS 2006).

Continuous vesicant infusions (e.g. parenteral nutrition or chemotherapy) should be administered via a tunnelled catheter (RCN 2005b; INS 2006). Extravasation is a potentially devastating complication of continuous vesicant infusions. Implanted ports are associated with an increased risk of extravasation and may not be appropriate for this type of therapy. *See* section on extravasation on page 417.

A cuffed, tunnelled CVC or PICC is recommended for therapies that necessitate frequent or continuous access. An implanted port is advocated in situations requiring long-term therapy that is infrequent and intermittent (Pratt *et al*, 2007).

A dual- or triple-lumen tunnelled CVC will be required to deliver multiple therapies that may incorporate concurrent infusions of incompatible solutions and accommodate the frequent blood sampling necessitated by a bone marrow transplant or intensive chemotherapy (Wiener & Albanese 1998). However, the device used should comprise the minimum number of lumens essential to manage the patient (CDC 2002; Pratt *et al*, 2007). The data regarding single- versus multilumen CVCs and infection rates in children are inconclusive (Kline 2005).

Duration of therapy

The anticipated duration of planned therapy may affect the choice of device. Once the decision has been made that central venous access rather than peripheral venous access is necessary to administer the treatment safely, then the duration of therapy should be considered (Bravery & Todd 2002).

Short-term i.v. therapy indicates the use of either a non-tunnelled catheter or a PICC. As these catheters are centrally placed, both are suitable for the administration of vesicant and irritant solutions. PICCs are advocated for intermediate-term i.v. therapy of greater than 2 weeks' duration. To date, no upper limit has been established for the length of time a PICC may remain *in situ* (Frey 2007). In practice, PICCs may remain *in situ* for months to years (CDC 2002). A PICC by virtue of its extended dwell time is now considered to be appropriate for intermediate-term therapies. The small gauge of some PICCs may lead to collapse on aspiration. If frequent blood sampling is a priority, a 3 French or larger PICC may be required (Frey 2007).

Percutaneous non-tunnelled catheters are made of polyurethane, a stiff material that makes catheter insertion easier. Catheter sizes range from 3 to 5 French and may have one to four lumens. In paediatrics, these catheters are often used in high-dependency settings where several weeks of i.v. access are required that may include parenteral nutrition. A potential problem associated with the use of these catheters placed in jugular and femoral veins is their occlusion by the movement of the baby's head or legs (Frey 2007).

Long-term i.v. therapy lasting months to years mandates a long-term CVAD, either an implanted port or tunnelled catheter. Some decisions regarding the most appropriate device are straightforward and are dictated by the type of therapy to be administered, frequency of venous access and whether a multilumen device is necessary.

Ability of child and family to care for the CVAD

An explanation of the main care required may be useful to aid decision-making for families. An implanted port with minimal maintenance care may appeal to some families, especially those who do not wish to be involved in the routine care of a device. Some families express concerns that a tunnelled catheter may 'fall out' or become damaged, especially in babies and small children. Safety concerns may influence a family's decision. If parents opt for a tunnelled catheter, they must be willing and able to participate in the routine care and prevention of damage or dislodgement of the device. Parents should be taught any techniques necessary to prevent infection and safely manage the CVAD at home (NICE 2003). This will include how to secure the device, cope with bathing and what to look out for (e.g. signs of infection or damage).

Child and family preference

A child who is to undergo long-term i.v. therapy and who does not require frequent venous access or continuous vesicant infusions may be offered a choice between a tunnelled catheter and an implanted port. This is dependent on the availability of both devices, a surgeon or interventional radiologist willing to place either, and skilled staff available to care for both devices in the hospital or community setting. Much of the routine care and detection of problems associated with the use of CVADs is now the responsibility of parents. It is vital that they receive adequate information to make an informed decision if a choice of CVAD is offered. The advantages and disadvantages of implanted ports and tunnelled catheters should be discussed with the child and family to facilitate an informed choice (Winslow *et al.* 1995). *See* Table 15.5 for the advantages and disadvantages of CVADs.

When parents are offered a choice, it may be pertinent to consider child and family preference, as evidence of major differences in complication rates is inconclusive. Quality-of-life issues and the impact of the CVAD on the child and family may be more appropriate factors to guide parents in their choice of device.

A study by Blakeley *et al.* (2000) investigated parent satisfaction with education, support and decision-making regarding their child's CVAD. Parents of children with cancer were given information about implanted ports and tunnelled catheters, including the advantages and disadvantages of each type. Parents had input into the choice of CVAD and were asked about their satisfaction with their decision. The findings indicated that not all parents take part in decisions about the type of device used, and that if offered a choice, they would choose implanted ports over tunnelled catheters, based on their experience. Whilst it is important that families are fully informed about CVADs available, staff involved in preparing families for CVAD insertion should be aware that not all families wish to be involved in this type of decision. It should also be remembered that a choice is not always possible and the type of CVAD used may in some circumstances be dictated by overriding therapy-related factors. For example, a single-lumen implanted port may not be appropriate for a child who is to undergo a bone marrow transplant or high-dose therapy as frequent, continuous venous access with a multilumen catheter would be required.

Munro *et al.* (1999) interviewed 64 families about their opinions of their child's CVAD (either an implanted port or a tunnelled catheter). More parents with tunnelled catheters felt that this device limited their child's activities compared with those with ports. More parents of children with ports were satisfied with the cosmetic appearance than those with a tunnelled catheter. Parents of children with either device said they worried about complications (blockage, infection, dislodgement). However, more parents worried about the risk of an infection with a tunnelled catheter than with a port. Both groups of parents felt that the CVAD greatly facilitated treatment, particularly by reducing the number of venepunctures and injections.

Complications

The CVAD selected should be the one with the lowest risk of complications (infectious and non-infectious) for the anticipated type and length of therapy. Implanted ports represent the lowest risk for catheter-related bloodstream infection compared to non-tunnelled CVCs, which account for the majority of infections. Both PICCs and tunnelled catheters have lower rates of infection than non-tunnelled CVCs (CDC 2002).

Most of the research in children with CVADs has focused on children with cancer and leukaemia. In this population, implanted ports (in children with acute lymphoblastic leukaemia) have a lower risk of infection, thrombosis and need for removal than tunnelled catheters (McLean *et al.* 2005). Implanted ports have lower overall complication rates, and less risk of dislodgement and occlusion when compared with tunnelled CVCs (Mirro *et al.* 1990; Wiener *et al.* 1992). Significantly lower rates of infection have also been reported (Mirro *et al.* 1990; Ingram *et al.* 1991; La Quaglia *et al.* 1992). Other studies have demonstrated lower infection rates in implanted ports, but these did not reach statistical significance (McGovern *et al.* 1985; Soucy 1987; Ross *et al.* 1988; Wurzel *et al.* 1988). Conversely, Wiener *et al.* (1992) found no difference in infection as a cause of removal when comparing the two devices. It should be noted that all of the above studies represent paediatric oncology patients and may not be applicable to other conditions.

McCloskey (2002) compared several paediatric studies that described complication rates in tunnelled catheters, PICCs and ports. Overall PICCs demonstrated the lowest rate of infection (1%), followed by ports (8%) and tunnelled catheters (18%). PICCs have a higher thrombosis rate (8%) compared to ports (4%) and tunnelled catheters (3%).

Routine care, use and maintenance of central venous access devices

There are many different catheter types and protocols for care. Wide variations exist in the care of CVADs at both a national and international level. Tweddle *et al.* (1997) describe differences in flushing techniques amongst paediatric oncology centres in the UK, Knue *et al.* (2006) identify differences in flushing and blood sampling practices for PICCs across the USA and finally Galway *et al.* (2003) highlight the variability of hand-washing techniques used for CVADs in Australia.

Several evidence-based guidelines now exist with the aim of reducing healthcare-associated infections occurring in CVADs. Whilst none of the guidelines were devised solely for paediatric use, some aspects of the recommendations can be applied to paediatric practice. Indeed, many aspects of CVAD care in children and neonates are not researched adequately and it is therefore difficult to make specific recommendations for care in children (Garland *et al.* 2002). A systematic review was undertaken in 2005 with the intention of presenting the best available evidence for the effective management of CVADs and catheter sites in the prevention of catheter-related complications in paediatric patients in hospital. This review highlighted a lack of quality research for optimal management of CVADs in children. The authors concluded that it would be extremely difficult to develop evidence-based policies or guidelines in order to improve CVAD-related outcomes for paediatric patients. In addition, there remain many issues relating to the management of CVADs in children that are unresolved (Lee & Johnston 2005). It is suggested that in the absence of evidence-based guidelines that relate specifically to children, adult guidelines are reviewed and adapted where appropriate. For example, many recommendations, such as the use of aseptic technique and hand-washing, are applicable regardless of the age of the patient.

The standard principles of preventing infection associated with CVADs are the same for all patient groups (Pratt *et al,* 2007). Compliance with infection control guidelines such as ensuring effective hand hygiene and optimal staffing levels, practising aseptic techniques and taking appropriate care of devices, can reduce the number of healthcare-associated infections (MacQueen 2005). Hand-washing and aseptic techniques are accepted worldwide as cornerstones for the prevention of infection (Foster *et al.* 2002).

Section 3

Adherence to policies/protocols and training for the handling of different catheter types will help to minimize potential problems (Hollis 1992; Wiener & Albanese 1998). Generally speaking, protocols for the care of CVADs should be based on manufacturers' guidelines, current research, experience with adults, and catheter type and volume (Frey 2007). Protocols for use in children should take into account the developmental level of the child and the unique problems associated with the use of CVADs.

Maintaining patency, blood sampling and medication administration

Catheter volume in children

The catheter volume of a paediatric-sized tunnelled CVC is 1 mL or less (Frey 2001). This should be accounted for when compiling protocols for maintaining patency, blood sampling and drug administration (*See* Table 15.6). However, adult-sized tunnelled CVCs and implanted ports may be placed in children to take advantage of the larger internal diameter of the lumen for blood administration and sampling. The catheter will be cut to size during placement and the catheter volume will be reduced accordingly. For example, a 10 French dual-lumen tunnelled catheter cut during insertion will result in a catheter volume of approximately 1 mL (MacGeorge *et al.* 1988). It is important to know what size of catheter is placed in a child as catheter volumes may vary if both adult and paediatric sizes are used. The manufacturers should be consulted if the catheter volume is unknown.

Maintaining patency

CVADs should be flushed at established intervals to maintain patency and prevent the mixing of incompatible medications or solutions (RCN 2005b; INS 2006). There is however, controversy as to the exact amount of flush solution to use, the type of solution, and the frequency of flushing. The volume of flush solution should be twice the volume of the catheter and add-on devices (RCN 2005b; INS 2006). Refer to Table 15.6 for guidance on amounts to use. There are two solutions commonly used to maintain patency: 0.9% sodium chloride and heparinized saline. There have been very few studies comparing these two solutions (Dougherty 2006). The efficacy of using heparin flushes in between use of CVCs to prevent thrombus formation and prolong catheter patency is unproven (Randolph *et al.* 1998). Current guidelines advocate the use of heparinized saline for open-ended catheters and implanted ports (NICE 2003; RCN 2005b; INS 2006; Pratt *et al.* 2007). The concentration of heparinized saline should be the lowest possible to maintain patency (RCN 2005b; INS 2006). Whilst 100 units/mL is recommended as a monthly flush for implanted ports this concentration is too high if the port is used frequently (e.g. to administer i.v. antibiotics). A weaker solution of 10 units/mL is suggested in this situation (Bravery & Hannan 1997; Frey 2001; Frey 2007). For adults there are recommendations that tunnelled catheters may be flushed weekly when not in use (Kelly *et al.* 1992; Dougherty 2006). In a survey of paediatric oncology centres in the UK, 45% report flushing Hickman catheters weekly. The RCN (2005b) suggests that weekly flushing is sufficient for long-term CVADs, unless occlusive problems dictate otherwise. In contrast, the Infusion Nurses Society (INS) (2006) makes no recommendation on the frequency of flushing. Valved catheters can be flushed with 0.9% sodium chloride to maintain patency, according to manufacturer's instructions (RCN 2005b; INS 2006).

Safety Aspects of Paediatric Intravenous Medication Administration

The administration of i.v. medication to children is now commonplace in both the hospital and community setting (RCN 2005c). Intravenous medications may be administered

Table 15.6 Flushing and heparinization of central venous access devices.

CVAD type	Catheter volume (mL)	Heparin			Sodium chloride 0.9% (mL)	
		Routine hepariniza-tion (mL)	Heparinized saline (Units per mL)	Frequency	After blood sampling	Before and after drug administration
Tunnelled catheter: small bore 2.7–6.6 Fr (a)	0.15–0.7 (a)	1.5 (a)	10*	Weekly	3 (a)	1–2 (a)
Tunnelled catheter: large bore	1 ml or less paediatric sized catheter (e) 0.6–1.3 (a)	2–5 (d, e)	10*	Daily – Weekly (d, e)	5–10 (e)	3 (e)
Implantable port Reservoir Catheter	0.2–0.6 (b) 0.6–1.5 (b)	2–5 (d, e)	100 (d) 10* for child receiving one or more drugs daily (d)	Monthly** (d)	5–10 (e)	2–5 (e)
PICC Open ended	0.15–0.42 (a)	1–2 (d, e)	10* for child receiving one or more drugs daily (d)	Once or twice daily (d,e)	5–10 (e)	2–3 (e)
Valved	0.3–0.62 (c)	2 mL sodium chloride 0.9% (a)	N/A	Weekly (a)	3 (a)	2 (a)
Non-tunnelled catheter	0.3 per lumen (e)	1–2 (d,e)	10*	Once or twice daily (d)	5–10 (e)	3 (e)

Information from : (a) Bard Access Systems, Inc.www.bardaccess.com accessed 18.06.06, (b) Bard Access Systems, Inc. www.accessabillty-bybard.co.uk accessed 10.06.06, (c) Bard Access Systems, Inc. 2003; (d) Frey 2007; (e) Frey 2001.
* Lowest possible concentration of heparin.
This table should be used as a guide only. It is based on the references listed above. Where a range is specified, it is intended to reflect variations in flushing protocols. More research is needed to establish the optimum flush volumes required to maintain patency of the wide range of CVADs in use. Always consult the manufacturers of the device for information on catheter volumes.

to children by direct bolus injection or by means of intermittent/continuous infusion via peripheral or central venous access devices (Dyer *et al.* 2006; Frey 2006). There are several factors to consider to ensure safe practice. The *Guidelines for the Administration of Medicines* (NMC 2004a), *Code of Conduct* (NMC 2004b) and *Guidelines for Records and Record Keeping* (NMC 2005) along with the local hospital policy should be adhered to when administering medicines to children (Hutton & Gardner 2003; Watt 2003a; Dyer *et al.* 2006). Intravenous medications must be prepared according to the manufacturer's instructions (Dyer *et al.* 2006).

Medication error in children

The preparation and administration of i.v. medications may create opportunities for error. Dosages of i.v. drugs vary widely in children of different sizes and frequently require dilution, giving rise to miscalculations (Clayden 2004). Errors in the preparation and administration of i.v. medications involving children have been described in practice. Ross *et al.* (2000) in a study of medication errors in a British paediatric teaching hospital found that errors involving the i.v. route were the most frequent (56%).

Kaushal *et al.* (2001) in a study of medication errors and adverse drug events in paediatric inpatients in two North American hospitals found that dosing errors and errors involving the i.v. route were the most frequent. In addition, an analysis of claims against the NHS relating to i.v. therapy demonstrated that 42.6% of incidents occurred in paediatric settings—three times more than in any other specialty (Quinn & Upton 2006). In hospital settings although medication errors in children occur at similar rates when compared to adults, the error has three times the potential to cause harm. In children the risk of error is frequently compounded by the need for additional calculations to determine the dose. In addition, complex manipulations may be required in the preparation of doses for small babies (DH 2004a).

A common source of error in paediatric practice is misplacement of the decimal point in dose calculations (DH 2004b). Misplaced decimal points can lead to 10- or 100-fold dosing errors, often involving digoxin or opiates, which may prove fatal (DH 2004a).

Recommendations to reduce the risk of i.v. medication errors include:

- carefully checking and documenting the dose, volume and rate calculations prior to the administration of medicines (DH 2004b)
- double-checking dose calculations before administration (DH 2004a)
- use of standardized charts, aide-memoirs or validated computer software for calculating doses and infusion rates for potent medicines such as digoxin and opiates (DH 2004a)
- standardization of concentrations and diluents to simplify the calculation processes for continuous infusion diluents (DH 2004a).

Calculating drug dosages

Prescriptions for i.v. infusions in children involve more than one calculation, as both the dose and rate of administration need to be calculated. Safe administration of i.v. medication to children requires careful calculation of dosage. Drug dosing for children is more complex because of the need to account for body weight/surface area and variations in the metabolism or elimination of drugs by the child (DH 2004a).

Drug dosage in children is commonly calculated in milligrams or micrograms per kilogram of body weight (mg/kg or mcg/kg) (Hutton & Gardner 2003; Frey 2007). However, medications may be prescribed in grams, milligrams, micrograms or even nanograms. In addition drug dosages may be based on surface area (Hutton & Gardner 2003). Paediatric nurses are frequently required to convert grams (g) to milligrams (mg) and milligrams to micrograms (mcg). Care should be taken to ensure that no mistakes are made during conversions. Giving a dose of 100 mg when 100 mcg is what is required can have grave consequences.

The following formula is commonly used to calculate the amount of drug to be administered to a child:

$$\text{Dose (what you give)} = \frac{\text{what you want/require}}{\text{what you've got/have}} \times \text{what it's in (dilution)}$$

(Hutton & Gardner 2003; Watt 2003b).

For example, if the dose of amikacin to be administered is 80 mg and the drug is available in a vial containing 100 mg in 2 mL, then the amount to be given is:

$$\frac{80}{100} \times 2 = 1.6 \; mL$$

Because of the wide variation in volumes required for doses needed in children all doses should be double-checked against the milligram per kilogram dose. Guidance on dosages for children should be checked using a paediatric formulary (Hutton & Gardner 2003). The first *British National Formulary for Children* (BNFC) was published in 2005 and aims to provide up-to-date information on the use of medicines for treating children (Royal Pharmaceutical Society of Great Britain 2005). All staff involved in paediatric medication therapy should have access to a paediatric formulary (DH 2004a).

Displacement values/volumes

Awareness of displacement values/volumes is important as children are often prescribed a small dose that is part-drawn from a vial (Dyer *et al.* 2006). Some drugs are available as a powder and require reconstitution with an appropriate diluent before administration. The powder adds volume, which is known as the displacement value (Hutton & Gardner 2003). This must be accounted for when reconstituting drugs for administration to children. Failure to account for the displacement volume will lead to an incorrect dose of the drug being given (Ellis 1995).

The displacement volume of a 1-g vial of chloramphenicol is 0.8 mL. To reconstitute the drug, 9.2 mL of water is added to a 1-g vial of chloramphenicol. A volume of 10 mL of solution will be present in the vial after reconstitution. Conversely, if 10 mL is added to the vial and 10 mL of the reconstituted solution is given to the child, 0.8 mL will remain in the vial. As a consequence, the child will not have received the total dose of 1 g (Ellis 1995).

In adults, it is common practice to administer a complete ampoule or vial of a drug. Only a portion of an ampoule or vial is required in paediatrics. If the dose to be administered to a child exceeds one ampoule or vial, it should be confirmed by consulting the medical staff or pharmacy department (Frey 2007).

Administration of Intravenous Medications

Syringe size and central venous access devices

Large amounts of pressure can cause catheter fracture or rupture and the manufacturer's guidelines for syringe size or maximum pound per square inch (psi) recommendations should be followed when using CVADs (Hadaway 1998a). It is generally recommended that 10-mL syringes are used routinely for all procedures involving CVADs. Instillation, aspiration and flushing of CVADs should be done using a method that does not exceed the catheter manufacturer's maximum pressure limits of psi (RCN 2005b). When attempting to clear a catheter of an occlusion a syringe size smaller than 10 mL should not be used, to avoid catheter rupture (Conn 1993).

Small syringes are often necessary to ensure accuracy of drug dosage in children. Small syringes can be used if absolutely necessary, after catheter patency has been established (Moureau 1999). It is recommended that the patency of the device is established using a 10-mL syringe before a smaller syringe is used to avoid the risk of damaging the CVAD (Bravery & Hannan 1997; Hadaway 1998a). However, it is vital that the injection is stopped if any resistance is encountered whilst administering an injection manually to avoid catheter rupture or fracture (Hadaway 1998a).

Methods of intravenous medication administration

Intravenous medications may be administered using an infusion device or syringe pump. Some medications require further dilution before administration. This is achieved by adding the drug to a bag of fluid, a syringe (for use with a syringe pump) or to a burette (in-line calibrated chamber). The burette is commonly used in paediatric practice. Medication added to the burette is infused at the prescribed rate. On completion of the infusion, the burette is flushed with a volume of compatible solution (Frey 2007). Small volumes of i.v. medications (< 3 mL) may require further dilution with a compatible solution according to the manufacturer's recommendations. This will prevent retention of the drug within the infusion tubing.

Avoidance of fluid overload

A problem frequently encountered when administering i.v. medications to children is the need to limit the amount of fluid used to administer and flush the drug through the infusion tubing (Frey 2007). The method of administration should be carefully chosen to avoid excessive administration of fluid. Intravenous drugs for infusion may be added to the burette of an administration set, and this can be used in older children, who are more able to tolerate the extra 20–30 mL needed to clear the administration set of drug. Once added to the burette, the drug should be further diluted in accordance with the manufacturer's instructions. When calculating the rate of the infusion, the flush volume should be added to the drug volume after dilution to give the total amount to be infused. This burette method may not be suitable for use with neonates as the infusion tubing volume may be too great (Frey 2007).

A syringe pump should be used for i.v. drug administration in infants, toddlers and older children who are fluid-restricted (Watt 2003a). The tubing (microbore) used with a syringe pump has a lower priming volume and ensures that less fluid is administered. The syringe containing the drug may be 'piggybacked' via an extension tubing to the primary set or connected directly to the venous access device. Luer-lock connections must be used to achieve this connection to avoid the risk of disconnection. If the drug is incompatible with the primary solution, a flush of compatible solution will be given before and after the drug is administered.

Flushing

All i.v. medications should be followed immediately with a sodium chloride 0.9% flush or other compatible solution to clear the drug from the access device. The priming volume of all i.v. tubing that the drug is administered through should be considered when calculating the amount of compatible solution required, to ensure that the total drug dose is administered to the child (Watt 2003a; Frey 2007). Ford *et al.* (2003) suggest that using two times the volume of the dead space of the i.v. tubing is the most effective way to ensure that the full dose of medication is delivered. The flush must be administered at the same rate as the drug, as some of the drug will be retained in the infusion tubing (Axton & Hall 1994). If the flush rate is increased, the retained drug will be given rapidly and may result in speedshock and increased risk of side-effects (Hicks-Keen 1995; Whitman 1995).

When administering i.v. medications directly via CVADs, it is important that the device is flushed with sufficient amounts of sodium chloride 0.9% to effectively clear the device of drug (*See* Table 15.6). When administering i.v. drugs, the catheter volume of the access device should be accounted for to avoid retention of the drug within the device. Failure to clear a drug from the access device may have serious consequences if the retained drug is inadvertently flushed into the child at a later date. Ben-Arush and Berant (1996) reported the retention of an anaesthetic drug cocktail within an implanted port in a 2-year-old child following sedation for radiotherapy. Failure to flush the device led to collapse of the child when the device was reheparinized on return to the ward.

Electronic infusion devices

Accuracy and safety are of the utmost importance when selecting an electronic infusion device for use in children (Frey 2007). An accurate infusion device is now considered essential to deliver i.v. therapies safely and effectively. This is particularly so in paediatrics where children and neonates require precise volumes, often at low flow rates (Brown 2002).

The Medicines and Healthcare products Regulatory Agency (MHRA) classifies infusion devices according to four categories of infusion risk: neonatal risk, high risk, low risk and ambulatory. These classifications apply to both volumetric and syringe pumps. Neonatal devices can be used for neonatal risk infusions in paediatric and neonatal intensive care settings, whereas high-risk devices are considered more suitable for use in older children and adults for the administration of high-risk infusions (Quinn 2000). Syringe pumps are often used to deliver small-volume medications accurately in intensive care settings (Frey 2007).

When choosing an infusion device, neonatal risk infusions dictate the need for:

- high accuracy/consistency of flow
- infusion rates of 0.1 mL/hour upwards
- low-pressure occlusion settings
- fast alarm times
- low bolus on release of occlusion
- alarm identification to alert the clinician to specific problems.

High-risk devices have many of the features described above for neonatal devices with one main difference. The neonatal device is more accurate in the short term, especially when infusing at very low rates (< 5 mL/hour) (Quinn 2000).

A syringe pump is the preferred choice for low-volume, low-rate infusions. A volumetric pump can be set to infuse at rates below 1 mL/hour and will perform satisfactorily at rates down to 5 mL/hour. However, these pumps are not recommended for delivery of medications at such low rates (MHRA 2003).

Blood sampling

When obtaining blood samples from CVADs, care should be taken to ensure that blood loss is minimal, the potential for infection is minimized and an accurate sample is obtained.

Minimizing blood loss

Blood sampling is one of the major causes of anaemia in infants and children (Wilson & Gaedeke 1996). Collecting more blood than required can lead to iatrogenic anaemia in hospitalized patients (Dale & Ruby 2003). Circulating blood volume decreases in proportion to body weight from a neonate (80–90 mL/kg) to an adolescent (65–70 mL/kg). The greater proportion of blood volume to lower body weight of a neonate/infant means that the blood loss percentage is much higher in this group, even with relatively small losses. For example, a 25-mL blood loss in a 5-kg infant represents 6% of the infant's circulating blood volume of 400 mL (Frey 2007). Neonates, infants and children requiring frequent blood sampling from CVADs are particularly at risk of blood loss. Anaemia and bleeding are common complications of bone marrow transplant, and paediatric bone marrow transplant patients may have blood samples drawn daily or more frequently (MacGeorge *et al.* 1988). It is essential to minimize blood loss in these patients. Blood replacement may be necessary if the cumulative blood loss exceeds 5–10% of the circulating blood volume (Hazinski 1992; Wilson & Gaedeke 1996).

Blood sampling should be coordinated and limited to once daily in high-risk patients. A running total should be kept of discard and waste volume, and this should be documented in the patient record (Wilson & Gaedeke 1996; Frey 2003; RCN 2005b; INS 2006).

Methods employed to conserve blood loss in infants and children include daily evaluation to ensure all tests are necessary, recording blood volumes withdrawn and discarded, ensuring correct techniques for blood sampling are adhered to, avoiding contamination from parenterally administered fluids and subsequent repeat sampling, ensuring the least amount of blood is collected that is required by the laboratory, using paediatric-sized collection tubes, and using microchemistry techniques (Wilson & Gaedeke 1996; Hadaway 2003).

Minimizing the risk of infection

Frequent blood sampling from CVADs may be associated with an increased risk of infection (Keller 1994; Long *et al.* 1996; Frey 2003). This may be a particular concern in immunocompromised paediatric patients.

Obtaining accurate blood samples

To obtain an accurate sample for laboratory analysis, the catheter must be cleared of heparinized saline and infusion fluid (MacGeorge *et al.* 1988; Keller 1994). The removal of three times the catheter volume is advocated to clear the catheter of infusate (Frey 2003, 2007). The amount of blood withdrawn from the CVAD to obtain accurate samples will reflect the smaller catheter volume—3 mL is sufficient for tunnelled CVCs and implanted ports (MacGeorge *et al.* 1988; Keller 1994).

Methods of blood sampling

There are three methods (discard, reinfusion, and push–pull or mixing) currently used for blood sampling via CVADs although little research exists to support any particular method. In practice, there appear to be variations both in the techniques for obtaining blood samples and in the rationale for each method. In a survey of 34 paediatric bone marrow transplant units in the USA, Keller (1994) found that 75% used the discard method, 14% used the reinfusion method and only one unit used the mixing method. There were wide variations in the volume of blood discarded: 61%, 4–6 mL; 29%, 7–10 mL; and 32%, 0.5–3 mL. Only four of the units surveyed cited catheter volume as the rationale for the discard volume.

Discard method   Using this method, 3–10 mL of blood is withdrawn and discarded before the sample is taken in a separate syringe (Keller 1994). Holmes (1998) suggests that the discard method involves flushing the catheter first with sodium chloride 0.9% and without removing this syringe aspirating 6 mL of blood, which is then discarded. If this method is used, care should be taken to minimize blood loss, the risk of blood exposure for the operator and the potential to confuse the discard syringe with the blood sample (Frey 2003).

Reinfusion method   A volume of 6 mL is withdrawn from the CVAD, the sample taken and the withdrawn fluid replaced (McGeorge *et al.* 1988). This method theoretically reduces the amount of blood withdrawn from the child. However, this method involves a risk of blood exposure for the operator, the potential to confuse the discard syringe with the blood sample, potential contamination of the catheter/fluid withdrawn and possible clots being reinfused (Cosca *et al.* 1998). No research to date has been carried out to confirm that reinfusion of the waste blood actually minimizes blood loss.

Push–pull or mixing method   McGeorge *et al.* (1988) describe the mixing method as attaching a syringe to the catheter, withdrawing 6 mL and immediately reinfusing this into the patient. This procedure is repeated four times without disconnecting the syringe. A new syringe is then attached and the sample taken. Holmes (1998) varies this approach slightly by flushing first with 5 mL of sodium chloride 0.9%. This syringe remains attached to the catheter and 6 mL of blood is aspirated and pushed back into the catheter. This step is repeated for a total of three times in all. The empty syringe is removed and a new syringe or vacutainer attached to collect the sample.

This method requires good blood flow on aspiration to be effective. Small-lumen silicone catheters may collapse on aspiration and may not be appropriate for this method of blood sampling. The mixing method may eliminate the potential blood loss from frequent blood sampling in high-risk patients (i.e. neonates or bone marrow patients). In addition, this method may reduce the risk of catheter contamination or blood exposure (Frey 2003). Further research is required to confirm the accuracy of blood samples obtained by this method.

Despite the recommendation by manufacturers and clinicians that 3 French PICCs are not suitable for blood sampling, this practice is widespread in the USA, with 76% of institutions using these catheters for blood sampling (Knue *et al.* 2006). A recent study by Knue *et al.* (2005) confirms the effectiveness and feasibility of blood sampling from 3 French PICCs in children.

Blood samples for coagulation tests may be inaccurate if drawn from CVADs (Pinto 1994; Mayo *et al.* 1996; Hinds *et al.* 2002; RCN 2005b). Limited data regarding antibiotic blood level sampling from a CVAD indicate conflicting results as regards aminoglycoside levels. It has been proposed that antibiotic blood levels may be safely drawn via a PICC but not other types of CVAD (McBeth *et al.* 2004). Other research on drug levels suggests that when administered intermittently, drug levels for cyclosporine A (CSA) may be obtained safely via the CSA-naive lumen of a dual-lumen catheter (Senner *et al.* 2005). There has not yet been enough research to safely advocate the routine taking of drug levels from CVADs in children.

Dressings and exit site care

There is a tendency to use research based on adult populations when devising protocols for the care of exit sites in children, but this may not always be appropriate. Chlorhexidine has been found to be superior to povidone iodine for the prevention of microbial colonization of the central venous catheter insertion site/tip and reducing the risk of local site infection (Carson 2004). Chlorhexidine 2% is recommended as the preferred solution for catheter site care. However, no recommendation can be made for the use of chlorhexidine in infants less than 2 months of age (CDC 2002).

Alcoholic or aqueous chlorhexidine gluconate solutions are advocated in UK guidelines for site care (Pellowe *et al.* 2004; RCN 2005b; Pratt *et al.* 2007). In low birth weight infants (< 1000 g), chlorhexidine gluconate has been associated with localized contact dermatitis (Garland *et al.* 2001). However, Irving (2001a) suggests that aqueous chlorhexidine can be safely used on preterm infants. The use of chlorhexidine is advocated for catheter site care in the USA, along with povidone iodine. In order to prevent systemic absorption of chlorhexidine in neonates, it is recommended that the solution is completely removed after the procedure, using sterile water or sodium chloride 0.9% (Association for Women's Health, Obstetric and Neonatal Nurses 2001; INS 2006). In recent years, it has become common practice in the UK to use chlorhexidine 0.5% in 70% alcohol with caution in paediatric practice (MacQueen 2005).

Recommendations about dressings are frequently extrapolated to paediatrics from adult studies (Kline 2005). A systematic review conducted by Lee and Johnston was unable to make any recommendations on type of dressing or frequency of dressing change based on paediatric research evidence available (Lee & Johnston 2005). The use of adult guidelines will continue unless further high-quality research is undertaken in paediatric populations.

Current adult guidelines suggest that either a sterile gauze or transparent semipermeable dressing can be used to cover the catheter site (CDC 2002; NICE 2003; RCN 2005b; INS 2006; Pratt *et al.* 2007). A transparent semipermeable polyurethane dressing is the preferred option (NICE 2003; Pratt *et al.* 2007). Gauze dressings should be used in patients who are diaphoretic or have oozing/bleeding catheter sites (CDC 2002; NICE 2003; RCN 2005b; Pratt *et al.* 2007). Transparent dressings should be changed every 7 days or sooner if the integrity of the dressing is compromised (CDC 2002; NICE 2003;

RCN 2005b; Pratt *et al.* 2007). Gauze dressings should be changed every 48 hours or replaced when the dressing becomes damp, loose or soiled or site inspection is necessary (NICE 2003; RCN 2005b).

If a non-coring needle is left *in situ* the implanted port access site should be covered with a sterile transparent semipermeable dressing (RCN 2005b; INS 2006). Gauze may be placed under the needle wings and sterile paper strips used to secure the wings to the chest, under the dressing. The dressing should be changed weekly with the needle.

Complications of Central Venous Access Devices used in Children

Accidental dislodgement of central venous catheters

Accidental dislodgement of tunnelled catheters has been described as a major and frequent problem in paediatric oncology patients (Mirro *et al.* 1990; Wiener *et al.* 1992). This may reflect poor tissue in growth into the cuff due to poor nutritional status and delayed healing in this group of patients (Wiener *et al.* 1992). The incidence of dislodgement is greater in children less than 3 years of age and significantly associated with a cuff to exit site distance of less than 2 cm (Wiener *et al.* 1992). A unique consideration in toddlers and babies is that they may tug at the catheter and unintentionally subject it to traction, thus increasing the likelihood of dislodgement.

To reduce the risk of dislodgement, catheters should be looped and taped securely to the chest wall using an adherent tape (Frey 2007). Other measures include keeping the catheter out of reach of the baby or toddler by taping it over the shoulder, or around the side of the torso to the back. Ensuring that the catheter remains under clothing may help to deter inquisitive fingers. Babygros and vests that are fastened between the legs are useful in babies. It is recommended that a baby or toddler with the catheter free should never be left unattended. Education of the child and family to avoid traction on the catheter and to exercise caution when infusions are in progress is vital.

PICC dislodgement is one of the more frequently reported complications in children. Dislodgement may occur if the child or carer pulls on the PICC, or from tension exerted by the weight of the tubing and attachments. There may be an increased likelihood of dislodgement occurring if the catheter is not trimmed to fit the child and excess catheter remains looped outside the insertion site (Frey 1999). Thiagarajan *et al.* (1997) maintain that dislodgement is more likely to occur in older infants and children aged 31 days–5 years in comparison with neonates less than 30 days old and children older than 5 years. Securement devices can be used to reduce the potential for PICC dislodgment. These include sterile skin closure strips, transparent semipermeable dressings, sutures or catheter-specific securement devices. Often several products are used to maintain security. There are no studies that compare securement methods for PICCs in children. Failure to secure a PICC adequately may lead to delays in treatment and the discomfort of an additional PICC insertion. If the PICC appears to have migrated out of the insertion site the tip position should be confirmed by chest X-ray. The PICC should not be used until tip position has been verified (Frey 2001).

A problem unique to children is that of rapid growth. The growth of the torso may dislodge the catheter upwards out of the SVC (Reed & Philips 1996). This will be identified by a chest X-ray. If this situation arises, the catheter will require replacement.

Infection and central venous catheters

The risk of infection in children varies with age, birth weight, underlying disease (e.g. cystic fibrosis, cancer, AIDS, prematurity or short bowel syndrome), medications, type of device and the nature of the infusate (e.g. lipids) (Mermel *et al.* 2001). As in adults the majority of nosocomial bloodstream infections (BSIs) are associated with the use of an intravascular catheter (CDC 2002). Most of the data on catheter-related infection are derived from paediatric/neonatal intensive care or oncology settings (Mermel *et al.* 2001). Rates of catheter-related BSI are higher in intensive care settings than in less acute or ambulatory care settings (Kline 2005). As in adults, most catheter-related infections are caused by coagulase-negative staphylococci, followed by *S. aureus*. In neonates, coagulase-negative staphylococci account for just over half of catheter-related infections, followed by *Candida* species, enterococci and Gram-negative bacilli (Mermel *et al.* 2001).

The management of catheter-related infection in children is challenging and there are some differences to adults. Children with infected catheters are often treated without catheter removal (Mermel *et al.* 2001). Removal of the catheter for diagnostic purposes may not be indicated as catheter replacement can be associated with a high risk of complications or reinsertion difficulties. It is considered more prudent to try and eradicate the infection. Peripheral blood cultures are often not undertaken, as venepuncture is more difficult in children (Mermel *et al.* 2001; Randolph *et al.* 2005).

Use of antibiotics should be based on the expected identity and susceptibility of the isolate and modified once culture results are known. Treatment for suspected infection should include an agent effective against Gram-positive and Gram-negative bacteria, and antifungal treatment when a yeast is isolated or highly suspected. The optimum length of treatment of catheter-related infections in children has yet to be established with or without catheter removal. Children treated without catheter removal require careful monitoring and removal of the device if the child's condition deteriorates (Mermel *et al.* 2001).

Thrombosis

The incidence of symptomatic venous thromboembolism in neonates (birth–28 days, corrected for gestational age) is reported to be 2.4 per 1000 admissions to neonatal ICUs. More than 80% of cases of venous thromboemboli in neonates are secondary to the placement of a CVC. In this age group this includes CVCs placed in umbilical veins or into the upper venous system through peripheral veins or major veins (jugular veins). CVCs are used in neonates for administration of fluids, medications or TPN. The mechanisms thought to cause thromboembolic events associated with CVC use include damage to vessel walls, disrupted blood flow, infusion of TPN that damages the endothelial cells and thrombogenic catheter materials. In children (28 days–16 years) the estimated incidence of symptomatic venous thromboembolism is 5.3 per 10 000 hospital admissions. In children 95% of venous thromboemboli are secondary to cancer, trauma/surgery, congenital heart disease and systemic lupus erythematosus. More than 50% of venous thromboemboli occur in the upper venous system in children secondary to the use of CVCs. The incidence of CVC-related venous thromboembolism varies according to underlying condition, use of diagnostic tests and different indices of suspicion. For example, the incidence of venous thromboembolism in children receiving long-term TPN varies from 1% (based on clinical diagnosis) to 35% (based on ventilation–perfusion scans or echocardiography) to 75% (based on venography) (Monagle *et al.* 2004).

Recommendations for treatment of thromboembolic events have been based mostly on data from adult studies. Whilst there have been attempts to undertake multicentre randomized controlled trials, these have failed due to poor recruitment and consent rates. Current advice for the management of CVC-related thrombosis includes the following.

- Remove the CVC if it is non-functioning or no longer required. Give 3–5 days' anticoagulation therapy prior to removal.
- If the CVC is still required for access and is functioning the CVC should remain *in situ* and anticoagulation therapy should be administered (*See* Monagle *et al.* 2004 for details of anticoagulation therapy).

- For children with a first CVC-related deep vein thrombosis after the initial 3 months of therapy, use prophylactic doses of vitamin K antagonists or low molecular weight heparin (LMWH) until the CVC is removed.
- For children with recurrent CVC-related thromboembolic events after the initial 3 months of therapy, use prophylactic doses of vitamin K antagonists or LMWH until removal of the CVC. If recurrence occurs whilst on prophylactic therapy use continuing therapeutic doses until CVC removal or for a minimum of 3 months.
- Routine primary prophylaxis for children with CVCs is not recommended.
- For children receiving long-term home TPN antithrombotic prophylaxis is advocated using vitamin K antagonists either continuously or for the first 3 months after each CVC is inserted (Monagle *et al.* 2004).

Catheter occlusion

The causes of catheter occlusion can be divided into three categories: mechanical, non-thrombotic and thrombotic (Bagnall-Reeb 1998). Occlusion may be classified in two ways: complete occlusion, i.e. inability to infuse fluids or withdraw blood; or partial occlusion (withdrawal occlusion), i.e. catheter flushes but blood return is sluggish or absent (McCloskey 2002).

Catheter occlusions occur frequently with the long-term usage of CVADs. In children, slower infusion rates may cause reflux of blood in the catheter and subsequent catheter occlusion. In addition, parenteral nutrition solutions used may contain more calcium and phosphorus which may lead to precipitate occlusions, particularly in neonates (Reed & Philips 1996). Occlusion occurs more frequently in small catheters and may be more problematic in paediatric-sized PICCs.

Management

Once the position of the catheter has been confirmed by chest X-ray or dye studies, attempts can be made to relieve the occlusion using an appropriate agent (Reed & Philips 1996). Dye studies are advocated in preference to chest X-ray as they will identify fibrin sheath formation which may result in extravasation if undiagnosed (Mayo & Pearson 1995; Masoorli 2005). Some occluded CVADs will not allow instillation of the medication. Excessive force may cause rupture of the catheter or clot dislodgement. When instilling medications to relieve catheter obstruction, the use of syringes smaller than 10 mL is contraindicated to avoid the risk of catheter rupture (Reed & Philips 1996). The so-called 'stopcock method' can be used to create a vacuum to pull the medication into the catheter (Hooke 2000) (*See* page 34 for details). Frey (1999) reports modifying this procedure for use with paediatric PICCs. The stopcock is somewhat bulky when attached to a PICC and may be replaced with a T-connector. Using this method, air is first withdrawn from the hub end of the connector. The T-connector is then clamped and then the medication is given via the port on the T-connector.

Agents used to relieve catheter occlusion

It is important to ascertain the cause of the catheter occlusion to enable the appropriate agent to be used to relieve the obstruction. Clues as to the cause of the obstruction can be elicited from the history of the occlusion. Lipid occlusion generally takes several days or weeks for the catheter to become totally obstructed (Pennington & Pithie 1987), whereas an occlusion caused by a drug precipitate often occurs suddenly and may be caused by insufficient flush volumes between drugs or between drugs and parenteral nutrition (Holcombe *et al.* 1992). Precipitate may be visible in the infusion tubing or catheter (Duffy *et al.* 1989). In practice, it may be difficult to identify the cause of the catheter occlusion. If unsure, urokinase or alteplase should be tried first to relieve the occlusion before trying other means (Holcombe *et al.* 1992). Since the withdrawal of urokinase

Table 15.7   Agents used to relieve catheter occlusion in children (Reed & Phillips 1996; Hadaway 1998b; Harris & Macguire 1999; Andris & Krzywda 1999; Fisher *et al.* 2004).

Cause of occlusion	Agent / method of administration
Blood, fibrin	Urokinase bolus: 5000 units per mL Use amount equivalent to catheter volume (small-bore tunnelled catheter 0.2–0.5 mL, tunnelled catheter 1 mL, implanted port 2 mL to accommodate larger priming volume and extension tubing of needle). Leave *in situ* for 30–120 minutes. May be repeated to a total of three doses
	Tissue plasminogen activator— Alteplase 1 mg/mL solution give 2mL for child ≥ 30 kg, give 110% of catheter lumen volume for child < 30 kg (maximum 2 mL). Leave *in situ* 30–120 minutes. Two doses may be given
Fibrin sheath resistant to bolus urokinase	Urokinase infusion: 200 units per kg per hour for 24 hours
Drug precipitate	Sodium bicarbonate 8.4% (1 mEq/mL): dose 1 ml or equivalent to catheter volume. Leave *in situ* for 60 minutes. For precipitated drugs formulated with a high pH.
	0.1 N solution of hydrochloric acid: dose 1 mL or equivalent to catheter volume. 0.2–1 mL has been used. Leave *in situ* for 20–60 minutes. Aspirate to avoid adverse reactions. May be repeated to a total of three doses. For precipitated drugs with a low pH
Lipid	Ethyl alcohol 70%: dose 1 mL or equivalent to catheter volume. Leave *in situ* for 60–120 minutes

from use in the USA alteplase has been identified as an effective alternative. Several studies have concluded that alteplase can be safely used in children (Hooke 2000; Choi *et al.* 2001; Jacobs *et al.* 2001; Fisher *et al.* 2004) *See* Table 15.7 for more information on agents used to relieve catheter occlusion.

A study by Gordon and Dearmun (2003) highlighted occlusion as a cause of distress for parents of children with CVCs *in situ*. Parents' concerns about occlusion were dominated by the fear of venepuncture and potential need for a replacement CVC. Many parents felt that they were not informed about the potential for occlusion and that the problem was not taken seriously by staff when dealing with the catheter. Catheter occlusion has been identified as a common phenomenon, experienced by 89% of parents of children with CVCs *in situ*, with 87% reporting multiple incidences of occlusion (Gordon & Lloyd 2003). Staff who deal with catheter occlusions should take parental concerns about occluded catheters seriously.

Catheter damage

Children can and invariably do damage CVCs. Catheters can be bitten, or even cut with scissors. The incidence of catheter damage in children has been reported to be 6.2–27.5% (Cameron 1987; Bagnall-Reeb & Ruccione 1990). Catheter damage may occur above the bifurcation as a result of catheter fatigue and persistent twisting, or below the bifurcation in the lower portion of the catheter due to wear and tear (Bagnall-Reeb & Ruccione 1990). Education of staff and parents caring for children is vital to prevent catheter damage. Children should be encouraged to keep the catheter covered with clothing to minimize the risk of damage. Crop tops are popular with girls as the ends can be tucked up and secured within the top. If damage occurs at home, parents should be taught to clamp the catheter above the damaged portion, seal the catheter with an occlusive dressing and return to the hospital for repair. Atraumatic, non-toothed clamps should always be available wherever the child is cared for.

PICCs used in children are small and fragile and may break either inside or outside the body. Blood or fluid leaking under the dressing may indicate catheter damage. If the catheter fractures completely, the broken part can migrate within the child's circulation and lodge in the pulmonary artery, SVC, hepatic vein, innominate vein, and right or left atrium. If this occurs the migrated portion of catheter should be retrieved urgently by an interventional radiologist. If a PICC breaks internally a tourniquet can be placed at the axilla or groin above the insertion site to reduce the risk of catheter embolus. If the PICC breaks externally the catheter may be repaired using a repair kit. Other causes of PICC fracture described include the use of a 1-mL syringe with an occluded PICC, and being cut by sterile tape thread (Frey 1999). A review by Chow *et al.* (2003) of 1650 paediatric PICCs identified 11 cases of PICC fracture necessitating retrieval. Duration of placement and a PICC complication (occlusion or leaking at the insertion site) were significantly associated with catheter fracture. In all cases the embolized PICC fragment was successfully retrieved.

Air embolism and haemorrhage

The child with a CVAD is at risk of air embolism and haemorrhage if the integrity of the infusion system is interrupted (Marcoux *et al.* 1990). Air may be introduced if the administration set is incorrectly primed and contains air, or when a stopcock or connection is open to the environment. Laskey *et al.* (2002) describe how a mother forgot to prime an administration set before connecting the tubing to administer an antibiotic in the home setting. The child collapsed immediately and was fortunately resuscitated by her mother.

Children are curious and may fiddle with infusion tubing and caps attached to the catheter. Infusion pump controls and tubing should be kept out of the reach of small hands. Luer-lock connections and caps should be used and all connections regularly checked at intervals. Currently there is no completely child-proof connection system or cap available!

Swimming and central venous catheters

Swimming is an important part of normal life for a child. Although some centres do restrict swimming in children with CVCs, there is little research to support this approach. A study by Robbins *et al.* (1999) found that swimming does not increase the risk of catheter-related infection in children with tunnelled catheters. A more recent study by Smith *et al.* (2002) found that paediatric haematology/oncology outpatients with tunnelled catheters were at a greater risk of infection during the summer. This was thought to be related to recreational exposure to water in the summer and occurred despite parents being advised to avoid this type of exposure. The authors advise that greater attention should be paid to keeping the catheter site clean and free of potentially contaminated water by reducing contact with water from lakes, rivers, swimming pools and lawn sprinklers. Further research undertaken by Robbins *et al.* (2000) demonstrated that there was no greater incidence of catheter-related infection rates in children who swam than in those who did not. This study led the authors to change practice and allow swimming for children with tunnelled catheters.

If swimming/water activities are allowed the exit site should be healed and the cuff firmly fixed. An adherent, waterproof occlusive dressing is advised to protect the exit site. The dressing should be changed, the site cleaned and a new dressing applied immediately after swimming. If swimming is important to the child an implanted port should be considered as there are no restrictions on water activities with this device when not accessed.

Needle dislodgement and extravasation associated with implanted ports

Needle dislodgement has been identified as the most common cause of extravasation associated with the use of implanted ports in adult patients (Bothe *et al.* 1984; Reed *et al.* 1985; Strum *et al.* 1986; Moore *et al.* 1986; Brothers *et al.* 1988; Schulmeister 1989; Ramirez *et al.* 1993; Ingle 1995). Early rates of extravasation associated with port use ranged from 3 to 50%. Later studies with larger patient groups indicate rates of 0.3–4.7%, in adult studies. Four mechanisms of action have been reported as common causes of extravasation associated with implanted port use. These are incomplete needle placement and dislodgment, thrombus or fibrin sheath formation at the catheter tip, perforation of the SVC by the catheter, and catheter fracture/catheter-port separation (Schulmeister & Camp-Sorrell 2000). Although the potential for needle dislodgement would seem greater in active children, there are few published reports of occurrence of this problem. At the author's institution needle dislodgement occurs infrequently, usually the result of an accidental tug or pull on the infusion tubing whilst the child is attached to an infusion pump. In a series of 149 ports placed in paediatric oncology patients Munro *et al.* (1999) reported one occurrence of needle dislodgement involving epirubicin. Needle dislodgement may be hard to recognise as the needle may dislodge from the port and remain under the skin, giving the illusion that the needle is still *in situ* (Cunningham & Bonam-Crawford 1993). This is compounded by the fact that the extravasation may not become apparent until enough fluid has infused to cause swelling and discomfort (Sauerland *et al.* 2006). Rapid assessment and intervention is vital to identify extravasation and reduce morbidity (Hallquist Viale 2003).

Prevention

- When placing the needle do not rock or tilt the needle after insertion as this may cause fluid leakage (Gullo 1993).
- Always use a needle of adequate length (Schulmeister & Camp-Sorrell 2000). If the needle does not reach the base of the port reservoir, a longer needle should be used. A needle length of 0.75 inches (20 mm) is appropriate for most children (Bravery & Hannan 1997). If the needle is too short, it will compress the tissue over the port; as the tissue expands the needle may be pushed out of the port reservoir when the patient moves (Wood & Gullo 1993). If a child gains weight, a longer needle may be needed.
- Insert the needle with the bevel up, facing the shoulder, and tape the tubing to the shoulder. This will reduce traction on the tubing (Bagnall & Ruccione 1987).
- Secure the needle with sterile paper strips and a transparent dressing to allow visualization of the site during infusion. Use a dressing that does not obscure the site (Sauerland *et al.* 2006).
- Loop and tape the infusion tubing to the child's chest so that a tug on the tubing will be felt at the taped portion of tubing rather than directly on the needle. Ensure there is sufficient length to allow movement (Schulmeister & Camp-Sorrell 2000). This is vital to prevent direct traction on the needle.
- Parents should be told that extravasation is a known risk when vesicant medications are infusing. They should be taught how to move the child safely during the infusion and to prevent 'pulls' and traction on the infusion tubing. Vigorous activity should be avoided during the infusion such as trying to ride a bike whilst attached to an infusion with the parent struggling to keep up, pushing the pump along! Parents should be advised to report immediately any signs of pain or unusual sensations felt by the child (at the port site, tunnel or neck), leakage of fluid or swelling. A baby or toddler may be unable to verbalize pain or burning associated with vesicant extravasation (Sauerland *et al.* 2006). The child in this situation may become irritable, restless and cry. Parents can be taught how to stop the pump if they witness a 'pull' on the tubing/needle or any signs of extravasation.

Section 3

Before administration of vesicant drugs and infusions

- Confirm the correct needle position and catheter tip position by feeling the needle hit the base of the port and aspiration of free-flowing blood (Schulmeister & Camp-Sorrell 2000; Masoorli 2002, 2003). Aspiration of free-flowing blood (i.e. 3–5 mL) will indicate that the catheter tip is properly positioned within a vein (Masoorli 2005).
- If blood return is absent, gently flush the port with sodium chloride 0.9% using a push–pull technique. Obtaining a 'flash' of blood or a pink-tinged fluid is not indicative that the catheter is functioning correctly in a vein (Schulmeister & Camp-Sorrell 2000; Masoorli 2003, 2005).
- If blood return is still not obtained after flushing, an antithrombolytic agent can be administered (Schulmeister & Camp-Sorrell 2000; Masoorli 2002). Dye studies may be indicated if blood return remains unsuccessful (Mayo & Pearson 1995; Schulmeister & Camp-Sorrell 2000; Masoorli 2002). This will confirm the position of the catheter tip and the presence of thrombosis or fibrin sheath, either of which may cause extravasation (Lokich *et al.* 1985; Moore *et al.* 1986; Mayo & Pearson 1995).

During infusion of vesicant infusions

- Frequent assessment of needle position is advised, especially during vesicant infusions. This can be achieved by gently pressing on the needle or by aspiration of blood every 4 hours (Cunningham & Bonam-Crawford 1993; Wood & Gullo 1993).
- Observe the port site and chest wall for any signs of swelling. Check dressing for leakage as this may indicate extravasation (Schulmeister 1992). The site should be observed at least hourly (MacDonald 2001; Masoorli 2003). More frequent observation of the site (i.e. every 30 minutes) is advised during vesicant infusions (Masoorli 2003).
- If extravasation occurs, stop the infusion and follow the hospital's extravasation policy.
- Alarms on infusion pumps may sound when needles dislodge, but some will continue to infuse the vesicant into the subcutaneous tissue or onto the skin surface if complete needle dislodgement occurs (Schulmeister & Camp-Sorrell 2000). Infusion pumps cannot be relied to indicate extravasation, as the infiltration of fluid does not cause sufficient pressure to trigger an alarm (Marders 2005). Some infusion pumps allow the user to alter the occlusion alarm pressure. The occlusion alarm pressure should be set low to reduce the time it takes for the pump to alarm. The pressure can be set at approximately 30 mmHg higher than the pumping pressure (Amoore & Adamson 2003). It is important to note that whilst the occlusion alarm pressure system will protect against occlusions, it is not sufficiently sensitive to protect the child from extravasation (Irving 2001c). Venous pressure rises of as little as 30 mmHg have been known to lead to extravasation (Amoore & Adamson 2003). The importance of observing the site for signs of extravasation and the child for signs of pain/distress cannot be stressed enough. The nurse should not rely solely on the infusion pump to indicate extravasation. The pressure reading should be monitored and recorded hourly (MacDonald 2001).

Methods to Reduce Pain and Anxiety Associated with Intravenous Therapy Procedures

The requirement to help children cope with painful procedures related to i.v. therapies has been discussed by a number of authors (Duff 2003; Franck 2003; Willock *et al.* 2004; The Royal Australasian College of Physicians 2005). Children may experience pain and anxiety during a number of procedures associated with i.v. therapy, such as venepuncture, cannulation, capillary blood sampling (heel/finger prick), insertion of a PICC/midline catheter and implanted port access. All of these procedures involve the use of a needle to puncture the skin. Such procedures are particularly distressing for both children and those who assist in or witness the procedure, i.e. parents and staff. Venepuncture has been described as one of the most frightening aspects of hospital care (Duff 2003; Willock *et al.* 2004). Whether a child's reaction to needles can be labelled needle phobia has been challenged. Duff (2003) proposes that what is seen when a child is confronted with a needle is not a fear or phobia of needles per se, but anticipatory fear and distress. Furthermore, it is rare for a child to become frightened and upset on seeing needles outside the context of the procedure. In addition, fear ratings tend to be higher before insertion of the needle and decrease after insertion. Anticipatory or procedural distress necessitates the routine use of effective psychological techniques to avoid conflict, reduce unnecessary anticipation and promote effective coping strategies in children.

There is evidence that children's pain, including procedure-related pain, may be inadequately assessed and treated in hospital settings (DH 2003b; Franck 2003). Duff (2003) maintains that the continuing focus on replicating research findings in reducing venepuncture-related distress has meant that actually changing clinical practice has been neglected. He suggests that the problem is too big to be delegated solely to psychologically trained professionals, and that other staff such as play specialists and nurses should be supported and trained in psychological approaches to reduce distress. An example of a strategy employed to improve practice in performing venepuncture in an ambulatory care setting is provided by Thurgate and Heppell (2005).

The nurse involved in paediatric i.v. therapy should be familiar with different methods and techniques designed to alleviate pain and anxiety in children undergoing painful procedures. An understanding of the developmental level of the child is needed to initiate the most appropriate intervention (*See* Table 15.8). Broadly speaking, methods/techniques to reduce pain and anxiety can be considered as pharmacological (involving the use of medicines) or non-pharmacological (psychological techniques/interventions). The RCN (RCN 2005a,d) proposes the following competencies for nurses undertaking venepuncture, capillary blood sampling and cannulation. It is suggested that these can be adapted and applied to all painful (needle-related) procedures associated with i.v. therapy. The nurse should be able to:

- demonstrate best practice in gaining informed consent from the child and family
- assess the child's physical and psychological needs before, during and after the procedure and use these to develop a plan of care
- demonstrate knowledge of pharmacological and non-pharmacological methods and techniques that can be employed to reduce pain
- demonstrate the safe application of the principles of 'restraining, holding still and containing children' (RCN 2003)
- use appropriate strategies to minimize pain and distress
- communicate with the child and family during the procedure using a manner that minimises anxiety and encourages compliance
- identify when other staff should be involved in the preparation of children and families (e.g. play specialist, child psychologist).

Pharmacological techniques employed in paediatric intravenous therapy procedures

Topical anaesthetic agents
The use of topical anaesthetic agents for needle-related procedures can be hailed as the single most important development in children's pain management. However, it should be remembered that these agents do not eliminate the behavioural distress associated

Table 15.8 Interventions to reduce anxiety associated with intravenous therapy procedures (Duff 2003;Doellman 2003, 2004; Ferguson & Costa; Willcock *et al.* 2004; Frey 2006).

Age	Developmental stage	Intervention
0–1 years	Fears separation from parents and strangers	Encourage parents' presence. Provide physical comfort and warmth during procedure Wrap in a blanket; use dummy. Give feed or oral glucose during procedure. Use visual and auditory stimulation to distract e.g. with bright, noisy toys, blowing bubbles. Prepare parents—describe what will happen and their role during the procedure
1–3 years	Limited concept of time Prone to fantasies; bargains and stalls to avoid procedures Unable to comply with commands to sit still and not touch equipment Short attention span Limited language skills Likes to say 'no'	Encourage parents' presence Prepare immediately prior to procedure. Provide simple explanations of what will happen Distract with blowing bubbles, 'pop up' books, books that make sounds, songs, stories and counting Allow favourite toy and comfort items (blanket, dummy) Offer reward immediately after procedure, e.g. stickers. Allow child to play with equipment used, e.g. syringes in the bath, stick plaster on a doll Do not offer a choice as the answer will be no!
4–6 years	Attention span 15 minutes Vivid imagination Fears bodily injury, loss of control, being alone, blood loss, invasive procedures and the dark May consider pain as a form of punishment Easily engages in distraction techniques	Encourage parents' presence Prepare prior to procedure. Allow security/comfort items. Use simple terminology in explanations Give control where possible, e.g. choice of plaster, help with cleaning the site Use dolls to explain what is happening and how it will feel. Use doll with a CVAD *in situ*. Use medical play. Use stories that involve the child or a super hero Distract by getting the child to blow away pain, blow feather off adult's hand, favourite video Praise cooperation. Reassure that it is OK to cry. Use positive reinforcement
6–12 years	Wants to participate in the procedure Grasps concept of time, including future and past Wants to understand what is happening Needs a sense of control Language skills improving Increasing awareness of body functions	Encourage parents' presence Prepare hours in advance of the procedure Offer choices Allow child to help as much as possible during the procedure Reassure that it is OK to cry. Offer unconditional praise Distract with games, counting, sums, telling jokes, favourite video Use dolls or models, photograph books or videos of procedure for explanations
12 + years	Fears loss of control, being different from peers, altered body image Peer group important to child Able to think and reason in the abstract Understands how the body functions Increasing independence from parents	Parental presence if requested by the child Prepare in advance Encourage participation and allow the child a part in their care. Offer choices, e.g. site of cannula, method of fixation, time of procedure Explanations using adult terminology Promote independence Provide privacy during procedure Use another child of the same age to explain procedure Use body diagrams and models to aid explanations Hypnosis, guided imagery, relaxation techniques. Distract using Walkman and favourite music, videos or computer games

with the fear of needles (Franck 2003). In many children's hospitals it has become standard practice to use a topical anaesthetic for all procedures that involve the use of a needle (Ellis *et al.* 2004). Topical anaesthetics used in practice include EMLA (eutectic mixture of local anaesthetics: lignocaine 2.5%, prilocaine 2.5%; 2 g), Ametop gel (amethocaine 4% w/w; 1 g) and ethyl chloride (Cryogesic™).

In a meta-analysis of 20 studies EMLA has been shown to significantly reduce the pain of venepuncture and cannulation in 85% of the population (Fetzer 2002). EMLA should not be used in children below 1 month of age, as it is associated with methaemo-globinaemia (Moureau & Zonderman 2000; The Royal Pharmaceutical Society of Great Britain 2005). Side-effects include transient paleness, redness and oedema (The Royal Pharmaceutical Society of Great Britain 2005). Vasoconstriction has been reported with the use of EMLA; applying the cream immediately below the preferred portion of vein will minimize this difficulty (Moureau & Zonderman 2000). For some children the application of EMLA or removing the dressing acts as a stimulus for distress and avoidance behaviours in the child. Some parents may choose not to use topical anaesthetic creams as the distress exhibited in the child outweighs the potential benefits of pain relief (Dahlquist *et al.* 2002a; Duff 2003; Ellis 2004).

EMLA has been used to numb the skin prior to PICC insertion. EMLA is placed directly below the vein in the area where the introducer will penetrate the skin to counteract the negative effects of vasoconstriction. In addition 1% lidocaine may be injected subcutaneously in the numb area where the EMLA cream has been, to further reduce the pain of PICC insertion (Doellman 2003). The use of EMLA has also been reported for midline catheter insertion in children with cystic fibrosis (Turner *et al.* 2002).

A more recent addition to the range of topical anaesthetic agents is Ametop gel. This has been compared with EMLA in several studies (Lawson *et al.* 1995; Morton 1996; Arrowsmith & Campbell 2000; O'Brien *et al.* 2005; Lander & Weltman 2006). Ametop is comparable to EMLA when used for venepuncture and accessing CVADs for paediatric pain. In addition, anaesthesia can be achieved more rapidly and with an extended duration of action using Ametop, thus making it more useful in busy clinical settings (O'Brien *et al.* 2005). Arrowsmith and Campbell (2000) found that both EMLA and Ametop produced adequate analgesia for cannulation. However, children in the Ametop group demonstrated significantly less pain than those in the EMLA group. A Cochrane review by Lander and Weltman (2006) confirms the superiority of Ametop for the prevention of pain associated with needle procedures in comparison to EMLA.

Limited research has been conducted into the pain and anxiety associated with implanted port access in children. The use of both EMLA and Ametop as a topical anaesthetic before insertion of a needle into an implanted port has been studied in children (Halperin *et al.* 1989; Miser *et al.* 1994; Bishai *et al.* 1999). Halperin *et al.* (1989) compared EMLA with placebo for port access in children aged 6–14 years. Using a visual analogue scale, the pain scores were significantly lower ($P< 0.04$) when EMLA was used. The children in this study rated the pain of accessing a port as 3.9 with placebo, and 1.8 with EMLA on a scale of 1–10 (0 = no pain, 10 = the worst pain imaginable). Miser *et al.* (1994) found a statistically significant reduction in pain intensity scores ($P< 0.002$) reported by children and investigators in a comparison of EMLA and placebo in children with cancer undergoing implanted port access. In a comparison of ELMA and Ametop, Bishai *et al.* (1999) found Ametop to be clinically equivalent to EMLA for the relief of pain during implanted port access. They advocated the use of Ametop on the basis of a shorter application time.

There are far fewer studies investigating the use of topical anaesthetics to relieve pain associated with implanted port access when compared to the wealth of research related to venepuncture and cannulation. Despite the lack of research into the efficacy of topical anaesthetics for the alleviation of the pain of port access, it has been described as routine in paediatric practice (Bravery & Hannan 1997; Ellis *et al.* 2004; Kurdahi Badr *et al.* 2006). Anecdotally, Ross *et al.* (1988) maintained that the level of pain felt during port access is dependent on who inserts the needle. This has implications for nurses not experienced in this procedure. Further research is needed to establish the efficacy of topical anaesthetics before port needle insertion and the effect of other factors such as operator experience and the role of non-pharmacological methods to reduce pain and anxiety.

Ethyl chloride spray temporarily numbs the skin on contact (Heckler-Medina 2006). It is a topical anaesthetic skin refrigerant, applied seconds before the needle insertion (Moureau & Zonderman 2000). It can be used to produce instant skin anaesthesia. There is some confusion over application techniques (distance from the skin when applying the spray and length of time to apply the spray), and no instruction is provided by the manufacturers on its administration for venepuncture (Davies & Molloy 2006). Its use in children has been described anecdotally as an alternative to EMLA and Ametop to relieve the pain associated with vascular access procedures (Moureau & Zonderman 2000; Heckler-Medina 2006). Zappa and Nabors (1992) described the use of ethyl chloride spray to reduce the pain of port access. Children aged 7–12 years received the greatest benefit from use of the spray. Younger children in the study perceived the spray as painful due to the intense cold feeling. A more recent study by Davies and Molloy (2006) compared ethyl chloride spray with Ametop for children undergoing venepuncture. Ethyl chloride spray was found to be comparable to Ametop, with lower self-reported pain scores. The authors suggest that it is fast acting, convenient and cheaper than topical anaesthetics and can be viewed as an alternative option to topical anaesthesia, although further research is needed to clarify the application technique.

Whatever topical anaesthetic agent is used it must be applied in accordance with the manufacturer's instructions for it to be effective.

Entonox

The use of nitrous oxide to manage procedural pain in children has expanded in recent years (Bruce & Franck 2000). Its use with respect to i.v. therapy procedures includes venepuncture and peripheral venous cannulation (Annequin *et al.* 2000; Bruce & Franck 2000; The Royal Australasian College of Physicians 2005), and midline catheter insertion (Turner *et al.* 2002). Nitrous oxide is a mixture of nitrous oxide and oxygen containing 50% of each gas (Entonox®, Equanox®) that can be used to produce analgesia without loss of consciousness (The Royal Pharmaceutical Society of Great Britain 2005). It is said to be effective when used in children aged 3 years or older, with few side-effects (Annequin *et al.* 2000). There are two methods of administration: continuous flow using a mask, or self-administration. Continuous flow may lead to deep sedation and necessitates close monitoring by trained healthcare professionals and immediate access to emergency equipment. In contrast, self-administration avoids the potential problem of over-sedation and the need for special monitoring or equipment. It can also involve the child in their own pain management, offering the child some control during the procedure. It is suggested that nitrous oxide is used as an adjunct to analgesia and psychological interventions and not in isolation (Bruce & Franck 2000).

Sedation

In paediatric i.v. therapy the use of sedation has been described for PICC insertion (Doellman 2004; Ferguson & Costa 2004), vascular access procedures such as venepuncture and cannulation (Scottish Intercollegiate Guidelines Network (SIGN) 2004), midline catheter insertion (Turner *et al.* 2002) and implanted port access (Ljungman *et al.* 2000). Sedation is defined as the drug-induced depression of consciousness during which patients respond purposefully to verbal commands, either alone or accompanied by light tactile stimulation (SIGN 2004). Intervention is not required to maintain a patent airway and spontaneous ventilation is adequate. Cardiovascular function is usually maintained. Sedation in children should only be performed in an environment where the facilities, personnel and equipment to manage emergency situations are immediately available. The response of a child to sedation is unpredictable. The child may progress in depth of sedation along the continuum to anaesthesia. This must be anticipated and managed safely whenever sedatives are given (SIGN 2004).

Sedation is not without risk and the decision to use sedation in children should not be taken lightly as it can be associated with drug-related adverse outcomes (Cote *et al.* 2000). In paediatric settings sedation is not routinely employed for i.v. therapy procedures such as venepuncture, cannulation and implanted port access. It should be reserved for situations/procedures where other more commonly utilized methods such as topical anaesthetics and non-pharmacological techniques have failed. Ljungman *et al.* (2000) maintain that sedation is indicated in paediatric settings when other means to overcome a child's fears fail. For short procedures gentle containment or restraint may reduce the requirement or need for sedation and is preferable to forcible restraint (SIGN 2004). Practitioners performing any procedure that requires the use of restraint of a child should perhaps consider performing the procedure under sedation (Ferguson & Costa 2004). Holding a child down and using physical restraint to facilitate a procedure has ethical, legal and safety implications for the staff, parents and child involved (Tomlinson 2004). The RCN has produced guidelines for restraining, holding still and containing children, and these should be used to guide practice in such situations (RCN 2003).

When choosing a drug or technique for sedation, consideration should be given as to whether the procedure is painless or painful (SIGN 2004). For a painful procedure a sedative may be given in combination with a local anaesthesia (topical or as a nerve block) (The Royal Pharmaceutical Society of Great Britain 2005). Topical anaesthetics should be used for techniques that involve the use of a needle during sedation (SIGN 2004). Benzodiazepines can be employed to sedate a child. Whilst these drugs have an anxiolytic and amnesic effect, they have no analgesic properties. Thus drugs used for sedation may not provide adequate analgesia. Benzodiazepines are particularly useful for short procedures or during procedures where a local anaesthetic is used (The Royal Pharmaceutical Society of Great Britain 2005). Examples of benzodiazepines commonly used for sedation include midazolam, diazepam, and lorazepam (Ferguson & Costa 2004). Intranasal midazolam has been shown to relieve anxiety in children during implanted port access, venepuncture, and cannulation. Its use by this route is limited, particularly in young children who dislike the associated nasal discomfort (Ljungman *et al.* 2000). Oral chloral hydrate and triclofos are other drugs that may be used to sedate children, particularly school-aged children (The Royal Pharmaceutical Society of Great Britain 2005).

If deep sedation/general anaesthesia is required, propofol, ketamine, or a potent opioid such as fentanyl may be used. In the UK, deep sedation is considered to be part of the spectrum of general anaesthesia. Drugs used for general anaesthesia should only be administered in a hospital setting by an appropriately trained anaesthetist (SIGN 2004). General anaesthesia may be necessary for prolonged procedures that may be painful or distressing. In paediatric i.v. therapy the insertion of a tunnelled central venous catheter or implanted port usually requires the use of a general anaesthetic. However, older children and adolescents may tolerate central venous catheter insertion with sedation and analgesia. This is dependent on the child's psychological coping skills, preparation level and patient/family choice (The Royal Australasian College of Physicians 2005). PICC insertion can be achieved successfully using sedation in children. The insertion technique used during PICC placement may indicate the need for sedation. A modified Seldinger or microintroducer technique is more invasive than using a peel-away catheter and may dictate the requirement for sedation. In addition, sedation may be necessary if ultrasound is used to locate the vein and to ensure the child remains still and cooperative (Doellmann 2004). It may be feasible for the child to have a PICC placed whilst undergoing another procedure under general anaesthesia; for example lumbar puncture and intrathecal chemotherapy in a child with leukaemia, or bronchoscopy in a child with cystic fibrosis.

Section 3

The use of pharmacological techniques in neonates

The use of pharmacological treatments in neonates has been avoided because of concerns over adverse side-effects (Carbajal *et al.* 2003). There is a risk of methaemoglobinaemia associated with the use of EMLA. More current advice indicates that these risks can be minimized by using EMLA no more frequently than daily, on intact skin, and avoiding the use of other medicines known to cause methaemoglobinaemia (American Academy of Pediatrics and Canadian Paediatric Society 2006). The efficacy of Ametop for venepuncture and cannulation in neonates has been studied in two randomized controlled trials. Jain and Rutter (2000) found that Ametop provides effective pain relief for venepuncture in newborns. Moore (2001) found Ametop to be an effective local anaesthetic for the relief of pain associated with cannulation in neonates. In contrast, Ametop has been shown to be ineffective for pain relief associated with PICC insertion in term and preterm infants (Ballantyne *et al.* 2003; Lemyre *et al.* 2006). Lemyre *et al.* (2006) suggest that the length of the procedure (up to 30 minutes), restraint of the infant, and application of a tourniquet may all contribute to the pain felt by the infant. PICC insertion is not just a simple skin puncture. It is suggested that a longer application time and the addition of oral sucrose may increase the effectiveness of Ametop when used for PICC insertion.

Non-pharmacological techniques employed in paediatric intravenous therapy procedures

A number of psychological interventions to manage the pain and distress associated with the use of needles in i.v. therapy in children are available. Most of these are cognitive behavioural interventions (Uman *et al.* 2005) (*See* Table 15.9). Cognitive behavioural

Table 15.9   Cognitive behavioural interventions for needle-related procedural pain in children (Duff 2003; Uman *et al.* 2005).

Intervention	Description
Modelling	Using a demonstration of positive coping behaviours during a mock procedure by another child. Often a film/video. Observing another child going through the procedure and overcoming it may help child to utilize coping skills
Relaxation training— includes progressive muscle relaxation and breathing exercises	Teaching the child to gain control over symptoms of psychological arousal by breathing slowly and deeply and releasing muscle tension. Can be used with guided imagery (*see* below) Breathing exercises—using party blowers or blowing bubbles
Guided imagery	Cognitive technique used to encourage the child to cope with pain/distress by imagining a pleasant object/experience
Distraction	Cognitive distraction—techniques to shift attention away from procedure-related pain or specific counter activities e.g. counting, listening to music, non-procedure related talk Behavioural distraction—techniques to shift attention away from procedure-related pain or specific counter activities e.g. videos, games, interactive books
Graded exposure/active behavioural rehearsal	Graded exposure to the feared stimulus e.g. the needle. May involve the development of a hierarchy of tasks related to the feared stimuli and successfully overcoming progressively more difficult tasks Elements of the procedure are rehearsed, quickly building up to full behavioural rehearsals in a treatment room
Reinforcement/incentive scheduling	Each accomplishment in a graded exposure hierarchy is rewarded, thus focusing on what the child is actually achieving as opposed to what remains to be achieved

therapy is a well-established intervention for procedure-related pain in children and adolescents. It encompasses breathing exercises and other forms of relaxation/distraction, imagery and other forms of cognitive coping skills, filmed modelling (depicting a coping peer model), reinforcement/incentives, behavioural rehearsal, and active coaching by a psychologist, parent and/or healthcare professional (Powers 1999). When choosing specific non-pharmacological interventions for children, consideration should be given to the child's age/cognitive level, type of pain and any contributing factors highlighted during pain assessment (McGrath 1999).

Nurses, play specialists and parents have an important role to play in employing various techniques to help children cope with painful procedures in i.v. therapy. Parents and staff may require training to undertake psychological interventions effectively. The technique should be rehearsed before the procedure takes place. Duff (2003) maintains that more emphasis should be given to training nurses and play specialists in psychological techniques, as they already possess skills in this area. Healthcare professionals should be able to use psychological techniques to improve the management of procedure-related pain, regardless of whether pharmacological methods are used. Psychological techniques have the advantage that they can be used in the anticipatory phase as well as before, during and after the procedure (The Royal Australasian College of Physicians 2005). Nurses may be more effective than parents in helping children cope with painful procedures. Thus nurses should be encouraged to take the lead during procedures. This approach will enable the parent to focus on comforting the child and clarify the roles of parents and nurses (Cohen *et al.* 2002).

The role of parents

A systematic review conducted in 2005 showed that the evidence is mixed as to the helpfulness to the child of parental presence during painful procedures. Whilst parental presence may not have a clear, direct influence on the child's distress and behavioural outcomes, there are potential advantages for parents. Parents' perception is that being there during a painful procedure is helpful for their child. This may give parents a sense of control, which should not be underestimated (Piira *et al.* 2005). Excluding parents during painful procedures may not be in the best interests of the child's family and is incongruent with a family-centred approach to care (Cohen *et al.* 2002).

Parents can be trained in both cognitive and behavioural interventions, the goal being to reduce the parent's distress which in turn can help relieve the child's distress and/or pain. Parents may also act as coaches for their child and verbally encourage their child to use a coping strategy throughout the procedure (Uman *et al.* 2005). If parents are able to learn coping strategies such as distraction and relaxation, they will be more able to effectively support their child during painful procedures (Christensen & Fatchett 2002). A study by Cavender *et al.* (2004) taught parents how to position and use distracters whilst their child underwent venepuncture or cannulation. This intervention was tested against standard care, which included a full explanation of the procedure and parental presence. The children whose parents used the positioning/distraction intervention demonstrated significantly less fear than children receiving standard care. Levels of self-reported fear and pain and observed distress, although not statistically different, tended to be lower in the intervention group. No topical anaesthesia was used in this study. The study concludes that if parents are given a clear role, guidance and coaching it will maximize their presence and facilitate child coping. The positioning/distraction intervention is an age-appropriate, inexpensive, easy-to-use non-pharmacological adjunct to conventional standards of care.

It should be remembered that not all parents are able to be there whilst their child undergoes a painful procedure, and some will prefer not to watch. The parent may have a fear of needles, and these fears may be transmitted to the child, thus increasing the distress (Sclare & Waring 1995). Parents in this situation will need help from staff to overcome their own fears in order to help their child. If parents choose not to participate, their wishes should be respected. Parents should not be involved in restraining their child during a procedure (Duff 2003).

Distraction techniques

Distraction is a simple, practical, inexpensive, psychological pain management technique that has the potential to remain effective over several repeated procedures (Dahlquist 2002a). Distraction is described as an active process that involves diverting attention away from the hurt, pain, fear and anxiety to something incompatible with those experiences. Other techniques, such as relaxation and imagery, can be employed to augment the effect of distraction interventions (Blount *et al.* 1999). The aim of this technique is to capture the child's interest during the procedure. It will only be effective if the child's age, developmental level and interests are taken into account (Sclare & Waring 1995). The distracter used must be appealing and of interest to the child. The more interactive and varied the distraction technique, and the more active processing and motor responses used by the child, the greater the chance of a reduction in distress (Dahlquist *et al.* 2002b). The distracter must be variable enough to continue to be interesting to the child for repeated procedures; electronic games are ideal. Distraction should involve the child in an activity he enjoys. This may include singing, counting, story-telling, games, telling jokes, as well as the use of television, favourite videos and electronic games. The school-age child may enjoy a story that involves either themselves or a TV superhero, especially when they can add their own contribution to the story. The involvement of a play specialist to facilitate distraction is invaluable and allows the nurse or doctor to concentrate on the procedure. Tools for distraction have perhaps become increasingly more sophisticated and technological over time. Initial research described simple measures such as party blowers and bubbles to distract children during painful procedures. More recent research has focused on the use of interactive multisensory computer games, the use of computer-taught coping skills (Franck & Jones 2003) and the use of virtual reality (Gershon *et al.* 2004; Uman *et al.* 2005) as tools for distraction.

There are however, times when distraction may prove to be ineffective; children may have bad days when nothing will distract them. It should also be remembered that not all children respond to distraction (Dhalquist *et al.* 2002a).

The use of non-pharmacological techniques in neonates

Heel lance and venepuncture are the most common painful procedures performed on healthy infants. There is a tendency to avoid the use of pharmacological treatments due to concerns about adverse side-effects in neonates (Carbajal *et al.* 2003). However, topical anaesthetics have been shown to be ineffective for these procedures in this age group (American Academy of Pediatrics and Canadian Paediatric Society 2006). The technique employed when obtaining blood samples from neonates has been shown to be important. Statistically significant lower pain scores are achieved if venepuncture is the method used for blood sampling (Shah & Ohlsson 2004).

In neonates sucrose, non-nutritive sucking and breastfeeding have been shown to reduce pain during venepuncture and heel lancing (Carbajal *et al.* 2003; Stevens *et al.* 2004). The administration of sucrose with or without non-nutritive sucking (use of a dummy) is the most frequently studied non-pharmacological intervention for the relief of procedural pain in neonates. Current recommendations indicate that a combination of oral sucrose/glucose and other non-pharmacological pain reduction methods (sucking, skin-to-skin contact, facilitated tuck, swaddling and developmental care) should be used for minor painful procedures in neonates. Attempts should be made by staff to reduce the overall number of painful procedures experienced in this age group (American Academy of Pediatrics and Canadian Paediatric Society 2006). Dummies should only be used in accordance with the parent's wishes and consent.

Play

Therapeutic play is structured by adults for children. Its aims to help the child achieve emotional and physical well-being by engaging in various activities, in order to achieve therapeutic ends (Stebbings 2006). Play can be used as a means of helping a child assimilate new information, adjust to and gain control over a potentially frightening environment, and prepare for/cope with procedures and investigations (DH 2003b). Children can be prepared through the use of play and education when painful procedures are planned (DH 2004c).

'Needle play' can be used to help children cope with fears associated with procedures that involve the use of needles. This type of play is usually undertaken on a one-to one basis with the child and involves using real needles in a controlled manner. It is recommended that only a hospital play specialist or nurse who has received training in 'needle play' should undertake this activity (Stebbings 2006). For more information about needle play refer to the National Association of Hospital Play Staff website www.nahps.org.uk/needle.html (NAHPS 2000).

Play preparation is an invaluable tool for parents and nurses to help children cope with painful procedures associated with i.v. therapy. The language of play is understood by all children, whereas information conveyed verbally may be misunderstood or forgotten (Collier *et al.* 1993).

Dolls and puppets can be used to demonstrate, in a non-threatening manner, what will happen during a procedure (Frey 2006; Stebbings 2006). A doll with a CVC *in situ* can be used to explain what will happen during a dressing change or drug administration. A puppet can 'tell' the child what will happen during venepuncture, what it will feel like, how long it will last and how the child should respond.

Photographic books and videos that detail a child undergoing the planned procedure are useful to prepare older children. These can convey information about the actual procedure and can be used by the adult as a focus for discussion. Story books centring on a child coping with the procedure have the advantage that they can be used in advance and repeatedly at the child's own pace.

Integrated approaches (pharmacological and non-pharmacological)

Interventions that combine behavioural and pharmacological approaches may be more effective than the use of medicines alone. An integrated approach is advocated that involves combining pharmacological and non-pharmacological approaches to procedure-related pain in children. (Powers 1999; Duff 2003; The Royal Australasian College of Physicians 2005). An integrated approach may also be more effective in reducing anxiety in the child. Although pain can be treated effectively with the use of medications, anxiety before and during the procedure may continue to be a problem, especially for younger children or during a child's first encounter with a procedure (Manne 1999). Examples of integrated approaches employed in children requiring venepuncture are described by Kolk *et al.* (2000) and Schiff *et al.* (2001).

Conclusion

There are many factors to consider when caring for children with venous access devices *in situ*. The nurse should be knowledgeable of the complications and risks associated with the care and use of venous access devices and the most effective management strategies.

Section 3

Safety in the administration of i.v. therapies to children is paramount. In addition, the nurse involved in caring for children receiving i.v. therapies should consider the child's developmental level and emotional needs, and actively seek to minimize the pain and anxiety associated with i.v. therapy procedures. This chapter has highlighted a lack of research in paediatric i.v. therapy practices and has identified variations in practice at both a national and international level. As a consequence, research from and guidelines created for adult populations are often adapted for use in paediatric practice. There is a pressing need for high-quality research to establish the optimal management of venous access devices in paediatric populations.

References

Aitken ML, Tonelli MR (2000) Complications of indwelling catheters in cystic fibrosis. A 10-year review. *Chest* 118(6): 1598–1602.

American Academy of Pediatrics and Canadian Paediatric Society (2006) Prevention and management of pain in the neonate: an update. *Pediatrics* 118(5): 2231–2241.

Amoore J, Adamson L (2003) Infusion devices: characteristics, limitations and risk management. *Nursing Standard* 17(28): 45–52.

Andris DA, Krzywa EA (1999) Central venous catheter occlusion: successful management strategies *Medsurg Nursing* 8(4): 229–236.

Annequin D, Carbajal R, Chauvin P *et al.* (2000) Fixed 50% nitrous oxide oxygen mixture for painful procedures: a French survey. *Pediatrics* 105(4): E47–E52.

Arrowsmith J, Campbell C (2000) A comparison of local anaesthetics for venepuncture. *Archives of Disease in Childhood* 82(4): 309–310.

Association for Women's Health, Obstetric and Neonatal Nurses (2001) *Neonatal Skin Care. Evidence-based Clinical Practice Guideline.* AWHONN, Washington.

Axton SE, Hall B (1994) An innovative method of administering IV medications to children. *Pediatric Nursing* 20(4): 341–344.

Bagnall H, Ruccione K (1987) Experience with a totally implanted venous access device in children with malignant disease. *Oncology Nursing Forum* 14(4): 51–55.

Bagnall-Reeb H (1998) Diagnosis of central venous access device occlusion. *Journal of Intravenous Nursing* 21(5S): S115–S121.

Bagnall-Reeb HA, Ruccione K (1990) Management of cutaneous reactions and mechanical complications of central venous access devices in pediatric patients with cancer: algorithms for decision making. *Oncology Nursing Forum* 17(5): 677–681.

Ballantyne M, McNair C, Ung E *et al.* (2003) A randomized controlled trial evaluating the efficacy of tetracaine gel for pain relief from peripherally inserted central catheters in infants. *Advances in Neonatal Care* 3(6): 297–307.

Banta C (1992) Hyaluronidase. *Neonatal Network* 11(6): 103–104.

Barber JM, Booth DM, King JA *et al.* (2002) A nurse-led peripherally inserted central catheter line insertion service is effective with radiological support. *Clinical Radiology* 57(5): 352–354.

Bard Access Systems Inc. (2003) *Groshong NXT PICC Nursing Procedure Manual.* Available from www.bardaccess.com (accessed 4 January 2007).

Ben-Arush M, Berant M (1996) Retention of drugs in venous access port chamber: a note of caution. *British Medical Journal* 312: 496–497.

Bishai R, Taddio A, Bar-Oz B *et al.* (1999) Relative efficacy of amethocaine gel and lidocaine-prilocaine cream for port-a-cath puncture in children. *Pediatrics* 104(3): 31–33.

Blakeley JA, Ribeiro V, Crocker J (2000) Parent satisfaction with education, support, and decision-making regarding their children's central venous access devices. *Canadian Oncology Nursing Journal* 10(1): 8–10.

Blount RL, Schaen ER, Cohen LL (1999) Commentary: current status and future directions in acute pediatric pain assessment and treatment *Journal of Pediatric Psychology* 24(2): 150–152.

Bothe A, Piccione W, Ambrosino JJ, Benotti PN, Lokich JJ (1984) Implantable central venous access system. *The American Journal of Surgery* 147: 565–569.

Bravery K, Hannan J (1997) The use of long term central venous access devices in children. *Paediatric Nursing* 9(10): 29–37.

Bravery K, Todd J (2002) The AccessAbility™ Programme. Bard Limited, London. Available from www.accessabilitybybard.co.uk (accessed 10 December 2006).

Bravery KA, Wright L (1998) Practical considerations of peripheral blood stem cell collection in children with solid tumours. *European Journal of Oncology Nursing* 2(2): 123–128.

Brothers TE, Niederhuber JE, Roberts JA, Ensminger WD (1988) Experience with subcutaneous infusion ports in three hundred patients. *Surgery, Gynecology and Obstetrics* 166(4): 295–301.

Broviac JW, Cole JJ, Schribner BH (1973) A silicone rubber atrial catheter for prolonged parenteral alimentation. *Surgery, Gynecology and Obstetrics* 136(4): 602–606.

Brown P (2002) Volumetric infusion pumps: the challenge of change. *Paediatric Nursing* 14(1): 14–18.

Bruce E, Franck L (2000) Self-administered nitrous oxide (Entonox) for the management of procedural pain. *Paediatric Nursing* 12(7): 15–19.

Callaghan S, Copnell B, Johnston L (2002) Comparison of two methods of peripheral intravenous cannula securement in the pediatric setting. *Journal of Infusion Nursing* 25(4): 256–264.

Cameron GS (1987) Central venous catheters for children with malignant disease: surgical issues. *Journal of Pediatric Surgery* 22(8): 702–704.

Carbajal R, Veerapen S, Couderc S *et al.* (2003) Analgesic effect of breast feeding in term neonates: randomized controlled trial, *British Medical Journal* 326(7379): 13–15.

Carson SM (2004) Chlorhexidine versus povidone-iodine for central venous catheter site care in children. *Journal of Pediatric Nursing* 19(1): 74–80.

Cavender K, Goff MD, Hollon EC *et al.* (2004) Parents' positioning and distracting children during venepuncture. *Journal of Holistic Nursing* 22(1): 32–56.

Centers for Disease Control and Prevention (CDC) (2002) Guidelines for the prevention of intravascular catheter-related infections. *Morbidity and Mortality Weekly Report* 51(RR10): S35–S63.

Choi M, Massicotte P, Marzinotto V *et al.* (2001) The use of alteplase to restore patency of central venous lines in pediatric patients: a cohort study, *Journal of Pediatrics* 139(1): 152–156.

Chow LML, Friedman JN, MacArthur C *et al.* (2003) Peripherally inserted central catheter (PICC) fracture and embolisation in the pediatric population. *Journal of Pediatrics* 142(2): 141–144.

Christensen J, Fatchett D (2002) Promoting parental use of distraction and relaxation in pediatric oncology patients during invasive procedures. *Journal of Pediatric Oncology Nursing* 19(4): 127–132.

Clayden G (2004) Care of the sick child. In: Lissauer T, Clayden G, eds. *Illustrated Textbook of Paediatrics*, 2nd edn, pp. 39–51. Mosby, Edinburgh.

Cohen LL, Bernard RS, Greco LA *et al.* (2002) A child-focused intervention for coping with procedural pain: are parent and nurse necessary? *Journal of Pediatric Psychology* 27(8): 749–757.

Collier J, Mackinlay D, Watson AR (1993) Painful procedures: preparation and coping strategies for children. *Maternal and Child Health* 18(9): 282–286.

Conn C (1993) The importance of syringe size when using implanted vascular access devices. *Journal of Vascular Access Networks* 3(1): 11–18.

Cosca PA, Smith S, Chatfield S *et al.* (1998) Reinfusion of discard blood from venous access devices. *Oncology Nursing Forum* 25(6): 1073–1076.

Cote CJ, Karl HW, Notterman DA *et al.* (2000) Adverse sedation events in pediatrics: an analysis of medications used for sedation. *Pediatrics* 106(4): 633–644.

Crowley JJ (2003) Vascular access. *Techniques in Vascular and Interventional Radiology* 6(4): 176–181.

Cunningham RS, Bonam-Crawford D (1993) The role of fibrinolytic agents in the management of thrombotic complications associated with vascular access devices. *Nursing Clinics of North America* 28(4): 899–909.

Dahlquist LM, Busby SM, Slifer KJ *et al.* (2002a) Distraction for children of different ages who undergo repeated needle sticks. *Journal of Pediatric Oncology Nursing* 19(1): 22–34.

Dahlquist LM, Shroff Pendley J, Landthrip DS *et al.* (2002b) Distraction intervention for preschoolers undergoing intramuscular injections and subcutaneous port access. *Health Psychology* 21(1): 94–99.

Dale JC, Ruby SG (2003) Specimen collection volumes for laboratory tests. *Archives of Pathology and Laboratory Medicine* 127(2): 162–168.

Danek GD, Noris EM (1992) Pediatric IV catheters: efficacy of saline flush. *Paediatric Nursing* 18(2): 111–113.

Davies EH, Molloy A (2006) Comparison of ethyl chloride spray with topical anaesthetic in children experiencing venepuncture. *Paediatric Nursing* 18(3): 39–43.

Dawson D (2002) Midline catheters in neonatal patients. Evaluating a change in practice. *Journal of Vascular Access Devices* 7(2): 17–19.

De Backer A, Otten VJ, Deconinck P (1993) Totally implantable central venous access devices in pediatric oncology—our experience in 46 patients. *European Journal of Pediatric Surgery* 3:101–106.

Decker MD, Edwards KM (1988) Central venous catheter infections. *Pediatric Clinics of North America* 35(3): 579–612.

Department of Health (DH) (2001) *Seeking Consent: Working with Children*. Department of Health, London.

Department of Health (2003a) *Winning Ways: Working Together to Reduce Healthcare Associated Infection in England*. Department of Health, London.

Department of Health (2003b) *Getting the Right Start: National Service Framework for Children. Standard for Hospital Services*. Department of Health, London.

Department of Health (2004a) *Building a Safer NHS for Patients. Improving Medication Safety*. Department of Health, London.

Department of Health (2004b) *National Service Framework for Children, Young People and Maternity Services. Medicines for Children and Young People*. Department of Health, London.

Department of Health (2004c) *National Service Framework for Children, Young People and Maternity Services. Children and Young People who are Ill.* Department of Health, London.

Doellman D (2003) Pharmacological versus non-pharmacological techniques in reducing venepuncture psychological trauma in pediatric patients. *Journal of Infusion Nursing* 26(2): 103–109.

Doellman D (2004) Pediatric PICC insertions easing the fears in infants and children. *Journal of the Association of Vascular Access* 9(2): 68–71.

Dougherty L, ed. (2006) *Central Venous Access Devices. Care and Management.* Blackwell Publishing, Oxford.

Drewett S (2000) Central venous catheter removal: procedures and rationale. *British Journal of Nursing* 9(22): 2304–2306, 2308, 2310.

Duck S (1997) Neonatal intravenous therapy. *Journal of Intravenous Nursing* 20(3): 121–128.

Duff AJA (2003) Incorporating psychological approaches into routine paediatric venepuncture. *Archives of Disease in Childhood* 88(10): 931–937.

Duffy LF, Kerzner B, Gebus V, Dice J (1989) Treatment of central venous catheter occlusions with hydrochloric acid. *Journal of Pediatrics* 114(6): 1002–1004.

Dyer L, Furze C, Maddox C *et al.* (2006) Administration of medicines. In: Trigg E, Mohammed TA, eds. *Practices in Children's Nursing. Guidelines for Hospital and Community,* 2nd edn, pp. 45–74. Elsevier Churchill Livingstone, Edinburgh.

Egan-Sansivero G (1995) Why pick a PICC? *Nursing* 25(7): 35–42.

Ellis J (1995) Administering drugs. *Paediatric Nursing* 7(4): 29–39.

Ellis JA, Sharp D, Newhook K *et al.* (2004) Selling comfort: a survey of interventions for needle procedures in a pediatric hospital. *Pain Management Nursing* 5(4): 144–152.

Ewenstein BM, Valentino LA, Journeycake JM *et al.* (2004) Consensus recommendations for use of central venous access devices in haemophilia. *Haemophilia* 10(5): 1365–2516.

Ferguson E, Costa N (2004) Pediatric sedation: it's more than just the drugs. *Journal of the Association of Vascular Access* 9(2): 73–77.

Fetzer SJ (2002) Reducing venepuncture and intravenous insertion pain with eutectic mixture of local anesthetic: a meta analysis. *Nursing Research* 51(2): 119–124.

Few BJ (1987) Hyaluronidase for treating intravenous extravasations. *American Journal of Maternal and Child Nursing* 12(1): 23.

Fisher AA, Deffenbaugh C, Poole RL *et al.* (2004) The use of alteplase for restoring patency to occluded central venous access devices in infants and children. *Journal of Infusion Nursing* 27(3): 171–174.

Fitzsimons R (2001) Intravenous cannulation. *Paediatric Nursing* 13(3):21–23.

Flemmer L, Chan JSL (1993) A pediatric protocol for management of extravasation injuries. *Pediatric Nursing* 19(4): 355–358, 424.

Flint A, McIntosh D, Davies MW (2005) Continuous infusion versus intermittent flushing to prevent loss of function of peripheral catheters used for drug administration in newborn infants. *Cochrane Database of Systematic reviews* 4 (CD004593.pub2): 1–12.

Ford NA, Drott HR, Cieplinski-Robertson JA (2003) Administration of IV medications via soluset. *Pediatric Nursing* 29(4): 283–319.

Foster L, Wallis M, Paterson B, James H (2002) A descriptive study of peripheral intravenous catheters in patients admitted to a pediatric unit in one Australian hospital. *Journal of Infusion Nursing* 25(3): 159–167.

Franck L (2003) Nursing management of children's pain: current evidence and future directions for research. *Nursing Times Research* 8(5): 330–353.

Franck L, Jones M (2003) Computer-taught coping techniques for venepuncture: preliminary findings from usability testing with children, parents and staff. *Journal of Child Health Care* 7(1): 41–54.

Frey AM (1998) Success rates for peripheral IV insertion in a children's hospital. *Journal of Intravenous Nursing* 21(3): 160–165.

Frey AM (1999) PICC complications in neonates and children. *Journal of Vascular Access Devices* 4(1): 17–26.

Frey AM (2000) Pediatric I.V. insertion. *Nursing* 30(12): 54–56.

Frey AM (2001) Intravenous therapy in children. In: Hankins J, Walderman Lonsway RA, Hedrick C, Perdue MB, eds,. *Infusion Therapy in Clinical Practice,* 2nd edn, pp. 561–591. WB Saunders, Philadelphia.

Frey AM (2002) Peripherally inserted central catheters in neonates and children. Modified Seldinger (microintroducer) technique. *Journal of Vascular Access Devices* 7(2): 9–19.

Frey AM (2003) Drawing blood samples from vascular access devices. *Journal of Infusion Nursing* 26(5): 285–293.

Frey AM (2007) Pediatric intravenous therapy. In: Weinstein SM, ed. *Plumer's Principles and Practice of Intravenous Therapy,* 8th edn, pp. 613–685. Lippincott Williams and Wilkins, Philadelphia.

Galway R, Harrod ME, Crisp J *et al.* (2003) Central venous access and handwashing: variability in policies and practices. *Paediatric Nursing* 15(10): 14–8.

Garland JS, Dunne WM, Havens P *et al.* (1992) Peripheral intravenous catheter complications in critically ill children: a prospective study. *Pediatrics* 89(6): 1145–1150.

Garland JS, Alex CP, Mueller CD *et al.* (2001) A randomized trial comparing povidone-iodine to a chlorhexidine gluconate-impregnated dressing for prevention of central venous catheter infections in neonates. *Pediatrics* 107(6): 1431–1436.

Garland JS, Henrickson K, Maki DG (2002) The 2002 Hospital Infection Control Practices Advisory Committee Centers for Disease Control and Prevention guideline for prevention of intravascular device-related infection. *Pediatrics* 110(5): 1009–1013.

Gault DT (1993) Extravasation injuries. *British Journal of Plastic Surgery* 46: 91–96.

Gault D (2006) *Extravasation Flush-Out Technique. The National Extravasation Information Service.* Available from www.extravasation.org.uk (accessed 4 December 2006).

Gershon J, Zimand E, Pickering M *et al.* (2004) A pilot and feasibility study of virtual reality as a distraction for children with cancer. *Journal of The American Academy of Child and Adolescent Psychiatry* 43(10): 1243–1249.

Gordon K, Dearmun AK (2003) Occlusion problems in central venous catheters: the child and family perspective. *Journal of Child Health Care* 7(1): 55–69.

Gordon K, Lloyd A (2003) An exploration of the possible causes of occlusion problems in skin-tunnelled catheters used in paediatric oncology. *Nursing Times Research* 8(5): 380–388.

Gordon B, Crisp J, Nagy S *et al.* (2002) Children's efforts to make sense of intravenous cannulation. *Australian Nursing Journal* 10(4): 27–29.

Goren A, Laufer J, Yativ N *et al.* (2001) Transillumination of the palm for venepuncture in infants. *Pediatric Emergency Care* 17(2): 130–131.

Gullo SM (1993) Implanted ports: technologic advances and nursing care issues. *Nursing Clinics of North America* 29(4): 850–871.

Gyr P, Smith K, Pontious S, Burroughs T, Mahl C, Swerczek L (1995) Double blind comparison of heparin and saline flush solutions in maintenance of peripheral infusion devices. *Pediatric Nursing* 21(4): 383–389.

Hacking MB, Brown J, Chisholm DG (2003) Position-dependent ventricular tachycardia in two children with peripherally inserted central catheters (PICCs). *Paediatric Anaesthesia* 13(6): 527–529.

Hadaway L (1998a) Catheter connection—are large syringes necessary? *Journal of Vascular Access Devices* 3(3): 40.

Hadaway L (1998b) Major thrombotic and nonthrombotic complications. *Journal of Intravenous Nursing* 21(5S): S143–S160.

Hadaway L (1999) Catheter connection. *Journal of Vascular Access Devices* 4(1): 41.

Hadaway L (2002) IV infiltration. *Nursing* 32(8): 36–42.

Hadaway L (2003) Catheter connection—blood sampling from catheters, *Journal of the Association for Vascular Access* 8(3): 38.

Hallquist Viale P (2003) Complications associated with implantable vascular access devices in the patient with cancer. *Journal of Infusion Nursing* 26(2): 97–102.

Halperin DL, Koren G, Attias D, Pellegrini E, Greenberg ML, Wyss M (1989) Topical skin anesthesia for venous, subcutaneous drug reservoir and lumbar punctures in children. *Pediatrics* 84(2): 281–284.

Hanrahan KS, Kleiber C, Loebig Fagan C (1994) Evaluation of saline for IV locks in children. *Pediatric Nursing* 20(6): 549–552.

Harris JL, Maguire D (1999) Developing a protocol to prevent and treat pediatric central venous catheter occlusions. *Journal of Intravenous Nursing* 22(4): 194–198.

Hatchard L, O'Leary S (1999) Pre-operative awareness for children with implantable ports. *Journal of Child Health Care* 3(2): 20–23.

Hazinski MF (1992) Children are different. In: Ladig D, Van Schaik T, eds. *Nursing Care of the Critically Ill Child*, 2nd edn. pp. 1–17 Mosby, St Louis.

Heckler-Medina GA (2006) The importance of child life and pain management during vascular access procedures in pediatrics. *Journal of the Association of Vascular Access* 11(3): 144–151.

Hicks-Keen J (1995) Drug update. Slow down. *Journal of Emergency Nursing* 21(4): 323–326.

Hinds PS, Quargnenti A, Gattuso *et al.* (2002) Comparing the results of coagulation tests on blood drawn by venepuncture and through heparinized tunnelled venous access devices in pediatric patients with cancer. *Oncology Nursing Forum* 29(3): E26–E34.

Hockenberry M, Wilson D, Barrera P (2006) Implementing evidence-based nursing practice in a pediatric hospital. *Pediatric Nursing* 32(4): 371–377.

Hodge D, Puntis JWL (2002) Diagnosis, prevention, and management of catheter-related bloodstream infection during long term parenteral nutrition. *Archives of Disease in Childhood*. Fetal and neonatal edition, 87(1): F21–F24.

Holcombe BJ, Forloines-Lynn S, Garmhausen LW (1992) Restoring patency of long-term central venous access devices. *Journal of Intravenous Nursing* 15(1): 36–41.

Holden C, Brook G, Wills J *et al.* (1996) Home parenteral nutrition: present management, future options. *British Journal of Community Health Nursing* 1(6): 347–353.

Hollis R (1992) Central venous access in children. *Paediatric Nursing* 4(2): 18–21.

Holmes KR (1998) Comparison of push–pull versus discard method from central venous catheters for blood testing. *Journal of Infusion Nursing* 21(5): 282–285.

Hooke C (2000) Recombinant tissue plasminogen activator for central venous access device occlusion. *Journal of Pediatric Oncology Nursing* 17(3): 174–178.

Hutton M, Gardner H (2003) Calculation skills. *Paediatric Nursing* 17(2): 1–17.

Infusion Nurses Society (INS) (2006) *Infusion Nursing Standards of Practice*. Infusion Nurses Society, Norwood.

Ingle RJ (1995) Rare complications of vascular access devices. *Seminars in Oncology Nursing* 11(3): 184–193.

Ingram J, Weitzman S, Greenberg ML *et al.* (1991) Complications of indwelling venous access lines in the pediatric haematology patient: a prospective comparison of external venous catheters and subcutaneous ports. *Journal of Pediatric Haematology/Oncology* 13(2): 130–136.

Irving V (2001a) Caring for and protecting the skin of pre-term infants. *Journal of Wound Care* 10(7): 253–256.

Irving V (2001b) Reducing the risk of epidermal stripping in the neonatal population: an evaluation of an alcohol free barrier film. *Journal of Neonatal Nursing* 7(1): 5–8.

Irving V (2001c) Managing extravasation injuries in preterm neonates. *Nursing Times Plus* 97(35): 42–46.

Jacobs BR, Haygood M, Hingl J (2001) Recombinant tissue plasminogen activator in the treatment of central venous catheter occlusion in children. *Journal of Pediatrics* 139(4): 593–596.

Jain A, Rutter N (2000) Does topical amethocaine gel reduce the pain of venepuncture in newborn infants? A randomized double blind controlled trial. *Archives of Disease in Childhood*. Fetal and neonatal edition 83(3): F207–F210.

Kassner E (2000) Evaluation and treatment of chemotherapy extravasation injuries. *Journal of Pediatric Oncology Nursing* 17(3): 135–148.

Kaushal R, Bates DW, Landrigan C *et al.* (2001) Medication errors and adverse drug events in pediatric inpatients. *Journal of the American Medical Association* 285(16): 2114–2120.

Keller CA (1994) Methods of drawing blood samples through central venous catheters in pediatric patients undergoing bone marrow transplant: results of a national survey. *Oncology Nursing Forum* 21(5): 879–884.

Keller S (1995) Small gauge needles promote safe blood transfusions. *Oncology Nursing Forum* 22(4): 718.

Kelly C, Dumenko L, McGregor *et al.* (1992) A change in flushing protocols of central venous catheters. *Oncology Nursing Forum* 19(4): 599–605.

Kleiber C, Hanrahan K, Loebig Fagan C, Zittergruen MA (1993) Heparin vs. saline for peripheral IV locks in children. *Pediatric Nursing* 19(4): 405–409.

Kleidon T (2004) *Insertion of central venous access devices in children by a paediatric clinical nurse specialist.* Abstract presented at Royal College of Nursing Intravenous Therapy Forum conference—Raising the standards in infusion therapy, York, 5th and 6th November.

Klenner AF, Fusch C, Rakow A *et al.* (2003) Benefit and risk of heparin for marinating peripheral venous catheters in neonates: a placebo-controlled trial. *Journal of Pediatrics* 145(6): 741–745.

Kline AM (2005) Pediatric catheter-related bloodstream infections: latest strategies to decrease risk. *AACN Clinical Issues* 16(2): 185–198.

Knue M, Doellman D, Rabin K *et al.* (2005) The efficacy and safety of blood sampling through peripherally inserted central catheter devices in children. *Journal of Infusion Nursing* 28(1): 30–35.

Knue M, Doellman D, Jacobs BR (2006) Peripherally inserted central catheters in children. A survey of practice patterns. *Journal of Infusion Nursing* 29(1): 28–33.

Kolk AM, Van Hoof R, Dop MJ *et al.* (2000) Preparing children for venepuncture. The effect of an integrated intervention on distress before and during venepuncture. *Child Care Health and Development* 26(3): 251–160.

Kurdahi Badr L, Puzantian H, Abboud M *et al.* (2006) Assessing procedural pain in children with cancer in Beirut, Lebanon. *Journal of Pediatric Oncology Nursing* 23(6): 311–320.

Lander JA, Weltman BJ (2006) EMLA and amethocaine for reduction of children's pain associated with needle insertion. *Cochrane Database of Systematic Reviews* 3 (CD004236).

La Quaglia MP, Lucas A, Thaler HT, Friedlander-Klar H, Exelby PR, Groeger JS (1992) A prospective analysis of vascular access device-related infections in children. *Journal of Pediatric Surgery* 27(7): 840–842.

Laskey AL, Dyer C, Tobias JD (2002) Venous air embolism during home infusion therapy. *Pediatrics* 109(1): E15.

Lawson RA, Smart NG, Gudgeon AC, Morton NS (1995) Evaluation of an amethocaine gel preparation for percutaneous analgesia before venous cannulation in children. *British Journal of Anaesthesia* 75: 282–285.

LeDuc K (1997) Efficacy of normal saline versus heparin solution for maintaining patency of peripheral intravenous catheters in children. *Journal of Emergency Nursing* 23(4): 306–309.

Lee OKE, Johnston L (2005) A systematic review for effective management of central venous catheters and catheter sites in acute care paediatric patients. *Worldviews on Evidence-Based Nursing* 2(1): 4–13.

Lemyre B, Sherlock R, Hogan D *et al.* (2006) How effective is tetracaine 4% gel, before a peripherally inserted central catheter, in reducing procedural pain in infants: a randomized double-blind placebo controlled trial. *BMC Medicine* 4(11): 1–9.

Liesner RJ, Vora AJ, Hann IM, Lilleymann JS (1995) Use of central venous catheters in children with severe congenital coagulopathy. *British Journal of Haematology* 91: 203–207.

Linden N, Davidovitch, Reichman B *et al.* (1997) Topical iodine-containing antispetics and subclinical hypothyroidism in pre-term infants. *Journal of Pediatrics* 131(3): 434–439.

Livesley J (1996) Peripheral IV therapy in children. *Paediatric Nursing* 8(6): 29–33.

Ljungman G, Kreuger A, Andreasson S *et al.* (2000) Midazolam nasal spray reduces procedural anxiety in children. *Pediatrics* 105(1): 73–78.

Lokich JJ, Bothe A, Benotti P, Moore C (1985) Complications and management of implanted venous access catheters. *Journal of Clinical Oncology* 3(5): 710–717.

Lombardi TP, Gunderson B, Zammett LO, Walters K, Morris BA (1998) Efficacy of 0.9% sodium chloride injection with or without heparin sodium for maintaining patency of intravenous catheters in children. *Clinical Pharmacy* 7: 832–836.

Long CA, Stashinko EE, Byrnes K *et al.* (1996) Central line associated bacteremia in the pediatric patient. *Pediatric Nursing* 22(3): 247–51.

Lorenz JM, Funaki B, Van Ha T *et al.* (2001) Padiologic placement of implamtable chest ports in pediatric patients. *American Journal of Roentgenology* 176(4): 991–994.

Lund C (1999) Neonatal skin care: the scientific basis for practice. *Neonatal Network* 18(4): 15–25.

MacDonald A (2001) Record keeping in intravenous therapy: do yours meet the standards? *Paediatric Nursing* 13(2): 31–34.

MacGeorge L, Steeves L, Steeves RH (1988) Comparison of the mixing and reinfusion methods of drawing blood from a Hickman catheter. *Oncology Nursing Forum* 15(3): 335–338.

Macklin D (2003) Phlebitis. *American Journal of Nursing* 103(2): 55–60.

MacQueen S (2005) The special needs of children receiving intravenous therapy. *Nursing Times* 101(8):59–64.

Manne S (1999) Commentary: well-established treatments for procedure related pain: issues for future research and policy implications. *Journal of Pediatric Psychology* 24(2): 147–149.

Marcoux C, Fisher S, Wong D (1990) Central venous access devices in children. *Pediatric Nursing* 16(2): 123–133.

Marders J (2005) Sounding the alarm for I.V. infiltration. *Nursing* 35(4): 18, 20.

Mason Wyckoff M (1999) Midline catheter use in the premature and full-term infant. *Journal of Vascular Access Devices* 4(3): 26–29.

Masoorli S (2002) Blood return issues related to central vascular access devices. *Journal of Vascular Access Devices* 7(3): 18–19.

Masoorli S (2003) Legally speaking. Pediatrics: small children at high risk. *Journal of the Association of Vascular Access* 8(3): 42–43.

Masoorli S (2005) Legal issues related to vascular access devices and infusion therapy. *Journal of Infusion Nursing* 28(3S): S18–S21.

Mayo DJ, Pearson DC (1995) Chemotherapy extravasation: a consequence of fibrin sheath formation around venous access devices. *Oncology Nursing Forum* 22(4): 675–680.

Mayo DJ, Dimond EP, Kramer W *et al.* (1996) Discard volumes necessary for clinically useful coagulation studies from heparinised hickman catheters. *Oncology Nursing Forum* 34(4): 671–675.

McBeth CL, McDonald RJ, Hodge MB (2004) Antibiotic sampling from central venous catheters versus peripheral veins. *Pediatric Nursing* 30(3): 200–202.

McCloskey DJ (2002) Catheter-related thrombosis in pediatrics. *Pediatric Nursing* 28(2): 97–106.

McGovern B, Solenberger K, Reed K (1985) A totally implantable venous access system for long-term chemotherapy in children. *Journal of Pediatric Surgery* 20: 725–727.

McGrath PA (1999) Commentary: psychological interventions for controlling children's pain: challenges for evidence-based medicine. *Journal of Pediatric Psychology* 24(2): 172–174.

McInally W (2005) Whose line is it anyway? Management of central venous catheters in children. *Paediatric Nursing* 17(5): 14–18.

McIntosh N (2006) Intravenous therapy. In: Trigg E, Mohammed TA, eds. *Practices in Children's Nursing. Guidelines for Hospital and Community*, 2nd edn, pp. 211–224. Elsevier Churchill Livingstone, Edinburgh.

McLean TW, Fisher CJ, Snively BM *et al.* (2005) Central venous lines in children with lesser risk acute lymphoblastic leukaemia: optimal type and timing of placement. *Journal of Clinical Oncology* 23(13): 3024–3029.

McMahon C, Smith J, Khair K, Liesner R, Hann IM, Smith OP (2000) Central venous access devices in children with congenital coagulation disorders: complications and long-term outcome. *British Journal of Haematology* 110(2): 461–468.

McMullen A, Dutko Fioravanti I, Pollack V, Rideout K, Sciera M (1993) Heparinized saline or normal saline as a flush solution on intermittent intravenous lines in infants and children. *American Journal of Maternal and Child Nursing* 18(2): 78–85.

Medicines and Healthcare products Regulatory Agency (MHRA) (2001) SN 2001(20) *Blood Sampling from Small Infants*. Medicines and Healthcare products Regulatory Agency, London.

Medicines and Healthcare products Regulatory Agency (MHRA) (2003) Device Bulletin (02) *Infusion systems*. Medicines and Healthcare products Regulatory Agency, London.

Mermel LA, Farr BM, Sheretz RJ *et al.* (2001) Guidelines for the management of intravascular catheter-related infections. *Clinical Infectious Diseases* 32(9): 1249–1272.

Miall LS, Das A, Brownlee KG, Conway SP (2001) Peripherally inserted central catheters in children with cystic fibrosis. Eight cases of difficult removal. *Journal of Infusion Nursing* 24(5): 297–300.

Mirro J, Rao BN, Kumar M *et al.* (1990) A comparison of placement techniques and complications of externalized catheters and implantable port use in children with cancer. *Journal of Pediatric Surgery* 25(1): 120–124.

Miser AW, Goh TS, Dose AM *et al.* (1994) Trial of a topically administered local anesthetic (EMLA cream) for pain relief during central venous port accesses in children with cancer. *Journal of Pain and Symptom Management* 9(4): 259–264.

Monagle P, Chan A, Massicotte P *et al.* (2004) Antithrombotic therapy in children. *Chest* 126(3): 645S–687S.

Moore J (2001) No more tears: a randomized controlled double-blind trial of amethocaine gel vs. placebo in the management of procedural pain in neonates. *Journal of Advanced Nursing* 34(4): 475–482.

Moore CL, Erikson KA, Yanes LB, Franklin M, Gonsalves L (1986) Nursing care and management of venous access ports. *Oncology Nursing Forum* 13(3): 35–39.

Morton NS (1996) A comparison of ametop gel with EMLA cream in venous cannulation in children. In: Woolfson AD, McCafferty DFM, eds. *Amethocaine Gel, a New Development in Effective Percutaneous Local Anaesthesia*. Royal Society of Medicine Press, London.

Moureau N (1999) Focus on prevention of vascular access device complications. *Journal of Vascular Access Devices* 4(2): S1–S4.

Moureau N, Zonderman A (2000) Does it always have to hurt? Premedications for adults and children for use with intravenous therapy. *Journal of Intravenous Nursing* 23(4): 213–219.

Munro FD, Gillett PM, Wratten JC (1999) Totally implantable central venous access devices for paediatric oncology patients. *Medical and Pediatric Oncology* 33(4): 377–381.

National Association of Hospital Play Staff (2000) *Guidelines for professional practice. Number 6 Needle Play*. Available from www.nahps.org.uk/needle.htm (accessed 26 November 2006).

National Association of Neonatal Nurses (2001) *Peripherally Inserted Central Catheters. Guidelines for Practice*. National Association of Neonatal Nurses, Glenview.

National Association of Vascular Access Networks (1998) Tip location of peripherally inserted central catheters. *Journal of Vascular Access Devices* 3(2): 2–4.

National Institute for Clinical Excellence (NICE) (2002) *Guidance on the Use of Ultrasound Locating Devices for Placing Central Venous Catheters*. National Institute for Health and Clinical Excellence, London.

National Institute for Clinical Excellence (2003) *Infection Control. Prevention of Healthcare-Associated Infection in Primary and Community Care*. National Institute for Health and Clinical Excellence, London.

National Institute for Health and Clinical Excellence (2005) *Guidance on Cancer Services. Improving Outcomes in Children and Young People with Cancer*. National Institute for Health and Clinical Excellence, London.

National Kidney Foundation (2006) *Clinical Practice Recommendations for Vascular Access*. Available from www.kidney.org (accessed 6 January 2007).

Nosher JL, Bodner LJ, Ettinger LJ *et al.* (2001) Radiologic placement of a low profile implantable venous access port in a pediatric population. *Cardiovascular and Interventional Radiology* 24(6): 395–399.

Nursing and Midwifery Council (NMC) (2004a) *Guidelines for the Administration of Medicines*. Nursing and Midwifery Council, London.

Nursing and Midwifery Council (2004b) *The NMC Code of Conduct: Standards for Conduct, Performance and Ethics*. Nursing and Midwifery Council, London.

Nursing and Midwifery Council (2005) *Guidelines for Records and Record Keeping*. Nursing and Midwifery Council, London.

O'Brien L, Taddio A, Lyszkiewicz DA *et al.* (2005) A critical review of the topical local anesthetic amethocaine (Ametop) for pediatric pain. *Pediatric Drugs* 7(1): 41–54.

Oishi LA (2001) The necessity of routinely replacing peripheral intravenous catheters in hospitalized children. *Journal of Intravenous Nursing* 24(3): 174–179.

Pellowe CM, Pratt RJ, Loveday HP *et al.* (2004) The Epic project. Updating the evidence-base for national evidence-based guidelines for preventing healthcare-associated infections in NHS hospitals in England: a report with recommendations. *British Journal of Hospital Infection* 5(6): 10–16.

Pennington CR, Pithie AD (1987) Ethanol lock in the management of catheter occlusion. *Journal of Parenteral and Enteral Nutrition* 11(5): 507–508.

Pettit J (2000) Challenges to providing vascular access in neonatal patients. *Journal of Vascular Access Devices* 5(1): 16–21.

Pettit J, Hughes K (1993) Intravenous extravasation: mechanisms, management, and prevention. *Journal of Perinatal and Neonatal Nursing* 6(4): 69–79.

Philip RK, Beckett M (2000) Neonatal blood sampling: time for safer devices. *Journal of Neonatal Nursing* 6(3): Insert 1–3.

Philpot P, Griffiths V (2003) The peripherally inserted central catheter. *Nursing Standard* 17(44): 39–46.

Piira T, Sugiura T, Champion GD *et al.* (2005) The role of parental presence in the context of children's medical procedures: a systematic review. *Child Care Health and Development* 31(2): 233–243.

Pinto KM (1994) Accuracy of coagulation values obtained from a heparinised central venous catheter. *Oncology Nursing Forum* 21(3): 573–575.

Powers SW (1999) Empirically supported treatments in pediatric psychology: procedure-related pain. *Journal of Pediatric Psychology* 24(2): 131–145.

Pratt RJ, Pellowe C, Wilson JA *et al.* (2007) Epic 2: national evidence-based guidelines for preventing healthcare-associated infections in NHS hospitals in England. *Journal of Hospital Infection* 655(Suppl): S1–S64.

Quinn C (2000) Infusion devices: risks, functions and management. *Nursing Standard* 14(26): 35–41, 43.

Quinn C, Upton D (2006) A review of claims against the NHS relating to intravenous infusion therapy. *Healthcare Risk* March: 15–17.

Ramage IJ, Bailie A, Tyerman KS, McColl JH, Pollard SG, Fitzpatrick MM (2005) Vascular access survival in children and young adults receiving long-term hemodialysis. *American Journal of Kidney Diseases* 45(4): 708–714.

Ramirez JM, Miguelena JM, Guemes A, Moncada E, Cabezali R, Sousa R (1993) Fully implantable venous access systems. *British Journal of Surgery* 80: 347–348.

Randolph AG, Cook DJ, Gonzales CA *et al.* (1998) Benefit of heparin in central venous and pulmonary artery catheters. A meta-analysis of randomized controlled trials. *Chest* 113(1): 165–171.

Randolph AG, Brun-Buisson C, Goldman D (2005) Identification of central venous catheter-related infections in infants and children. *Pediatric Critical Care Medicine* 6(3) (Suppl): S19–S24.

Reed T, Philips S (1996) Management of central venous catheter occlusions and repairs. *Journal of Intravenous Nursing* 19(6): 289–294.

Reed WP, Newman KA, Applefeld MM, Sutton FJ (1985) Drug extravasation as a complication of venous access ports. *Annals of Internal Medicine* 102(6): 788–789.

Robbins J Cromwell P, Korones D (1999) Swimming and central venous catheter-related infections in the child with cancer. *Journal of Pediatric Oncology Nursing* 16(1): 51–6.

Robbins J, Cromwell P, Korones DN (2000) Swimming and central venous catheter-related infections in children with cancer. In: Nolan MT, Mock V, eds. *Measuring Patient Outcomes*, pp. 169–184. Sage Publications, Inc., Thousand Oaks.

Ross M, Haase GM, Poole MA *et al.* (1988) Comparison of totally implanted reservoirs with external catheters as venous access devices in pediatric oncology patients. *Surgery, Gynecology and Obstetrics* 167: 141–144.

Ross LM, Wallace J, Paton JY (2000) Medication errors in a paediatric teaching hospital in the UK: five years operational experience. *Archives of Disease in Childhood* 83(6): 492–497.

Roth D (2003) Extravasation injuries of peripheral veins a basis for litigation? *Journal of Vascular Access Devices* 8(1): 13–19.

Roth D (2006) Legally speaking—pediatric infiltration and extravasation. *Journal of the Association of Vascular Access* 11(1): 14.

Royal Australasian College of Physicians (2005) *Guideline Statement: Management of Procedure-Related Pain in Children and Adolescents*. Royal Australasian College of Physicians, Sydney.

Royal College of Nursing (RCN) (2001) *Administering Intravenous Therapy to Children in the Community*. Royal College of Nursing, London.

Royal College of Nursing (2003) *Restraining, Holding Still and Containing Children and Young People*. Royal College of Nursing, London.

Royal College of Nursing (2005a) *An Education and Training Competency Framework for Peripheral Venous Cannulation in Children and Young People*. Royal College of Nursing, London.

Royal College of Nursing (2005b) *Standards for Infusion Therapy*. Royal College of Nursing, London.

Royal College of Nursing (2005c) *Competencies: An Education and Training Competency Framework for Administering Medicines Intravenously to Children and Young People*. Royal College of Nursing, London.

Royal College of Nursing (2005d) *Competencies: An Education and Training Competency Framework for Capillary Blood Sampling and Venepuncture in Children and Young People*. Royal College of Nursing, London.

Royal Pharmaceutical Society of Great Britain, Royal College of Paediatrics and Child Health (2005) *British National Formulary for Children*. BMJ Publishing Group, London.

Sauerland C, Engelking C, Wickham R, Corbi D (2006) Vesicant extravasation part 1: mechanisms, pathogenesis, and nursing care to reduce risk. *Oncology Nursing Forum* 33(6): 1134–1141.

Schiff WB, Holtz KD, Peterson N *et al.* (2001) Effect of an intervention to reduce procedural pain and distress for children with HIV infection. *Journal of Pediatric Psychology* 26(7): 417–427.

Schulmeister L (1989) Needle dislodgement from implanted venous access devices: inpatient and outpatient experiences. *Journal of Intravenous Nursing* 12(2): 90–92.

Schulmeister L (1992) An overview of continuous infusion chemotherapy. *Journal of Intravenous Nursing* 15(6): 315–321.

Schulmeister L, Camp-Sorrell C (2000) Chemotherapy extravasation from implanted ports. *Oncology Nursing Forum* 27(3): 531–538.

Sclare I, Waring M (1995) Routine venepuncture: improving services. *Paediatric Nursing* 7(4): 23–27.

Scottish Intercollegiate Guidelines Network (SIGN) (2004) Safe sedation of children undergoing diagnostic and therapeutic procedures. Scottish Intercollegiate Guidelines Network, Edinburgh.

Seemann S, Reinhardt A (2000) Blood sample collection from a peripheral catheter system compared with phlebotomy. *Journal of Intravenous Nursing* 23(5): 290–297.

Senner AM, Johnston K, McLachlan AJ (2005) A comparison of peripheral and centrally collected cyclosporine A blood levels in pediatric patients undergoing stem cell transplant. *Oncology Nursing Forum* 32(1): 73–77.

Shah PS, Ng E, Sinha AK (2005) Heparin for prolonging peripheral intravenous catheter use in neonates. *Cochrane Database of Systematic Reviews* 4 (CD002774): 1–10.

Shah V, Ohlsson A (2004) Venepuncture versus heel lance for blood sampling in term neonates. *Cochrane Database of Systematic Reviews* 4 (CD001452).

Shimandle RB, Johnson D, Baker M *et al.* (1999) Safety of peripheral intravenous catheters in children. *Infection Control and Hospital Epidemiology* 20(11): 736–740.

Sliwa CM (1997) A comparative study of hematocrits drawn from a standard venepuncture and those drawn from saline lock device. *Journal of Emergency Nursing* 23(3): 228–231.

Smith TL, Pullen GT, Crouse V *et al.* (2002) Bloodstream infections in pediatric oncology outpatients: a new healthcare systems challenge. *Infection Control and Hospital Epidemiology* 23(5): 239–243.

Section 3

Soucy P (1987) Experiences with the use of the Port-a-Cath in children. *Journal of Pediatric Surgery* 22(8): 767–769.

Stebbings J (2006) Play. In: Trigg E, Mohammed TA, eds. *Practices in Children's Nursing. Guidelines for Hospital and Community,* 2nd edn, pp. 457–463. Elsevier Churchill Livingstone, Edinburgh.

Stevens B, Yamada J, Ohlsson A (2004) Sucrose for analgesia in newborn infants undergoing painful procedures. *Cochrane Database of Systematic Reviews* 3 (CD001069): 1–52.

Strum S, McDermed J, Korn A, Joseph C (1986) Improved methods for venous access: the Port-a-Cath, a totally implanted catheter system. *Journal of Clinical Oncology* 4(4): 596–603.

Sundquist Beauman S (2001) Didactic components of a comprehensive pediatric competency program. *Journal of Infusion Nursing* 24(6): 367–374.

Taylor MJ (2000) A fascination with phlebitis. *Journal of Vascular Access Devices* 5(3): 24–28.

Thiagarajan RR, Ramamoorthy C, Gettmann T *et al.* (1997) Survey of the use of peripherally inserted central venous catheters in children. *Pediatrics* 99(2): E4–E7.

Thurgate C, Heppell S (2005) Needle phobia—changing venepuncture practice in ambulatory care. *Paediatric Nursing* 17(9): 15–18.

Tomlinson D (2004) Physical restraint during procedures: issues and implications for practice. *Journal of Pediatric Oncology Nursing* 21(5): 258–263.

Turner MA, Unsworth V, David TJ (2002) Intravenous long-lines in children with cystic fibrosis: a multidisciplinary approach. *Journal of the Royal Society of Medicine* 95 (Suppl 41): 11–21.

Tweddle DA, Windebank KP, Barrett AM *et al.* (1997) Central venous catheter use in UKCCSG oncology centres. *Archives of Disease in Childhood* 77(1): 58–59.

Uman LS, Chambers CT, McGrath PJ *et al.* (2005) Psychological interventions for needle-related procedural pain and distress in children and adolescents (Protocol). *Cochrane Database of Systematic Reviews* 1 (CD005179): 1–20.

Valentino LA, Ewenstein B, Navickis RJ, Wilkes MM (2004) Central venous access devices in haemophilia. *Haemophilia* 10(2): 134–146.

Watt S (2003a) Safe administration of medicines to children: part 2. *Paediatric Nursing* 15(5): 40–44.

Watt S (2003b) Safe administration of medicines to children: part 1. *Paediatric Nursing* 15(4): 40–43.

Weinstein SM (2007a) Complications and interventions. In: Weinstein SM, ed. *Plumer's Principles and Practice of Intravenous Therapy,* 8th edn, pp. 152–186. Lippincott Williams and Wilkins, Philadelphia.

Weinstein SM (2007b) Central venous access. In: Weinstein SM, ed. *Plumer's Principles and Practice of Intravenous Therapy,* 8th edn, pp. 277–330. Lippincott Williams and Wilkins, Philadelphia.

Whitman M (1995) Delivering medications safely by I.V. bolus. *Nursing* 25(8): 52–54.

Wiener ES, Albanese CT (1998) Venous access in pediatric patients. *Journal of Intravenous Nursing* 21(5S): S122–S133.

Wiener ES, McGuire P, Stolar CJH *et al.* (1992) The CCSG prospective study of venous access devices: an analysis of insertions and causes for removal. *Journal of Pediatric Surgery* 27(2): 155–164.

Willock J, Richardson J, Brazier A, Powell C, Mitchell E (2004) Peripheral venepuncture in infants and children *Nursing Standard* 18(2): 43–50.

Wilson J, Gaedeke MK (1996) Blood conservation in neonatal and pediatric populations. *AACN Clinical Issues* 7(2): 229–237.

Wiltgen-Trotter C (1996) Percutaneous central venous catheter-related sepsis in the neonate: an analysis of the literature from 1990 to 1994. *Neonatal Network* 15(3): 15–28.

Winslow MN, Trammell L, Camp-Sorrell D (1995) Selection of vascular access devices and nursing care. *Seminars in Oncology Nursing* 11(3): 167–173.

Wood LS, Gullo SM (1993) IV vesicants: how to avoid extravasation. *American Journal of Nursing* 93(4): 42–46.

Wurzel CL, Halom K, Feldman JG, Rubin LG (1988) Infection rates of Broviac–Hickman catheters and implantable venous devices. *American Journal of Diseases of Children* 142: 536–540.

Zappa SC, Nabors SB (1992) Use of ethyl chloride topical anesthetic to reduce procedural pain in pediatric oncology patients. *Cancer Nursing* 15(2): 130–136.

Zenk KE, Dungy CI, Greene GR (1981) Nafcillin extravasation injury. Use of hyaluronidase as an antidote. *American Journal of Diseases in Children* 135(12): 1113–1114.

CHAPTER 16

Safe Handling and Administration of Intravenous Cytotoxic Drugs

Janice Gabriel

Introduction

Cytotoxic drugs target dividing cells so therefore they can damage normal cells as well as cancer cells. The word cytotoxic means quite literally 'toxic to cells'. It refers to a group of drugs used mainly in the treatment of cancer to prevent proliferation and destroy abnormal cells, although some cytotoxic drugs can be administered for non-malignant conditions such as psoriasis, rheumatoid arthritis and other autoimmune conditions (Knight 2004). There are also other drugs such as monoclonal antibodies used to treat cancer that do not fall into the 'cytotoxic' category, e.g. trastuzumab (Herceptin), and these will be discussed later in this chapter (Modjtahedi 2004).

The primary action of a cytotoxic drug is to destroy as many dividing cells as possible and prevent cancerous cells from dividing further. Since cancer cells exhibit rapid and uncontrolled cell division, they are very receptive to the action of cytotoxic drugs (Robinson 1993; Knight 2004). However, certain structures, such as bone marrow, are also areas of rapidly dividing cells and as a result are affected by the cytotoxic action of the drug(s). This often results in the problems of toxicity that are associated with cytotoxic therapy. Cytotoxic drugs can be administered via a variety of routes, including oral, intramuscular, subcutaneous and intracavity, but the main route is intravenous, administered as bolus injection, or intermittent or continuous infusion (Dougherty 2006).

This chapter will focus mainly on how the practitioner manages intravenous cytotoxic therapy, focusing on the handling, administration and prevention of specific complications such as extravasation.

Classification and Types of Drugs

Normal cells require growth signals in order to proliferate. However, many cancer cells have the ability to synthesize growth factors and can replicate independently (Knight 2004). The 'normal' cell can undergo between 60–70 replications, after which it will come to the end of its life and die. Cancer cells do not behave in the same way. As a consequence of the enzyme telomerase they can continue to replicate independently (Knight 2004).

Understanding the complexity of the cell cycle and its components has enabled medical researchers to develop drugs (cytotoxic chemotherapy) that can interfere with the cell cycle and therefore prevent cancerous cells from replicating and ultimately destroy them (Knight 2004).

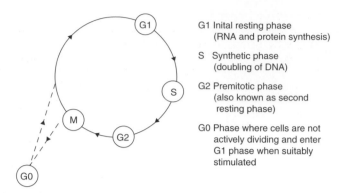

Figure 16.1   The five phases of the cell cycle: G0, G1, S, G2 and Mitosis.

Cytotoxic drugs are grouped according to their specific effects on the cell and the phase of the cell cycle upon which they are active. The cell cycle is a sequence of steps through which all cells grow and replicate and consists of five phases (Tortorice 1997; Knight 2004; Trevit & Phillips 2006) (Figure 16.1). Cell cycle phase-specific drugs are active only during a particular phase of the cell cycle. These give the greatest tumour 'kill' when administered in divided doses or as a continuous infusion with a short cycle time. Cell cycle phase non-specific drugs are active at any point in the cell cycle, including the G0 resting phase (Knight 2004; Trevit & Phillips 2006) (Figure 16.1). They are effective in the treatment of slow-growing tumours, and 'cell kill' is directly proportional to the amount of drug given. Ninety per cent of human tumour cells have cell cycle times within the range of 15–120 hours, with an average of 48 hours (Priestman 1989; Robinson 1993; Begg 2006).

Cytotoxic drugs are further classified according to their chemical structure, e.g. vinca alkaloids, antimetabolites, alkylating agents, anthracyclines, platinum compounds, taxanes, topoisomerase inhibitors. (*See* Table 16.1 for a summary of classification and mode of action.)

Other groups of drugs are being developed for the management of malignant disease and include monoclonal antibodies (mAbs) (Modjtahedi 2004). Cells produce proteins known as antigens and cancer cells produce tumour antigens. Understanding cancer biology has enabled medical scientists to look at developing new approaches for the treatment of cancer. Monoclonal antibodies are developed from mouse antibodies and transferred into a human IgG framework (Modjtahedi 2004). The mAbs have the potential to be developed against a wide range of antigens, including those produced by some cancers. For example, HER2, which is expressed by one type of breast cancer, can be 'switched off' by using the drug trastuzumab (Herceptin). These mAbs will block the receptor site and prevent protein interaction with the receptor, ultimately causing cell death. Although mAbs are not 'conventional' cytotoxic drugs, they are being used more widely in the management of malignant disease, for example rituximab (Rituxan) for non-Hodgkin's lymphoma and alemzutumab (Campath) for chronic lymphatic leukaemia (Modjtahedi 2004).

Rationale for Method of Delivery of Cytotoxic Therapy

Continuous infusional chemotherapy

If a single drug, or combination of drugs is administered as a continuous infusion, regardless of the length of cell cycle for individual tumour cells, the cytotoxic drug(s) will

Table 16.1 Classification of cytotoxic drugs.

Group of drugs	Mechanism of action	Names of drugs in category	Administration methods	Common side-effects
Cell cycle specific Anti-metabolites	Class II S phase action	Methotrexate	Intravenous bolus or infusion	Stomatitis, anorexia, malaise, eye irritation, bone marrow depression (BMD), renal failure, photosensitivity, pulmonary changes, fever, chills
		Fluorouracil	Bolus, infusion, continuous infusion	Diarrhoea, stomatitis, anorexia, palmar–plantar syndrome, hyperpigmentation, mild alopecia with high doses
		Raltitrexed	Intravenous infusion	Mucositis, nausea and vomiting, anorexia, diarrhoea, rash, fatigue
		Cytarabine	Intravenous infusion	Nausea and vomiting, flu-like syndrome, BMD, stomatitis, lethargy
		Cladrabine Capecitabine	Oral	Palmar–plantar syndrome, Diarrhoea
		Tegafur with uracil	Oral	Palmar–plantar syndrome, hyperpigmentation, mild alopecia
		Fludarabine	Intravenous bolus, short infusion	Mild nausea and vomiting, fatigue, anorexia
		Gemcitabine	Intravenous infusion over 30 minutes Oral	Rash, injection site reaction, flu-like syndrome, mild peripheral oedema, bronchospasm Stomatitis
		Hydroxycarbamide		
		6-Mercaptapurine		Nausea
		6-Thioguanine		Diarrhoea
Vinca alkaloids	Class II phase-specific occurs in S phase and shows in M phase, binds to tuberlin	Vincristine	Intravenous bolus or infusion (central venous route only)	Cold sensation along vein during injection, jaw or tumour pain, neurotoxicity—peripheral neuropathy, constipation, alopecia (high doses only), BMD
		Vinblastine		As above and phlebitis
		Vindesine		As above
		Vinorelbine		As above, severe injection site pain, in arm and back during injection, venous discoloration and phlebitis
Antitumour antibiotics	Class III Binds with DNA, active in S phase	Bleomycin	Intravenous bolus or infusion	Tumour pain, allergic reactions, fever, chills, skin reactions, nail ridging, stomatitis, pulmonary fibrosis
		Actinomycin D	Slow i.v. bolus into side-arm of saline infusion	Nausea and vomiting, anorexia, stomatitis, skin changes, BMD, reactivation of radiation sites, alopecia
		Mitomycin C	Slow i.v. bolus	Pain on injection, nausea and vomiting, diarrhoea, anorexia, BMD, fatigue, nephrotoxic, phlebitis, stomatitis
Epipodo-phyllotoxins	Inhibits at metaphase; G2 and S phase also affected	Etoposide	Intravenous infusion over 30 minutes	Severe hypotension if infused rapidly, nausea and vomiting, alopecia, BMD
Taxanes	Effective in G2 and M phase; inhibits cell division	Paclitaxel	Intravenous infusion	Severe anaphylaxis, nausea and vomiting, diarrhoea, stomatitis, alopecia, BMD, hypotension, sensory perception loss, neuropathy
		Docetaxel	Intravenous infusion	Mild skin reaction, phlebitis, allergic reaction, nausea and vomiting, fluid retention, diarrhoea, stomatitis, rash, BMD, alopecia, myalgia, paraesthesia

Section 3

(*Continued*)

Table 16.1 (*Continued*)

Group of drugs	Mechanism of action	Names of drugs in category	Administration methods	Common side-effects
Anthracyclines		Daunorubicin	Slow i.v. bolus into side-arm of a fast-running infusion	Red venous flush, nausea and vomiting, fever, red discoloured urine, BMD, diarrhoea, alopecia, phlebitis, stomatitis, congestive cardiac failure
		Doxorubicin	Intravenous bolus or infusion (central venous route only)	Red flush 'flare reaction', aching along veins, nausea and vomiting, alopecia, stomatitis, red discoloured urine, BMD, thrombophlebitis, cardiotoxicity
		Epirubicin	Slow i.v. bolus into side-arm of a fast-running infusion	As above
		Idarubicin	Slow i.v. bolus	Venous pain, rash, nausea and vomiting, stomatitis, diarrhoea, BMD, alopecia, cardiotoxicity
		Mitozantrone	Slow i.v. bolus or infusion	Green discoloration of urine, anorexia, mild nausea and vomiting, blue discoloration of vein, minimal alopecia, fever, amenorrhoea
		Adarubicin	Intravenous bolus into fast running infusion	Mild phlebitis, nausea and vomiting, stomatitis, red urine, BMD, mild alopecia, cardiotoxicity
Miscellaneous	Inhibits intracellular protein synthesis	Asparaginase	Intravenous bolus	Severe anaphylaxis, malaise, anorexia, hepatotoxic, central toxicity, pancreatic dysfunction
Nitrosurea (alkylating)	Cell cycle non-specific	Carmustine	Intravenous infusion over 1–2 hours	Intense venous pain when given rapidly, facial flushing, BMD, nausea and vomiting, gynaecomastia
		Lomustine	Oral	Anorexia, nausea and vomiting, BMD
Alkylating	Class III, cell cycle non-specific Interferes with DNA replication	Cyclophospha-mide	Intravenous bolus or infusion	Hot flush, dizziness, metallic taste, nasal stuffiness—all during injection, nausea and vomiting, anorexia, BMD, alopecia, chemical haemorrhagic cystitis, sterility
		Busulphan	Oral	BMD, skin pigmentation, hyperuricaemia
		Chlorambucil	Oral	Nausea and vomiting in high doses, BMD, sterility, secondary malignancy
		Dacarbazine	Intravenous infusion	Pain along the vein if infusion too rapid, facial flushing, flu-like syndrome, anorexia, BMD, alopecia
		Ifosfamide	Slow i.v. bolus or infusion	Nausea and vomiting, haematuria, anorexia, chemical thrombophlebitis, alopecia, nephrotoxicity, haemorrhagic cystitis, lethargy, confusion
		Melphalan	Slow i.v. bolus, oral	Anaphylaxis, nausea and vomiting, BMD, alopecia, dermatitis, pulmonary fibrosis
		Thiotepa	Slow i.v. bolus or infusion	Pain at injection site, rare nausea, allergy, alopecia, BMD, amenorrhoea
		Treosulfan	Slow i.v. bolus	Nausea and vomiting, mild allergic reaction, BMD, alopecia
		Cisplatin	Infusion over 1–6 hours	Rare anaphylaxis, metallic taste, nausea and vomiting, nephrotoxic, BMD, otological and neurological toxicity
		Procarbazine	Oral	Nausea and vomiting, flu-like syndrome, diarrhoea, CNS toxicity, BMD, reacts with alcohol and certain foods
		Carboplatin	Intravenous infusion over 30–60 minutes	Rare allergic reaction, nausea and vomiting, BMD, nephrotoxicity

Up-to-date listings available in the *British National formulary*.

always be present when a sensitive phase of the cycle is reached. The transport of cyto-toxic drugs across a tumour cell membrane may depend not only on drug concentration, but also on the time the drug is available to the cell membrane. As many cytotoxic drugs have short pharmacological half-lives, the therapeutic action may be more effective if exposed to tumour cells for prolonged periods rather than given by intermittent bolus injections. When given continuously, the concentration of the drug in the plasma is far lower than levels seen immediately after bolus injections or short infusions. Many of the acute toxicities of the drug may therefore be avoided as the peaks and troughs of drug levels are eliminated (Priestman 1989; Knight 2004).

Intermittent chemotherapy

The 'normal' cell population is depleted by treatment with cytotoxic chemotherapy, but 'normal' cells recover more rapidly than cancerous cells. The rationale for giving repeated doses, or 'pulses', of cytotoxic drugs is to allow a period of recovery for 'normal' cells, but hopefully prevent the cancerous cells from replicating and thereby eradicate the tumour (Trevit & Phillips 2006).

The timing of the treatment is crucial in the design of the specific drug regimen. If the interval is too short, 'normal' stem cells will not have recovered sufficiently and cumula-tive toxicity will result. Side-effects such as bone marrow depression or mucositis may delay the next pulse of cytotoxic chemotherapy and thereby prevent adequate treatment. If, on the other hand, the interval between courses is too long, tumour cell recovery will be complete, allowing the tumour to remain static or even increase in size between treat-ments. The splitting of chemotherapy into short intensive intervals is known as intermit-tent chemotherapy and it has allowed multiple drug combinations to be used without causing irreversible toxicity and with a consequent increase in response rates (Priestman 1989; Knight 2004).

Combination chemotherapy

Cytotoxic drugs exert a variety of actions on the dividing cell. Therefore, a tumour cell that may be resistant to one drug with a particular mode of action might well be suscep-tible to a different agent with an alternative form of cytotoxicity. Combining drugs with different mechanisms of 'cell kill' reduces the risk of encountering resistant cells and tox-icity and increases fractional cell kill, thereby improving response rates (Tortorice 1997). The combined effects of two or more cytotoxic drugs can cause a synergistic effect; i.e. the sum of the effect of the drugs on the malignant cells is greater than if they are given separately.

The choice of drugs for combination chemotherapy is based on the following.

- All drugs in the combination should be of proven value against the disease they are intended to treat.
- The drugs should have different modes of cytotoxic action.
- If possible, the dose-limiting toxicities of the chosen agents should be different, so that the additive toxicity does not limit the dose intensity of treatment (Priestman 1989; Holmes 1990; Knight 2004).

High-dose chemotherapy (autologous bone marrow transplant)

A few drugs (those whose major toxicity is to the bone marrow) may be used in very high doses if bone marrow/stem cells are taken from the patient before treatment and returned later (autografting). In this way, doses of the cytotoxic drug that are severely toxic to the bone marrow may be given more safely. This is because the bone marrow autograft is not exposed to the drug, as it was harvested before treatment and then reinfused following treatment. When it is returned to the patient, the autograft will restore the blood count to normal within a few weeks. However, a bone marrow/stem cell autograft will not reduce the other toxicities that may result from high-dose chemotherapy. Autografting can be used for individuals with haematological malignancies who are too frail to undergo allogenic transplant, or for patients with solid tumours requiring treatment with higher doses of cytotoxic drugs which would result in bone marrow depression if the patient's bone marrow/stem cells had not been harvested and preserved before treatment (Robinson 1993; Richardson & Atkinson 2006).

Occupational Hazards

Cytotoxic drug handling by nursing, medical and pharmacy personnel is an acknowledged occupational hazard (Valanis *et al.* 1993; HSE 2002; DH 2004; Trevit & Phillips 2006). Concerns have increased in recent years as more cytotoxic drugs are used, and scientific evidence has come to light regarding the potential and actual hazards of exposure to cytotoxic drugs (Falck *et al.* 1979; Waksvik *et al.* 1981; Vennit *et al.* 1984; Selevan *et al.* 1985; Valanis *et al.* 1993; HSE 2002; DH 2004; Trevit & Phillips 2006). As these agents are administered to eradicate or control a patient's cancer, it is inevitable that any individual other than the patient who comes into contact with such drugs could potentially be adversely affected, especially if they are handling these agents on a regular basis.

The health risk associated with exposure to cytotoxic drugs is measured by the time, dose and route of exposure (Gabriel 2001; Polovich *et al.* 2004; Trevit & Phillips 2006). Primary routes for exposure include absorption through the skin, inhalation or ingestion. Exposure can occur during drug preparation and reconstitution, administration and handling. This can result from aerosolization of powder or liquid during reconstitution, contact with contaminated equipment used in preparing or administering the drugs, or contamination of food leading to oral ingestion (Valanis *et al.* 1993; Gabriel 2001; Trevit & Phillips 2006). Patients also excrete some level of the drugs in their urine or faeces, and other body fluids can also be affected such as vomit etc. Therefore staff are potentially exposed to these hazardous agents when handling and disposing of waste. Such waste should be treated as potentially hazardous for 48 hours after the patient receives/completes their cytotoxic chemotherapy (RCN 1998; Allwood *et al.* 2002; Trevit & Phillips 2006). Exposure has been reported to result in both local effects, caused by direct contact with the skin, eyes and mucous membranes, and systemic complaints from handling (*See* Box 16.1) (Valanis *et al.* 1993; Gabriel 2001; Sims 2005; Trevit & Phillips 2006; Weinstein 2007). A number of early studies looking at health professionals involved in reconstitution and administration have suggested that there are potential serious long-term effects of exposure. For example, some nurses exposed to cytotoxic agents have suffered spontaneous abortion or given birth to children with malformations, while others have shown increased mutagenic activity in their urine and blood serum (Falck *et al.* 1979; Hemminki *et al.* 1985; Selevan *et al.* 1985; Behamou 1986; Taskinan 1990). As a result of these studies, a number of safety measures have been introduced in order to protect all personnel who prepare, administer or handle cytotoxic drugs or waste products. In 1988, the Heath and Safety Executive introduced the *Control of Substances Hazardous to Health* (COSHH) regulations, and these are regularly updated (HSE 2002). These regulations cover a wide range of hazardous substances, but include guidance on the safe handling of cytotoxic drugs. Employers are now obliged to identify hazardous substances, the people who may be exposed to them, how they should be handled and what to do in the event of accidental exposure (RCN 1998; HSE 2002; DH 2004; MARCH Guidelines 2007). The literature supports the theory that the use of protective practices and equipment when handling cytotoxic drugs will provide

> **BOX 16.1**
>
> **Effects of cytotoxic drugs**
>
> **Local effects**
> - Dermatitis
> - Inflammation of mucous membranes
> - Excessive lacrimation
> - Pigmentation
> - Blistering
> - Other miscellaneous, allergic reactions
>
> **Systemic effects**
> - Light-headedness
> - Dizziness
> - Nausea
> - Headache
> - Alopecia
> - Coughing
> - Pruritus
> - General malaise
> - Infections
> (Adapted from Hyde 2004; Trevit & Phillips 2006)

adequate protection from their effects (Wiseman & Wachs 1990; RCN 1998, 2005). Work practice guidelines have focused on how the use of protective clothing can substantially reduce staff exposure levels, including levels and changes found in urine and serum (RCN 1998; Allwood *et al.* 2002; Trevit & Phillips 2006).

Nieweg *et al.* (1994) carried out a survey of Dutch nurses who were involved in caring for patients receiving cytotoxic drugs on a regular basis. They wanted to discover how many of these nurses made use of the protective measures provided. The majority of nurses wore gloves (91%) when preparing and administering drugs, but few wore masks, gowns or goggles, and use was even lower in those handling excreta and other bodily fluids. This was also the case in a survey carried out by Wiseman and Wachs (1990), who concluded that healthcare workers still did not use available protective equipment and procedures. Cardonick and Iacobucci (2004) identified that handling of cytotoxic agents during the second and third trimesters appeared to be safe, as staff were apparently aware of a potential risk and therefore wore protective clothing. However, as the first trimester poses the greatest risk to the fetus, due to the rapid cell division, staff should avoid exposure or reduce their exposure to the lowest level practicable.

All organizations using cytotoxic agents are subject to health and safety reviews and must develop and implement policies and procedures that will lower the risk to staff and the environment (HSE 2002; Sims 2005; Sewell 2007). In addition, organizations using cytotoxic agents for the management of patients with malignant disease are also subject to National Cancer Peer Reviews, which have specific measures (standards) relating to the health and safety aspects of cytotoxic chemotherapy (DH 2004). Christensen *et al.* (1990) found that the existence of a formal hospital policy for handling of cytotoxics positively influenced the use of personal protective equipment. The aim of such a policy should be to recognize the hazards of cytotoxic drugs and to prevent, or reduce to a minimum, exposure to these hazards in the workplace. This would be achieved by the provision of adequate protective equipment and clothing, regular staff monitoring, and effective written procedures and guidelines for dealing with preparation, administration, disposal and handling of spillage. It would also require ongoing staff training to ensure that these drugs are only administered by skilled, knowledgeable and experienced healthcare professionals (Mayer 1992; Allwood *et al.* 2002; Hyde 2004; Trevit & Phillips 2006). The publication of the *National Manual of Cancer Measures* (DH 2004) has put in place minimum standards to ensure that all acute hospital trusts treating cancer patients which undertake the preparation and administration of cytotoxic chemotherapy have written procedures which cover the prescribing, preparation, storage, transportation and administration of these agents, together with guidance on their disposal and management of waste products including spillage.

Safe Handling

Environment

All reconstitution of cytotoxic drugs must be conducted within a suitable safety cabinet or isolator such as a biological safety cabinet class II vertical laminar air flow. This equipment should meet national standards and be inspected and serviced regularly according to the manufacturer's recommendations. Cabinets should be situated within a specified or dedicated area with the access restricted to appropriately trained personnel. Standard operating procedures should be in place and strictly adhered to for maximum operator protection (Allwood *et al.* 2002; DH 2004; Trevit & Phillips 2006; Weinstein 2007).

Protective clothing

Protective clothing should be worn at all times when handling cytotoxics (Allwood *et al.* 2002; March Guidelines 2007; Trevit & Phillips 2006). There are minimum requirements for the degree of protective clothing to be worn and these are often based upon the amount of possible exposure and the situation in which the practitioner is handling the drug, e.g. controlled or uncontrolled preparation environment, administration or transportation. The requirements are usually based on local or nationally agreed guidelines (March Guidelines 2007; Trevit & Phillips 2006).

Gowns

This category includes gowns, suits, armlets and aprons. It has been suggested that gowns be made of a lightweight, low-linting, low-permeability material with a solid front and long cuffed sleeves; these may be either disposable or made of conventional fabric (Allwood *et al.* 2002; Polovich *et al.* 2004; Hayden & Goodman 2005; March Guidelines 2007; Weinstein 2007). There are many commercially available gowns and suits and these are commonly used by personnel who are reconstituting cytotoxic drugs. Allwood *et al.* (2001) suggested that disposable gowns made of polyurethane-coated Tyvek and Saranex-laminated Tyvek offered the maximum protection. In studies, the non-porous Tyvek did allow some drug penetration, but when used with armlets has proved suitable for all administration and waste disposal procedures, along with the use of plastic aprons. The practitioner should be provided with a protective water-resistant barrier to accidental spills or sprays. Tyvek aprons provide added protection in an uncontrolled environment.

As long ago as the mid-1990s, the negative effect that all this protective clothing could have on the patient has been highlighted. Each organization should undertake a risk assessment for the extent of protective clothing that is required for each procedure. A patient receiving intravesicular chemotherapy will require the health professional administering the treatment to wear more extensive protective clothing than that required for a patient receiving a single bolus injection of vincristine. The protective clothing is not only for the benefit of the health professional but also for their colleagues and other patients in the wider environment, which also has the potential to be contaminated. Hayden and Goodman (2005) suggested that education regarding cytotoxic drug handling was the answer, so that patients and their family members understand why gloves and gowns etc. are being worn and do not feel alienated by the practice.

Masks

The standard surgeons' masks are not suitable for procedures carried out in a contained environment. A FFP2 or FFP3 filtered face piece respirator should be used (March Guidelines 2007). The further risk of inhalation should be reduced by use of a correct and safe technique when reconstituting drugs and by the use of equipment such as 0.2-mm filtered venting needles. If there is a possibility of inhalation, a suitable dust mask should be worn, e.g. BS EN 149: 1992 6016 (Allwood *et al.* 2002; Trevit & Phillips 2006).

Eye protection

Goggles should be used to protect the eyes from splashes and any dust particles and should fully enclose the eye. March Guidelines (2007) recommend such eye protection should meet British Standard EN 166. Goggles should be worn whenever reconstituting or dealing with a spillage (Allwood *et al.* 2002; Trevit & Phillips 2006).

Gloves

There is little doubt that disposable gloves should be worn at all times when reconstituting, administering or handling cytotoxic agents (March Guidelines 2007). They should also be worn when handling the excreta of patients receiving these drugs. It is the one piece of protective clothing that most practitioners wear when dealing with any aspect of cytotoxic therapy. The type of disposable glove is still open to debate. Allwood *et al.* (2002) concluded that no glove material is completely impermeable to every cytotoxic agent. The major factors affecting penetration rates include glove thickness, molecular weight of the drug, lipophilicity, the nature of the solvent in which the drug is dissolved and glove material composition (Allwood *et al.* 2002).

When selecting gloves, the material should be of a suitable thickness and integrity to maximize protection whilst maintaining manual dexterity. Certainly, the use of poor-quality, low-cost gloves is neither safe nor cost-effective (Allwood *et al.* 2002). Some experts recommend the practice of double-gloving during reconstitution (Vandergrift 2001; Polovich *et al.* 2004; Weinstein 2007). However, this may be unnecessary if gloves are of good quality and is usually only required when cleaning up large spills (MARCH guidelines (2007). Nitrile gloves are now widely used because of their protection properties and also because they are latex free (MARCH Guidelines 2007). Regular changing of gloves is common, although the frequency varies from changing them every 30–60 minutes to changing them at each work session/individual patient contact. They should also be changed immediately following known contact with a cytotoxic agent or following puncture (Allwood *et al.* 2002; Hyde 2004; Polovich *et al.* 2004; Weinstein 2007).

Reconstitution

Cytotoxic drugs should be reconstituted:

- in a pharmacy-controlled centralized unit where reconstitution of cytotoxic drugs is only performed by specially trained individuals (Allwood *et al.* 2002; DH 2004)
- in a pharmacy-controlled satellite unit where work is centralized in designated hospital areas (DH 2004)
- in a ward/clinic-based isolator when the pharmacy service is unavailable
- using a commercial service where the drugs are bought in already prepared.

The use of a plastic absorbent pad or liner on the work surface or a plastic or stainless steel tray is recommended, to contain and minimize contamination (Polovich *et al.* 2004;

Hayden & Goodman 2005; Weinstein 2007). Protective clothing should be worn, i.e. gown/apron, gloves, goggles, mask and armlets. Aseptic technique should be used throughout the reconstitution procedure. Ampoules should be handled carefully and the neck of the ampoule disinfected before breaking with a dedicated ampoule breaker (Hyde 2004; Polovich *et al.* 2004; RCN 2005; Weinstein 2007).

When reconstituting drugs in powder form, care should be taken when adding diluents to vials or ampoules. The drug should be added slowly, and 'dribbled' down the side of the container so it gradually mixes with the powder and minimizes the formation of an aerosol (Hyde 2004; Polovich *et al.* 2004; RCN 2005). The use of filtered venting systems, large-bore needles or specifically designed needle-free systems will help to reduce the risk of aerosol formation by creating a negative pressure in the vial and filtering the air released (Allwood *et al.* 2002; Polovich *et al.* 2004; RCN 2005; Weinstein 2007). If air is present in the syringe, it should be held in such a way that the air is near the plunger and the practitioner should simply stop pushing on the plunger when all the drug is expelled and the air is reached. Luer-lock syringes should always be used to ensure that there is no risk of disconnection during the procedure (Hyde 2004; RCN 2005). Ideally, administration sets should be primed in the reconstitution unit (Polovich *et al.* 2004). However, where accidental spillage is possible, infusion bags should be connected to intravenous (i.v.) administration sets and primed before adding cytotoxic drug to the infusion solution. If this is not possible, then the bag should be laid flat and the administration set spike pushed firmly into it, as it would be potentially unsafe to spike a hanging bag because of the risk of splashing or puncturing the side of the bag. With the increasing range of needle-free devices available, and a greater awareness of the potential dangers to staff of needlestick injuries, needle-free and safer sharps should be used wherever possible (Gabriel 2006a).

Once reconstituted, the syringe or infusion bag/container must be labelled according to organizational policy—this usually includes the patient's name, their hospital number, time, name and dose of drug, volume of drug, expiration date and diluent fluid.

Administration

The Department of Health (DH) has produced guidance stating that cytotoxic drugs used in the treatment of oncology patients should only be administered by appropriately trained staff. This guidance also stipulates the training that is required for chemotherapy nurses (DH 2004).

Before commencing the administration of the chemotherapy, the nurse must be satisfied that the patient has given informed consent and has been given a full explanation regarding the potential side-effects that may occur during or following administration. Appropriate laboratory results, e.g. full blood count and renal function tests, should be within acceptable levels and the prescription should be dated, legible and signed. Protocols and dosage should also be checked and the appropriate premedication administered, e.g. prehydration or antiemetics (DH 2004; Hyde 2004; Polovich *et al.* 2004; Ellis *et al.* 2006; Weinstein 2007).

Patients who are beginning cytotoxic therapy often have minimal knowledge about what it involves and the possible side-effects. Many may have gleaned inappropriate information from the media or friends and family. Moreover, patients receiving therapy are repeatedly exposed to venepuncture and cannulation unless they have had a central venous catheter inserted at the beginning of treatment. All this can be stressful for patients and provoke a good deal of anxiety. In addition, practitioners should be aware that aspects of cytotoxic drug administration which they may dismiss as unimportant can also be causes of concern to patients (Colbourne 1995; Gabriel 2001).

A change in a patient's routine can also be upsetting. Back in 1983 Kaplan reported:

> One patient became anxious when her chemotherapy was administered in a different manner than it had been previously. The first time the drug was given by i.v., the nurse was at her side. The second time, the i.v. was begun and the patient was left unattended; she mistakenly assumed she was receiving the wrong drug.

These concerns and worries are as real today for patients as they were back in 1983. They must be addressed before starting treatment and an adequate explanation should be given, along with written information in the form of booklets or videotapes; cassettes or other teaching aids should be available to support verbal information, taking into account the specific needs of each individual patient. The *National Cancer Measures* (DH 2004) clearly state that patients must receive appropriate information before beginning treatment and throughout their patient journey. Patient information needs are also addressed in the various Improving Outcomes Guidances (IOGs) which have been published for cancer.

Appropriate protective clothing should be worn and its necessity explained to the patient. Aseptic technique should be followed throughout the administration procedure. All syringes and infusion bags should be checked for any leakage or contamination, the details on the labels should correspond with the prescription chart and the patient's identity should be checked immediately before administration. Only i.v. administration sets with luer-lock fittings should be used, to ensure there is minimal risk of accidental disconnection during administration (Gabriel 2001; RCN 2005).

Drugs may be administered via a winged infusion device, a peripheral cannula or a central venous access device (CVAD) depending on the prescribed therapy and patient's preference. A winged infusion device can be used for bolus injections of non-vesicant drugs, but is associated with an increased risk of infiltration (RCN 2005). Cannulae can also be used for both bolus and short-term infusions of non-vesicant drugs. The smallest gauge possible should be selected for the prescribed treatment to minimize the potential damage to the patient's vein (Box 16.2). Central venous access is preferred for patients who require long-term therapy, or require vesicant cytotoxic agents, or who have difficult venous access (RCN 2005; Weinstein 2007). The suggested order for site selection of winged infusion devices or cannulae is the forearm and the dorsum of the hand. The antecubital fossa should be avoided for the administration of cytotoxic agents (RCN 2005) (*See* Figure 16.2). If the patient has an established peripheral cannula *in situ*, the dressing should be removed and the site assessed for redness, pain or tenderness.

BOX 16.2

Needle/cannula gauge size

Favouring use of larger gauges
- Irritant drugs/infusates reach the general circulation faster, with a less irritating effect on the wall of peripheral veins
- Administration time is decreased, which reduces patient's exposure

Favouring use of smaller gauges
- Less likely to puncture posterior wall of small vein
- Less scar tissue formation
- Less pain on insertion
- Increased blood flow around the needle, increasing dilution of the drug
- Reduced risk of mechanical phlebitis
- Less trauma to the vein

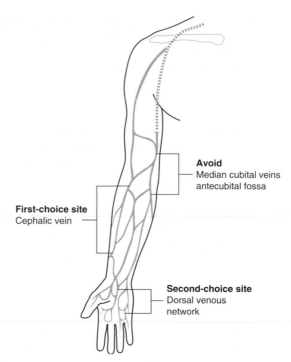

Avoid
Median cubital veins
antecubital fossa

First-choice site
Cephalic vein

Second-choice site
Dorsal venous
network

Figure 16.2   Sites for cannulation and administration of chemotherapy.

Patency of the cannula must be checked by withdrawing blood and then flushing using 5–10 mL of 0.9% sodium chloride to ensure there is no resistance to the flow of fluid. This also allows the practitioner to observe for any swelling or signs of pain or discomfort from the patient. If the practitioner is in any doubt regarding the patency of the device, it should be resited before administering the chemotherapy.

Cytotoxic drugs may be administered intravenously by:

- bolus injection.
- the side-arm of a fast running infusion of sodium chloride 0.9%.
- a continuous infusion.

The choice of vein should depend on the type of drug, the pharmacological considerations (such as stability or the need for dilution in a certain volume of fluid), the degree of potential venous irritation, whether the drug is a vesicant or not, and the type of device (Hadaway 2006).

Bolus injection

By administering a drug as a bolus injection, the integrity of the vein can be assessed and the early signs of extravasation can be noted more easily. Any observation of signs or symptoms of infiltration or extravasation must result in the immediate discontinuation of the injection, investigation of the signs and symptoms and the appropriate management. Bolus injections can increase the risk of venous irritation due to the continual contact of the drug with the vein wall. This can result in pain and make it difficult to distinguish between venous spasm and extravasation. The site must be monitored throughout the bolus injection to check for signs of infiltration, extravasation or leakage at the site. This will ensure the prompt recognition and management of any complication, thus minimizing local damage and preserving venous access for future treatment (Hyde 2004; RCN 2005). A gauze swab should be kept at connecting points in case of droplets (Hayden & Goodman 2005).

Via a side-arm

Bolus injections can also be administered via the side-arm of a free-flowing infusion of 0.9% sodium chloride. This ensures maximum dilution of the potentially irritant drugs and aids rapid circulation away from the insertion site. It can also allow the practitioner to observe for early signs of infiltration or extravasation. However, if the veins are small or the cannula is too small, there will still not be a brisk flow of the infusate and the drug may reflux up the tubing. The practitioner will need to clamp off the tubing to check for blood return and continually check flow of the infusate. If there is any suspicion that the infusion may be infiltrating/extravasating, the administration should cease immediately and prompt action be instigated (RCN 2005; Hadaway 2006).

Continuous infusion

Infusions allow increased dilution of the drug, thereby reducing the chemical irritation that can occur if drugs are given as a bolus injection. They may also be necessary depending on the side-effects of the medication, such as hypotension or hypoglycaemia. Vesicant cytotoxic drugs given as a continuous infusion into a peripheral vein should be avoided where possible, as the risk of extravasation is significant and if required, such an infusion should ideally be administered via a CVAD (RCN 2005; Gabriel 2006b; Weinstein 2007). Infiltration and extravasation may be subtle and difficult to detect until a large volume has infiltrated, and the patient may be sedated and unable to report any sensations associated with extravasation. The practitioner should not rely on the i.v. pump to alarm if an infusion begins to infiltrate. Initially, the flow is free and it is only when the pressure builds up in the tissues that the pump will alarm 'occlusion'. When vesicants are given as infusions via an implantable injection device (port), extra care must be taken to ensure the needle does not become dislodged. The incidence of extravasation in ports is significantly higher than with skin-tunnelled catheters and peripherally inserted central catheters (PICCs) (Hadaway 2006)

The drugs should be administered in the correct order, i.e. vesicants first, unless contraindicated with other medication (Hyde 2004; RCN 2005; Weinstein 2007) (Table 16.2). At least 5–10 mL of sodium chloride 0.9% (unless contraindicated) should be used to flush in between each drug, to avoid mixing as this could result in chemical interactions. Blood return should be checked regularly, especially when administering a vesicant, i.e. every 2–5 mL (RCN 2005; Weinstein 2007). If attaching an infusion, ensure that all the connections are luer-locked and secure, and the giving set is taped/secure so that the tubing cannot be pulled or the cannula dislodged. After all the drugs have been administered, a final flush of 5–10 mL of 0.9% sodium chloride should be given to ensure adequate flushing of the device, the tubing and the vein.

On completion, waste products should be disposed of according to the organization's policy. Documentation must be completed immediately after administration is complete, including any adverse reactions, to prevent duplication of treatment. The patient should be made comfortable and given appropriate information, especially if they are an outpatient or day-care patient (DH 2004).

Table 16.2 When to give vesicants.

When?	For	Against
First	Vascular integrity decreases over time Initially, practitioner observation is more accurate Patient may be sedated if antiemetic given first and less able to report pain	Vesicant is irritating and compromises integrity Venospasm may occur early, altering assessment of patency
Last	Venous spasm occurs early; less likely to be confused with pain of extravasation if vesicant given last Assumed that if vein can tolerate non-vesicant, it can tolerate vesicant	Vein may be irritated and not remain patent for vesicants
Between two non-vesicants	Cytotoxics are irritating to veins and non-vesicants are less irritant than vesicants	

Disposal of Waste

Each organization should have a clear and concise procedure for the safe handling and disposal of cytotoxic drugs and material contaminated by them (HSE 2002; DH 2004)— the recommended method is incineration. Sharps should be placed in designated sharps containers as complete needle–syringe units to prevent the risk of needlestick injury or contamination during disconnection. Protective clothing, administration sets and other contaminated material should be placed in leak-proof waste disposal bags/bins, and sealed and labelled according to the organization's policies. Contaminated linen should be bagged and labelled as contaminated to ensure that it is handled correctly by laundry staff. All reusable equipment, such as goggles or trays, should be washed with soap and water and dried thoroughly. Disposal via domestic sewerage systems should not be used for large quantities of pharmaceutical waste, but may be acceptable for small quantities (Gabriel 2001; Allwood *et al.* 2002; Hyde 2004). Cytotoxic drugs can be excreted as unchanged drug(s) or active metabolites in urine, faeces, blood, vomit and even saliva. In order to comply with safe technique and practice, universal precautions should be used and gloves worn when disposing of any excreta of patients receiving cytotoxic therapy for up to 48 hours following the patient's last infusion/administration of cytotoxic chemotherapy (Hyde 2004; Trevit & Phillips 2006; Weinstein 2007).

Dealing with a Spill

It is recommended that a spill kit is available wherever cytotoxic drugs are being reconstituted, administered or handled, and that staff are trained in its use (HSE 2002; DH 2004; Hyde 2004; Polovich *et al.* 2004). This enables staff to have immediate access to all the necessary equipment which will help to prevent further contamination of the environment and aid prompt cleaning. The contents of spill kits vary, but there are some basic requirements (Box 16.3).

In the event of a spill, the immediate area should be cleared where possible and the necessary protective clothing worn, i.e. two pairs of nitrile gloves, gown or apron, armlets, overshoes, goggles and, in the event of a powder spill, a face mask (*See* mask guidance above) (MARCH Guidelines 2007). Powder spills should be contained with dampened paper towels to prevent dispersal. All spills should be wiped up with absorbent towels, starting from the outside edge and working towards the centre to prevent spread of contamination to a larger area (Hyde 2004). All contaminated surfaces should

> **BOX 16.3**
>
> **Contents of a spill kit**
>
> - Plastic apron
> - Plastic overshoes
> - Disposable armlets
> - Disposable nitrile gloves (two pairs)
> - Face masks
> - Goggles
> - Disposable cytotoxic waste bags
> - Paper towels
> - Eye irrigation kit
> - Instruction/documentation sheet
> - All contained within a large cardboard/plastic bucket/box

be cleaned with cold soapy water at least three times, and dried to remove residual contamination (Hyde 2004; Polovich *et al.* 2004; Weinstein 2007).

Powell (1996) does not recommend the use of chemical inactivation (with the exception of sodium thiosulphate) to absorb drug spills because of the potentially dangerous byproducts that may be produced.

Accidental exposure of patient or practitioner

If a cytotoxic drug is spilled onto the clothing of staff or the patient, the piece of clothing should be removed as soon as possible and treated as contaminated linen. If the spill has penetrated clothing and come into contact with the person's skin, the area must be thoroughly washed with soap and large amounts of water (Hyde 2004). In the case of exposure or splashing into the eye, the eye should be flooded with water or an isotonic eye wash solution for at least 5 minutes and medical attention sought (Hyde 2004; Weinstein 2007). In the event of any direct exposure of the practitioner, the incident should be reported to the occupational health department and documented according to the organization's policies.

Staff Monitoring/Surveillance

It is essential that a system of health surveillance is provided for staff directly involved in handling cytotoxic drugs. Allwood *et al.* (2002) recommended a programme which contains a medical history, physical examination, laboratory tests (FBC & differential) and biological monitoring (although the value of monitoring levels of drugs and their metabolites is limited due to the wide range of drugs and the, reliability, sensitivity and validation of the test methods available (Sims 2005). It has been suggested there are no data to support a cause and effect relationship between precautionary cytotoxic drug handling and abnormal physical and laboratory findings, and it is therefore less common for staff to undergo extensive testing (Sims 2005). In general, staff that are pregnant, planning a pregnancy or breast-feeding may elect to refrain from preparation or administration of cytotoxics and most organizations would support this, especially as there is no conclusive evidence that ongoing exposure to such agents during pregnancy has no adverse effect on the unborn child, particularly during the second and third trimesters (Polovich *et al.* 2004). (Individual organizations will have policies/guidance to inform staff and managers of the appropriate advice for individuals planning a pregnancy or who are pregnant and work with cytotoxic agents.)

Section 3

Side-Effects

Most side-effects are temporary and usually result from the action of the cytotoxic drug on the rapidly dividing cells, such as stomatitis, nausea and vomiting, alopecia and bone marrow suppression (Dougherty & Bailey 2001). Some toxicity may be permanent, such as when an organ is affected, for example cardiac myopathy, pulmonary fibrosis or sterility (Dougherty & Bailey 2001). Side-effects can be further categorized in relation to their onset as follows (*See* also Table 16.3):

- immediate: occur within 30 minutes of commencing treatment
- short-term: occur between 3 and 7 days after treatment
- long-term: manifested later than 7 days; many are cumulative in nature.

The practitioner administering i.v. cytotoxic therapy will need the knowledge to be aware of the immediate effects or those that may affect the choice of veins when establishing venous access. Nurses must be accountable for their own actions and able to recognize and differentiate the side-effects from more serious complications and respond appropriately (Box 16.4).

Pain at the insertion site

A number of cytotoxic drugs are irritants or vesicants. During administration, chemical irritation by the drug can lead to venous spasm, resulting in an ache or pain at the insertion site.

Table 16.3   Side-effects of cytotoxic drugs.

Immediate effects	Short-term effects	Long-term effects
Cold sensation along vein	Anorexia	Bone marrow depression
Pain at insertion site	Nausea and vomiting	Alopecia
Red flush along vein	Stomatitis	Skin reactions
Metallic taste	Potentiation of radiation	Nail ridging
Nasal stuffiness	skin reactions	Thrombophlebitis
Anticipatory nausea	Pain at tumour site/jaw	Pulmonary fibrosis
and vomiting	Malaise	Congestive cardiac failure
Allergic reaction	Flu-like syndrome	Renal toxicity
Hot flush	Chemical cystitis	Liver dysfunction
Dizziness	Haematuria	Neurological problems
Hypotension	Discoloration of urine	CNS toxicity
Hypoglycaemia	Constipation	Sexual dysfunction
	Diarrhoea	

BOX 16.4

Side-effects and nursing interventions (adapted from Eli Lilley 2005)

Dermatological

1. Venous sensations, e.g. cold or pain
   - Distinguish from extravasation
   - Explain to patients the possibility of it occurring
   - Administer drug slowly with fast-running infusion of sodium chloride 0.9% (unless contraindicated)
   - Use local heat to aid vasodilation
   - Dilute drugs where possible

(Continued)

BOX 16.4 (*Continued*)

2. Skin pigmentation/venous discoloration
   - Explain to patients the possibility of it occurring
   - Reassure that it is only temporary
   - Advise against prolonged exposure to sunlight
3. Palmar–plantar syndrome
   - Explain to the patient the possibility of it occurring and when to report to medical/nursing team
   - Encourage patient to use moisturizer on hands and feet and to avoid any damage
4. Dermatitis/rash
   - Explain to patients the possibility of it occurring
   - Administer antihistamine where appropriate
   - Seek dermatology opinion
5. Flushing along the vein
   - Advise patients of the possibility at the time of administration
   - Apply local steroid cream when necessary
6. Body and facial flushing
   - Administer drug slowly
   - Reassure patients that the effect is short-lived
7. Alopecia
   - Explain to patients the possibility of it occurring
   - Reassure that hair will regrow
   - Advise on hair care and order wig before hair loss
   - Use scalp cooling where appropriate

Gastrointestinal
1. Taste aberration
   - Advise patients that it may occur during injection or at any time during the course of treatment
   - Encourage sipping of drinks and sucking of sweets
   - Encourage different food/addition of seasoning
2. Anorexia
   - Encourage small, frequent meals
   - Monitor the patient's weight
   - Refer to dietician for advice and food supplements where necessary
3. Stomatitis
   - Regular observation of mouth
   - Teach patients good oral care and to avoid hot, spicy and citrus foods, alcohol and smoking
   - Administer analgesics and/or antifungals as required
4. Nausea and vomiting
   - Administer effective antiemetics and encourage patients to take them regularly
   - Encourage patients to use distraction, meditation, relaxation and other therapies such as acupuncture or aromatherapy
   - Observe for symptoms of fluid and electrolyte imbalance and treat as required
5. Diarrhoea
   - Encourage low-fibre diet and good perianal care
   - Observe for symptoms of dehydration and electrolyte imbalance, and treat as required
   - Administer antidiarrhoeal agents as required
6. Constipation
   - Inform patients of the possibility of it occurring and encourage high-fibre diet with plenty of fluids
   - Administer prophylactic aperients

Haematological
1. Anaemia
   - Observe for pallor, dizziness and shortness of breath
   - Check full blood count on regular basis
   - Encourage high dietary iron intake, e.g. red meat, green vegetables, etc.
   - Administer blood transfusions and/or haematopoetic agents as prescribed
2. Leucopenia
   - Prevent/minimize exposure of patients to known infections
   - Teach patients to perform meticulous hygiene and recognize early symptoms of infection such as fever or cough, and supplement with written information, including 24-hour contact details

(*Continued*)

BOX 16.4   Continued

- Check full blood count on a regular basis
- Administer antibiotics and GCSF as required (either prophylactically or for treatment)

3. Thrombocytopenia
- Inform patients of the necessity to avoid physical injury (while shaving, brushing teeth, gardening, etc.)
- Avoid drugs which further interfere with platelet function, e.g. aspirin
- Observe for signs of bleeding, including petechiae and haematoma
- Check full blood count on regular basis
- Administer platelet transfusions as prescribed

Organs

1. Hepatic
- Observe for signs of jaundice
- Monitor liver function tests and report abnormalities

2. Cardiac
- Ensure baseline ECG and/or echocardiogram/MUGA scans before treatment if appropriate
- Observe for cumulative effects

3. Pulmonary
- Ensure baseline chest X-ray if appropriate for prescribed regime
- Observe for onset of symptoms, e.g. shortness of breath and wheezing, and report

4. Renal
- Monitor renal dysfunction if appropriate for prescribed regime
- Record all fluid intake and output
- Test urine for pH and blood
- Administer mesna for protection of bladder if appropriate
- Inform and reassure patients of the possibility of discoloration of urine if appropriate, e.g. administration of doxourubicin

5. CNS
- Observe for abnormal signs and symptoms
- Reassure patients about. peripheral neuropathy and report—drug may be changed

6. Sexual dysfunction
- Advise female patients of possibility of amenorrhoea, early menopause and potential sterility
- Discuss pretreatment sperm banking with male patients
- Advise both sexes on contraception

Miscellaneous

1. Malaise/fatigue
- Inform patients of the possibility of it occurring, when it may occur and for how long
- Advise patients to plan actions and have regular rest periods

2. Cold induced paraesthesia
- Inform the patient of when and how this may occur e.g. following cold drinks, muscle tightness in throat and jaw, leg and arm cramps
- Encourage patient to wear hats and gloves and wrap scarf around mouth when out and to avoid eating and drinking any cold foods/fluids

3. Flu-like syndrome
- Inform patients of the possibility of fever, chills and headache and that it is only temporary
- Administer prophylactic steroids if indicated

4. Allergic reactions
- Be prepared if anaphylaxis is a possibility
- Carry out regular observations during administration of treatment
- Administer prophylactic drugs as required as per prescription

5. Pain, e.g. in tumour, jaw
- Reassure patients that it is only temporary
- Administer analgesics as required

6. Hyperglycaemia/hypotension
- Observe for signs and symptoms
- Administer infusion slowly (unless contraindicated)

It is important that the practitioner can distinguish between this venous spasm and extravasation. Knowledge of the drugs that are likely to cause pain is vital, as well as methods to prevent, minimize and relieve the pain. Drugs which are known to cause pain include:

- doxorubicin
- epirubicin
- dacarbazine
- oxaliplatin
- cytosine
- vinorelbine
- thiotepa
- streptocozin
- Carmustine.

(Rittenberg *et al.* 1995; Polovich *et al.* 2004; Eli Lilley 2005; Weinstein 2007)

Where possible, and unless contraindicated by the manufacturer, the drug should be diluted and either given as an infusion, preferably via a central venous catheter, or administered slowly via the side-arm of a fast-running infusion of 0.9% sodium chloride (RCN 2005). Heat can be applied above the peripheral cannula to relieve the spasm. The application of a glyceryl trinitrate (GTN) patch below the cannula has been demonstrated to encourage vasodilation and results in better dilution and more rapid circulation away from the insertion site (Hecker 1988).

Local allergic reaction or 'flare reaction'

Some drugs cause a red streak or flush from the insertion site along the vein. This is known as a flare reaction and is caused by a venous inflammatory response to subsequent histamine release (Curran *et al.* 1990). This reaction is characterized by redness and blotchiness, and may result in the formation of small wheals, having a similar appearance to a nettle rash. It is usually associated with red-coloured drugs, such as doxorubicin and epirubicin, and occurs in a small percentage of cases (Allwood *et al.* 2002). It does not cause pain, although the area may feel itchy, and it usually subsides within 30–45 minutes with or without treatment (Hyde 2004). Flare does respond well to the application of a topical steroid or an i.v. injection of hydrocortisone (Weinstein 2007). Prevention includes dilution of the drug, administering via the side-arm of an infusion, or administration via a CVAD.

Discoloration of the veins/hyperpigmentation

This is not a progressive side-effect and may influence the practitioner's choice of veins. There is an increased incidence in individuals with darker skin pigmentation, and it may be associated with exogenous trauma/postinflammatory changes or areas of increased vasodilation (Polovich *et al.* 2004). This side-effect is associated with a number of cytotoxic drugs, but the incidence is highest with alkylating and antitumour antibiotics, such as 5 Fluorouracil, vinblastine, mustine and dactinomycin. The exact mechanism is unknown, but it may result in direct stimulation of the melanocytes. It usually disappears 2–3 months after completion of treatment and causes no other adverse effects. Powell (1996) suggested the avoidance of the use of heating pads or warm compresses to aid vasodilation during the administration of the causative drugs, as these may exacerbate the problem.

Cold sensation

The patient may complain of a cold sensation along the vein during the administration of their treatment. This is often related to the difference between the temperature of the

Section 3

drug and that of the patient. However, some drugs specifically cause a cold sensation, such as vinca alkaloids and oxaliplatin, and the patient should be informed and reassured that this is normal and nothing to be concerned about. However, it should be emphasized that they were right to mention this discomfort to the practitioner as it could have been a sign of extravasation.

Chemical phlebitis and thrombophlebitis

This can result from administration of irritant drugs and can make it more difficult for the practitioner when locating suitable veins for subsequent cannulation and cytotoxic drug administration due to the resulting chemical phlebitis, i.e. irritation to the tunica intima by a chemical (Gabriel 2006b) The incidence is increased when combinations of drugs are administered. Early signs include pain, erythema, oedema, a sensation of warmth and protracted discoloration of the venous pathway. The patient will experience discomfort, in some extreme cases the skin becomes taut and stretched and the vein becomes cord-like, and, depending on the location, it can lead to restricted use of the limb. Knowing which drugs have the potential for this will enable the practitioner to apply all preventative measures at the time of administration. Diluting the drugs (if pharmaceutically acceptable), administering the drug slowly with frequent flushing with sodium chloride 0.9%, and application of heat to the area to aid vasodilation may all reduce the incidence. The use of a small-gauge cannula in a large vein with good blood flow can also help, but if the veins are deep, difficult to visualize or extremely small, it may be necessary to reassess the patient's venous access and opt for a CVAD from the outset of treatment (Gabriel 2006b).

Anaphylactic reaction

According to Weinstein (2007): 'the practitioner should be prepared for anaphylactic reaction at any time with any drug in any patient'. Some cytotoxic drugs are known to cause anaphylaxis, e.g. asparaginase, the taxanes, trastuzumab and other monoclonal antibodies, and the practitioner should be aware of which drugs are more likely to cause the reaction, how to administer the drugs safely and what to do in the event of a reaction (Trevit & Phillips 2006). The patient should be monitored for signs of flushing, shaking, sudden agitation, nausea, urticaria, hypotension, generalized pruritus or wheezing and shortness of breath. If undetected, this reaction can progress to cardiac arrest. To comply with the *Manual of Cancer Measures* (DH 2004), all NHS organizations administering cytotoxic drugs for the treatment of oncology patients are required to have anaphylaxis guidelines.

Extravasation

Extravasation comes from the Latin word *vesicare*, meaning 'to blister', and is defined as the inadvertent administration of a vesicant drug into the surrounding tissues (infiltration is the inadvertent administration of a non-vesicant drug into the tissues) (Hadaway 2006; Trevit & Phillips 2006). A vesicant is a drug which has the potential to cause blistering, severe tissue damage and even necrosis if extravasated, and usually requires some form of management (Trevit & Phillips 2006). An irritant drug can cause local sensitivity and if it infiltrates it can cause local inflammation and discomfort but no long-term damage (How & Brown 1998).

Extravasation is one of the most serious complications associated with the administration of i.v. cytotoxic drugs (Beason 1990). The incidence of cytotoxic drug extravasation has been estimated to range from 0.1 to 6% in patients receiving peripheral chemotherapy, but it is difficult to be accurate and this may not reflect the true rate, as incidents of extravasation may not be recognized or be under-reported (Cox *et al.* 1988; Polovich *et al.* 2004; Masoorli 2005). The incidence appears to be higher in children than in adults, and in central venous catheters it appears to occur more commonly in implantable port devices, often as a result of needle dislodgement (Polovich *et al.* 2004; Masoorli 2005; Hadaway 2006).

Risk factors

Risk factors for extravasation are as follows.

- Patient-related risk factors: the inability to communicate appropriately, e.g. neonates, infants, young children, comatosed or sedated patients, confused patients, very restless patients (Rudolph & Larson 1987; Masoorli 2005; Hadaway 2006).
- Patients with vascular impairment and reduced vascular integrity, e.g. elderly patients, Raynaud's disease, irradiated areas, multiple attempts at venepuncture, cardiac disease, obstructed venous drainage and lymphoedema, superior vena cava syndrome, fragile, sclerosed, thrombosed and small veins (Banerjee *et al.* 1987; Masoorli 2005; Hadaway 2006)
- Skill level of the person performing cannulation and administering the drugs (Beason 1990; Masoorli 2005; Hadaway 2006).

Selection of vein and device

Veins on the dorsum of the hand are unsatisfactory because of the lack of subcutaneous tissue and the proximity of tendons and joints to the overlying skin, which could be damaged if extravasation occurs. Severe problems have been reported with ulceration in this area (Banerjee *et al.* 1987; Rudolph & Larson 1987; Wood & Gullo 1993; Masoorli 2005). Veins in the antecubital fossa are in close proximity to nerves, arteries and tendons and therefore this area should be avoided for administration of cytotoxic drugs (Masoorli 2005). Extravasation is often difficult to detect in this region and it is best left for venepuncture and collection of blood samples (RCN 2005) (Table 16.4).

The ideal location is the proximal forearm over the flexor and extensor muscle bulk, but these veins are often not available or visible or have already been used extensively (Rudolph & Larson 1987; Wood & Gullo 1993; Masoorli 2005; Hadaway 2006). Veins that have been used recently for blood sampling or recently subjected to multiple punctures are not suitable because of the risk of leakage of the drug/infusion from the previous venepuncture sites. If cannulation has been unsuccessful, then a different vein, if

Table 16.4 Use of antecubital fossa.

For	Against
Larger veins allow rapid infusion of drug	Mobility is restricted
Larger veins allow irritant drugs to reach general circulation more quickly and with less irritation than small veins	Risk of extravasation increased if patient tends to be mobile
Easier to palpate and therefore increases successful insertion of device	Early recognition of extravasation is difficult due to the deeper veins—less chance of observing swelling and could go undetected; delayed response to pain
	Damage can result in loss of structure and function; ulceration and fibrosis. Can ultimately result in amputation of limb

possible one in the opposite limb, should be used. If none is available, then a site in the same vein may be selected, but it should be above the previous puncture site (Wood & Gullo 1993).

A vesicant drug should never be administered via a winged infusion device, as it has been demonstrated that the incidence of extravasation is greater when steel needles are used compared with plastic cannulae (Masoorli 2005; RCN 2005).

The cannula must be securely fixed to the patient's skin and it is essential that the insertion site is visible throughout the administration of the drug(s) or infusion. Venous patency must always be checked with at least 5–10 mL of 0.9% sodium chloride before administration of a vesicant, the area assessed for pain and swelling, and the patient asked to inform the practitioner of any discomfort. Should the patency be in any doubt, the device should be removed and resited (RCN 2005).

Use of an existing device

Weinstein (2007) and Masoorli (2005) recommended that a pre-existing peripheral device should not be used for vesicant drug administration in the following circumstances:

- the i.v. cannula was placed more than 12–24 hours earlier
- the area/insertion site is red, swollen or painful, or there is evidence of infiltration
- the site is over or around the wrist (or over a joint)
- blood return is sluggish or absent
- the infusion fluid is flowing erratically and appears positional
- the i.v. cannula is sited in an antecubital fossa vein.

If the fluid runs freely, there is a good and consistent blood return, the site is free of swelling, pain and redness, and the patient has exhausted or has limited potential cannulation sites, then it is up to the practitioner to make the decision to use the device based on their experience, knowledge of the drug(s) to be administered and risk assessment for the patient (Hadaway 2006). All the steps taken to assess the patient should be clearly documented in the notes (RCN 2005; Hadaway 2006).

Skill of the practitioner

The key to preventing extravasation is good venous assessment and using methods to improve and maintain venous access. The practitioner should be proficient in performing cannulation (Masoorli 2005) before attempting to cannulate for vesicant drug administration, as well as being knowledgeable about the signs and symptoms of extravasation. Multiple attempts after failure to cannulate a vein should be discouraged, and inexperienced practitioners should not attempt to cannulate a patient with difficult veins (Cox *et al.* 1988; Masoorli 2005). If the practitioner does not feel confident in their ability or is unsuccessful after one or two attempts at cannulation, they should seek the assistance of an experienced colleague. It is the individual nurse who is ultimately accountable for their own actions (NMC 2004). Any patient who consistently requires frequent attempts to successfully obtain vascular access should be considered for a CVAD.

Preparation of the patient

Patients should be informed about the drugs being given, any anticipated side-effects and the potential risks of extravasation (How & Brown 1998; DH 2004). They should be advised not to move the limb that has the cannula *in situ* during the bolus drug administration and should be asked to report immediately any pain, burning or unusual sensations during the injection. If patients cannot verbalize discomfort, the practitioner should observe them closely for any non-verbal signs of pain, such as facial expressions. The dressing used to cover the cannulation site and secure the device to the patient's skin should be transparent, to ensure adequate visualization of the site at all times during the administration of the drug(s) (RCN 2005). The device should then be checked for patency immediately before beginning administration of the drug(s) (RCN 2005; Hadaway 2006).

Signs and symptoms

Pain

Pain and stinging can be the first signs of an extravasation. However, extravasation can occur in the absence of pain and any sensations must be distinguished from venous spasm or the feeling of cold that can occur with some cytotoxic drugs (Trevit & Phillips 2006). Pain can be indicative of both peripheral and central venous extravasation. Patients may complain of pain along the catheter tunnel for a skin-tunnelled catheter, along the upper arm for a PICC, or around the port site. The latter may result from needle dislodgement from the port, poor needle placement, a split catheter or a fibrin sheath. It is rare that extravasation results from the disconnection of the catheter from the portal body (Schulmeister 1992; Wood & Gullo 1993; Masoorli 2005; Hadaway 2006). Fibrin sheath is a phenomenon that can affect any vascular access device. It is a condition where fibrin completely envelopes the outer wall of the vascular access device (VAD). When the drug/infusion is administered, it cannot be delivered into the venous circulation as its exit point is blocked. Instead the drug/infusion flows backwards between the external wall of the VAD and the internal wall of the fibrin sheath, exiting where it can find a break in the fibrin. For skin-tunnelled catheters this can be in the subcutaneous tissue and therefore result in extravasation (Gabriel 2006b).

Leaking, swelling or induration

The practitioner should be constantly assessing the patient's i.v. site for signs of swelling. Observation of this problem may be delayed if the patient has a cannula sited in an area of subcutaneous fat or if the leak is via the posterior wall, deep into subcutaneous tissue (Hadaway 2006).

Redness and blanching

Skin blanching can occur if the drug infiltrates/extravasates into the surrounding tissue.

Redness is not usually present at the time of extravasation and often occurs later as a delayed effect. Redness at the site may also be indicative of flare.

Blood return

The return of blood should be checked at regular intervals, although blood return does not guarantee vein/device patency, and any change should be investigated (RCN 2005; Hadaway 2006). If lack of blood return is the only sign, it should not automatically be regarded as an indication of a non-patent vein/device. A vein may not bleed back for a number of reasons; for example the device may be situated in a small vein which collapses when the syringe plunger is pulled back, or excess fluid from an infusion may have prevented blood from pooling at the tip of the cannula. A CVAD may not readily bleed back, if the catheter tip is not placed centrally. This is commonly a consequence of syringe aspiration (negative pressure) causing the tip of the CVAD to 'suck' against the vein's wall. It can also be a result of intraluminal or extraluminal occlusion, pinch-off or fibrin sheath formation (Gabriel 2006b).

Other signs

Other signs of extravasation include a reduction or absence of flow rate during an infusion and any resistance felt on the plunger of the syringe when administering a bolus injection. If any signs or symptoms are present or if there is any doubt in the practitioner's mind whether the drug is being administered correctly, administration should be discontinued immediately (Polovich *et al.* 2004; Masoorli 2005; RCN 2005; Weinstein 2007). If unsure of an extravasation, the practitioner may check with a solution of 0.9% sodium chloride; however, if an extravasation has occurred this may cause the drug to spread further into the tissues, so therefore any flushing of the i.v. device should be undertaken with caution.

Pathogenesis of extravasation

When an extravasation occurs:

1. Fluid leaks into the tissue.
2. The tissue is compressed due to the restricted blood flow.
3. This in turn reduces the amount of oxygen to the site and lowers the cellular pH.
4. There is loss of capillary wall integrity, an increase in oedema and eventual cellular death.

This is further compounded by the chemistry of an extravasation and by whether or not the drug binds to DNA.

Drugs that do not bind to DNA   These drugs tend to inhibit mitosis and often cause immediate damage. However, they are quickly metabolized and inactivated. The type of injury that occurs is similar to a burn, and ulceration can result. These drugs tend not to erode down to deeper structures and healing occurs within 3–5 weeks if the extravasation is detected early (Trevit & Phillips 2006).

Drugs that bind to DNA   These drugs do not always cause any immediate damage but lodge in the tissues, binding to the DNA, preventing the fibrostem cells from replicating and reproducing, and resulting in the cells losing their ability to heal spontaneously, which explains the prolonged effect. Drugs in this group include mustine (nitrogen mustard), which tends to bind rapidly to the tissues and cause immediate injury, and the drugs in the antibiotic family, e.g. doxorubicin, daunorubicin (Trevit & Phillips 2006).

Clinically, the majority of experience has been gained from doxorubicin, which is the most widely used of the cytotoxic drugs, and the majority of extravasation studies have been carried out on this drug. A correlation has been found between the degree of concentration of doxorubicin and the degree of ulceration. Active drug has been isolated from wounds between 3 and 5 months after a doxorubicin extravasation (Banerjee *et al.* 1987; Rudolph & Larson 1987; Vandergrift 2001; Masoorli 2005). Under ultraviolet light, tissue containing doxorubicin glows a dull red and this helps to identify the area of injured tissue (Rudolph & Larson 1987).

Stages of damage

The first suggestion of an extravasation of doxorubicin may be the patient complaining of a burning sensation around the area of the infusion, although local discomfort does not always occur. This pain can be quite severe and last minutes, hours or even days, but will eventually subside.

In the weeks following the extravasation, the tissue will become reddened and firm (*See* Figure 16.3). The skin may blanch when pressure is applied and necrosis may become obvious as early as a few days post administration, depending on the size of the area of extravasation (Figure 16.4). If the area is small, the redness gradually reduces over a few weeks. If the extravasation is large, a small necrotic area will appear in the centre of the red, painful skin and once necrosis occurs then surgical debridement is indicated. If this is not performed, a thick black eschar will result, surrounded by a rim of red painful skin. When this is removed, deep subcutaneous necrosis is found. The key feature of doxorubicin ulceration is that it is often progressive and may lead to extensive joint stiffness and neuropathy (Rudolph & Larson 1987; El Saghir *et al.* 2004; Masoorli 2005).

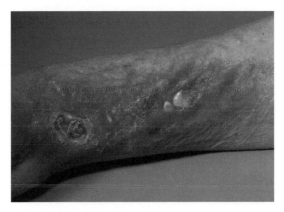

Figure 16.3 Blistering following vincristine extravasation.

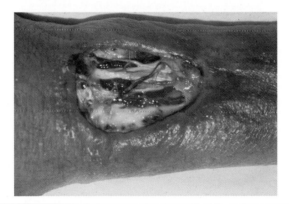

Figure 16.4 Extensive damage following an extravasation of doxorubicin.

Extravasation syndrome

Allwood *et al.* (2002) have suggested that there is a three-part syndrome of extravasation, although the management of types I and II is the same.

- *Pre-extravasation syndrome* often involves little or no leakage of vesicants, but particularly severe phlebitis and/or local hypersensitivity, together with a number of other local risk factors such as difficulty cannulating. This is an indication that patients may be more susceptible to extravasation and may be candidates for early central venous access. In the USA, CVADs are recommended and inserted for all patients requiring the administration of vesicant cytotoxic agents (Hadaway 2006).
- *Type I extravasation* injuries cause a blister and have a defined area of firmness around the site of injury. They are usually associated with bolus injections where pressure is applied by the person administering the drugs.
- *Type II extravasations* are differentiated by a diffuse, 'soggy' type of tissue injury, where dispersal into intracellular space has occurred. These injuries are associated with gravity-fed infusions or bolus injections through the side-arm of an infusion.

Management of extravasation

One of the main aims when administering vesicant cytotoxic drugs is to prevent extravasation. However, despite the skill of the practitioner, extravasations do occur and the

Section 3

emphasis should be on immediate recognition and prompt management to minimize complications. It is these two factors that will prevent the serious consequences of an extravasation injury. Sometimes it is difficult to detect whether an extravasation has actually occurred, but the literature stresses that in the event of a suspected extravasation it is better to assume it has occurred and act accordingly (Masoorli 2005; Weinstein 2007).

Comprehensive treatment and expert advice must be available as early as possible following an extravasation. Ideally, this should occur within 10 minutes of the event, certainly within 1 hour and definitely within 24 hours (Allwood *et al.* 2002; Masoorli 2005). The aim of this initial (emergency) treatment should be to remove as much of the drug as is possible from the subcutaneous tissue, but at the same time aimed at preventing further subcutaneous damage (Allwood *et al.* 2002). After 24 hours, the management will no longer be aimed at preventing injury, but will be more an exercise in damage limitation. Whatever form of treatment is chosen, it should not cause further damage or, in the case of misdiagnosis of an extravasation, any damage at all (Allwood *et al.* 2002; Masoorli 2005). All management, including advice/information given to the patient, should be documented in their notes (RCN 2005; Hadaway 2006).

The issues related to the management and treatment of extravasation are complex and controversial. There has been a lack of controlled clinical trials, for a number of reasons. First, while there are serious implications for untreated extravasations, the incidence is relatively small and thus the number of patients available for entry into studies is low (Cox *et al.* 1988; Langer *et al.* 2000). Secondly, there are moral and ethical considerations with having a treatment arm and a control arm where patients sustaining injuries are offered no treatment. Some studies performed on animals have demonstrated both effective and ineffective antidotes, but extrapolation from animals to humans has its limitations (Langer *et al.* 2000; Polovich *et al.* 2004).

Once an extravasation is suspected, clinicians agree that the infusion or administration should be stopped immediately, followed by aspiration of any remaining drug in order to reduce the size/volume of the extravasation (Rudolph & Larson 1987; Cox *et al.* 1988; Allwood *et al.* 2002; Masoorli 2005; Weinstein 2007).

Back in 1980, Ignoffo and Friedman described a protocol where, following cessation of the injection, an attempt to aspirate 3–5 mL of blood was carried out. However, in the majority of cases the device is displaced or the vein damaged and the likelihood of withdrawing any blood is small, and the practitioner may waste valuable time attempting to achieve this.

It is here that the first dilemma arises: should the peripheral device be removed or remain *in situ*? Cox *et al.* (1988) advocated that the device be left *in situ* in order to instil an antidote through it and into the surrounding tissues, thus infiltrating the area where the extravasation has occurred. This view is supported by Ignoffo and Friedman (1980), Powell (1996) and Weinstein (2007). However, Rudolph and Larson (1987) recommended that the device be removed and felt that the evidence for leaving it *in situ* was anecdotal. However, there is still no conclusive evidence to support either. Allwood *et al.* (2002) stress initial (emergency) treatment should remain simple in order to avoid confusion and cause no further damage.

Hot packs or cold packs?

There appear to be two main courses of treatment (Allwood *et al.* 2002):

- localize and neutralize
- spread and dilute.

Localize and neutralize   In order to localize the extravasated drug, the recommended course would be to apply a cold pack to the area. This would result in vasoconstriction, which reduces the locally destructive effects by minimizing the local uptake of the drug by the tissues, decreasing local oedema and slowing the metabolic rate of the cells. It has also been suggested that the reduced blood supply and the cooling effect may help to reduce local pain (Beason 1990; Langer *et al.* 2000; Vandergrift 2001; Weinstein 2007). There is still no decision as to how long the pack should be left *in situ*, although some suggest periods of 15 minutes (Rudolph & Larson 1987) or 20–40 minutes (Cox *et al.* 1988) four times a day for up to 24–48 hours. The use of cold packs is recommended for a number of vesicant drugs, but in the treatment of vinca alkaloid extravasation the use of heat packs has been particularly advocated. However, it is important that heat is not used inappropriately. Dorr *et al.* (1983) found experimentally that, while cooling could be helpful in preventing ulcers due to doxorubicin extravasation, heat could be harmful. Allwood *et al.* (2002) stress the importance of applying treatments for extravasation in the correct order to avoid the potential for catastrophic consequences.

Spread and dilute   It appears that heat is beneficial in non-DNA-binding vesicant drugs and it is used once the antidote is given with the aim of increasing blood supply and therefore increasing dispersal and absorption of the antidote into the subcutaneous tissues. Also, the increased blood supply may help to promote healing by increasing metabolic demands and reducing cellular destruction (Weinstein 2007). The use of heat is recommended for vinca alkaloid extravasation (Powell 1996; Allwood *et al.* 2002; Hyde 2004). Allwood *et al.* (2002) also recommend the application of heat for up to 24 hours post injury for specific vesicant cytotoxic drugs including cisplatinum, docetaxel, paclitaxel and the vinca alkaloids, i.e. vincristine, vinblastine and vindesine.

Elevation of the extremity

The elevation of the extremity is recommended, the aim being to minimize swelling. Both Rudolph and Larson (1987) and Powell (1996) stress the importance of elevation, following the application of an ice pack, for up to 48 hours. Movement should also be encouraged to prevent adhesion of damaged areas to underlying tissue, which could result in restriction of future movement (Hyde 2004).

'Antidotes'

There are two main types of 'antidote':

- those with the aim of diluting the drug, such as sodium chloride 0.9% and hyaluronidase
- those with the aim of neutralizing the drug and reducing subsequent local inflammation, such as steroid cream.

Some organizations have a list of antidotes for specific vesicant drugs. For example, sodium bicarbonate 8.4% can be used in carmustine extravasations (however, Allwood *et al.* 2002 pointed out the documented risks associated with using sodium bicarbonate 8.4% which itself can be a causative agent of extravasation injuries). Sodium theosulphate (useful with mustine or cisplatinum) was evaluated in a study by Tsavaris *et al.* back in 1992 (Tsavaris *et al.* 1992). They found that healing time was reduced by using sodium theosulphate with hydrocortisone and dexamethasone in extravasated drugs such as doxorubicin, epirubicin, vincristine and mitomycin-c. They concluded this may reduce the need for extensive surgery. Topical antidotes aim to minimize skin inflammation and erythematous reactions. Application of dimethyl sulphoxide (DMSO) of between 50 and 99% has been found to be beneficial in treating doxorubicin and mitomycin C extravasations (Hammond & Bachur 1987; Allwood *et al.* 2002). The recommended application is 1–2 mL applied to the site every 6 hours (Polovich *et al.* 2004), although this could delay healing.

Hyaluronidase is an enzyme that destroys tissue cement, aiding in the reduction or prevention of tissue damage by allowing rapid diffusion of the extravasated fluid and promoting drug absorption. The usual dose is 1500 IU administered following vinca alkaloid extravasations. However, 0.9% sodium chloride has also been used successfully to limit the effects of vinca alkaloid extravasation, by diluting the concentration of the drug, and a combination of both of these drugs has been reported to be effective in the reduction of local ulceration (Masoorli 2005).

Recently dexrazoxane, a topoisomerase II catalytic inhibitor used clinically to minimize the cardiotoxicity of doxorubicin, has been tested in animal models and a small number of patients for its use in extravasation. It was given i.v. 3–6 hours after the extravastion and it appears to reduce the wound size and duration with anthracyclines. Triple dosage appears to be more effective than a single dose (Langer *et al.* 2000; El Saghir *et al.* 2004). A consensus opinion in its use in the treatment of anthracycline extravasation provided the following guidance.

For anthracycline extravasation resulting from peripheral administration, a site expert or team should be consulted to determine the use of dexrazoxane (Savene) but if the extravasated volume exceeds 15 mL it was agreed that this would be an absolute indication and also in the case of extravasation from a CVAD. Intravenous dexrazoxane should be administered as soon as possible after extravasation of anthracyclines (doxorubicin; epirubicin and daunarubicin) and then again on day 2 and day 3 (Jackson 2007).

Surgery

When is surgical intervention necessary? Some centres suggest that a plastic surgery consultation be performed as part of the management procedure (Weinstein 2007). Early surgical intervention with excision of the area (particularly with doxorubicin) has been demonstrated to stop progression of cellular destruction, thereby minimizing damage (Heckler 1989; Langer *et al.* 2000; Hadaway 2006; Goolsby & Lombardo 2006). However, the requirement for surgery is probably related to the size and location of the extravasation as well as the type of drug that has been extravasated. Goolsby and Lombardo (2006) stress that surgery should not be the initial treatment for extravasation of chemotherapy agents, other than anthracyclines. As anthracyclines can often cause tissue necrosis, surgical intervention is felt to be worthwhile in limiting the degree of tissue damage. El Saghir *et al.* (2004) have reported how the administration of dexrazoxane 1 hour following extravasation of doxorubicin and again at 5 and 24 hours later prevented the immediate breakdown of the site, but 4 months later the patient did require surgery for removal of necrotic tissue. The use of 0.9% sodium chloride flushing conducted within the first 24 hours following an extravasation has been suggested as a less traumatic procedure. This technique involves several small 'stab' incisions, which facilitates the flushing out of any drug from the subcutaneous tissues, and is advocated for use with drugs such as doxorubicin (How & Brown 1998; Wickham *et al.* 2006).

Rudolph and Larson (1987) and Goolsby and Lombardo (2006) have concluded that once ulceration and pain occur, surgery is often indicated as it can relieve the discomfort and pain for the patient. However, if pain, erythema and swelling persist, it may be necessary to intervene before ulceration occurs. Linder *et al.* (1981) found a high incidence of residual joint stiffness and sympathetic dystrophy related to delay in excision of necrotic tissue. Excision should include removal of all indurated, reddened, oedematous and pale tissue with a margin of normal-appearing tissue (Banerjee *et al.* 1987). Identification and demarcation of the area can be achieved by the use of fluorescence microscopic analysis (Dahlstrom *et al.* 1990). Photographs and/or diagrams are also useful, as is marking the area of extravasation with a pen to observe for an increase or decrease in swelling and redness (Allwood *et al.* 2002; Goolsby & Lombardo 2006).

Patient feedback

Patients should always be informed when an extravasation has occurred and an explanation should be provided of what has happened as well as what is required in order to manage the situation. Following the management of the extravasation, the patient should be advised as to what signs and symptoms to observe for, and whom to contact and when during the follow-up period. All treatment and advice given to the patient (written and verbal) should be clearly documented in their notes (Allwood *et al.* 2002; DH 2004; Masoorli 2005).

Consequences of poor or no treatment

The consequences of an untreated or poorly managed extravasation can be extensive, but such occurrences can be greatly minimized through careful preparation, administration and monitoring by a practitioner experienced in cannulation and chemotherapy administration.

Physical defect (Figure 16.5)

Patients may already have undergone surgery (e.g. a mastectomy or stoma formation) and may have suffered side-effects from treatment (e.g. loss of hair), all of which will have had an impact on body image and self-esteem. A necrotic, ulcerated injury as a result of extravasation could therefore be devastating and have an additional impact on the patient's ability to work and function normally, both socially and emotionally. This is particularly difficult if the extravasation has occurred over a joint, limiting mobility and even resulting in permanent disability. As a result of the injury the patient may suffer from pain, which in turn may lead to problems with working, sleeping and generally coping with treatment (Ellis *et al.* 2006; Hadaway 2006).

Disease control

Various aspects of an extravasation injury may affect the patient's long-term prognosis. A patient may not be able to continue treatment as the wound may need time to heal, and if they become myelosuppressed during treatment, the wound is a potential area for infection. This is also the case for patients waiting to undergo intensive or high-dose chemotherapy. If the patient is debilitated through the injury, this could lead to secondary medical problems, which may also impact on the patient's ability to receive and cope with further treatment (Masoorli 2005).

Cost

There are costs in time and money and to the patient's overall health and quality of life. If a patient cannot resume work due to disability or the need to take time off for plastic surgery, then it may impact on both the patient and their family. There may be costs involved in surgery both to treat the injury and to repair the damage cosmetically, and repeated hospitalization may be necessary (Masoorli 2005; Weinstein 2007). There are

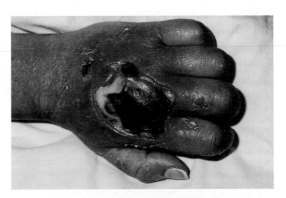

Figure 16.5 Necrotic area as a result of doxorubicin extravasation.

BOX 16.5

Contents of an extravasation kit

- Hot/cold packs
- Injectable antidotes as per organizational policy
- Steroid cream
- Syringes
- Needles
- Alcohol swabs
- Copy of extravasation management procedure
- Documentation forms

---

also potential costs to the organization and individual practitioner if negligence can be proved (Hadaway 2006).

The use of extravasation kits

The availability of an extravasation kit and policy is now recommended in all NHS hospitals where cytotoxic chemotherapy is used to treat oncology patients (DH 2004). An extravasation kit is particularly useful in areas where staff routinely administer vesicant cytotoxic drugs as it gives them immediate access to a step-by-step guide to management, as well as having all the required equipment to hand (*See* Box 16.5).

The kit should remain simple in order to avoid confusion (especially as the practitioner will be anxious), but comprehensive enough to meet all reasonable needs (Gabriel 2001; Allwood *et al.* 2002). The instructions should be clear and easy to follow and the use of a flow chart is an easy way to help staff follow the management procedure (*See* Figure 16.6). Kits should be assembled according to the particular needs of the individual organization/department and be readily available in all areas where cytotoxic agents are administered. If chemotherapy is administered in the patient's home the practitioner should also have access to a kit there.

Documentation and reporting

Documentation of an extravasation is vital for a number of reasons.

- An extravasation is an adverse incident and must be reported, fully documented and investigated.
- The patient will require follow-up care and the documentation must be available to all practitioners involved in the follow-up.
- The information will be used for statistical purposes/audit.
- It may be required in the case of litigation.
  The documentation should contain the following aspects:
- patient details
- date and time of incident
- the drug given
- who was administering the drug(s)
- the method used, e.g. bolus or infusion
- type of device, e.g. cannula, CVAD
- who sited the device and where it was anatomically sited
- a diagram or photograph to indicate the location and size of the injured area
- the appearance of the area
- any signs and symptoms experienced by the patient/observed by the practitioner
- how the procedure was performed step by step

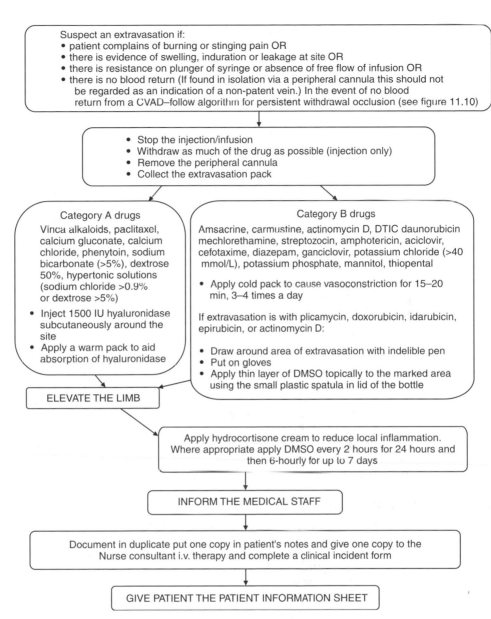

Figure 16.6 Treatment of extravasation.

- whether photographs were taken
- any referrals to plastic surgeons/oncologists
- information given to patient
- follow-up appointment/arrangements
- section for follow-up documentation
- date and signature of practitioner.

There is a scheme for the collation and analysis of extravasation events called the 'green card scheme', which is organized by St Chad's Hospital, Birmingham (Allwood *et al.* 2002). The aim is to obtain accurate statistics of the number of incidents, the treatment methods and the outcome. All staff who encounter an extravasation should be

Section 3

encouraged to use this scheme. Extravasation injury is obviously an unwanted occurrence for both the patient and the health professional involved. The health professional should receive support from their colleagues and have an opportunity to discuss the event so that any lessons learned can be shared and hopefully reduce the risk of such an injury for future patients.

Conclusion

The preparation and administration of cytotoxic drugs is a procedure which must be undertaken by skilled and competent practitioners, as it is associated with hazards for both the individual patient and staff. Knowledge of protective measures and of the immediate, short- and long-term side-effects of the drugs to be administered will enable the practitioner to handle the drugs safely, as well as provide the necessary teaching and support for the individual patient. Being a recipient of cytotoxic chemotherapy is obviously a very anxious experience for any patient. A practitioner who is knowlegeable and skilled in this area will be able to support their patient by reducing their anxiety levels and ultimately help them through their patient pathway.

References

Allwood M, Stanley A, Wright P (2002) *The Cytotoxic Handbook*. Radcliffe Medical Press, Oxford.

Banerjee A, Brotherson TM, Lamberty BGH, Campbell RC (1987) Cancer chemotherapy agent induced perivenous extravasation injuries. *Postgraduate Medical Journal* 63: 5–9.

Beason R (1990) Antineoplastic vesicant extravasation. *Journal of Intravenous Nursing* 13(92): 111–114.

Begg AC (2006) *Growth and Kinetics of Human Tumours* [www document]. www.oup.co.uk [accessed 26 November 2006]

Behamou S (1986) Mutagenicity in urine from nurses handling cytotoxic drugs. *European Journal of Cancer and Clinical Oncology* 22: 1489–1493.

Cardonick E, Iacobucci I (2004). Use of chemotherapy during human pregnancy. *The Lancet Oncology* 5: 283–291.

Christensen CJ, Le Masters GK, Wakeman MA (1990) Work practices and policies of hospital pharmacists preparing antineoplastic agents. *Journal of Occupational Medicine* 32(6): 508–512.

Colbourne L (1995) Patients' experiences on chemotherapy treatment. *Professional Nurse* 10(7): 439–442.

Cox K, Stuart-Harris RA, Addini G, Grygiel J, Raghavan D (1988) The management of cytotoxic drug extravasation: guidelines drawn up by a working party for the Clinical Oncological Society of Australia. *The Medical Journal of Australia* 148: 185–189.

Curran CF, Luce JK, Page JA (1990) Doxorubicin-associated flare reactions. *Oncology Nursing Forum* 17: 387–389.

Dahlstrom KK, Chenoufi HL, Daugaard S (1990) Fluorescence microscopic demonstration and demarcation of doxorubicin extravasation. *Cancer* 65: 1722–1726.

Department of Health (DH) (2004) *Manual of Cancer Measures*. HMSO, London.

Dorr RT, Alberts AS, Salmons SE (1983) Cold protection from intradermal doxorubicin ulceration in the mouse. *Proceedings of the Annual Meeting of the American Association Cancer Research* 24: 255.

Dougherty L (2006) Managing complications. In: *Central Venous Access Devices: Care and Management*, pp. 135–173. Blackwell Publishing, Oxford.

Dougherty L, Bailey C (2001) Chemotherapy. In: Corner J, Bailey C, eds. *Cancer Nursing Care in Context*, pp. 179–221. Blackwell Publishing, Oxford.

El Saghir N, Otrock Z, Mufarri A *et al.* (2004) Dexrazoxane for anthracycline extravasation and GM-CSF for skin ulceration and wound healing. *Lancet Oncology* 5: 320–321.

Ellis M, Woodcock C, Rawlings E, Bywater L (2006). Psychological issues. In: Grundy M, ed. *Nursing in Haematological Oncology*, 2nd edn, pp. 457–474. Ballière Tindall Elsevier, Edinburgh.

Eli Lilley (2005) *Cytotoxic Chemotherapy*. Lilley Oncology, Hampshire.

Falck G, Rohn P, Sorsa M, Vainio H, Heinenon E, Holsti L (1979) Mutagenicity in urine of nurses handling cytotoxic agents. *The Lancet* 1: 1250.

Gabriel J (2001) Understanding cytotoxic chemotherapy In: Gabriel J, ed. *Oncology Nursing in Practice*, pp. 30–50. Whurr Publishers, London.

Gabriel J (2006a) Needlestick injuries: how we can minimize our risk. *Journal of Vascular Access* 7: 1–4.

Gabriel J (2006b) Vascular access. In: Grundy M, ed. *Nursing in Haematological Oncoclogy*, 2nd edn, pp. 295–320. Balliere Tindall Elsevier, Edinburgh.

Goolsby TV, Lombardo FA (2006) Extravasation of chemotherapeutic agents: prevention and treatment. *Seminars in Oncology* 33: 139–143.

Hadaway L (2006) *Infiltration and Extravasation from Vascular Access Devices*. Oral presentation, 20th Annual Assocation of Vascular Access (AVA) Conference, Indianapolis USA.

Hammond K, Bachur N (1987) Evaluation of dimethyl sulfoxide and local cooling as antidotes for doxorubicin extravasation in a pig model. *Oncology Nursing Forum* 14(1): 39–44.

Hayden BK, Goodman M (2005) Chemotherapy: principles of administration. In: Henke Yarbro C *et al.*, eds. *Cancer Nursing – Principles and Practice*, 6th edn, pp. 351–411. Jones and Bartlett, Massachusetts.

Health and Safety Executive (HSE) (2002) *The Control of Substances Hazardous to Health Regulations*. HMSO, London.

Heckler FR (1989) Current thoughts on extravasation injuries. *Clinics in Plastic Surgery* 16(3): 557–563.

Hecker J (1988) Improved techniques in IV therapy. *Nursing Times* 84(34): 28–33.

Hemminki K, Kyyronen P, Linbohm M (1985) Spontaneous abortions and malformations in the offspring of nurses exposed to anaesthetic gases, cytostatic drugs and other potential hazards in hospitals based on registered information of outcome. *Journal of Epidemiological Community Health* 39: 141–147.

Holmes S (1990) *Cancer Chemotherapy*. Austin Cornish, London.

How C, Brown J (1998) Extravasation of cytotoxic chemotherapy from peripheral veins. *European Journal of Oncology Nursing* 2(1): 51–58.

Hyde L (2004) Cytotoxic drugs: handling and administration. In: Dougherty L, Lister S, eds. *The Royal Marsden Hospital Manual of Clinical Nursing Procedures*, 6th edn, pp. 228–258. Blackwell Publishing, Oxford.

Ignoffo RJ, Friedman MA (1980) Therapy of local toxicities caused by extravasation of cancer chemotherapeutic drugs. *Cancer Treatments Review* 7: 17–27.

Jackson G (2007) *Consensus Opinion on the Use of Dexrazoxane (Savene) in the Treatment of Anthracycline Extravasation*. Topotarget.

Kaplan M (1983) Viewpoint: the cancer patient. *Cancer Nursing* 6: 103–107.

Knight L (2004) The cell. In: Gabriel J, ed. *The Biology of Cancer*, pp. 33–49. Whurr, London.

Langer S, Sehested M, Jensen P (2000) Treatment of anthracycline extravasation with dexrazoxane. *Clinical Cancer Research* 6: 3680–3686.

Linder RM, Upton J, Osteen R (1981) Management of extensive doxorubicin hydrochloride extravasation injuries. *Journal of Hand Surgery* 8: 32–38.

MARCH Guidelines (2007) management and awareness of risks of cytotoxic handling[www document]. www. marchguidelines.com [accessed 20th July 2007]

Masoorli S (2005) *Infusion Therapy Standards: Clinical and Legal Implications*. Royal College of Nursing IV Conference, Brighton Metropole Hotel, 5th November.

Mayer DK (1992) Hazards of chemotherapy—implementing safe handling practices. *Cancer* 70: 988–992.

Modjtahedi H (2004) Monoclonal antibodies. In: Gabriel J, ed. *The Biology of Cancer*, pp. 109–124. Whurr, London.

Nieweg RM, De Boer M, Dubbleman RC *et al.* (1994) Safe handling of antineoplastic drugs: results of a survey. *Cancer Nursing* 17(6): 501–511.

Nursing and Midwifery Council (NMC) (2004) *Code of Professional Conduct*. Nursing and Midwifery Council, London.

Polovich M, White JM and Kelleher LO, ed. (2004) *Chemotherapy and Biotherapy Guidelines and Recommendations for Practice*, 2nd edn. Oncology Nursing Press, Pittsburgh.

Powell L, ed. (1996) *Cancer Chemotherapy Guidelines and Recommendations for Practice*, Oncology Nursing Press, Pittsburgh.

Priestman TJ (1989) *Cancer Chemotherapy: an Introduction*, 3rd edn. Springer-Verlag, Berlin.

Richardson C, Atkinson J (2006). Blood and marrow transplantation. In: Grundy M, ed. *Nursing in Hematological Oncology*, 2nd edn, pp. 265–292. Balliere Tindall Elsevier, Edinburgh.

Rittenberg CN, Gralla RJ, Rehmeyer TA (1995) Assessing and managing venous irritation with vinorelbine tartrate. *Oncology Nursing Forum* 22(4): 707–710.

Robinson S (1993) Principles of chemotherapy. *European Journal of Cancer Care* 2: 55–65.

Royal College of Nursing (RCN) (1998) *Clinical Practice Guidelines: the Administration of Cytotoxic Chemotherapy. Technical Report*. Royal College of Nursing, London.

Royal College of Nursing (RCN) (2005) *Standards for Infusion Therapy*. Royal College of Nursing, London.

Rudolph R, Larson DL (1987) Etiology and treatment of chemotherapeutic agent extravasation injuries: a review. *Journal of Clinical Oncology* 5(7): 1116–1126.

Schulmeister L (1992) An overview of continuous infusion chemotherapy. *Journal of Intravenous Nursing* 15(6): 315–321.

Selevan SG, Lindbohm M, Horning R, Hemminki K (1985) A study of occupational exposure to antineoplastic drugs and foetal loss in nurses. *New England Journal of Medicine* 19: 1173–1178.

Sewell, G (2007) Cytotoxic contamination in the workplace, Paper given Hazardous Drugs: managing the risks, UKONS/bopa, June 14th, Kings College , London

Sims, J (2005) Risk management In: Brighton D & Wood M, eds. *The Royal Marsden Hospital Handbook of Cancer Chemotherapy*, pp. 31–42. Elsevier, Edinburgh.

Taskinen HK (1990) Effects of parental occupational exposures on spontaneous abortion and congenital malformation. *Scandinavian Journal of Work and Environmental Health* 16: 297–314.

Tortorice PV (1997) Chemotherapy: principles of therapy. In: Groenwald SL, Frogge MH, Goodman M, Henke Yarbro C, eds. *Cancer Nursing—Principles and Practice*, pp. 283–316. Jones & Bartlett, Boston.

Trevit S, Phillips K (2006) Chemotherapy. In: Grundy M, ed. *Nursing in Hematological Oncology*, 2nd edn, pp. 173–200. Balliere Tindall Elsevier, Edinburgh.

Tsavaris NB, Komitsopoulou P, Karagiaouris P *et al.* (1992) Prevention of tissue necrosis due to accidental extravasation of cytostatic drugs by a conservative approach. *Cancer Chemotherapy Pharmacology* 30: 330–333.

Valanis BG, Vollmer WM, Labuhn KT, Glass AG (1993) Acute symptoms associated with antineoplastic drug handling among nurses. *Cancer Nursing* 16(4): 288–295.

Vandergrift KV (2001) Oncologic therapy. In: Hankin J *et al.*, eds. *Infusion Therapy in Clinical Practice*, 2nd edn, pp. 248–275. Saunders, Philadelphia.

Vennit S, Crofton-Sleigh C, Speechley V, Briggs K (1984) Monitoring exposure of nursing and pharmacy personnel to cytotoxic drugs: urinary mutation assays and urinary platinum as markers of absorption. *The Lancet* 1: 74–76.

Waksvik H, Klepp O, Brogger A (1981) Chromosome analysis of nurse handling cytostatic agents. *Cancer Treatment Reports* 65: 607–610.

Weinstein SM (2007) Antineoplastic therapy. In: *Plumer's Principles and Practice of IV therapy*, 8th edn, pp. 486–575. JB Lippincott, Philadelphia.

Wickham R, Engelking C, SauerlandC, Corbi D (2006) Vesicant extravasation part II: Evidence-based management and continuing controversies. *Oncol Nurs Forum* Nov 27; 33(6): 1143–1150.

Wiseman KC, Wachs JE (1990) Policies and practices used for the safe handling of antineoplastic drugs. *American Association of Occupational Health Nursing Journal* 38(11): 517–523.

Wood LS, Gullo SM (1993) IV vesicants: how to avoid extravasation. *American Journal of Nursing* 4: 42–45.

Index